THE HARRIET LANE HANDBOOK OF PEDIATRIC ANTIMICROBIAL THERAPY

THE HARRIET LANE HANDBOOK OF PEDIATRIC ANTIMICROBIAL THERAPY

Julia A. McMillan, MD
Vice Chair for Education, Department of Pediatrics
Professor of Pediatrics
Johns Hopkins University School of Medicine
Baltimore, MD

George K. Siberry, MD, MPH
Assistant Professor of Pediatrics
Johns Hopkins University School of Medicine
Baltimore, MD

James D. Dick, PhD
Department of Pathology
Director, Bacteriology Section, Division of Medical Microbiology
Associate Professor of Pathology, Molecular Microbiology and Immunology
Johns Hopkins School of Medicine
Baltimore, MD

Carlton K.K. Lee, PharmD, MPH
Assistant Professor of Pediatrics
Johns Hopkins University School of Medicine
Clinical Pharmacy Specialist in Pediatrics
Director, Pediatric Pharmacy Residency Program
The Johns Hopkins Hospital
Baltimore, MD

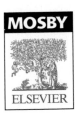

MOSBY

ELSEVIER

MOSBY
ELSEVIER

1600 John F. Kennedy Blvd.
Ste 1800
Philadelphia, PA 19103-2899

THE HARRIET LANE HANDBOOK OF
PEDIATRIC ANTIMICROBIAL THERAPY

ISBN: 978-0-323-05334-1

Notice

Knowledge and best practice in this field are constantly changing. As new research and experience broaden our knowledge, changes in practice, treatment, and drug therapy may become necessary or appropriate. Readers are advised to check the most current information provided (i) on procedures featured or (ii) by the manufacturer of each product to be administered, to verify the recommended dose or formula, the method and duration of administration, and contraindications. It is the responsibility of the practitioner, relying on his or her own experience and knowledge of the patient, to make diagnoses, to determine dosages and the best treatment for each individual patient, and to take all appropriate safety precautions. To the fullest extent of the law, neither the Publisher nor the Editors assume any liability for any injury and/or damage to persons or property arising out or related to any use of the material contained in this book.

ISBN: 978-0-323-05334-1

Acquistitions Editor: Jim Merrit
Developmental Editor: Marybeth Thiel
Project Manager: Mary B. Stermel
Design Direction: Karen O'Keefe Owens
Marketing Manager: Courtney Ingram

Printed in the United States of America.

Last digit is the print number: 9   8   7   6   5   4   3   2   1

Dedication

This First Edition of *The Harriet Lane Handbook of Pediatric Antimicrobial Therapy* is dedicated to all **practitioners** who treat infectious diseases in children; to our **patients**, who help us understand that treatment decisions must be made in recognition of the needs, risks, and clinical context of the individual; and to our **teachers**, who led us to the challenges and excitement of identifying the pathogen and determining appropriate therapy. In addition, we dedicate this Handbook to our **spouses—Nancy Dick, Joanne Lee, Jed Dietz, and Uma Reddy, and children—Kelly, Catherine, Laura, Brendan, Edith, Robert, Elihu, Vikram, and Vinod**—whose support has made this book possible.

James D. Dick, PhD
Carlton K. K. Lee, PharmD, MPH
Julia A. McMillan, MD
George K. Siberry, MD, MPH

EDITORS

Julia A. McMillan, MD
Vice Chair for Education, Department of Pediatrics
Professor of Pediatrics
Johns Hopkins University School of Medicine

George K. Siberry, MD, MPH
Assistant Professor of Pediatrics
Johns Hopkins University School of Medicine

James D. Dick, PhD
Department of Pathology
Johns Hopkins University School of Medicine

Carlton K.K. Lee, PharmD, MPH
Assistant Professor of Pediatrics
Johns Hopkins University School of Medicine
Clinical Pharmacy Specialist in Pediatrics
Director, Pediatric Pharmacy Residency Program
The Johns Hopkins Hospital

CONTRIBUTORS

Allison G. Agwu, MD
Assistant Professor
Divisions of Adult & Pediatric Infectious Diseases
Johns Hopkins University

Michelle C. Caruso, PharmD
Clinical Pharmacy Specialist, Emergency Medicine
Cincinnati Children's Hospital Medical Center

Sanjay K. Jain, MD
Assistant Professor of Pediatrics
Pediatric Infectious Diseases and Center for Tuberculosis Research
Johns Hopkins University

Aaron M. Milstone, MD
Department of Pediatrics
Division of Infectious Diseases
Johns Hopkins University

Kara L. Murray, PharmD, BCPS
Clinical Pharmacy Specialist, Neonatal and Women's Health
Centennial Medical Center

Susanna Sowell, PharmD
Clinical Pharmacy Specialist for Women's Services
Winnie Palmer Hospital for Women and Babies

Jeffrey L. Wagner, PharmD, BCPS
Clinical Pharmacy Specialist, Critical Care
Texas Children's Hospital

Preface

The Harriet Lane Handbook was first published commercially in 1969, and since then, every third year, the chief residents and senior residents of the Harriet Lane Pediatric Residency Program, assisted by faculty advisors, have revised and updated the information they find most essential for providing medical care for infants and children. As pharmacologic options for treatment have increased and become more complex, the Formulary has become an increasingly important resource, and since the 12th Edition in 1990, Carlton Lee, PharmD, MPH, has been the source of pharmacologic knowledge and expertise for the *Handbook*.

This first edition of the *Harriet Lane Handbook for Pediatric Antimicrobial Therapy* embraces the principles of the original *Handbook*, recognizing that those on the front lines of providing care (in this case pediatric infectious diseases fellows) are in the best position to determine the information that will be most helpful, as well as its format. All three of the fellows who contributed to this *Handbook* (Allison G. Agwu, MD, Sanjay K. Jain, MD, and Aaron M. Milstone, MD) have since joined the faculty of the Infectious Diseases Division of the Department of Pediatrics at Johns Hopkins. In addition to Dr. Lee's Formulary, former Pediatric Pharmacy residents have contributed tables for chapters describing "Drug Dosing in Special Circumstances," "Therapeutic Drug Monitoring," "Adverse Effects," and "Antimicrobial Desensitization Protocols." Every infectious disease practitioner recognizes the invaluable help provided by the microbiology laboratory in sorting out identification and susceptibilities of microbial pathogens, and for many years James Dick, PhD, has been a valued consultant and advisor for the pediatric infectious diseases service at Johns Hopkins. Through this *Handbook* his expertise is being made available to others in chapters describing "Mechanism of Action and Routes of Administration of Antimicrobial Agents" and "Mechanisms of Drug Resistance."

Together, we've sorted through the pediatric infectious diseases literature in an attempt to provide evidence-based recommendations for antimicrobial therapy appropriate for infants, children, and adolescents. We have considered data regarding safety, likely antimicrobial resistance, pharmacokinetics and distribution, as well as efficacy. When they were available, we consulted current guidelines promulgated by the American Academy of Pediatrics, the Centers for Disease Control and Prevention, and other authoritative sources. We recognize that microbes will always find pathways that defy our attempts to eradicate or control them, and we understand that new evidence and, hopefully, new therapies, will supersede some of the recommendations we make today. With all that in mind, however, we provide this resource in the hope that pediatric patients will receive effective, safe, and individualized antimicrobial therapy.

Julia A. McMillan, MD
George K. Siberry, MD, MPH
Carlton K. K. Lee, PharmD, MPH
James D. Dick, PhD
Allison G. Agwu, MD
Sanjay K. Jain, MD
Aaron M. Milstone, MD
Michelle C. Caruso, PharmD
Kara L. Murray, PharmD
Susanna Sowell, PharmD
Jeffrey L. Wagner, PharmD

Contents

Chapter 1: Infectious Agents and Drugs of Choice 1
Julia A. McMillan, MD, George K. Siberry, MD, MPH, and James D. Dick, PhD

    I. *Recommended Treatment for Bacterial Infections 2*

    II. *Recommended Treatment for Mycobacterial Infections 38*

    III. *Recommended Treatment for Viral Infections 48*

    IV. *Recommended Treatment for Fungal Infections 54*

    V. *Recommended Treatment for Parasitic and Protozoal Infections 74*

Chapter 2: Recommended Empiric Antimicrobial Therapy for Selected Clinical Syndromes 107
Aaron M. Milstone, MD, Allison G. Agwu, MD, and Sanjay K. Jain, MD

Chapter 3: Drug Dosing in Special Circumstances 151
Jeffrey L. Wagner, PharmD, and Carlton K.K. Lee, PharmD, MPH

    I. *General Pediatric Drug Dosing 151*

    II. *Developmental Dosing Considerations (Developmental Pharmacology) 153*

    III. *Drug Dosing in Renal Insufficiency 156*

    IV. *Drug Dosing in Hepatic Insufficiency 170*

    V. *Drug Dosing in Obesity 170*

    VI. *Antimicrobial Tissue Distributed by Key Organ Systems 191*

Chapter 4: Mechanisms of Action and Routes of Administration of Antimicrobial Agents 217
James D. Dick, PhD

    Antibacterial 218
    Antimycobacterial 222
    Antifungal 222
    Antiviral 223
    Antiparasitic 225

Chapter 5: Mechanisms of Drug Resistance 227
James D. Dick, PhD

    I. *Common Mechanisms of Microbial Resistance 227*

    II. *Discordance Between In Vitro Susceptibility and In Vivo Efficacy 228*

Chapter 6: Therapeutic Monitoring 231
Michelle C. Caruso, PharmD, and Carlton K.K. Lee, PharmD, MPH

    I.   General Principles 231
    II.   Antimicrobials Requiring Therapeutic Drug Monitoring 233
    III.   Special Topics in Antimicrobial Therapeutic Drug Monitoring 239
    IV.   Pharmacokinetic Monitoring in Therapeutic Drug Monitoring 240
    V.   Pharmacokinetic/ Pharmacodynamic (PK/PD) Antimicrobial Relationships 244
    VI.   Drug Interactions 247

Chapter 7: Adverse Effects 261
Kara L. Murray, PharmD, Susanna Sowell, PharmD, and Carlton K. K. Lee, PharmD, MPH

    I.   Blood 261
    II.   Cardiovascular 262
    III.   Central Nervous System 263
    IV.   Skin 266
    V.   Gastrointestinal 267
    VI.   Endocrine/ Metabolic 271
    VII.   Renal/ Genitourinary 271
    VIII.   Respiratory 272
    IX.   Hepatic 272
    X.   Ocular 273
    XI.   Musculoskeletal 273
    XII.   Hypersensitivity 273
    XIII.   Other 274

Chapter 8: Recommended Antimicrobial Prophylaxis for Selected Infectious Agents and Conditions 275
Julia A. McMillan, MD, and George K. Siberry, MD, MPH

    Situational 276
    Prevention of Infection Due to Specific Bacterial Pathogens 281
    Prevention of Infection Due to Specific Viral Pathogens 284
    Prevention of Infection Due to Specific Fungal Pathogens 287
    Prevention of Infection Due to Specific Parasitic Pathogens 287

Chapter 9: Antimicrobial Desensitization Protocols 291
Kara L. Murray, PharmD, Carlton K. K. Lee, PharmD, MPH

    I.   Penicillin 291
    II.   Cephalosporins 294
    III.   Trimethoprim/ Sulfamethoxazole (TMP/SMX) Oral 295
    IV.   Fluoroquinolone 297
    V.   Vancomycin 298
    VI.   Aminoglycosides 300

Chapter 10: Formulary 305
Carlton K. K. Lee, PharmD, MPH

    I.   Note to Reader 305
    II.   Sample Entry 306
    III.   Explanation of Breast-Feeding Categories 307

IV. Explanation of
     Pregnancy
     Categories   307
V.   Drug Index   307

VI. Drug Doses   317

Index   497

Infectious Agents and Drugs of Choice

Julia A. McMillan, MD, George K. Siberry, MD, MPH, and James D. Dick, PhD

I. RECOMMENDED TREATMENT FOR BACTERIAL INFECTIONS

TABLE 1-1
RECOMMENDED TREATMENT FOR BACTERIAL INFECTIONS*

Pathogen	Host Category	Indication/Type of Infection	Recommended Treatment	Duration	Alternative Treatment	Duration	Comments
Acinetobacter spp	All	Respiratory, bacteremia	Carbapenem + AG	≥14 days (depending on site of infection)	Pip/tazo + AG *or* Amp/sulb + AG *or* Pceph + AG *or* Gatifloxacin	≥14 days (depending on site of infection)	Variably but often highly resistant; colistin or sulbactam used in some highly resistant cases
Actinobacillus spp	All	Any	3rd Ceph	Variable (endocarditis, 4-6 wk)	Penicillin + gentamicin *or* Ampicillin + gentamicin *or* Ciprofloxacin	Variable endocarditis, 4-6 wk	Common coinfection with *Actinomyces*. May add AG or rifampin to 3rd Ceph for endocarditis.
Actinomyces israeli and other spp	All	Any	IV PenG Ampicillin, then oral amoxicillin	4-6 wk 6-12 mo	PCS3 or IV Pceph Oral: erythro-, doxy-, or clindamycin	3 wk 4 wk 6-12 mo	Surgical debridement. Prolonged antibiotics essential. Failure of erythro-, doxycycline, or clindamycin may be due to presence of *Actinobacillus*.
Aeromonas hydrophila	All	Gastroenteritis	TMP/SMX	5 days?	FQ Tetracycline	5 days? 5 days?	Unclear benefit of antimicrobial treatment.

Organism		Drug	Duration	Drug	Duration	Comments
	Invasive	3rd ceph + gentamicin	≥10 days (depending on site of infection)	Carbapenem or TMP/SMX or Tetracycline or Ciprofloxacin	≥10 days (depending on site of infection)	Debridement
Achromobacter xylosoxidans	All	Ceftazidime	≥10 days (depending on site of infection)	Meropenem or TMP/SMX	≥10 days (depending on site of infection)	Variable activity of Pip/tazo, Tic/clav, FQ
Anaplasma phagocytophila (formerly *Ehrlichia phagocytophila*)	Disseminated	Doxycycline	≥7 days *and* 3 days afebrile	Tetracycline	≥7 days *and* 3 days afebrile	Doxycycline is drug of choice regardless of age. No evidence of teeth staining after ≤2 wk course of doxycycline. CHL not recommended.
	Pregnant	Rifampin	≥7 days *and* 3 days afebrile	Doxycycline	≥7 days *and* 3 days afebrile	Limited clinical data about efficacy of rifampin vs potential negative effect on bones and teeth of fetus
Arcanobacterium haemolyticum	Pharyngitis	Erythromycin	Unknown	Clindamycin or Tetracycline or Penicillin	Unknown	TMP/SMX resistant Test for penicillin susceptibility and tolerance.
	Invasive disease	PenG + AG	10 days?	Clindamycin or Ceph or Macrolide	Variable	

INFECTIOUS AGENTS AND DRUGS OF CHOICE

1

TABLE 1-1

RECOMMENDED TREATMENT FOR BACTERIAL INFECTIONS—cont'd

Pathogen	Host Category	Indication/Type of Infection	Recommended Treatment	Duration	Alternative Treatment	Duration	Comments
Bacillus anthracis (potential bioterrorism [BT] agent)	All	Cutaneous	Doxycycline *or* Ciprofloxacin	7-10 days (60 days if bioterrorism)			Potential bioterrorism agent. Penicillin or amoxicillin can be used to complete therapy for children <8 yr old with naturally acquired anthrax or proven penicillin-susceptible after initial treatment with doxycycline or ciprofloxacin.
		Gastrointestinal; pulmonary; invasive	[Doxycycline *or* ciprofloxacin] + [Rifampin *or* vancomycin *or* clinda]	60 days			Potential bioterrorism agent. Cephalosporins and TMP/SMX not reliable
Bacillus cereus	All	Food poisoning	None				Supportive care only
		Invasive	[Vancomycin *or* clinda] ± AG	Variable	Ciprofloxacin *or* Meropenem *or* Imipenem	Variable	Debridement and hardware removal. Uniformly resistant to beta-lactams

Bacteroides: fragilis group	All	Above diaphragm	Pip/tazo *or* Tic/clav *or* A/C *or* Amp/sulb *or* Clindamycin	Depends on site and ability to drain/debride	Debridement/drainage important for therapy
		Below diaphragm	Metronidazole	Depends on site and ability to drain/debride	Clindamycin *or* Pip/Tazo *or* Carbapenem *or* Cefoxitin	Depends on site and ability to drain/debride	Debridement/drainage important for therapy
		Intracranial	Metronidazole	Unknown	Carbapenem?	Unknown
Bartonella henselae (cat scratch disease)	Immunocompetent	Adenitis	None *or* Azithromycin	5 days			Modest reduction in lymph node with azithromycin. Needle aspiration of suppurative lymph node for relief.
		Severe systemic cat scratch disease	TMP/SMX *or* Rifampin *or* Azithromycin *or* Ciprofloxacin *or* IV gentamicin	Unknown			Preferred therapy unclear

INFECTIOUS AGENTS AND DRUGS OF CHOICE   1

TABLE 1-1

RECOMMENDED TREATMENT FOR BACTERIAL INFECTIONS—cont'd

Pathogen	Host Category	Indication/Type of Infection	Recommended Treatment	Duration	Alternative Treatment	Duration	Comments
Bartonella henselae or *quintana*	Immunocompromised	Bacillary peliosis (liver, other RE sites) Bacillary angiomatosus	Erythromycin ± rifampin *or* Doxycycline ± rifampin	2 mo (angiomatosus) 4 mo (peliosis)	Azithromycin ± rifampin *or* ciprofloxacin	2 mo (angiomatosus) 4 mo (peliosis)	
Bartonella bacilliformis (Bartonellosis or Carrion's disease)	All	Acute (Oroya fever)	CHL (preferred because also treats Salmonella)	Unknown	Penicillin *or* Tetracycline *or* Streptomycin	Unknown	Seen in the Andes mountains
		Chronic (Verruga peruana)	Tetracycline *or* Rifampin *or* Ciprofloxacin				Seen in the Andes mountains. Unclear benefit of treatment. Surgery.
Bordetella pertussis, parapertussis	All	Respiratory	Erythromycin or estolate Azithromycin *or* Clarithromycin	14 days 5 days 7 days	TMP/SMX	14 days	Increased pyloric stenosis with erythromycin use <2 wk old; not studied for other macrolides
Borrelia burgdorferi	Nonpregnancy, ≥8 yr old	Early localized disease/EM	Doxycycline *or* Amoxicillin	14-21 days 14-21 days	Cefuroxime *or* Erythromycin	14-21 days 14-21 days	
		Multiple EM	Doxycycline *or* Amoxicillin	21 days	Cefuroxime *or* Erythromycin	21 days	
		Isolated facial palsy	Doxycycline *or* Amoxicillin	21-28 days	Cefuroxime *or* Erythromycin	21-28 days	Steroids not helpful

	Condition					Comments
	Arthritis—initial	Doxycycline or Amoxicillin	28 days	Cefuroxime or Erythromycin	28 days	There is no clear option for patients intolerant of penicillin and ceftriaxone
	Arthritis—recurrent or persistent	Repeat initial rx or Ceftriaxone or Penicillin IV	28 days / 14-21 days / 14-28 days			
Child <8 yr old, or pregnancy	Early localized disease/EM	Amoxicillin	14-21 days	Cefuroxime or Erythromycin	14-21 days / 14-21 days	
	Multiple EM	Amoxicillin	21 days	Cefuroxime or Erythromycin	21 days	
	Isolated facial palsy	Amoxicillin	21-28 days	Cefuroxime or Erythromycin	21-28 days	Steroids not helpful
	Arthritis—initial	Amoxicillin	28 days	Cefuroxime or Erythromycin	28 days	NSAIDs helpful adjunctive therapy
	Arthritis—recurrent or persistent	Repeat initial rx or Ceftriaxone or Penicillin IV	28 days / 14-21 days / 14-28 days	—	—	No clear option for patients intolerant of penicillin and ceftriaxone
All	Carditis	Ceftriaxone or Penicillin IV	14-21 days / 14-28 days	—	—	
	Meningitis or encephalitis	Ceftriaxone or Penicillin IV	28 days		28 days	Repeated or prolonged antibiotic course not helpful

INFECTIOUS AGENTS AND DRUGS OF CHOICE

1

TABLE 1-1

RECOMMENDED TREATMENT FOR BACTERIAL INFECTIONS—cont'd

Pathogen	Host Category	Indication/Type of Infection	Recommended Treatment	Duration	Alternative Treatment	Duration	Comments
Borrelia recurrentis, hermsii, and *turicate*	<8 yr old, or pregnant	Relapsing fever —louseborne (*recurrentis*)	Erythromycin	5-7 days	Penicillin *or* CHL	5-7 days	Give additional starting dose of penicillin (PO or IV) if febrile
	Nonpregnant, ≥8 yr old	—tickborne (others)	Doxycycline	5-7 days	Erythromycin Penicillin CHL	5-7 days	
Brucella abortus and other spp	Nonpregnant, ≥8 yr old	Brucellosis	Doxycycline + gentamicin *or* Doxycycline + rifampin	6 wk 2 wk 6 wk 2-3 wk	Doxycycline + streptomycin	6 wk 2 wk	
	<8 yr old, or pregnant		TMP/SMX + gentamicin *or* TMP/SMX + rifampin	4-8 wk 2 wk 6 wk 6 wk	—		
	Nonpregnant, ≥8 yr old	Meningitis or endocarditis	Doxycycline + rifampin + (Streptomycin *or* gentamicin)	4-6 mo 4-6 mo 2-3 wk	—		
	<8 yr old, or pregnant		TMP/SMX + rifampin + (Streptomycin *or* gentamicin)	4-6 mo 4-6 mo 2-3 wk			

Organism		Disease	Drug of Choice	Duration	Alternative	Duration	Comments
Burkholderia cepacia (potential BT agent)	All	Any	Meropenem	14 days?	TMP/SMX or Minocycline or Piperacillin or 3rd Ceph or Quinolones	14 days	Meropenem + 1 or 2 agents from alternative list may be best.
Burkholderia mallei (potential BT agent)	All	Glanders	Sulfadiazine	Unknown	Doxycycline or AG or FQ or Streptomycin or gentamicin or Imipenem or ceftazidime or TMP/SMX	Unknown	
Burkholderia pseudomallei (Potential BT agent) (SE Asia, Australia, India, Central America)		Meliodosis	Ceftazidime or Imipenem, followed by oral doxycycline	10-14 days 4-6 mo	TMP/SMX or Doxycycline or CHL or Ciprofloxacin or Piperacillin	Unknown (Alternative regimens are less effective.)	After IV therapy, give prolonged oral therapy.
Calymmatobacterium granulomatis		Granuloma inguinale; donovanosis	Doxycycline TMP/SMX	≥3 wk	Ciprofloxacin or Erythromycin or Azithromycin (weekly)	≥3 wk	Should have response within 7 days; if not, add gentamicin.
Campylobacter jejuni	Children	Gastroenteritis	Erythromycin or Azithromycin	5-7 days	Doxycycline (≥8 yr old)	5-7 days	
	Adults		Erythromycin or Ciprofloxacin or Azithromycin	5-7 days	Doxycycline	5-7 days	FQ resistance is increasing.

INFECTIOUS AGENTS AND DRUGS OF CHOICE

1

TABLE 1-1

RECOMMENDED TREATMENT FOR BACTERIAL INFECTIONS—cont'd

Pathogen	Host Category	Indication/Type of Infection	Recommended Treatment	Duration	Alternative Treatment	Duration	Comments
All *Campylobacter* spp	All	Invasive	Carbapenem *and/or* AG	Variable	—	Variable	Human oral flora
Capnocytophaga ochracea	All	Any	Clindamycin *or* Imipenem	Variable	Doxycycline A/C FQ	Variable	
Capnocytophaga canimorsus	All	Any	Penicillin	Variable	A/C *or* Clindamycin *or* Erythromycin *or* Doxycycline	Variable	Dog oral flora. Consider splenic dysfunction. Susceptible to penicillin but may prefer A/C for coinfection with other oral dog flora.
Cardiobacterium hominis			(Penicillin *or* 3rd ceph) + gentamicin	Variable			PCS3/gentamicin until penicillin susceptibility confirmed
Chlamydophila (Chlamydia) Pneumoniae	<8 yr old	Pneumonia	Erythromycin *or* Azithromycin	10-21 days 5 days	Clarithromycin	10 days	
	≥8 yr old	Pneumonia	Doxycycline *or* Erythromycin *or* Azithromycin	14 days 10-21 days 5 days	FQ *or* Clarithromycin	10 days 10 days	
Chlamydophila (Chlamydia) psittaci	<8 yr old	Psittacosis	Erythromycin	10-14 days after fever resolved	Azithromycin *or* Clarithromycin	10-14 days after fever resolved	
	≥8 yr old	Psittacosis	Doxycycline		Erythromycin *or* Azithromycin *or* Clarithromycin		

Chlamydia trachomatis	Infant	Conjunctivitis or pneumonia	Erythromycin _or_ Azithromycin	14 days 5 days	Clarithromycin _or_ Sulfonamide	14 days 14 days?	Increased risk of pyloric stenosis with Erythromycin in <6 wk old. Avoid sulfonamides <4 wk old.
	All	Urethritis, cervicitis, proctitis	Doxycycline _or_ Azithromycin	7 days 1 dose (1 g)	Erythromycin _or_ Ofloxacin _or_ Levofloxacin	7 days	6 mo–12 yr: Erythromycin or azithromycin Pregnancy: Erythromycin, azithromycin, or amoxicillin
	All	PID					See PID treatment recommendations in Chapter 2 (includes recommendations for _C. trachomatis_)
	All	Epididymitis	Doxycycline	10 days			
Chryseobacterium spp	All	Health-care associated invasive	Vancomycin + rifampin	Unknown	[TMP/SMX or FQ _or_ Minocycline] + rifampin		Formerly _Flavobacterium_; susceptibility testing may be unreliable.
Chromobacterium violaceum	All	Any	[TMP/SMX or FQ _or_ imipenem] _then_ [TMP/SMX PO or doxycycline PO or CHL PO]	2-3 wk 2-3 wk 2-3 wk 4 wk to several mo			R/O CGD. Erythromycin resistant, even if appears susceptible in vitro. Preferred treatment not well established. Two drugs from list (±TMP/SMX) used by some for first 2-3 wk. Relapse common

TABLE 1-1

RECOMMENDED TREATMENT FOR BACTERIAL INFECTIONS—cont'd

Pathogen	Host Category	Indication/Type of Infection	Recommended Treatment	Duration	Alternative Treatment	Duration	Comments
Citrobacter spp	All	Non-CNS	Imipenem or Meropenem	Variable	PCS3 or Pip/tazo or TMP/SMX or FQ	Variable	
		CNS	PCS3 + aminoglycoside	≥21 days; ≥4-6 wk if abscesses	Imipenem or Cefotaxime or Ceftriaxone	≥21 days; ≥4-6 wk if abscesses	
Clostridium botulinum	Infant	Infant botulism	Human botulism immune globulin intravenous (BG-IV) as soon as possible. Ordering info at http://www.infantbotulism.org/ or 510-231-7600				Do *not* use aminoglycosides!
	All	Wound or foodborne botulism	Equine botulinin antitoxin from local health department or CDC. [If local health department unavailable, contact CDC Drug Service at 404-639-3670 during business hours or 404-639-2888 after hours.]				
Clostridium difficile	All	Colitis	Oral metronidazole	7-10 days	Oral vancomycin or IV metronidazole or Nitazoxanide	7-10 days	Stop other antibiotics. Positive toxin in infant may not signify disease.
Clostridium tetani	All	Tetanus	Metronidazole + antitoxin	10-14 days	PenG IV + antitoxin	10-14 days	Human tetanus immunoglobulin (TIG) 3000-6000 units IM. Some experts infiltrate part of TIG into wound.

Clostridium perfringens, other spp	All	Food poisoning (perfringens)	None (supportive)		
		Septicemia, necrotizing myositis/fasciitis	PenG + clindamycin + surgery	Variable	[Clindamycin or metronidazole or carbapenem] + surgery	Variable	Surgery essential. Hyperbaric oxygen may be helpful.
Corynebacterium diphtheriae	All	Any	Antitoxin + [Erythromycin or penG aq or penG procaine]	14 days		Before IV antitoxin is given, a scratch test with 1:1000 dilution of antitoxin in saline solution should be performed, followed by an intradermal test if the scratch test is negative. Dose of antitoxin depends on severity of clinical presentation. Antitoxin and specific instructions available from the CDC (404-639-3311 or 404-639-2888). Document eradication by 2 consecutive negative cultures at least 24 hours after beginning treatment. Repeat erythromycin if culture is positive.

INFECTIOUS AGENTS AND DRUGS OF CHOICE 1

TABLE 1-1
RECOMMENDED TREATMENT FOR BACTERIAL INFECTIONS—cont'd

Pathogen	Host Category	Indication/Type of Infection	Recommended Treatment	Duration	Alternative Treatment	Duration	Comments
Corynebacterium jeikeum, other spp	All	Any	Vancomycin	Variable	Clindamycin or Erythromycin	Variable	Use vancomycin until specific susceptibilities are known.
Coxiella burnetti	All	Q fever	Doxycycline	10-14 days	FQ CHL TMP/SMX	10-14 days	May not need treatment in mild illness; TMP/SMX in pregnancy.
		Endocarditis	Doxycycline + hydrochloroquine	≥18 mo	[Doxycycline or ofloxacin] + rifampin	3 yr	
Edwardsiella tarda	All	Gastroenteritis	None				Similar to *Salmonella*. More common in warm climates.
		Invasive	PCS3	≥10-14 days	FQ (adults)	≥10-14 days	
Ehrlichia chafeensis	All	Any	Doxycycline	5-10 days and afebrile ≥3 days	Rifampin (pregnancy only)	5-10 days and afebrile ≥3 days	Doxycycline is drug of choice even in children <8 yr old. Consider alternative only for pregnant women.
Eikenella corrodens	All	Any	Ampicillin or Penicillin or A/C	7-10 days	Ureidopen or TMP/SMX or 2nd Ceph or 3rd Ceph or Carpapenem	7-10 days	A/C better than penicillin or ampicillin for occasional strain that produces beta-lactamase. All resistant to clindamycin and metronidazole.

Organism		Infection type		Duration		Duration	Comments
Enterobacter spp	All	Any	Ureidopen + aminoglycoside	≥10-14 days	Carbapenem or FQ (adult) or Tic/clav or Pip/tazo	≥10-14 days	Nosocomial strains may be multiresistant. Laboratory should test for ESBL.
Enterococcus faecalis and *faecium (not* vancomycin resistant)	All	Urinary tract	Ampicillin or Nitrofurantoin	7-14 days	Vancomycin	7-14 days	Add gentamicin for complicated or serious UTI.
		Sepsis, meningitis, endocarditis,	Ampicillin + gentamicin *or* Penicillin + gentamicin	≥2 wk (sepsis) 2-3 wk (CNS) 4-6 wk (endocarditis)	Vancomycin + gentamicin	≥2 wk (sepsis) 2-3 wk (CNS) 4-6 wk (endocarditis)	No gentamicin if high-level resistance, in which case longer course (8-12 wk for endocarditis).
Enterococcus, vancomycin resistant (VRE) (usually *E. faecium)*	All	Urinary tract	Linezolid *or* Quinupristin/ dalfopristin	7-14 days	Nitrofurantoin *or* FQ (if susceptible)	7-14 days	Most VRE are *E. faecium.* Quinupristin/ dalfopristin NOT active against *E. faecalis.*
		Sepsis, meningitis endocarditis, other invasive infection	Linezolid	≥2 wk (sepsis) 2-3 wk (CNS) ?8-12 wk (endocarditis)			Quinupristin/dalfopristin *not* active against *E. faecalis.* Expect higher relapse rate for endocarditis.
Erysipelothrix rhusiopathiae	All	Sepsis *or* Endocarditis	PenG *or* Amp	4-6 wk	PCS3 *or* FQ (adults) *or* Imipenem	4-6 wk	Oral antibiotics and shorter course for erysipiloid. Intrinsic vancomycin resistance.

INFECTIOUS AGENTS AND DRUGS OF CHOICE

1

TABLE 1-1

RECOMMENDED TREATMENT FOR BACTERIAL INFECTIONS—cont'd

Pathogen	Host Category	Indication/Type of Infection	Recommended Treatment	Duration	Alternative Treatment	Duration	Comments
Escherichia coli	All	Meningitis	PCS3	≥21 days	Meropenem or Cefepime	≥21 days	Treat for at least 21 days *and* at least 14 days from first negative CSF culture. Carbapenem if ESBL suspected.
		Sepsis	PCS3	≥14 days	FQ (adult) or Pip/Tazo or Carbapenem	≥14 days	Carbapenem if ESBL suspected.
		Cystitis	Amoxicillin or TMP/SMX	7-10 days	Sulfisoxazole or Nitrofurantoin or Oral ceph	7-10 days	Many oral options, based on susceptibility, including amoxicillin.
		Pyelonephritis	PCS 3 or OCS3	14 days	Ampicillin + gentamicin or FQ (adult) or TMP/SMX or Gentamicin or BL/BLI	14 days	Transition to oral antibiotics to complete 14-day course.
		Intra-abdominal	PCS3 or BL/BLI	≥14 days Longer courses for secondary peritonitis, abdominal abscesses	Carbapenem or FQ (adult) or Cefoxitin	≥14 days Longer courses for secondary peritonitis, abdominal abscesses	Carbapenem if ESBL suspected. If polymicrobial (gut florae) infection likely, add clindamycin or metronidazole to PCS3 or FQ to improve anaerobic coverage.

Escherichia coli—Enterohemorrhagic (STEC)	All	Diarrhea (risk of HUS)	None		Antibiotic therapy has no proven benefit and may increase risk of HUS.
Escherichia coli—Enteroinvasive	All	Dysentery	FQ (adult) or Azithromycin	3 days 5 days	TMP/SMX	3 days	TMP/SMX resistance common
Escherichia coli—Enterotoxigenic	All	Traveler's diarrhea	FQ (adult) or Azithromycin	3 days 5 days	TMP/SMX	3 days	TMP/SMX resistance common
Francisella tularensis	All	Tularemia	Streptomycin or gentamicin or amikacin	7 days (longer if more severe illness)	Imipenem or Ciprofloxacin or CHL	7 days (longer if more severe illness)	More relapses with tetracyclines. 3rd Ceph poor despite in vitro susceptibility.
		Tularemia with meningitis	CHL + [Streptomycin or gentamicin or amikacin]	≥10-14 days	Doxycycline + [Streptomycin or gentamicin or amikacin]	≥14 days	Recommendations based on very few cases.
Fusobacterium spp	All	Bacteremia (Septic jugular vein thrombosis/Lemierre syndrome)	PenG IV or Metronidazole or carbapenam	4-6 wk?	Clindamycin IV	4-6 wk?	Can switch IV to PO if ≥14 days, stable and good response. Penicillin is not appropriate for beta-lactamase + strains.

INFECTIOUS AGENTS AND DRUGS OF CHOICE

1

TABLE 1-1

RECOMMENDED TREATMENT FOR BACTERIAL INFECTIONS—cont'd

Pathogen	Host Category	Indication/Type of Infection	Recommended Treatment	Duration	Alternative Treatment	Duration	Comments
Gardenerella vaginalis—see Bacterial Vaginosis in Chapter 2							
Haemophilus ducreyi		Chancroid	Ceftriaxone or Azithromycin	1 dose 1 dose	Ciprofloxacin or Erythromycin	3 days 7 days	
Haemophilus influenzae—type b, occasionally other types, rarely nontypeable	All	Meningitis	Ceftriaxone or Cefotaxime	10 days	CHL FQ2	10 days	
		Other invasive, non-CNS	PCS3 or Amp/sulb IV	10 days 10 days	PCS2 or FQ IV	10 days 10 days	
Haemophilus influenzae—nontypeable		Ottitis, ottitis-conjunctivitis, sinusitis	A/C	10 days	OCS2 or OCS3 or Azithromycin or Clarithromycin or FQ or Ceftriaxone	10 days 10 days 5 days 10 days 10 days 1 dose	Some experts treat for only 5 days in children ≥6 yr
Haemophilus influenzae—aegypticus, other nontypeable	All	Conjunctivitis	FQ ophthalmic or Polymyx/TMP	5-10 days?	Gentamicin or Tobramycin	5-10 days?	
Haemophilus parainfluenza, haemolyticus, aphrophilus, other spp	All	Endocarditis	Ceftriaxone	4 wk	Ampicillin + gentamicin or Amp/sulb + gentamicin	4 wk	Use amp/sulb/gentamicin instead of ampicillin + gentamicin for beta-lactamase producers.

Organism	Type	Infection	Regimen 1	Duration	Regimen 2	Duration	Comments
Helicobacter pylori	All	Gastritis, gastric, and duodenal ulcers	Ampicillin + clarithromycin + [omeprazole or lansoprazole]	14 days	Metronidazole + clarithromycin + bismuth/ranitidine	14 days	
Kingella kingae, other spp	All	Osteomyelitis, arthritis	PCS 1/2/3 or PenG* or BL/BLI	≥21 days ≥21 days ≥21 days	AG or FQ or TMP/SMX or Oxacillin	≥21 days ≥21 days ≥21 days ≥21 days	*PenG drug of choice if no beta-lactamase. Longer course if osteo.
		Endocarditis	*PenG + gentamicin or *Amp + gentamicin or Ceftriaxone	28 days 28 days 28 days	Amp/Sulb + gentamicin or Other BL/BLI + gentamicin	28 days 28 days	*PenG or ampicillin only if no beta-lactamase. For regimens with gentamicin, use gentamicin for all 28 days.
Klebsiella spp	All	Cystitis, other minor infections	OCS 1/2/3 or A/C	7-10 days 7-10 days	TMP/SMX or FQ	7-10 days 7-10 days	For ESBL-positive strains, carbapenem usually drug of choice. Can use FQ if susceptible in vitro. Failure of BL/BLI (e.g., Pip/tazo) for ESBL-positive strains despite in vitro susceptibility. Meningitis: CSF cultures may be positive up to 2 wk despite treatment. Treat CNS infection ≥21 days *and* ≥10-14 days from first negative CSF culture.
		Pyelonephritis, bacteremia, sepsis (NO CNS)	PCS3 or FQ	≥14 days ≥14 days	Gentamicin Carbapenem BL/BLI	≥14 days ≥14 days	
		Meningitis	PCS3 ± AG	≥21 days	FQ Meropenem Pip/Tazo	≥21 days ≥21 days ≥21 days	
		ESBL-positive	Imipenem or Meropenem	As above for type of infection	FQ	As above for type of infection	

TABLE 1-1

RECOMMENDED TREATMENT FOR BACTERIAL INFECTIONS—cont'd

Pathogen	Host Category	Indication/Type of Infection	Recommended Treatment	Duration	Alternative Treatment	Duration	Comments
Legionella pneumophila	Healthy	Mild to moderate illness	Azithromycin or FQ	5-10 days 14-21 days	Doxycycline or TMP/SMX or Erythromycin or Clarithromycin	14-21 days 14-21 days 14-21 days 14-21 days	
	Immunocompromised and/or severe illness		Azithromycin + rifampin or FQ	≥10 days 14-21 days	Same as for less severe illness	14-21 days	
Leptospira interrogans	All	Mild illness	Amoxicillin or Doxycycline	7-14 days	—		Jarisch-Herxheimer reaction common after therapy initiation.
		Hospitalized or severe illness	PenG	14 days	Doxycycline	14 days	
Leuconostoc spp	All	Any	PenG ± AG or Ampicillin	Variable	Macrolide or Tetracycline or Carbapenem or CHL	Variable	Intrinsic vancomycin resistance. High rates of resistance to FQ and quinupristin/dalfopristin.
Listeria monocytogenes	ANY	Meningitis	Ampicillin + gentamicin	≥21 days	TMP/SMX	≥21 days	Intrinsic ceph resistance. No good alternative for neonates and late pregnancy.
	Neonatal	Non-CNS	Ampicillin + gentamicin	14-21 days			Failures reported with vancomycin and CHL; FQ and linezolid—minimal clinical data.
	Older	Sepsis, pneumonia	Ampicillin + gentamicin	14 days	TMP/SMX	14 days	
Moraxella catarrhalis	All	Noninvasive	A/C or TMP/SMX or OCS 2,3	≥10 days ≥10 days ≥10 days	Azithromycin or Clarithromycin or FQ or Doxycycline	≥10 days ≥10 days ≥10 days ≥10 days	Duration depends on site of infection

Organism		Infection	Drug	Duration	Drug	Duration	Comments
Morganella	All	Cystitis; other less serious infections	OCS3 or FQ	Variable	TMP/SMX or Amikacin	7–10 days for UTI, others, variable	Durations depends on site of infection
		Invasive and/or severe illness	PCS3, PCS4 + AG / FQ / Carbapenem	≥10 days / ≥10 days / ≥10 days		≥10 days / ≥10 days	
Mycobacterium TB and others—see Section II of this chapter							
Mycoplasma pneumoniae	All	Respiratory/ pulmonary	Azithromycin	5 days	Doxycycline or Erythromycin or Clarithromycin or FQ	7–10 days / 7–10 days / 7–10 days / 7–10 days	Best reponse if started within first 3–4 days of illness. Appropriate therapy for extrapulmonary disease not well defined.
Mycoplasma hominis	All	Any	Doxycycline or Clindamycin	≥10 days / ≥10 days	Rifampin or CHL	≥10 days / ≥10 days	Duration depends on site of infection. *M. hominis* is intrinsically resistant to macrolides. ?IVIG for agammaglobulinemics.
Neisseria gonorrhea	All	Urethritis, pharyngitis, proctitis, epididymitis	Ceftriaxone or Cefixime	Once / Once	Spectinomycin or Cefoxitin or Cefizoxime or Cefotaxime	Once / Once / Once / 7 days	Test and/or treat for *C. trachomatis.* Treatment failure more likely for pharyngitis. Fluoroquinolones *not* recommended unless susceptibility of infecting strain is documented.
		Conjunctivitis	Ceftriaxone	Once	Cefotaxime	7 days	Plus local irrigation. Add treatment for *C. trachomatis.*

INFECTIOUS AGENTS AND DRUGS OF CHOICE

1

TABLE 1-1
RECOMMENDED TREATMENT FOR BACTERIAL INFECTIONS—cont'd

Pathogen	Host Category	Indication/Type of Infection	Recommended Treatment	Duration	Alternative Treatment	Duration	Comments
		PID	See PID treatment recommendations in Chapter 2 (includes treatment for gonorrhea)				Add treatment for C. trachomatis.
		Disseminated, arthritis	Ceftriaxone then [Cefixime or Cefpodoxime]	≥24-48 hr after some clinical response 7 days	[Spectinomycin or Ceftizoxime or Cefotaxime] then [Cefixime or Cefpodoxime]	≥24-48 hr after some clinical response 7 days	Test and/or treat for C. trachomatis.
		Meningitis	Ceftriaxone	10-14 days	—		
		Endocarditis	Ceftriaxone	≥4 wk	—		
		Exposed infant	Ceftriaxone	Once			125 mg IM in term infant; 25-50 mg/kg (max 125 mg) IM in preterm infant
Neisseria meningitidis	All	Meningitis, sepsis, pneumonia	PenG	5-7 days	Ampicillin or PCS 3 or CHL	5-7 days 5-7 days 5-7 days	Some experts use PCS3 until susceptibilities known because of increasing penicillin resistance in some areas (especially Spain). CHL only if very severe β-lactam allergy.

Organism	Host	Type	Drug of choice	Duration	Alternative	Duration	Comments
Nocardia brasiliensis, asteroids, other spp	Normal	Noninvasive	TMP/SMX	6-12 wk	Minocycline or A/C	6-12 wk	High in vitro susceptibility to linezolid but minimal clinical data.
	Immunocompromised and/or invasive		TMP/SMX	≥6-12 mo		≥6-12 mo	
	All	CNS or severe	[TMP/SMX + Amikacin ± ceftriaxone]	≥6-12 mo / 1-3 mo / 1-3 mo	Amikacin + [Imipenem or ceftriaxone] or [Imipenem + amikacin ± ceftriaxone] or [TMP/SMX + imipenem + amikacin]	≥6-12 mo / 1-3 mo / 1-3 mo	
Pasteurella multocida	All	Localized	PenVK Amoxicillin	7-10 days 7-10 days	Azithromycin TMP/SMX OCS2 Doxycycline FQ	5 days 10-14 days 10-14 days 10-14 days 10-14 days	PCS3 susceptible in vitro but clinical data lacking
		Invasive or severe	PenG Ampicillin	10-14 days 10-14 days	PCS2 FQ Doxycycline	10-14 days 10-14 days 10-14 days	
Pediococcus spp	All	Any	PenG ± AG	Variable	Other beta-lactam or Erythromycin or CHL or Imipenem or Linezolid or Daptomycin	Variable	Intrinsic vancomycin resistance. High rates of resistance to quinupristin/dalfopristin.
Plesiomonas shigelloides	All	Diarrhea	TMP/SMX or FQ	3 days	A/C or CS 1/2/3 or Carbapenem	3 days 3 days 3 days	Probable diarrheal pathogen.

TABLE 1-1

RECOMMENDED TREATMENT FOR BACTERIAL INFECTIONS—cont'd

Pathogen	Host Category	Indication/Type of Infection	Recommended Treatment	Duration	Alternative Treatment	Duration	Comments
Plesiomonas shigelloides—cont.		Invasive	PCS3	Unknown			Definitive antibiotic therapy should be guided by susceptibility testing.
Prevotella spp	All	Oral, respiratory	Clindamycin	≥10 days	Penicillin *or* Ampicillin *or* APPN	≥10 days ≥10 days ≥10 days	BL/BLI if BL + strain. Longer duration if undrainable abscesses.
		GI, genitourinary	Metronidazole	≥10 days	Clindamycin *or* CHL *or* Cefoxitin *or* Carbapenem *or* BL/BLI	≥10 days ≥10 days ≥10 days ≥10 days ≥10 days	Longer duration if undrainable abscesses
Propionobacterium acnes	All	Acne vulgaris (inflammatory)	Erythromycin topical *or* Clindamycin topical	Many wk	Doxycycline PO *or* Minocycline PO	Many wk	Plus nonantibiotic topical anti-acne. Oral agents used for nonresponse to topicals or severe acne.
		Invasive	PenG (high dose)	Variable	Clindamycin Doxycycline Ceph		Usually associated with hardware.
Proteus mirabilis	All	Cystitis, other nonserious	Ampicillin	5-7 days	TMP/SMX *or* OCS *or* FQ	5-7 days 5-7 days 5-7 days	Proteus UTI associated with urolithiasis.

		Pyelonephritis, other invasive	Ampicillin or FQ	≥10 days ≥10 days	PCS3 or AG or Carbapenem	≥10 days ≥10 days ≥10 days	Isolates from urine/blood/CSF should be tested for ESBL.
Proteus vulgaris and other indole-positive spp	All	Cystitis, other nonserious	PCS3 or FQ	5-7 days 5-7 days	A/C	5-7 days	Dual treatment of invasive indole-positive Proteus to prevent emergence of resistance.
		Pyelonephritis, other invasive	PCS3 + AG or FQ + AG	≥10 days ≥10 days	[Carbapenem or BL/BLI + gentamicin]	≥10 days ≥10 days ≥10 days	
Providencia spp	All	Cystitis, other nonserious	TMP/SMX or A/C	5-7 days	OCS3	5-7 days	
		Pyelonephritis, other invasive	PCS3 + AG FQ	≥10 days ≥10 days	Amikacin BL/BLI	≥10 days ≥10 days	
Pseudomonas aeruginosa, other spp	All	Uncomplicated UTI, other nonserious	FQ (Ciprofloxacin) APCS APPN	≥10 days ≥10 days ≥10 days	AG Carbapenem	≥10 days ≥10 days	
		Pneumonia, bacteremia, sepsis	APCS3/4 + AG APPN + AG	≥14 days ≥14 days	Carbapenem + AG	≥14 days	
		Meningitis	APCS3/4 + AG APPN + AG	≥14 days ≥14 days	Carbapenem + AG	≥14 days	Cultures negative at least 10 days.
Rickettsia rickettsii	All	Rocky Mountain Spotted Fever (RMSF)	Doxycycline	7-10 days	CHL	7-10 days	Treat until at least 3 days afebrile. Doxycycline drug of choice even <8 yr old.
Rickettsia akari	All	Rickettsialpox	Doxycycline	3-5 days	CHL	3-5 days	Treat until at least 3 days afebrile.

TABLE 1-1

RECOMMENDED TREATMENT FOR BACTERIAL INFECTIONS—cont'd

Pathogen	Host Category	Indication/Type of Infection	Recommended Treatment	Duration	Alternative Treatment	Duration	Comments
Rickettsia prowazekii	All	Epidemic typhus	Doxycycline	7-10 days	CHL *or* FQ	7-10 days 7-10 days	Treat until at least 3 days afebrile. Doxycycline drug of choice even <8 yr old.
Rickettsia typhi	All	Endemic typhus	Doxycycline	5-10 days	CHL	5-10 days	Treat until at least 3 days afebrile. Doxycycline drug of choice even <8 yr old.
Rickettsia—other spp	All		Doxycycline	7-10 days	CHL	7-10 days	Treat until at least 3 days afebrile.
Salmonella typhi (type D)	All	Typhoid fever	PCS3 *or* FQ IV	10-14 days 10-14 days			High rates of FQ resistance in some geographic areas. Dexamethasone may be appropriate adjunctive therapy. May switch to oral therapy to complete course once improvement established. Clinical failure despite in vitro activity of 1st ceph and 2nd ceph, AG, furazolidone.
		Typhoid fever—mild	Azithromycin PO *or* PCS3 *or* FQ PO	7 days 7-14 days 7-14 days	Amoxicillin PO *or* TMP/SMX PO *or* CHL PO	10-14 days 10-14 days 10-14 days	Shorter courses for milder disease in non-immunocompromised host may be effective.

Organism	Host	Disease	Drug	Duration	Alternative	Duration	Comments
Salmonella, non-typhi	All	Enteric fever, bacteremia	Same as for typhoid fever				
		Localized, non-meningeal disease (osteomyelitis, abscess)	PCS3	≥4 wk			May change to ampicillin IV if isolate proven susceptible.
		Meningitis	PCS3	6 wk			May change to ampicillin IV if isolate proven susceptible.
	Normal	Gastroenteritis	NO antibiotics				Supportive treatment only
	Infant <3 mo; sickle cell; splenic dysfunction	Gastroenteritis	PCS 3 or Amoxicillin or TMP/SMX	5 days 5 days 5 days	FQ	5 days	FQ may be first choice in adults. Avoid amoxicillin and TMP/SMX in areas of prevalent resistance unless susceptibility proven.
Serratia marcescens	All	Invasive (bacteremia, meningitis, pneumonia)	[Imipenem or meropenem] + AG	Variable, ≥21 days for meningitis	[PCS3/4 or APPN] + AG	Variable, ≥21 days for meningitis	For neonatal meningitis perform daily CSF cultures until sterile. Treat 10-14 days after first sterile CSF culture. Susceptibility testing should guide therapy. Consider CGD evaluation for non-neonates.
Shigella sonnei, Shigella dysenteriae, Shigella boydii, Shigella flexneri	Child	Gastroenteritis, dysentery	TMP/SMX or Cefixime or FQ	3 days 3 days 5 days	Azithromycin or Ceftriaxone or Nalidixic acid or	5 days 2-5 days 5 days	TMP/SMX resistance high in many areas. Mixed results for efficacy of cefixime. Treat for 7-10 days in immunocompromised hosts.

INFECTIOUS AGENTS AND DRUGS OF CHOICE

1

TABLE 1-1

RECOMMENDED TREATMENT FOR BACTERIAL INFECTIONS—cont'd

Pathogen	Host Category	Indication/Type of Infection	Recommended Treatment	Duration	Alternative Treatment	Duration	Comments
	Adult	Gastroenteritis, dysentery	FQ	5 days	Azithromycin	5 days	Invasive disease is uncommon.
			TMP/SMX	5 days	Nalidixic acid	5 days	
				2 days	Ceftriaxone	2 days	
	All ages	Bacteremia, invasive	Ceftriaxone	≥10 days	FQ	≥10 days	
Staphyloccus aureus; Methicillin-susceptible *S. aureus* (MSSA)	All	Superficial	1st ceph or SS-pen or BL/ BLI or Macrolide	10 days 10 days 10 days 10 days	Clindamycin or TMP/SMZ or Linezolid	10 days 10 days 10 days	
		Osteomyelitis	SS-pen IV or 1st ceph IV	4-6 wk	Clindamycin IV or Vancomycin IV	4-6 wk	Switch from IV to PO when good clinical response.
		Arthritis	SS-pen IV or 1st ceph IV	3-4 wk	Clindamycin IV or Vancomycin IV	3-4 wk	
		Bacteremia/sepsis pneumonia/empyema	SS-pen IV	≥3 wk	Vancomycin IV	≥3 wk	Some experts add rifampin and/or gentamicin in selected cases.
		Endocarditis (native valve)	SS-pen IV + gentamicin	4-6 wk (gentamicin 3-5 days)	Vancomycin + gentamicin	4-6 wk (gentamicin 3-5 days)	
		CNS	SS-pen IV ± rifampin	10 days from negative culture	Vancomycin IV ± rifampin	10 days from negative culture	
		Toxic shock syndrome	SS-pen IV + clindamycin	10 days	Vancomycin + clindamycin	10 days	Eliminate either antibiotic; once stable can complete PO Some experts recommend adding IVIG.

Organism	Type		Duration		Duration	Comments
All	Superficial	Clindamycin or TMP/SMZ	10 days 10 days	Vancomycin IV or Doxycycline (≥8 yr) or Linezolid	10 days 10 days 10 days	Switch from IV to PO when good clinical response. Confirm clindamycin susceptibility with D-test.
	Osteomyelitis, arthritis	Clindamycin IV or Vancomycin IV	6 wk (osteomyelitis) 3-4 wk (arthritis)	Linezolid or Daptomycin	6 wk (osteomyelitis) 3-4 wk (arthritis)	May add rifampin and/or gentamicin. No daptomycin for pneumonia.
	Bacteremia/sepsis pneumonia/empyema	Vancomycin IV	≥3 wk	Linezolid IV Daptomycin	≥3 wk ≥3 wk	Gentamicin sometimes recommended for synergy
	Endocarditis (native valve)	Vancomycin IV	4-6 wk	Linezolid	4-6 wk	Add rifampin for shunt infections
	CNS	Vancomycin IV ± rifampin	10 days from negative culture			Confirm clindamycin susceptibility with D-test if erythromycin resistant
	Toxic shock syndrome	Vancomycin + clindamycin	10 days			
Stenotrophomonas maltophilia	All	TMP/SMX or Tic/clav	≥10 days ≥10 days	[Tic/clav + TMP/SMX] Minocycline or Doxycycline or Ceftazidime	≥10 days ≥10 days ≥10 days ≥10 days	Duration depends on site and severity of infection
Streptobacillus moniliformis	All	PenG procaine IM or penG IV	7-10 days for all regimens	Ampicillin IV or Cefuroxime IV or PCS3 or Erythromycin or Doxycyline or Streptomycin	7-10 days for all regimens	Course can be completed orally once patient stable and with good response.

INFECTIOUS AGENTS AND DRUGS OF CHOICE

1

TABLE 1-1

RECOMMENDED TREATMENT FOR BACTERIAL INFECTIONS—cont'd

Pathogen	Host Category	Indication/Type of Infection	Recommended Treatment	Duration	Alternative Treatment	Duration	Comments
Streptococcus pneumoniae	All	Sinopulmonary infections, otitis media (non-CNS, noninvasive)	Amoxicillin, high-dose Cefuroxime Cefdinir Cefpodoxime	10 days for all regimens	Azithromycin Clindamycin PCS3	5 days 10 days 10 days (1 day for otitis media)	Parenteral choices for more severe illnesses. Can switch to PO when stable in many cases. Susceptibility testing guides antibiotic options.
		Bacteremia, severe pneumonia (invasive, non-CNS)	PCS3	≥10 days (longer if focus of infection, e.g., bone)	Vancomycin IV or Clindamycin IV or Linezolid IV or Carbapenem IV	All ≥10 days (longer if focus of infection, e.g., bone)	Susceptibility testing guides antibiotic options.
		Meningitis, penicillin and PCS3 susceptible	PCS3 or AqPenG	14 days	Carbapenem IV or Vancomycin + rifampin	14 days	Susceptibility testing guides antibiotic options.
		Meningitis, penicillin nonsusceptible, and PCS3 susceptible	PCS3	14 days	Carbapenem IV or Vancomycin + rifampin	All 14 days	Susceptibility testing guides antibiotic options.
		Meningitis, penicillin, and PCS3 nonsusceptible	Vancomycin + PCS3 ± rifampin	14 days	CHL or Vancomycin + rifampin or Linezolid	All 14 days	Susceptibility testing guides antibiotic options. Repeat LP 48-72 hrs, especially if inadequate clinical improvement.

Group A *Streptococcus*		Pharyngitis	PenVK PO or Amoxicillin PO or PenG benzathine IM	10 days 10 days 10 days	OCS1 or Erythromycin or Azithromycin or Clarithromycin	5-10 days 10 days 5 days 10 days	PenVK bid and amoxicillin bid or once daily acceptable. Some data for 5 days OCS1.
		TSS, necrotizing fasciitis, other invasive	PenG IV + clindamycin	≥10 days	Ceftriaxone + clindamycin or Vancomycin + clindamycin	≥10 days ≥10 days	Simplify to 1 antibiotic when patient stable. Adjunctive sugery often needed. Duration depends on site of infection.
Group B *Streptococcus*	All	Invasive (nonmeningitis, not sepsis)	Ampicillin or PenG	≥10 days, depending on site of infection	PCS3 or Vancomycin	≥10 days, depending on site of infection	
		Meningitis, sepsis	[Ampicillin or penicillin] + gentamicin	14-21 days 2-3 days	PCS3 or Vancomycin	14-21 days 14-21 days	High-dose ampicillin or penicillin used for meningitis. Gentamicin used until clinical response and CSF/ blood sterile.
Group C, G *Streptococcus*	All	Pharyngitis; other noninvasive	PenVK PO	10 days	OCS1, OCS2, or TMP/SMX	10 days 10 days	
	All	Invasive, nonendocarditis	PenG IV	>10 days	PCS 1, 2, 3 or Vancomycin	>10 days >10 days	May add gentamicin if tolerance suspected

INFECTIOUS AGENTS AND DRUGS OF CHOICE 1

TABLE 1-1

RECOMMENDED TREATMENT FOR BACTERIAL INFECTIONS—cont'd

Pathogen	Host Category	Indication/Type of Infection	Recommended Treatment	Duration	Alternative Treatment	Duration	Comments
	All	Endocarditis	[PenG IV or ceftriaxone] + gentamicin	4-6 wk 4-6 wk 2 wk	Vancomycin	4-6 wk	Once-daily gentamicin not studied in pediatric endocarditis. If prosthetic valve/material or less susceptible organism, use 6 wk instead of 4. For highly resistant isolate, use 6 wk of [penicillin or ceftriaxone] *plus* 6 wk of gentamicin. Vancomycin *only* if penicillin and ceftriaxone contraindicated.
Viridans streptococci	All	Dental, soft tissue, noninvasive	Penicillin PO or Amoxicillin or Ampicillin	Variable	OCS or PSC or Vancomycin or CHL	Variable	Ceftriaxone preferred PCS. Must consider possible polymicrobial infections.
	Usually neonate, altered immunity or intravascular catheter	Bacteremia, other invasive	Penicillin ± gentamicin IV or Ampicillin ± gentamicin IV or Ceftriaxone ± gentamicin IV	10-14 days 10-14 days 10-14 days	Vancomycin ± gentamicin IV	10-14 days	Streptomycin may be substituted for gentamicin. Increasing penicillin-resistant strains, especially in oncology patients.

Condition	Drug of choice	Duration	Alternative	Duration	Comments
Native valve endocarditis, highly susceptible (Pen MIC ≤0.1)	PenG IV or Ceftriaxone IV or Penicillin + gentamicin IV or Ceftriaxone + gentamicin IV	4 wk 4 wk 2 wk 2 wk	Vancomycin IV	4 wk	Vancomycin only if intolerant of other regimen
Native valve endocarditis, relatively resistant (Pen MIC>0.12 g/mL–≤0.5 g/mL)	PenG IV/gentamicin IV or Ceftriaxone/gentamicin IV	4 wk/2 wk 4 wk/2 wk	Vancomycin IV	4 wk	Vancomycin only if intolerant of other regimen.
Native valve endocarditis, resistant	Ampicillin + gentamicin IV or Penicillin + gentamicin IV or Vancomycin + gentamicin IV	4-6 wk 4-6 wk 6 wk	—	—	Same as for enterococcal endocarditis. Vancomycin only if intolerant of other regimen.
Prosthetic valve endocarditis, susceptible (Pen MIC ≤0.12)	Pen G or Ceftriaxone ± gentamicin	6 wk 6 wk 2 wk	Vancomycin IV	6 wk	Vancomycin only if intolerant of other regimen.
Prosthetic valve endocarditis, relatively or fully resistant (Pen MIC >0.12)	Pen G or Ceftriaxone + gentamicin	6 wk 6 wk	Vancomycin IV	6 wk	Vancomycin only if intolerant of other regimen.

TABLE 1-1
RECOMMENDED TREATMENT FOR BACTERIAL INFECTIONS—cont'd

Pathogen	Host Category	Indication/Type of Infection	Recommended Treatment	Duration	Alternative Treatment	Duration	Comments
Treponema pallidum (syphilis)	Infants	Proven or probably congenital syphilis	PenG IV 50,000 units/kg/dose q12 hr (<8 days old) or q8hr (>7 days old)	10 days	PenG procaine IM 50,000 units/kg once daily	10 days	Close clinical and serologic follow-ups essential, especially if single dose regimen used
		Mother's treatment or response inadequate but infant evaluation normal	PenG IV *or* PenG procaine IM *or* PenG benzathine IM	10 days 10 days Once			Close clinical and serologic follow-ups essential, especially if single dose regimen used
		Mother adequately treated and infant evaluation normal	PenG benzathine IM *or* No antibiotic	Once			Close clinical and serologic follow-ups essential, especially if no treatment given.
	Beyond infancy	Primary; secondary; latent <1 year	PenG benzathine IM	Once	Doxycycline *or* Tetracycline	14 days 14 days	Doxycycline and tetracycline only used for penicillin-allergic, nonpregnancy patients. Penicillin-allergic pregnant women **must** be desensitized and treated with penicillin.

	Population	Condition	Drug	Duration	Alternative	Duration	Comments
	Beyond infancy	Latent 1 yr or greater; latent unknown duration; tertiary *without* neurosyphilis	PenG benzathine IM	Once weekly for 3 wk	Doxycycline *or* Tetracycline	28 days / 28 days	
	Beyond infancy	Neurosyphilis; Syphilitic eye disease	AqPenG IV	10-14 days	[PenG procaine IM + probenicid] *or* Ceftriaxone	10-14 days / 10-14 days	Penicillin-allergic pregnant women **must** be desensitized and treated with penicillin. Ceftriaxone only in nonpregnant women if penicillin cannot be used
Ureaplasma urealyticum	All	Urethritis	Doxycycline PO	7 days	Erythromycin PO / Azithromycin PO	7 days / 1 dose	Erythromycin ×14 days preferred for children <8 yr old.
	Preterm neonates	Symptomatic respiratory	Erythromycin IV/PO	10 days	Azithromycin(?) PO/IV	10 days	Route depends on degree of illness. Pyloric stenosis risk with erythromycin. Scant data for azithromycin treatment.
		Symptomatic CNS	Doxycycline IV	10-14 days	CHL IV	10-14 days	Very limited data.

INFECTIOUS AGENTS AND DRUGS OF CHOICE

1

TABLE 1-1

RECOMMENDED TREATMENT FOR BACTERIAL INFECTIONS—cont'd

Pathogen	Host Category	Indication/Type of Infection	Recommended Treatment	Duration	Alternative Treatment	Duration	Comments
Vibrio cholera	All	Moderate to severe illness	TMP/SMX PO or Doxycycline PO or Tetracycline PO or Ciprofloxacin PO	3 days 1 dose 3 days 1 dose	Furazolidone PO or Erythromycin PO or Azithromycin PO or Ofloxacin PO	3 days Unknown 1 dose Unknown	Fluid/electrolyte most important part of Rx. Tetracycline and doxycycline preferred for ≥8 yr old. Ciprofloxacin if ≥18 yr old. Variable resistance. Furazolidone preferred during pregnancy.
Vibrio vulnificus, Vibrio parahemolyticus, other spp	All	Bacteremia/sepsis Wound	Tetracycline + AG or Doxycycline + ceftazidime	Variable Variable	FQ or TMP/SMX or PCS3	Variable Variable Variable	Prompt debridement for wound infections and necrotizing fasciitis
Yersinia enterocolitica, Yersinia pseudotuberculosis	Normal	Enterocolitis Pseudoappendicitis Mesenteric adenitis	None				Antibiotics may limit duration of shedding but no clinical benefit
	Immunocompromised	Enterocolitis	TMP/SMX or AG or Cefotaxime or FQ or Tetracycline or Doxycycline or Piperacillin	Variable	CHL	Variable	Tetracycline and doxycycline for ≥8 yr old. FQ for ≥18 yr old. *Y. enterocolitica:* consider iron overload syndromes

All	Sepsis or other invasive illness	TMP/SMX or AG or Cefotaxime or FQ or Tetracycline or Doxycycline or Piperacillin	Variable	CHL	Variable	Treat until afebrile several days.
Yersinia pestis (plague)	Bubonic/ pneumonic plague	Streptomycin IM Gentamicin IM/IV	≥7-10 days ≥7-10 days	Tetracycline IV or Doxycycline IV or CHL IV	≥7-10 days ≥7-10 days ≥7-10 days	Variable
	Meningitis, endophthalmitis, or shock	CHL IV	≥7-10 days	—	—	

*Some recommendations are for antibiotics that are not approved by the Food and Drug Administration for use in children, and some may not be approved for treatment of the pathogen listed. Recommendations are based on published evidence of efficacy.

A/C, amoxicillin/clavulanic acid (Augmentin); AG, aminoglycoside; Amp/sulb, ampicillin/sulbactam (Unasyn); APCS, anti-Pseudomonal cephalosporin; APPN, anti-Pseudomonal penicillin; aq, aqueous; BL/BLI, beta-lactam + beta-lactamase; inhibitor combination; CDC, Centers for Disease Control and Prevention; Ceph, cephalosporin; 1st Ceph, first-generation cephalosporin; 2nd Ceph, second-generation cephalosporin; 3rd Ceph, third-generation cephalosporin; CGD, chronic granulomatous disease; CHL, chloramphenicol; Clinda, clindamycin; CNS, central nervous system; CSF, cerebrospinal fluid; EM, erythema marginatum; ESBL, extended-spectrum beta-lactamase producer; FQ, fluroquinolone; GI, gastrointestinal; HUS, hemolytic uremic syndrome; IM, intramuscular; IV, intravenous; IVIG, intravenous immunoglobulin; MIC, minimum inhibitory concentration; NSAID, nonsteroidal anti-inflammatory drug; OCS, oral cephalosporin; OCS1, first-generation oral cephalosporin; OCS2, second-generation oral cephalosporin; OCS3, third-generation oral cephalosporin; PCS, parenteral cephalosporin; PCS1, first-generation parenteral cephalosporin; PCS2, second-generation parenteral cephalosporin; PCS3, third-generation parenteral cephalosporin; PCS4, fourth-generation parenteral cephalosporin PID, pelvic inflammatory disease; Pen G, penicillin G; Pen VK, penicillin VK (oral); Pip/tazo, piperacillin/tazobactam (Zosyn); PO, by mouth; PPI, proton pump inhibitor; R/O, rule out; RE, reticuloendothelial; Rif, rifampin; Rx, treatment; SS-Pen, semi-synthetic penicillin (nafcellin, oxacillin); Tic/clav, ticarcillin/clavulinic acid (Timentin); TMP/SMX, trimethoprim/sulfamethoxazole; Ureidopen, ureidopenicillin (e.g., ticarcillin, piperacillin); UTI, urinary tract infection; Vanco, vancomycin.

INFECTIOUS AGENTS AND DRUGS OF CHOICE

1

II. RECOMMENDED TREATMENT FOR MYCOBACTERIAL INFECTIONS*

TABLE 1-2

RECOMMENDED TREATMENT FOR MYCOBACTERIAL INFECTIONS

Pathogen	Host Category	Indication/Type of Infection	Recommended Treatment	Duration	Alternative Treatment	Duration	Comments
Mycobacterium tuberculosis[1]	Immunocompetent	Latent infection (positive TST, no disease); isoniazid-susceptible	Isoniazid	9 mo			
		Latent infection, isoniazid-resistant	Rifampin	6 mo			
		Latent infection; isoniazid and rifampin-resistant	Treat only after consultation with a tuberculosis specialist				
	Pregnancy and breast feeding	Latent infection	Isoniazid + pyridoxine	9 mo			Treatment with **isoniazid** should *not* begin *before* the first trimester. **Isoniazid** is secreted in human milk but no adverse effects to infants have been detected.

Immunocompromised, HIV-infected	Latent infection	Same as for immunocompetent		Induction of ≥5 mm indicates a positive TST in immunocompromised individuals Consultation with a specialist is recommended.
Immunocompetent	Pulmonary and extra-pulmonary, **drug-susceptible disease** (excluding meningitis or disseminated/miliary tuberculosis)	[Isoniazid + rifampin + pyrazinamide] *followed by* [Isoniazid + rifampin]	2 mo 4 mo	DOT is advised. Six-month course of **isoniazid** and **rifampin** is sufficient for treatment of hilar adenopathy without additional site(s) of involvement. **Corticosteroids** may be considered as adjunctive therapy for 4-6 wk for patients with pleural and pericardial effusions, endobronchial disease, and abdominal tuberculosis.

TABLE 1-2

RECOMMENDED TREATMENT FOR MYCOBACTERIAL INFECTIONS—cont'd

Pathogen	Host Category	Indication/Type of Infection	Recommended Treatment	Duration	Alternative Treatment	Duration	Comments
		Pulmonary and extrapulmonary disease (excluding meningitis or disseminated/miliary tuberculosis)—**possibly drug resistant**	[Isoniazid + rifampin + pyrazinamide] + [Ethambutol or aminoglycoside[2]] *followed by* [Isoniazid trifampin] to complete a 6 month course	4 mo Until susceptibilities are known			DOT is advised. Determine susceptibilities from patient isolate when possible. If not available, infer susceptibility from suspected source. If that is not available, consider local endemic rates of drug resistance or use initial 4-drug regimen. **Corticosteroids** may be considered as adjunctive therapy for 4-6 wk for patients with pleural and pericardial effusions, endobronchial disease, and abdominal tuberculosis.

| Pulmonary and extrapulmonary disease—**possibly multidrug resistant or extensively drug resistant (XDR) isolate** | | Treat only after consultation with a tuberculosis specialist |
| Meningitis or disseminated/ miliary tuberculosis | 2 mo

7-10 mo | [Isoniazid + rifampin + pyrazinamide + [Ethionamide *or* aminoglycoside[2]] *followed by* [Isoniazid + rifampin] | If susceptibility to **isoniazid, rifampin, and pyrazinamide** is confirmed, the fourth drug can be discontinued. **Corticosteroid** (2 mg/ kg/day of prednisone, maximum 60 mg/day for 4-6 wk followed by taper) is also indicated for meningitis once anti-tuberculosis therapy is begun. |

TABLE 1-2

RECOMMENDED TREATMENT FOR MYCOBACTERIAL INFECTIONS—cont'd

Pathogen	Host Category	Indication/Type of Infection	Recommended Treatment	Duration	Alternative Treatment	Duration	Comments
	Pregnancy	Pulmonary and extrapulmonary disease	[Isoniazid + rifampin + ethambutol + pyridoxine]	9 mo	[Isoniazid + rifampin + pyrazinamide + pyridoxine]	6 mo	Although teratogenicity data are not available, **pyrazinamide** can probably be used safely during pregnancy and is recommended by the World Health Organization and the International Union against Tuberculosis and Lung Disease. If **pyrazinamide** is not included in initial treatment regimen, treatment should be for at least 9 mo.
	Congenital infection	Pulmonary and extrapulmonary disease	Isoniazid + rifampin + pyrazinamide + amikacin		Treat as above for tuberculosis disease, depending on antibiotic susceptibility		Add corticosteroid if meningitis is confirmed. Send placenta for TB culture and pathologic exam.

Mycobacterium bovis	All	Pulmonary and extrapulmonary disease, excluding meningitis	Isoniazid + rifampin	9-12 mo	Recommended treatment for *M. bovis* is based on treatment trials for *M. tuberculosis*. All strains of *M. bovis* are resistant to **pyrazinamide**.
		Meningitis	[Isoniazid + rifampin] + [Ethionamide *or* aminoglycoside²] *followed by* [Isoniazid + rifampin]	At least 9-12 mo	

Nontuberculous mycobacteria: Recommendations are for presumptive therapy and no recommendation for duration is provided. Controlled trials are limited, and susceptibility testing may not correlate with clinical response. Guidance from a specialist in treating mycobacterial infection is recommended.

Mycobacterium avium complex	Immunocompetent	Lymphadenitis	Excision of affected node(s)		Pharmacologic therapy is recommended if excision is incomplete or if disease recurs.
			[Clarithromycin *or* azithromycin] + [Ethambutol *and/or* (Rifampin *or* rifabutin)]		

INFECTIOUS AGENTS AND DRUGS OF CHOICE

1

TABLE 1-2

RECOMMENDED TREATMENT FOR MYCOBACTERIAL INFECTIONS—cont'd

Pathogen	Host Category	Indication/Type of Infection	Recommended Treatment	Duration	Alternative Treatment	Duration	Comments
	Immunocompetent or immunocompromised	Pulmonary infection	[Clarithromycin or azithromycin] + Ethambutol + [Rifampin or rifabutin]				Amikacin or streptomycin can be added initially for severe disease.
		Disseminated disease	Treat only in consultation with an expert. Initial recommended therapy with 3-4 drugs, including [Clarithromycin or azithromycin] + Ethambutol				

Mycobacterium kansasii	All	Pulmonary infection	[Rifampin + ethambutol + isoniazid]
		Osteomyelitis	Surgical debridement + rifampin + ethambutol + isoniazid
Mycobacterium marinum	All	Cutaneous infection	[Rifampin + TMP/SMX + [Clarithromycin or doxycycline[3]]	Minor infection may heal without therapy. Extensive lesions may require surgical debridement.
Mycobacterium ulcerans	All	Cutaneous and bone infection	Excision of tissue	**Rifampin + streptomycin** is under study for treatment of infections caused by this organism.

TABLE 1-2

RECOMMENDED TREATMENT FOR MYCOBACTERIAL INFECTIONS—cont'd

Pathogen	Host Category	Indication/Type of Infection	Recommended Treatment	Duration	Alternative Treatment	Duration	Comments
Mycobacterium fortuitum	All	Cutaneous infection	Excision of tissue				
		Serious infection	Amikacin + meropenem *followed by* [Clarithromycin *or* Doxycycline[3] *or* TMP/SMX *or* Ciprofloxacin]				Duration of therapy should be determined in consultation with an infections disease specialist.
		Catheter infection	Catheter removal + amikacin + meropenem *followed by* [Clarithromycin *or* Doxycycline[3] *or* TMP/SMX *or* Ciprofloxacin]				Definitive therapy should be based on susceptibility testing. Duration of therapy should be determined in consultation with an infectious disease specialist.

Mycobacterium abscessus	All	Otitis media	Clarithromycin + amikacin + cefoxitin	May require debridement. Susceptibility testing should be performed—**amikacin** resistance occurs in 50% of isolates.
	Patients with cystic fibrosis	Pulmonary infection	Clarithromycin + amikacin + cefoxitin	Surgical resection may be required. Susceptibility testing should be performed.
Mycobacterium chelonae	All	Catheter infection	Catheter removal + tobramycin + clarithromycin	
		Disseminated cutaneous infection	[Tobramycin + (Meropenem or Linezolid) + clarithromycin]	

*Some recommendations are for antibiotics that are not approved by the Food and Drug Administration for use in children, and some may not be approved for treatment of the pathogen listed. Recommendations are based on published evidence of efficacy.

1. Public health authorities should be notified if an individual with newly diagnosed latent infection is detected.
2. IM streptomycin is usually recommended; if not available, kanamycin, amikacin, or capreomycin can be used.
3. Doxycycline should be prescribed for children <8 years old only if the benefits outweigh the risks.

DOT, directly observed therapy; TMP/SMX, trimethoprim-sulfamethoxazole; TST, tuberculin skin test.

INFECTIOUS AGENTS AND DRUGS OF CHOICE   1

III. RECOMMENDED TREATMENT FOR VIRAL INFECTIONS*

TABLE 1-3

RECOMMENDED TREATMENT FOR VIRAL INFECTIONS

Pathogen	Host Category	Indication	Recommended Treatment	Alternative Treatment	Comment
Cytomegalovirus	Immunocompromised	GI tract, lungs, viremia	Ganciclovir, IV for 14-21 days	Foscarnet, IV or Cidofovir, IV or Valganciclovir, PO	For treatment of pulmonary or GI infection, immune globulin may be used along with ganciclovir. Long-term suppressive therapy is used to prevent relapse in patients with HIV infection. Cidofovir should be administered with probenecid and hydration.
		Ocular infection	Ganciclovir IV	Valganciclovir PO or Ganciclovir IV or Foscarnet IV or Cidofovir IV	Additional therapy using intraocular ganciclovir or fomivirsen may be used, depending on location of lesion(s) and degree of immunocompromise.
		Long-term suppression of ocular infection	Ganciclovir, IV indefinitely	Foscarnet, IV or Cidofovir, IV or Valganciclovir, PO	Cidofovir should be administered with probenecid and hydration.

Neonate	Symptomatic neurologic congenital infection ≤28 days of life	Ganciclovir, IV for 6 wk	Data to support optimal use and duration of ganciclovir for this indication are controversial.
Hepatitis B	Chronic disease, ≥2 years old	Interferon alpha or pegylated interferon alpha, subcutaneously, for 6 mo if HBeAG positive; for 12 mo or longer if HBeAG negative	Lamivudine for minimum of 12 mo or 6 mo after HBeAG seroconversion or Adefovir dipiroxil or Entecavir or telbivudine	Definition of "chronic disease" varies depending on the protocol used. Treatment of chronic hepatitis B infection in children is under continued investigation, and some drugs used to treat adults are not approved for children. Specialists in hepatology should be consulted. If lamivudine is used to treat children coinfected with HIV and hepatitis B, the lamivudine dose used should be the approved dose for treating HIV infection.
Hepatitis C	Chronic infection, ≥3 years old	Interferon alpha or pegylated interferon alpha, subcutaneously + ribavirin, PO, for 12-48 wk depending on virologic response and virus genotype		Children with symptomatic hepatitis C disease or histologically advanced pathologic features should be considered for treatment in consultation with a gastroenterologist or infectious disease consultant.

INFECTIOUS AGENTS AND DRUGS OF CHOICE

1

TABLE 1-3

RECOMMENDED TREATMENT FOR VIRAL INFECTIONS—cont'd

Pathogen	Host Category	Indication	Recommended Treatment	Alternative Treatment	Comment
Herpes simplex (HSV)	Immunocompetent	Genital (first episode)	Acyclovir PO for 5-10 days or Famciclovir PO or Valacyclovir PO or Acyclovir IV for 5-7 days		Famciclovir and valacyclovir are licensed only for adolescents and adults. May switch to PO to complete.
		Genital (recurrent)	Acyclovir PO for 5 days or Famciclovir PO or Valcyclovir PO or Acyclovir IV for 5-7 days		Famciclovir and valacyclovir are licensed only for adolescents and adults. May switch to PO to complete.
		Suppression of recurrent mucocutaneous outbreaks	Acyclovir PO or Famciclovir PO or Valacyclovir PO for as long as 12 mo continuously		Famciclovir and valacyclovir are licensed only for adolescents and adults

CNS (encephalitis)	Acyclovir IV for at least 21 days Higher dose for neonatal CNS/disseminated disease—see formulary	
Neonate	Any	Acyclovir IV for 14 (skin, eye, mucous membrane involvement) to 21 days (disseminated or CNS involvement)	
Immunocompromised	Any non-CNS site	Acyclovir IV for 7-14 days	Foscarnet IV	Use foscarnet for HSV infection resistant to acyclovir. Treat until infection resolves.
	Mucocutaneous	Acyclovir PO for 7-14 days or Famciclovir PO or Valacyclovir PO	Foscarnet IV	Use foscarnet for HSV infection resistant to acyclovir.
All	Keratoconjunctivitis	Trifluridine or Iododeoxyuridine or Vidarabine		Consult an ophthalmologist.

INFECTIOUS AGENTS AND DRUGS OF CHOICE 1

TABLE 1-3
RECOMMENDED TREATMENT FOR VIRAL INFECTIONS—cont'd

Pathogen	Host Category	Indication	Recommended Treatment	Alternative Treatment	Comment
Influenza	≥1 year of age	Treatment	Oseltamivir PO for 5 days		Most effective if treatment is initiated within 48 hours of onset of symptoms. Amantadine and rimantadine have been used to treat influenza A, but most isolates since 2006 have been resistant.
	≥7 yr of age	Treatment	Zanamivir, inhalation, for 5 days *or* Oseltamivir PO for 5 days		Most effective if treatment is initiated within 48 hours of onset of symptoms. Amantadine and rimantadine have been used to treat influenza A, but most isolates since 2006 have been resistant.
Respiratory syncytial virus (RSV)	Bronchiolitis/pneumonia, severe		Ribavirin, aerosol via small-particle generator, 18 hrs/day for 3-7 days		Longer treatment may be required for some patients. Effectiveness has been questioned. Not routinely recommended.

Varicella	Immunocompetent	Varicella	Acyclovir PO or IV for 5 days		Begin within 24 hours of symptoms
		Zoster	Acyclovir PO or IV for 5-7 days	Famciclovir PO *or* Valacyclovir PO	Famciclovir and valacyclovir are licensed only for adolescents and adults.
	Immunocompromised	Varicella	Acyclovir IV for 7-10 days	Foscarnet IV	Use of oral acyclovir instead of, or to complete an IV therapy course, is used by some experts for patients thought to be at low risk of severe disease.
		Zoster	Acyclovir PO or IV for 7-10 days	Famciclovir PO *or* Valacyclovir PO *or* Foscarnet IV	Famciclovir and valacyclovir are licensed only for adolescents and adults.
Parvovirus	Immunocompromised with persistent anemia		IVIG		

*Some recommendations are for antibiotics that are not approved by the Food and Drug Administration for use in children, and some may not be approved for treatment of the pathogen listed. Recommendations are based on published evidence of efficacy.
HBeAG, hepatitis B e antigen; IV, intravenous; PO, by mouth.

INFECTIOUS AGENTS AND DRUGS OF CHOICE   1

IV. RECOMMENDED TREATMENT FOR FUNGAL INFECTIONS*

Fungal pathogens are listed according to clinical and laboratory presentation on pp. 72-73.

A. SYSTEMIC TREATMENT

TABLE 1-4

RECOMMENDED TREATMENT FOR FUNGAL INFECTIONS: SYSTEMIC TREATMENT

Fungus	Host Category	Indication	Recommended Treatment	Duration§	Alternative Treatment	Duration§	Comment
Alternaria sp (Phaeohyphomycosis)	Immunocompromised	Locally invasive infection (mycotic keratitis, paranasal sinusitis, osteomyelitis, cutaneous infection)	Liposomal amphotericin B	≥10 wk	Itraconazole for localized cutaneous disease		Surgical debridement with or without granulocyte transfusion may be helpful additional modes of therapy.
Aspergillus sp	Immunocompromised	Invasive infection (pulmonary, sinus, disseminated, CNS)	Voriconazole	≥10 wk	Liposomal amphotericin B *or* Caspofungin	≥10 wk	Surgical debridement for sinusitis. Consult infectious disease specialist regarding possible combination therapy.

			Itraconazole may be helpful to reduce need for corticosteroid
Immunocompetent	Allergic bronchopulmonary aspergillosis	Corticosteroid	
	Allergic sinusitis	Surgical drainage, antibiotic for secondary bacterial infection, topical corticosteroid	
	Pulmonary aspergilloma	Surgical removal may be required; endobronchial instillation of amphotericin B or itraconazole has been used	
	Otomycosis	Debridement; topical clotrimazole or econazole nitrate	
Bipolaris sp	Immunocompromised or post trauma	Disseminated infection; sinusitis	Amphotericin B or lipid-formulation of amphotericin B; surgical excision or debridement may be required	Itraconazole for cutaneous infection

TABLE 1-4

RECOMMENDED TREATMENT FOR FUNGAL INFECTIONS: SYSTEMIC TREATMENT—cont'd

Fungus	Host Category	Indication	Recommended Treatment	Duration§	Alternative Treatment	Duration§	Comment
Blastomyces dermatitidis (Blastomycosis)	All	Disseminated, life-threatening disease	Amphotericin B (total dose: 15 mg/kg; max, 1.5-2.5 g) followed by itraconazole or fluconazole	2 wk of amphotericin B, followed by 6 mo of itraconazole or fluconazole	Fluconazole		Consider fluconazole therapy only for patients unable to tolerate amphotericin B. If oral therapy is used, serum concentration should be measured and adherence should be assessed. Treatment recommendations for children are extrapolated from adult studies. Consultation with infectious disease specialist is advised.
		CNS disease	Amphotericin B	Daily for 4-6 wk (total dose 30-40 mg/kg) followed by amphotericin B, 3 times weekly for 1-3 mo			

Immunocompromised	Cutaneous, pulmonary, bone disease	Amphotericin B (total dose: 15 mg/kg; max, 1.5-2.5 g) followed by itraconazole or fluconazole	2 wk of amphotericin B, followed by 6 mo of itraconazole or fluconazole. Bone infection should be treated for a total of 12 mo	Fluconazole or itraconazole	6 mo. Bone infection should be treated for a total of 12 mo	If oral therapy is used, serum concentration should be measured and adherence should be assessed. Treatment recommendations for children are extrapolated from adult studies. Consultation with infectious disease specialist is advised.
Immunocompetent	Mild to moderate skin, pulmonary, or bone infection	Itraconazole	6-12 mo (12 mo recommended for bone infections)	Fluconazole	Observation alone may be appropriate for mild or resolving disease
	Severe pulmonary disease	Amphotericin B (total dose 1.5-2.5 g) or amphotericin B (total dose 15 mg/kg over 2 wk) followed by itraconazole or fluconazole	If azole is used, it should be continued for 6-12 mo	Fluconazole	If oral therapy is used, serum concentration should be measured and adherence should be assessed

TABLE 1-4

RECOMMENDED TREATMENT FOR FUNGAL INFECTIONS: SYSTEMIC TREATMENT—cont'd

Fungus	Host Category	Indication	Recommended Treatment	Duration[6]	Alternative Treatment	Duration[6]	Comment
Candida sp[1]	Immunocompromised	Oropharyngeal (thrush)	Fluconazole	7-21 days	Topical nystatin or clotrimazole or voriconazole	7-21 days	Alternative drugs should be used for refractory cases; prolonged therapy may be required. Intraperitoneal infusion of amphotericin B is alternative for patients with candidal peritonitis; flucytosine provides synergistic therapy for Candida albicans but not demonstrated for other Candida species; alternative agents should not be used until the infecting species is known to be susceptible.
		Esophagitis	Fluconazole or Amphotericin B	21 days (or at least 14 days after resolution of symptoms)	Caspofungin or micafungin or voriconazole		
		Catheter-associated infection (intravascular or peritoneal)	Catheter removal + amphotericin B	Until blood/peritoneal cultures are negative for at least 14 days; longer treatment course for granulocytopenic and severely immunocompromised patients; at least 14 days for peritonitis	Fluconazole or caspofungin or micafungin or anidulafungin	Until blood/peritoneal cultures are negative for 14 days; longer treatment course for granulocytopenic and severely immunocompromised patients; at least 14 days for peritonitis	

Condition	Drug	Duration	Alternative	Duration	Comments
Disseminated infection	Amphotericin B ± flucytosine	Varies with site of infection, clinical response, and presence or absence of neutropenia	Fluconazole or caspofungin or micafungin or anidulafungin	Varies with site of infection, clinical response, and presence or absence of neutropenia	Flucytosine provides synergistic therapy for C. *albicans* but not demonstrated for other *Candida* species; alternative agents should not be used until the infecting species is known to be susceptible; rifampin is thought to provide synergistic effect
Endocarditis	Valve replacement + amphotericin B + flucytosine	6 wk following valve replacement			Lifelong suppressive therapy with fluconazole may be an alternative if valve replacement is not possible.
Meningitis	Amphotericin B + flucytosine	At least 4 wk following resolution of signs and symptoms			Fluconazole has been used for follow-up therapy and long-term suppression. Data on success are limited.
Chronic mucocutaneous candidiasis	Fluconazole or itraconazole	Lifelong	Amphotericin B (0.3 mg/kg/day IV)	Lifelong	

INFECTIOUS AGENTS AND DRUGS OF CHOICE

1

TABLE 1-4

RECOMMENDED TREATMENT FOR FUNGAL INFECTIONS: SYSTEMIC TREATMENT—cont'd

Fungus	Host Category	Indication	Recommended Treatment	Duration[b]	Alternative Treatment	Duration[b]	Comment
		Congenital/ disseminated candidiasis of newborn	Amphotericin B	Total dose of 10-25 mg/kg	Fluconazole	Unknown	Experience with fluconazole in newborns is limited. Some lipid formulations of amphotericin B have questionable renal penetration and should not be used to treat disseminated disease.
	Immunocompetent	Oropharyngeal (thrush)	Nystatin or clotrimazole	7-10 days	Fluconazole	7-10 days	
		Vulvovaginal	Topical agents, including clotrimazole or miconazole or butoconazole or terconazole or tioconazole or nystatin or Fluconazole (oral), single dose	1-14 days, depending on the agent used	Oral agents, including itraconazole or ketoconazole for refractory cases	7-14 days	

Infectious agent	Therapy	Duration	Alternative	Duration	Comments
Diaper dermatitis	Nystatin, topical	7-10 days	Topical miconazole or clotrimazole or naftifine or ketoconazole or econazole or ciclopirox	7-10 days	Surgical drainage is important for paronychia.
Intertrigo, paronychia	Topical agents, including clotrimazole, miconazole, and nystatin	Prolonged therapy may be required			
IV catheter-associated candidemia	Catheter removal + fluconazole or caspofungin or amphotericin B	7-10 days if blood cultures are negative following catheter removal			
Coccidioides immitis (Coccidioidomycosis) Severe infection; immunocompromised patients	Amphotericin B (total dose, 10-100 mg/kg; max 1 g), followed by fluconazole or itraconazole	1-12 mo, total, depending on clinical and immunologic response; lifelong for HIV patients			The majority of immunocompetent patients with coccidioidomycosis do not require treatment. Absorption of itraconazole is unpredictable; serum concentrations should be measured.
Pulmonary disease			Itraconazole or fluconazole for milder disease	1-12 mo, depending on clinical and immunologic response; lifelong for HIV patients	
Nonmeningeal, extrapulmonary disease	Itraconazole	At least 12 mo and 3 mo beyond resolution of symptoms	Amphotericin B (total dose, 10-100 mg/kg; max 1 g) or fluconazole	12 mo	

TABLE 1-4

RECOMMENDED TREATMENT FOR FUNGAL INFECTIONS: SYSTEMIC TREATMENT—cont'd

Fungus	Host Category	Indication	Recommended Treatment	Duration§	Alternative Treatment	Duration§	Comment
		CNS infection	Fluconazole	Lifelong	Amphotericin B IV and in the intrathecal, ventricular, or cisternal space	Lifelong	Dose of fluconazole should be in the upper end of the recommended range. Periodic CSF exam should be performed for 2 yr. May be a cause of disseminated infection in neutropenia
Curvularia sp		Eumycotic mycetoma	Surgical excision and itraconazole or Amphotericin B	≥10 mo (or at least 3 mo after inflammation has resolved			Surgical excision may be required
		Phaeohyphomycosis	Amphotericin B or Itraconazole	Unknown; prolonged therapy required depending on the host and the site of infection	Voriconazole	Unknown; prolonged therapy required depending on the host and the site of infection	
Cryptococcus neoformans	Immunocompromised	Disseminated disease without CNS involvement	Fluconazole or [Fluconazole + flucytosine for 10 wk; then fluconazole alone]	Lifelong	Itraconazole or weekly amphotericin B for lifelong suppressive therapy		CSF should be examined to rule out occult meningitis; maintain flucytosine serum concentration at 40-60 µgm/mL

	Drug	Duration	Alternative	Duration	Comments
Meningitis	[Amphotericin B + flucytosine] for 2 wk; then fluconazole (12 mg/kg/d, max 400 mg/day) for 10 wk; then fluconazole (6 mg/kg/d, max 200 mg/d)	Lifelong	[Amphotericin B + flucytosine] for 6-10 wk; then fluconazole (200 mg/day); itraconazole or weekly amphotericin B may be used for lifelong suppressive therapy	Lifelong	Manage increased intracranial pressure (↑ ICP) with repeat lumbar puncture; reassess CSF after 2 wk of therapy; intrathecal amphotericin B may be required.
Immunocompetent — Pulmonary disease	Fluconazole or [Amphotericin B + flucytosine for 2 wk followed by fluconazole]	3-6 mo	Itraconazole	3-6 mo	CSF should be examined to rule out occult meningitis.
Meningitis	Amphotericin B + [Flucytosine or fluconazole] for 2 wk; then fluconazole for 10 wk		Amphotericin B + flucytosine	6-10 wk	Reassess CSF after 2 wk; if culture is positive, prolonged therapy is required.
Exophiala sp	Eumycotic mycetoma; sinusitis	Surgical excision and itraconazole or amphotericin B	≥10 mo (or at least 3 mo after inflammation has resolved)	Voriconazole	≥10 mo (or at least 3 mo after inflammation has resolved)
Exserohilum sp	Eumycotic mycetoma; sinusitis	Surgical excision and [Itraconazole or amphotericin B]	≥10 mo (or at least 3 mo after inflammation has resolved)	Voriconazole	≥10 mo (or at least 3 mo after inflammation has resolved)

TABLE 1-4

RECOMMENDED TREATMENT FOR FUNGAL INFECTIONS: SYSTEMIC TREATMENT—cont'd

Fungus	Host Category	Indication	Recommended Treatment	Duration[5]	Alternative Treatment	Duration[5]	Comment
Fusarium sp	Immunocompromised	Disseminated disease (fungemia, skin lesions, multiple organ involvement)	Voriconazole		High dose amphotericin B or lipid formulation of amphotericin B or posoconazole		Granulocyte transfusion and granulocyte colony-stimulating factor may be beneficial.
	Immunocompetent	Locally invasive infection (mycotic keratitis, endophalmitis, sinusitis, subcutaneous infection)	High-dose amphotericin B or lipid formulation of amphotericin B		Voriconazole		
Histoplasma capsulatum (Histoplasmosis)	Immunocompromised	Disseminated infection	Amphotericin B, 30 mg/kg (total) over 4 wk, followed by itraconazole	Lifelong	Itraconazole	Lifelong	Monitor urine or serum antigen concentration; should decrease with effective therapy
		Meningitis	Amphotericin B for 3 mo, then fluconazole for 12 mo	Lifelong suppressive fluconazole			
	Immunocompetent	Acute pulmonary disease with symptoms >4 wk	Amphotericin B followed by itraconazole	Total therapy: 12 wk or until urine *Histoplasma* antigen is <4 units	Amphotericin B followed by fluconazole	Total therapy: 12 wk or until urine *Histoplasma* antigen is <4 units	Primary pulmonary infection does not require treatment in most individuals.

		Drug of choice	Duration	Alternative	Duration	Comments
	Progressive disseminated histoplasmosis	Amphotericin B for 4-6 wk followed by itraconazole	Total therapy 6-18 mo			Surgical drainage may be required for large, necrotic masses, but excision of fibrotic pulmonary lesions risks uncontrolled hemorrhage.
	Granulomatous mediastinitis	[Corticosteroids + amphotericin B] followed by itraconazole	Total therapy 6 mo	Amphotericin B for 2-3 wk followed by itraconazole	Total therapy 6-18 mo	
	Pericarditis, erythema nodosum, arthritis	NSAID; antifungal therapy not required	2-12 wk			Pericardial drainage may be required.
Madurella sp (South Asia)	Eumycotic mycetoma	Surgical excision and [itraconazole or amphotericin B]	≥10 mo (or at least 3 mo after inflammation has resolved)			
Malassezia sp — Immunocompromised (including neonates)	Catheter-associated fungemia	Catheter removal; + discontinuation of intravenous lipid + fluconazole	Depends on persistence of fungemia, presence/absence of metastatic foci			
Immunocompetent	Pityriasis versicolor	Topical selenium sulfide (2.5%)	1-2 wk; then monthly	Oral itraconazole or ketoconazole		
Paracoccidioides brasiliensis	All; GI infection; disseminated disease	Itraconazole or Amphotericin B	6-12 mo	Ketoconazole	6-12 mo	Sulfonamides are used in resource-poor countries, but maintenance therapy must be used for 3-5 yr to avoid relapse

TABLE 1-4

RECOMMENDED TREATMENT FOR FUNGAL INFECTIONS: SYSTEMIC TREATMENT—cont'd

Fungus	Host Category	Indication	Recommended Treatment	Duration[§]	Alternative Treatment	Comment
Penicillium marneffei	Immunocompromised (HIV+)	Pneumonitis; disseminated infection	Itraconazole or Amphotericin B			Common in AIDS patients in S.E. Asia
Pneumocystis jiroveci	Immunocompromised	Severe pneumonia (pO₂ < 70 mm Hg or alveolar-arterial gradient of >35)	Trimethoprim-sulfamethoxazole + prednisone	21 days (prednisone should be administered for 5-7 days at 1 mg/kg, then tapered over 7-12 days)	Pentamadine	Prednisone should be started within 72 hours after starting specific antibiotic therapy.
		Mild-moderate pneumonia	Trimethoprim-sulfamethoxazole	21 days—Oral therapy may be substituted for IV therapy in mild-	[Dapsone + trimethoprim] or Atovaquone or [Trimetrexate + leucovorin] or [Primaquine + clindamycin]	
		Prophylaxis	Trimethoprim-sulfamethoxazole	Depends on age and CD4+ T-lymphocyte count	Dapsone or [Dapsone + pyramethamine + folinic acid] or atovaquone or aerosolized pentamadine monthly	HIV+ Adults/Adolescents can discontinue primary or secondary prophylaxis if CD4 > 200 for at least 3 mo. HIV+ children >12 mo old can stop primary prophylaxis if age-related CD4 no longer severely immunosuppressed for 3 mo.

Organism	Host	Infection	Treatment	Duration	Treatment	Duration	Treatment	Duration	Comments
Pseudallescheria boydii	Immunocompromised	Pneumonia; disseminated infection	Surgical excision *and* voriconazole	Indefinitely	Surgical excision *and* voriconazole	Indefinitely	Itraconazole	Indefinitely	Usually resistant to amphotericin B. If oral therapy is used, serum concentration should be measured and adherence should be assessed.
	Immunocompetent	Eumycotic mycetoma; other localized infections (pneumonia, septic arthritis, osteomyelitis, sinusitis)	Surgical excision *and* itraconazole	3-6 mo if local excision is possible; otherwise, years	Surgical excision *and* fluconazole *or* voriconazole	3-6 mo if local excision is possible; otherwise, years			Usually resistant to amphotericin B. If oral therapy is used, serum concentration should be measured and adherence should be assessed.
Trichosporon sp (Trichosporonosis)	Immunocompromised	Disseminated infection	Voriconazole	Varies with site of infection, clinical response, and presence, or absence of neutropenia	Itraconazole				
Wangiella sp	Immunocompromised	Sinusitis; cutaneous lesions; disseminated infection	Itraconazole *or* amphotericin B; surgical excision	Varies with site of infection, clinical response and presence or absence of neutropenia					

1

INFECTIOUS AGENTS AND DRUGS OF CHOICE

TABLE 1-4

RECOMMENDED TREATMENT FOR FUNGAL INFECTIONS: SYSTEMIC TREATMENT—cont'd

Fungus	Host Category	Indication	Recommended Treatment	Duration[§]	Alternative Treatment	Duration[§]	Comment
Zygomycetes (Mucormycosis)[‖]	Immunocompromised, diabetes mellitus, metabolic aciduria, renal failure, neutropenia	Rhinocerebral, pulmonary, cutaneous, GI, or disseminated infection	Amphotericin B at maximum tolerated dose (1-1.5 mg/kg/day) + surgical excision of infected necrotic tissue		Posaconazole		Important considerations in association with antifungal therapy include reduction or discontinuation of immunosuppressive medication, correction of acidosis, discontinuation of iron chelation therapy.

*Some recommendations are for antibiotics that are not approved by the Food and Drug Administration for use in children, and some may not be approved for treatment of the pathogen listed. Recommendations are based on published evidence of efficacy.

Unless specific recommendation is made, decisions regarding the appropriate formulation of amphotericin B should be made based on a need to reduce toxicity associated with amphotericin B deoxycholate. Lipid complex and liposomal formulations are associated with fewer adverse events but they do not enhance efficacy. Amphotericin B deoxycholate is the preferred formulation for treating neonates and other patients with renal involvement because lipid complex and liposomal forms do not achieve effective concentration in the kidneys.

[§]Recommendations for duration of treatment often cannot be provided, because optimal duration depends on disease severity and immune status of the patient.

[†]*Candida albicans* is generally susceptible to fluconazole; *C. krusei* is resistant to fluconazole; *C. glabrata* is often resistant to fluconazole, but may be susceptible to high doses; *C. lusitaniae* may be resistant to amphotericin B.

[‖]Includes *Absidia* spp, *Mucor* spp, *Rhizomucor* spp, *Rhizopus* spp, *Mortierella* spp, *Cunninghamella* spp, *Penicillium* spp, *Acremonium* spp, *Fusarium* spp.

B. THERAPY FOR SUPERFICIAL CUTANEOUS INFECTIONS

TABLE 1-5

RECOMMENDED TREATMENT FOR FUNGAL INFECTIONS: THERAPY FOR SUPERFICIAL CUTANEOUS INFECTIONS

Site of Infection	Common Fungal Cause	Recommended Treatment	Duration	Alternative Treatment	Duration	Comments
Scalp (tinea capitis)	Trichophyton tonsurans, Microsporum canis, Mirosporum audouinii, Microsporum gypseum, Trichophyton mentagrophytes, Trichophyton violacea, Trichophyton soudanenae	Griseofulvin (ultramicronized)	4-8 wk, or at least 2 wk after clinical resolution	Itraconazole or terbinafine or once-weekly fluconazole	2-4 wk	Selenium sulfide or ketoconazole shampoo may reduce infectivity, but they are not sufficient for treatment; corticosteroid treatment may enhance resolution of kerion if used in conjunction with antifungal therapy.
Tinea pedis	T. mentagrophytes, Trichophyton rubrum, Epidermophyton floccusum	Topical terbinafine (twice daily) or clotrimazole or miconazole or econazole (once or twice daily)	1-4 wk	Fluconazole weekly or griseofulvin	Fluconazole weekly for 1-4 wk; griseofulvin for 6-8 wk	Burrow solution can be used along with antifungal for vesicular lesions. For dry, scaly variant ("moccasin" type), use longer course of oral agents.

INFECTIOUS AGENTS AND DRUGS OF CHOICE 1

TABLE 1-5

RECOMMENDED TREATMENT FOR FUNGAL INFECTIONS: THERAPY FOR SUPERFICIAL CUTANEOUS INFECTIONS—cont'd

Site of Infection	Common Fungal Cause	Recommended Treatment	Duration	Alternative Treatment	Duration	Comments
Tinea corporis	T. rubrum, T. tonsurans, T. mentagrophytes, Microsporum canis, E. floccosum, M. gypseum	[Topical miconazole or clotrimazole or terbinafind or tolnaftate or naftifine or ciclopirox] (twice daily) or [topical ketoconazole or econazole or oxiconazole or butenafine or sulconazole] (once daily)	4 wk	Griseofulvin or itraconazole or fluconazole or terbinafine	4 wk	
Tinea cruris (jock itch)	T. rubrum, T. mentagrophytes, E. floccosum	[Topical clotrimazole or miconazole or terbinafine or tolnaftate or ciclopirox] (twice daily) or [topical econazole or ketoconazole or naftifine or oxiconazole or butenafine or sulconazole] (once daily)	4-6 wk	Griseofulvin or itraconazole or fluconazole or terbinafine	2-6 wk	Burrow solution should be used to dry weeping areas of skin; concomitant topical corticosteroid treatment should be avoided

Tinea favosa (chronic scalp infection)	*Trichophyton schoenleinii, Trichophyton violaceum, M. gypseum*	Griseofulvin (ultramicronized)	4-8 wk, or at least 2 wk after clinical resolution	Itraconazole *or* terbinafine *or* weekly fluconazole	2-4 wk	Selenium sulfide or ketoconazole shampoo may reduce infectivity, but they are not sufficient for treatment; corticosteroid treatment does not enhance resolution of kerion, and corticosteroids enhance clinical symptoms in the absence of antifungal treatment.
Tinea unguium	*T. mentagrophytes, T. rubrum, E. floccusum*	Griseofulvin	6-12 mo	Itraconazole *or* terbinafine *or* weekly fluconazole	4-6 mo	

GROUPINGS OF FUNGAL GENERA BY CLINICAL PRESENTATION*

CUTANEOUS: SUPERFICIAL, NOT INFLAMMATORY
Tinea versicolor (Pityriasis versicolor): *Malassezia (M. furfur)*

CUTANEOUS: INFLAMMATORY
Dermatophytes: *Trichophyton, Microsporum, Epidermophyton*
Primary cutaneous candidiasis: *Candida*

MUCOSAL
Candida

SUBCUTANEOUS
Sporotrichosis: *Sporothrix*
Phaeohyphomycosis: *Alternaria, Bipolaris, Curvularia, Exophiala, Exserohilum, Wangiella*
Chromomycosis: *Fonsecaea, Cladophialophora, Phialophora, Rhinocladiella*
Mycetoma: *Madurella, Pseudallescheria, Acremonium, Exophiala, Leptosphaeria*

PULMONARY ± DISSEMINATION
Abnormal cell-mediated immunity: *Cryptococcus, Histoplasma, Pneumocystis, Coccidioides, Penicillium (P. marneffei)*
Neutropenia/Neutrophil dysfunction: *Aspergillus, Fusarium, Pseudallescheria*

SINUSITIS
Zygomycosis: *Rhizopus, Mucor, Absidia, Rhizomucor, Cunninghamella*
Aspergillosis: *Aspergillus*
Phaeohyphomycoses: *Alternaria, Bipolaris, Curvularia, Exophiala, Exserohilum, Wangiella*

GROUPINGS OF FUNGAL GENERA BY LABORATORY REPORT

Direct Exam of Tissues (Pathology or Fungal Stain in Microbiology) Reveals the Following:
Yeast: *Candida, Sporothrix, Malassezia, Histoplasma, Cryptococcus, Saccharomyces, Blastomyces, Paracoccidioides, Penicillium (P. marneffei)*
Hyphae

> **No melanin**: *Aspergillus; Scedosporium; Pseudallescheria;* Hyalohyphomycoses agents (*Fusarium, Acremonium, Paecilomyces*)
> **Melanin (dark)**: Phaeohyphomycosis agents (*Alternaria, Bipolaris, Curvularia, Exophiala, Exserohilum, Wangiella*)

*Thanks to William G. Merz, PhD for his help in the development of this guide to classification of pathogenic fungi.

Hyphae and yeast: *Candida*
Grains or granules: *Mycetoma* (*Madurella, Pseudallescheria, Acremonium, Exophiala, Leptosphaeria*)
Pigmented (melanin) sclerotic cells/bodies: *Chromomycosis agents* (*Fonsecaea, Cladophialophora, Phialophora, Rhinocladiella*)
Spherules seen in tissue: *Coccidioides*
Cysts and Trophozoites: *Pneumocystis*

Laboratory Culture Reveals the Following:
   Yeast growing in culture
       Candida
       Cryptococcus
       Malassezia (*M. pachydermatis* only)
       Trichosporon
       Saccharomyces
   Dimorphic fungi (Recovered as a filamentous fungus but also displays yeast form):
       Paracoccidioides
       Blastomyces
       Histoplasma
       Sporothrix
       Penicillium (*P. marneffei* only)
   Fungi only as Filamentous fungi
       Darkly pigmented (melanin) hyphae (Dematiaceous):
       Phaeohyphomycoses agents (*Alternaria, Bipolaris, Curvularia, Exophiala, Exserohilum, Wangiella*) and Chromomycosis agents (*Fonsecaea, Cladophialophora, Phialophora, Rhinocladiella*)
       Pale or brightly colored hyphae lacking dark pigment:
       Aspergillus, Scedosporium, Pseudallescheria, Hyalohyphomycoses agents (*Fusarium, Acremonium, Paecilomyces*)
       Zygomycosis/Mucormycosis agents: *Rhizopus, Mucor, Absidia, Rhizomucor, Cunninghamella*
       Coccidioidomycosis: *Coccidioides* (also a dimorphic fungus but without a yeast form)
   Fungal growth from blood culture
       Yeast: *Candida* (especially *C. albicans, C. parapsilosis*), *Malassezia*; *Cryptococcus*[†], *Histoplasma*[†], *Paracoccidioides*[†], *Blastomyces*[†]
       Filamentous: *Fusarium, Pseudallescheria*

[†]Growth not reliably detected in broth blood culture systems that depend on abundant CO_2 production to detect growth of pathogen.

V. RECOMMENDED TREATMENT FOR PARASITIC AND PROTOZOAL INFECTIONS

Pathogen listing by category is provided on p. 106.

TABLE 1-6

RECOMMENDED TREATMENT FOR PARASITIC AND PROTOZOAL INFECTIONS

Parasite/Where Infection Acquired	Host Category	Indication	Recommended Treatment	Duration	Alternative Treatment	Duration	Comments
Acanthamoeba/ Worldwide	Immunosuppressed	Granulomatous amebic encephalitis, disseminated infection	Usually susceptible in vitro to pentamidine, ketoconazole, amphotericin B. Fluconazole, sulfadiazine, sulfamethoxazole, and rifampin have been used in combination.	Unknown			Therapy is rarely successful. Susceptibility testing is advisable. Combination IV and intraventricular therapy may be of benefit but should be undertaken only in consultation with an infectious diseases specialist.
	Immunocompetent	Keratitis	[Topical 0.1% propamidine isethionate (Brolene) + neomycin-polymixin B-gramicidin ophthalmic solution]	Wks to mo	[Topical 0.02% polyhexamethylene biguanide (PHMB)[1] ± chlorhexadine gluconate]	Wks to mo	Topical corticosteroids are sometimes recommended once clinical improvement is noted. Successful treatment depends on early diagnosis.
Ancylostoma braziliense (dog hookworm)/ Southeast Asia, Caribbean, Puerto Rico	Worldwide						
	Symptomatic patient	Cutaneous larva migrans	Thiabendazole (topical) *or* albendazole[2] *or* ivermectin[2]	Until lesions inactivated 3 days 1-2 days			Disease is usually self-limited, lasting wk to mo without therapy.

Organism/Geography	Condition		Drug	Dose	Comments
Ancylostoma caninum (Dog hookworm)/Worldwide	Eosinophilic enterocolitis		Mebendazole *or* Albendazole[2] *or* Pyrantel pamoate	100 mg bid × 3 days or 500 mg once 400 mg once 3 days	Endoscopic removal of the parasite may be required.
Ancylostoma caninum, Ancylostoma ceylanic, Ancylostoma duodenale (hookworm)/Worldwide (*A. caninum,* predominantly Australia and United States; *A. ceylanic,* predominantly Southeast Asia and India; *A duodenale,* worldwide)	Dermatitis, anemia, nonspecific GI complaints	Symptomatic patient	Mebendazole *or* Albendazole[2] *or* Pyrantel pamoate	100 mg bid × 3 days or 500 mg once 400 mg once 3 days	World Health Organization (WHO) recommends half the adult dose of **mebendazole or albendazole**[2] for children < 2 yrs.
Angiostrongylus cantonensis (visceral larva migrans)/Southeast Asia, Hawaii, Pacific Islands, Philippines, China, Taiwan	Eosinophilic meningitis	Symptomatic patient			No treatment is well established; most infections are self-limited. Corticosteroids and analgesics may be helpful

INFECTIOUS AGENTS AND DRUGS OF CHOICE

1

TABLE 1-6
RECOMMENDED TREATMENT FOR PARASITIC AND PROTOZOAL INFECTIONS—cont'd

Parasite/Where Infection Acquired	Host Category	Indication	Recommended Treatment	Duration	Alternative Treatment	Duration	Comments
Angiostrongylus costaricensis/ Central and South America	Symptomatic patient	Fever, eosinophilia, abdominal pain					No treatment is well-established. Mebendazole treatment has resulted in modest success in experimental animals. Corticosteroids may be helpful.
Anisakis/Japan	Symptomatic patient	Viscera larva migrans	Endoscopic removal of the parasite				
Ascaris lumbricoides/ Worldwide	All		Mebendazole or	100 mg bid × 3 days or 500 mg once			In the case of an obstructing bolus of worms, pyrantel pamoate is not recommended because it can worsen obstruction. Mineral oil or Gastrografin (orally or by nasogastric [NG] tube) may cause relaxation of the worms and allow passage without surgery. **Albendazole** or **mebendazole** can then be administered safely.
			Albendazole[2] or	400 mg once			
			Pyrantel pamoate[2]	11 mg/kg once			
Babesia microti/ United States and Europe	Asplenic or normal host	Parasitemia	[Quinine + clindamycin] or [Atovaquone + azithromycin]	7-10 days	Europe only: Pentamidine + TMP/SMX		Most infections acquired in the United States are self-limited and require no specific therapy. Exchange blood transfusion may be required in cases of rapidly increasing parasitemia and massive hemolysis.

Balamuthia mandrillaris/ Worldwide	Immunosuppressed	Granulomatous amebic meningoencephalitis	[Clarithromycin + fluconazole + sulfadiazine + flucytosine + pentamidine]	Unknown	Recommendation is based on limited clinical experience.
Balantidium coli/Worldwide	Symptomatic patient	Intestinal infection	Tetracycline[3]	10 days	Healthy infected individuals usually recover without treatment; malnourished or immunosuppressed hosts are more likely to suffer severe disease.
			Metronidazole *or* Iodoquinol	5 days 20 days	
Baylisascaris procyonis (raccoon ascaris)/ United States	Symptomatic patient	Eosinophilic meningitis; ocular infection			No effective treatment has been documented. Albendazole, mebendazole, thiabendazole, levamisole, or ivermectin might theoretically be helpful. Albendazole has been recommended as preventive therapy following known exposure. Steroid therapy has been used to reduce CNS and/or ocular inflammation. Laser photocoagulation has been used to destroy intraretinal larvae.
Blastocystis hominis/ Worldwide	Symptomatic patient	Intestinal infection	Metronidazole	10 days	*B. hominis* has not been established as a cause of symptoms. Treatment should be initiated only if all other more likely causes of symptoms have been investigated and ruled out. In vitro metronidazole resistance has been observed.
			Iodoquinol *or* Furazolidone *or* TMP/SMX *or* Nitizoxanide	20 days Not established Not established	

INFECTIOUS AGENTS AND DRUGS OF CHOICE

1

TABLE 1-6

RECOMMENDED TREATMENT FOR PARASITIC AND PROTOZOAL INFECTIONS—cont'd

Parasite/Where Infection Acquired	Host Category	Indication	Recommended Treatment	Duration	Alternative Treatment	Duration	Comments
Brachiola vesicularum (microsporidiosis)/ Not defined	All	Disseminated microsporidiosis	Albendazole[2]				There is no known effective therapy for microsporidial infection. Albendazole may reduce symptoms. HIV-positive patients may benefit from highly active antiretroviral therapy to improve their own immunity.
Brugia malayi (filariasis)/ Southeast Asia	All	Lymphatic infection	Diethylcarbamazine[4] Day 1: 1 mg/kg after a meal (max 50 mg) Day 2: 1 mg/kg tid (max 50 mg tid) Day 3: 1-2 mg/kg tid (max 100 mg) Day 4-14: 6 mg/kg in 3 doses (max 6 mg/kg/d in 3 doses)	14 days			Antihistamines or corticosteroids may be required to decrease allergic reaction to microfilarial disintegration. Full doses can be given from day 1 for patients with no microfilariae in the blood.
		Tropical pulmonary eosinophilia	Diethylcarbamazine[4] (6 mg/kg/day in 3 doses)	21 days			Antihistamines or corticosteroids may be required to decrease allergic reaction to microfilarial disintegration.

Infectious agent				Comments
Brugia timori (filariasis)/Indonesia	Lymphatic infection	Diethylcarbamazine[4] Day 1: 1 mg/kg (max 50 mg) Day 2: 1 mg/kg tid (max 50 mg tid) Day 3: 1-2 mg/kg tid (max 100 mg) tid Day 4-14: 6 mg/kg in 3 doses (max 6 mg/kg/d in 3 doses)	14 days	Antihistamines or corticosteroids may be required to decrease allergic reaction to microfilarial disintegration. Full doses can be given from day 1 for patients with no microfilariae in the blood.
	Tropical pulmonary eosinophilia	Diethylcarbamazine[4]	21 days	Antihistamines or corticosteroids may be required to decrease allergic reaction to microfilarial disintegration.
Capillaria philippinensis/Philippines, Thailand	Symptomatic patient	Mebendazole[2]	20 days	
	Intestinal capillariasis (diarrhea, protein-losing enteropathy)	Albendazole[2]	10 days	
Clonorchis sinensis (Chinese liver fluke)/Far East, Eastern Europe, Russian Federation	All	Praziquant el *or* Albendazole[2]	1 day 7 days	
	Biliary tract involvement			
Cryptosporidium/Worldwide	Immunocompromised patient	Nitazoxanide	3 days (based on studies in immunocompetent children)	Most infections in immunocompetent individuals are self-limited and do not require treatment. Effective antiretroviral therapy is the most important treatment for HIV-infected individuals.
	Diarrhea	Paromomycin alone *or combined with* Azithromycin	Unknown Unknown	

TABLE 1-6

RECOMMENDED TREATMENT FOR PARASITIC AND PROTOZOAL INFECTIONS—cont'd

Parasite/Where Infection Acquired	Host Category	Indication	Recommended Treatment	Duration	Alternative Treatment	Duration	Comments
Cyclospora/Nepal, Peru, Haiti, Guatemala, Indonesia	Immunocompetent patient	Diarrhea	TMP/SMX	7-10 days	Ciprofloxacin	7 days	
	Immunocompromised patient	Diarrhea	TMP/SMX	10 days	Ciprofloxacin	7-10 days	Recurrence can often be prevented using prophylactic **TMP/SMX** given 3 times per week.
Dientamoeba fragilis/Worldwide	Symptomatic patient	Diarrhea	Iodoquinol or Paromomycin or Tetracycline or Metronidazole	20 days 7 days 10 days 10 days			
Diphyllabothrium latum (fish tapeworm)/Worldwide	All	Diarrhea, abdominal pain, intestinal obstruction	Praziquantel[2]	1 dose	Niclosamide	1 dose	Cobalamin injections and oral folic acid are indicated for individuals with evidence of vitamin B_{12} deficiency.
Dipylidium caninum (dog tapeworm)/Worldwide	All	Proglottids in stool	Praziquantel[2]	1 dose	Niclosamide	1 dose	Retreatment is indicated if proglottids are evident in stools 1 week or more after initial therapy. Cobalamin injections and oral folic acid are indicated for individuals with evidence of vitamin B_{12} deficiency.

Organism/Location	Patient	Manifestation	Drug	Duration	Comments
Dracunculus medinensis (Guinea worm)/ Africa	Symptomatic patient	Emerging worm from cutaneous lesion	Metronidazole	10 days	There is no curative therapy other than gradual removal of the worm, but **metronidazole** reduces local inflammation and facilitates removal.
Echinococcus granulosus/South America, Eastern Africa, Eastern Europe, Middle East, Mediterranean, China, Central Asia, Australia, New Zealand, Southeastern United States	All	Hydatid cyst of the liver or other site	Albendazole[2]	3 to 6 mo	Surgical excision of cysts may be required. **Praziquantel** has been used perioperatively. In uncomplicated patients percutaneous aspiration, infusion of scolicidal agents, and reaspiration (PAIR) should be performed a few days after initiation of albendazole therapy.
Echinococcus multilocularis/ Europe, Russia, Central Asia, Western China, Northwest Canada, Western Alaska	All	Liver disease, alveolar echinococcosis	Albendazole[2] *or* Mebendazole	Prolonged therapy	Surgical excision provides the only reliable cure.

TABLE 1-6

RECOMMENDED TREATMENT FOR PARASITIC AND PROTOZOAL INFECTIONS—cont'd

Parasite/Where Infection Acquired	Host Category	Indication	Recommended Treatment	Duration	Alternative Treatment	Duration	Comments
Encephalitozoon hellem (Microsporidiosis)/ Not defined	All	Ocular microsporidiosis	Albendazole[2] + fumagillin[5] (eye drops)				There is no known effective therapy for microsporidial infection. **Fumagillin** is used to control microsporidial disease in honey bees; **fumagillin** eye drops have been helpful in some HIV-infected patients. **Albendazole** may reduce symptoms. HIV-positive patients may benefit from highly active antiretroviral therapy to improve their own immunity.
	All	Disseminated microsporidiosis	Albendazole[2]				There is no known effective therapy for microsporidial infection. **Albendazole** may reduce symptoms. HIV-positive patients may benefit from highly active antiretroviral therapy to improve their own immunity.

Encephalitozoon cuniculi (Microsporidiosis)/ Not defined	All	Ocular microsporidiosis	Albendazole[2] + fumagillin[5] (eye drops)	There is no known effective therapy for microsporidial infection. **Fumagillin** is used to control microsporidial disease in honey bees, and **fumagillin** eye drops have been helpful in some HIV-infected patients. **Albendazole** may reduce symptoms. HIV-positive patients may benefit from highly active antiretroviral therapy to improve their own immunity.
	All	Disseminated microsporidiosis	Albendazole[2]	There is no known effective therapy for microsporidial infection. **Albendazole** may reduce symptoms. HIV-positive patients may benefit from highly active antiretroviral therapy to improve their own immunity.
Encephalitozoon [Septata] intestinalis (Microsporidiosis)/ Not defined	All	Intestinal microsporidiosis	Albendazole[2]	There is no known effective therapy for microsporidial infection. **Albendazole** may reduce symptoms. HIV-positive patients may benefit from highly active antiretroviral therapy to improve their own immunity.

1

INFECTIOUS AGENTS AND DRUGS OF CHOICE

TABLE 1-6

RECOMMENDED TREATMENT FOR PARASITIC AND PROTOZOAL INFECTIONS—cont'd

Parasite/Where Infection Acquired	Host Category	Indication	Recommended Treatment	Duration	Alternative Treatment	Duration	Comments
Encephalitozoon—cont.		Disseminated microsporidiosis	Albendazole[2]				There is no known effective therapy for microsporidial infection. **Albendazole** may reduce symptoms. HIV-positive patients may benefit from highly active antiretroviral therapy to improve immunity.
Entamoeba dispar/Worldwide							No treatment is needed. This organism does not cause human disease.
Entamoeba histolytica (amebiasis)/ Worldwide	All	Asymptomatic cyst excreters (intraluminal infection)	Iodoquinol or Paromomycin	20 days 7 days	Diloxanide furoate[6]	10 days	These agents provide intraluminal therapy only. Corticosteroids and antimotility drugs can worsen symptoms and disease.
		Mild to moderate intestinal disease	Metronidazole followed by [Iodoquinol or paromomycin]	7-10 days 20 days 7 days	Tinidazole (50 mg/kg/ day; maximum 2 g/ day divided tid) followed by [Iodoquinol or paromomycin]	3 days 20 days 7 days	Corticosteroids and antimotility drugs can worsen symptoms and disease.
		Amebic colitis, liver abscess	Metronidazole ± chloroquine followed by [Iodoquinol or paromomycin]	7-10 days 20 days 7 days	Tinidazole (60 mg/kg/ day; maximum 800 mg 3 times per day) ± chloroquine followed by [Iodoquinol or paromomycin]	3 days 20 days 7 days	Corticosteroids and antimotility drugs can worsen symptoms and disease. Dehydroemetine followed by idoquinol or paromycin should be considered if other therapies fail.

Organism/Distribution		Drug	Dosing	Comments
Entamoeba polecki/Tropics	All	Metronidazole	10 days	
Enterocytozoon bieneusi (microsporidiosis)/Not defined	All	Intestinal microsporidiosis Fumagillin[5] (oral)		Octreotide may provide symptomatic relief for patients with large volume diarrhea. Treatment with oral **fumagillin** has resulted in thrombocytopenia. There is no known effective therapy for microsporidial infection. HIV-positive patients may benefit from highly active antiretroviral therapy to improve their own immunity.
Enterobius vermicularis (pinworm)/Worldwide	All	Pyrantel pamoate *or* Mebendazole *or* Albendazole[2]	Give 1 dose; repeat in 2 wk	When multiple or repeated symptomatic infections occur, family members should be treated as a group.
Fasciola buski (intestinal fluke)/Far East	All	Praziquantel[2]	3 doses in 1 day	
Fasciola hepatica (sheep liver fluke)/Tropics and temperate areas	All	Triclabendazole[8] 10 mg	Once	**Triclabendazole** is a veterinary medication that may be safe and effective, but there is limited information about its use in humans.
		Bithionol,[4] 30-50 mg/kg	Give on alternate days for 10-15 doses	

1

INFECTIOUS AGENTS AND DRUGS OF CHOICE

TABLE 1-6

RECOMMENDED TREATMENT FOR PARASITIC AND PROTOZOAL INFECTIONS—cont'd

Parasite/Where Infection Acquired	Host Category	Indication	Recommended Treatment	Duration	Alternative Treatment	Duration	Comments
Giardia lamblia/ Worldwide	Symptomatic patient	Diarrhea, abdominal pain, anorexia	Nitazoxanide or Metronidazole[2] or Tinidazole	3 days 5 days 1 dose	Furazolidone or Paromomycin or Quinacrine[6]	7-10 days 7 days 5 days	Treatment of asymptomatic patients is generally not recommended. Because **paromomycin** is not absorbed from the GI tract, it may be particularly useful to treat giardiasis in pregnant women.
Gnathostoma spinigerum/ Thailand, Asia, Mexico	All	Ocular larva migrans, eosinophilic meningitis, subcutaneous swelling	Albendazole[2] or Ivermectin[2]	21 days 2 days			Surgical removal of the worm is an alternative to pharmacotherapy.
Gongylonema sp/Worldwide	All		Albendazole[2]	10 mg/kg/day for 3 days			Surgical removal of the worm is an alternative to pharmacotherapy.
Heterophyes heterophyes (intestinal fluke)/ Egypt, Far East, Southeast Asia	All		Praziquantel[2]	3 doses in 1 day			
Hymenolepis nana (dwarf tapeworm)/Worldwide	All		Praziquantel[2]	1 dose	Nitazoxanide	3 days	Repeat treatment may be necessary.

Isospora belli / Tropical and subtropical climates	Immunocompetent	Diarrhea	TMP-SMX	10 days	Pyrimethamine *or*	75 mg/day ± folinic acid for 10 days followed by 25 mg/day for 7 days
					Ciprofloxacin	
	Immunocompromised	Diarrhea	TMP-SMX	Administer qid × 10 days, followed by bid × 3 wk	Pyrimethamine *or*	75 mg/day ± folinic acid for 10 days followed by 25 mg/day for 7 days	Prolonged therapy may be required to control symptoms.
					Ciprofloxacin	10 days?
Leishmania spp./Worldwide	All	Visceral leishmaniasis (kala-azar)	Sodium stibogluconate[4,9] *or* Meglumine antimonate[7]	Minimum of 4 wk	Amphotericin B *or*	1 mg/kg on alternate days for a total of 2 g (adults)	Side effects of pentavalent antimonial drugs are common. Serious side effects include hepatotoxicity, pancreatitis, and cardiotoxicity. Relapses should be treated for at least twice the time period of the initial course.
					Liposomal amphotericin B *or*	3 mg/kg/day on days 1 through 5, and days 14 and 21	
					Pentamidine	2-4 mg/kg/day or every 2 days IV or IM for up to 15 doses	

INFECTIOUS AGENTS AND DRUGS OF CHOICE

1

TABLE 1-6

RECOMMENDED TREATMENT FOR PARASITIC AND PROTOZOAL INFECTIONS—cont'd

Parasite/Where Infection Acquired	Host Category	Indication	Recommended Treatment	Duration	Alternative Treatment	Duration	Comments
Leishmania spp.—cont.		Cutaneous leishmaniasis	Sodium stibogluconate[4,9] or Meglumine antimonate[7]	20 days 20 days	Pentamadine Paromomycin (topical)	Daily or every other day for 4-7 doses Twice daily for 10-20 days	Treatment decision should be made after consultation with infectious disease specialist or with CDC (404-639-3670). Use topical paromomycin only in geographic regions where cutaneous leishmaniasis species have low likelihood for mucosal spread. Should not be used for treating *L. loraziliensis, L. guyanensis, L. panamensis, L. amazohensis,* or *L. aethiopica.*
Loa loa (filariasis)/ West and Central Africa	All		Diethylcarbamazine[4] Day 1: 1 mg/kg pc (max 50 mg) Day 2: 1 mg/kg tid (max 50 mg tid) Day 3: 1-2 mg/kg tid (max 100 mg) tid Day 4-21: 9 mg/kg in 3 doses		Ivermectin? Albendazole?		Antihistamines or corticosteroids may be required to decrease allergic reaction to microfilarial disintegration. Apheresis may reduce the risk of encephalopathy associated with rapid microfilarial killing if blood microfilarial burden is high. Full doses of therapy can be given beginning on day 1 for patients with no microfilariae in the blood.

Malaria—see Plasmodium

Infection/Geography	Stage	Drug	Duration			Comments
Mansonella ozzardi (filariasis)/South and Central America, Caribbean	All	Ivermectin 200 µg/kg	1 dose			Antihistamines or corticosteroids may be required to decrease allergic reaction to microfilarial disintegration. Most infected persons are asymptomatic.
Mansonella perstans (filariasis)/Africa, South and Central America	All	Mebendazole[2] *or* Albendazole[2]	30 days 10 days			Most infected persons are asymptomatic. Antihistamines or corticosteroids may be required to decrease allergic reaction to microfilarial disintegration.
Mansonella streptocerca (filariasis)/West and Central Africa	All	Diethylcarbamazine[4] 6 mg/kg *or* Ivermectin, 150 µg/kg	14 days 1 dose			Antihistamines or corticosteroids may be required to decrease allergic reaction to microfilarial disintegration. **Diethylcarbamazine** kills both microfilariae and adult worms; **ivermectin** kills only microfilariae.
Metagonimus yokogawai (intestinal fluke)/Far East, Spain, Greece, Balkans	All	Praziquantel[2]	1 day			
Metrochis conjunctus (North American liver fluke)/North America	All	Praziquantel[2]	1 day	Albendazole	10 days	

TABLE 1-6

RECOMMENDED TREATMENT FOR PARASITIC AND PROTOZOAL INFECTIONS—cont'd

Parasite/Where Infection Acquired	Host Category	Indication	Recommended Treatment	Duration	Alternative Treatment	Duration	Comments
Microsporidia/Not defined	Immunocompetent	Keratopathy, diarrhea, myositis, encephalitis	(See specific organisms.) No therapy has demonstrated consistent benefit. Albendazole is beneficial for some. Metronidazole, atovaquone, nitrazoxanide, fumagillin have been used with some success.				
Microsporidia spp./Worldwide	Immunocompromised (HIV-infected)	Keratopathy, diarrhea, myositis, encephalitis, disseminated disease, sinusitis, osteomyelitis, urinary tract infection, peritonitis	(See specific organisms.) No therapy has demonstrated consistent benefit. Albendazole is beneficial for some. Metronidazole, atovaquone, nitrazoxanide, fumagilin have been used with some success.				HIV+ patients may benefit from highly active antiretroviral therapy to improve their immune function.
Naegleria fowleri/Worldwide	All	Amebic meningoencephalitis	Amphotericin B[2]	Uncertain			Treatment is usually unsuccessful. Combined therapy with intravenous and intrathecal **amphotericin B**, intrathecal **miconazole**, and oral **rifampin** has been reported successful.

Infectious Agents and Drugs of Choice

Organism		Drug	Dose	Notes
Nanophyetus salmincola (fluke)/Pacific northwestern United States	All	Praziquantel[2]	1 day	
Necator americanus (hookworm)/Western hemisphere, sub-Saharan Africa, Southeast Asia, Pacific Islands	All	Mebendazole or Albendazole[2] or Pyrantel pamoate	100 mg bid × 3 days or 500 mg once 400 mg once 3 days	WHO recommends half the adult dose of **mebendazole** or **albendazole** for children < 2 yr.
Oesophagostomum bifurcum/Togo; Ghana	All	Albendazole[2] or Pyrantel pamoate		Efficacy of these drugs is uncertain.
Onchocerca volvulus (river blindness) (filariasis)/Africa, South and Central America	All	Ivermectin[10]	150 µg/kg × 1; repeat every 6 to 12 mo until asymptomatic	Prevention: annual treatment with **ivermectin**, 150 µg/kg. A 6-week course of **doxycycline** is sometimes used as adjunctive therapy for individuals ≥ 8 yrs and nonpregnant adults. Diethylcarbamazine should NOT be used to treat this infection.
Opisthorchis viverrini (Southeast Asian liver fluke)/Thailand, Kampuchea, Laos	All	Praziquantel[2]	2 days	Biliary tract involvement
Paragonimus westermani (lung fluke)/Worldwide, especially Far East	All	Praziquantel[2] Bithionol[7]	2 days 30-50 mg/kg on alternate days for 10-15 doses	Pulmonary, cardiac, CNS, cutaneous involvement. A short course of corticosteroids should be given along with **praziquantel** when treating CNS disease.

INFECTIOUS AGENTS AND DRUGS OF CHOICE

1

TABLE 1-6

RECOMMENDED TREATMENT FOR PARASITIC AND PROTOZOAL INFECTIONS—cont'd

Parasite/Where Infection Acquired	Host Category	Indication	Recommended Treatment	Duration	Alternative Treatment	Duration	Comments
Plasmodium falciparum/ Tropical areas worldwide	Uncomplicated or mild malaria	**Oral therapy** for infections acquired in areas where **chloroquine resistance** is reported	Quinine sulfate + [doxycycline[2,3] or tetracycline[2,3] or pyrimethamine-sulfadoxine or clindamycin] or Atovaquone/ proguanil	3-7 days 7 days 7 days Adults, 3 tablets at once on the last day of therapy; pediatric dose, ¼ tablet 5 days 3 days	Mefloquine or Halofantrine or [Artesunate[7] + mefloquine]	1 day 1 day; 1 wk later 3 days 1 day	The longer course of **quinine** (7 days) should be used for patients who acquired infection in Southeast Asia. **Clindamycin** is the preferred adjunct to quinine sulfate for pregnant individuals. **Atovaquone** should be taken at least 45 mins after eating. **Mefloquine** should not be used in pregnancy; it should not be given along with **quinine, quinidine** or **halofantrine.** Caution is required in treating patients with **quinine, quinidine,** or **halofantrine** if they have received **mefloquine** as prophylaxis. **Halofantrine** can cause conduction defects (cardiac monitoring is recommended); GI absorption is variable, and it should not be taken 1 hour before or 2 hours after meals; it should not be used in pregnancy. **If in doubt, consult CDC malaria hotline at 770-488-7788.**

Plasmodium vivax/ Tropical areas worldwide	Uncomplicated or mild malaria	Oral therapy for infection acquired where **chloroquine resistance** has been reported	[Quinine sulfate + doxycycline[2,3] + primaquine phosphate] or Mefloquine + Primaquine phosphate	3-7 days 7 days 14 days 1 day 14 days	Halofantrine[7] + Primaquine phosphate	1 day (3 doses); repeat in 1 week 14 days

The longer course of **quinine** (7 days) should be used for patients who acquired infection in Southeast Asia. **Mefloquine** should not be used in pregnancy; it should not be given along with **quinine, quinidine,** or **haofantrine.** Caution is required in treating patients with **quinine, quinidine,** or **halofantrine** if they have received **mefloquine** as prophylaxis.

Halofantrine can cause conduction defects (cardiac monitoring is recommended); GI absorption is variable, and it should not be taken 1 hour before or 2 hours after meals; it should not be used in pregnancy.

Primaquine is used to prevent relapse due to latent forms. Exclude G-6-PD deficiency before giving **primaquine.**

Primaquine should not be used during pregnancy.
Consult CDC malaria hotline at 770-488-7788.

TABLE 1-6

RECOMMENDED TREATMENT FOR PARASITIC AND PROTOZOAL INFECTIONS—cont'd

Parasite/Where Infection Acquired	Host Category	Indication	Recommended Treatment	Duration	Alternative Treatment	Duration	Comments
Plasmodium other than chloroquine-resistant P. falciparum and chloroquine-resistant P. vivax/ Tropical areas worldwide	Uncomplicated or mild malaria	Oral therapy	Chloroquine phosphate	3 days	Hydroxychloroquine sulfate	3 days	**Primaquine phosphate** should be given for 14 days if Plasmodium ovale or P. vivax is suspected. **Consult CDC malaria hotline at 770-488-7788.**
Plasmodium—all species in patients for whom parenteral therapy is warranted/ Tropical areas worldwide	Moderate, severe, or complicated malaria	Parenteral therapy	Quinidine gluconate[11] or Quinine dihydrochloride	Until oral therapy can be initiated / Until oral therapy can be initiated	Artemether[7]	5-7 days	**Quinidine or quinine:** Continuous monitoring of EKG, blood pressure, and serum glucose is recommended. Decrease or omit the loading dose for patients who have received **mefloquine or quinine.** Consider exchange transfusion for parasitemia >10%. **Consult CDC malaria hotline at 770-488-7788.**

P. vivax and P. ovale/Tropical areas worldwide	Previously infected	Prevention of relapse	Primaquine phosphate	Adults: 30 mg base/day for 14 days Children: 0.6 mg base/kg/day for 14 days	**Primaquine** should not be used during pregnancy. **Primaquine** can cause hemolysis, particularly in patients with G-6-PD deficiency. Relapses that occur despite this treatment should be treated with a second 14-day course of 30-mg base per day. **Consult CDC malaria hotline at 770-488-7788.**
Pleistophora sp (microsporidia)/Not well defined	All	Disseminated microsporidiosis	Albendazole[2]		There is no known effective therapy for microsporidial infection. **Albendazole** may reduce symptoms. HIV-positive patients may benefit from highly active antiretroviral therapy to improve their own immunity.
Pneumocystis jiroveci—see Table 1-4					

1

INFECTIOUS AGENTS AND DRUGS OF CHOICE

TABLE 1-6

RECOMMENDED TREATMENT FOR PARASITIC AND PROTOZOAL INFECTIONS—cont'd

Parasite/Where Infection Acquired	Host Category	Indication	Recommended Treatment	Duration	Alternative Treatment	Duration	Comments
Sappinia diploidea/Worldwide	All	Amebic meningoencephalitis	Azithromycin + pentamidine (IV) + itraconazole + flucytosine				This organism has been recently recognized as pathogenic. Successful treatment with this combined therapy has been reported.
Schistosoma haematobium/Africa, eastern Mediterranean	All		Praziquantel, 20 mg/kg/dose				**Praziquantel** does not kill developing worms; treatment given within 4-8 wk of exposure should be repeated 1-2 mo later.
Schistosoma japonicum/China, Philippines, Indonesia	All		Praziquantel, 20 mg/kg/dose	3 doses in 1 day			**Praziquantel** does not kill developing worms; treatment given within 4-8 wk of exposure should be repeated 1-2 mo later.
Schistosoma mansoni/Africa, Caribbean, Venezuela, Brazil, Suriname, Arabian peninsula	All		Praziquantel 20 mg/kg/dose	2 doses in 1 day	Oxamniquine	One dose	**Praziquantel** does not kill developing worms; treatment given within 4-8 wk of exposure should be repeated 1-2 mo later. **Oxamniquine** dose should be increased in East Africa to 30 mg/kg, and in Egypt and South Africa to 30 mg/kg/day for 2 days. **Oxamniquine** is contraindicated in pregnancy.

Infectious Agent (Geographic Distribution)	Manifestations	Drug of Choice	Duration	Alternative Drug	Duration	Comments
Schistosoma mekongi / Cambodia, Laos, Japan, Philippines, Central Indonesia	All	Praziquantel 20 mg/kg/dose	3 doses in 1 day			**Praziquantel** does not kill developing worms; treatment given within 4-8 wk of exposure should be repeated 1-2 mo later.
Strongyloides stercoralis / Tropical and temperate climates worldwide	All	Ivermectin	1-2 days	Thiabendazole or Albendazole	2 days / 7 days	Prolonged treatment may be required in immunocompromised patients or in patients with disseminated disease. The recommended dose of **thiabendazole** may have to be reduced if toxicity (nausea, vomiting, diarrhea) occurs.
Taenia saginata (beef tape worm) / Worldwide	Diarrhea, abdominal pain, intestinal obstruction / All	Praziquantel[2]	1 dose	Niclosamide	1 dose	Cobalamin injections and oral folic acid are indicated for individuals with evidence of vitamin B_{12} deficiency.
Taenia solium (pork tape worm)	Diarrhea, abdominal pain, intestinal obstruction	Praziquantil[2]	1 dose	Niclosamide	One dose	Cobalamin injections and oral folic acid are indicated for individuals with evidence of vitamin B_{12} deficiency.

TABLE 1-6

RECOMMENDED TREATMENT FOR PARASITIC AND PROTOZOAL INFECTIONS—cont'd

Parasite/Where Infection Acquired	Host Category	Indication	Recommended Treatment	Duration	Alternative Treatment	Duration	Comments
		Cysticercosis	Albendazole (see comment) or Praziquantel[2] (see comment)	8-30 days 30 days			Usefulness of treatment with **albendazole** or **praziquantel** has not been demonstrated. Seizures should be treated with anticonvulsants . Surgery is indicated for obstructing cysts. Corticosteroids have been used in conjunction with surgery or in conjunction with **albendazole** or **praziquantel** to treat arachnoiditis, vasculitis, or cerebral edema. Neither **albendazole** nor **praziquantel** should be used to treat ocular or spinal cysts, even in conjunction with corticosteroids; an ophthalmologic examination should be performed before treating with these agents.
Toxocara canis; Toxocara catis/Worldwide	All	Visceral larva migrans	Albendazole[2] or Mebendazole[2]	5 days 5 days			Optimal duration of therapy is not known. Some experts treat as long as 20 days.

	Ocular larva migrans	Albendazole[2] *or* Mebendazole[2]	5 days 5 days	Antihelmenthic treatment alone may not be effective. Additional treatment may include vitrectomy and corticosteroids.
Toxoplasma gondii/Worldwide	Chorioretinitis	Pyrimethamine + Sulfadiazine + Folinic acid	3-4 wk 3-4 wk 3-4 wk	Pyrimethamine + Clindamycin + Folinic acid	3-4 wk 3-4 wk 3-4 wk	Adjunctive therapy with corticosteroids is recommended for macular involvement. Folinic acid is used to minimize pyrimethamine-associated hematologic toxicity.
	Central nervous system infection	[Pyrimethamine + Sulfadiazine] + Folinic acid	3-4 wk 3-4 wk 3-4 wk	[(Pyrimethamine + clindamycin) *or* (Pyrimethamine + Atovaquone)] + Folinic acid *or* [Atovaquone + sulfadiazine]	3-4 wk 3-4 wk 3-4 wk 3-4 wk	Adjunctive therapy with corticosteroids is sometimes recommended. Repeated LPs may be necessary to manage intracranial increased pressure. HIV-infected individuals with encephalitis should receive lifelong therapy or until clinical disease is resolved and sustained (>6 mo) reconstitution has been achieved using antiretroviral therapy. Folinic acid is used to minimize pyrimethamine-associated hematologic toxicity.

INFECTIOUS AGENTS AND DRUGS OF CHOICE

1

TABLE 1-6

RECOMMENDED TREATMENT FOR PARASITIC AND PROTOZOAL INFECTIONS—cont'd

Parasite/Where Infection Acquired	Host Category	Indication	Recommended Treatment	Duration	Alternative Treatment	Duration	Comments
Toxoplasma gondii—cont.		Congenital infection	Pyrimethamine every 2-3 days + sulfadiazine daily + Folinic acid	1 year			Folinic acid is used to minimize pyrimethamine-associated hematologic toxicity. Appropriate duration of treatment is not known.
	Pregnant women	<18 wk of gestation	Spiramycin	Duration of pregnancy if fetal infection is excluded			**Spiramycin** is the treatment of choice for primary infection in pregnancy if transmission to the fetus has not occurred. **Spiramycin** is not sold in the United States, but it can be obtained from the manufacturer with permission from the FDA. If fetal infection is confirmed after the 17th wk of pregnancy, or if the mother acquires primary infection in the last trimester, pyrimethamine and sulfadiazine should be considered. **Pyrimethamine** is a potential teratogen, and it should not be used during the first trimester.
		Fetal infection confirmed by amniocentesis after first trimester	[Spiramycin + sulfadiazine + folinic acid]	Until delivery			

Organism/Distribution		Drug of Choice	Duration	Alternative	Duration	Comments
Trachipleistopora sp (microsporidiosis)/ Not well defined	All	Disseminated microsporidiosis Albendazole²				There is no known effective therapy for microsporidial infection. **Albendazole** may reduce symptoms. HIV-positive patients may benefit from highly active antiretroviral therapy to improve their own immunity.
Trichinella spiralis/ Worldwide	All	Mebendazole²	10 days	Albendazole²	8-14 days	Corticosteroids help alleviate the inflammatory reaction and should be coadministered with **mebendazole** or **albendazole** when symptoms are severe.
Trichomonas vaginalis/Worldwide	All	Metronidazole	7 days	Tinidazole	2 g once	Sexual partners should be treated. **Metronidazole-resistant** strains should be treated with daily doses of 2-4 mg for 7-14 days (adults) or with high-dose **tinidazole.**
Trichostrongylus/ Worldwide	All	Pyrantel pamoate²	1 dose (500 mg) or 100 mg/kg twice daily for 3 days	Mebendazole² or Albendazole²	3 days 1 dose	
Trichuris trichiura (whipworm)/ Worldwide	All	Mebendazole	1 dose	Albendazole² or Ivermectin	3 days 3 days	

INFECTIOUS AGENTS AND DRUGS OF CHOICE

1

TABLE 1-6

RECOMMENDED TREATMENT FOR PARASITIC AND PROTOZOAL INFECTIONS—cont'd

Parasite/Where Infection Acquired	Host Category	Indication	Recommended Treatment	Duration	Alternative Treatment	Duration	Comments
Trypanosoma cruzi (Chagas' disease, American trypanosomiasis)/ Temperate, subtropical, tropical regions of the Americas and West Indies	Acute infection, indeterminate phase infection, congenital infection, reactivation associated with immunosuppression, transfusion-related infection		Benznidazole[7]	30-90 days	Nifurtimox[4]	90-120 days	Effectiveness of treatment of chronic infection has not been established. Side effects of **benznidazole** treatment are common and include rash, peripheral neuritis, anorexia and hepatologic alterations.
Trypanosoma brucei gambiense (sleeping sickness, West African trypanosomiasis)/ Western and Central Africa	All	Non-CNS infection	Pentamidine isethionate[2] (IM)	10 days	Suramin[4,7] (IV) *or*	100-200 mg IV test dose followed by doses on days 1, 3, 7, 14, and 21	
					Eflornithine[4]	400 mg/kg/ day IV in 4 divided doses for 14 days	
						400 mg/kg/d in 4 doses for 14 days	

Organism/Disease	Stage	Drug	Duration	Alternative	Comments
Trypanosoma brucei rhodesiense (East African trypanosomiasis, sleeping sickness)/Eastern Africa	CNS involvement	Melarsoprol[10] 2.2 mg/kg/day	10 days	Eflornithine[4] 400 mg/kg/day in 4 doses for 14 days	Melarsoprol treatment may be initiated in small doses (18 mg) with progressive increase and/or preceded by treatment with suramin in debilitated patients. Corticosteroids have been used to prevent encephalopathy. CSF should be followed every 3-6 mo for 2 yr during therapy.
	Hemolymphatic stage	Suramin[4,7]	100-200 mg test dose IV followed by doses on days 1, 3, 7, 14, and 21 400 mg/kg/day IV in 4 divided doses for 14 days		
	CNS involvement	Melarsoprol[10]	2-3.6 mg/kg/day for 3 days; after 7 days, 3.6 mg/kg/day for 3 days; repeat again after 7 days	Eflornithine[4] 400 mg/kg/day in 4 doses for 14 days	Melarsoprol treatment may be initiated in small doses (18 mg) with progressive increase and/or preceded by treatment with suramin in debilitated patients. Corticosteroids have been used to prevent encephalopathy. CSF should be followed every 3-6 mo for 2 yr during therapy.
Uncinaria stenocephala (cutaneous larva migrans)/Worldwide	Symptomatic patient	Cutaneous larva migrans	Thiabendazole (topical) or Albendazole[2] or Ivermectin[2]	Until lesions inactivated 3 days 1-2 days	Disease is usually self-limited, lasting wk to mo without therapy.

INFECTIOUS AGENTS AND DRUGS OF CHOICE

1

TABLE 1-6

RECOMMENDED TREATMENT FOR PARASITIC AND PROTOZOAL INFECTIONS—cont'd

Parasite/Where Infection Acquired	Host Category	Indication	Recommended Treatment	Duration	Alternative Treatment	Duration	Comments
Vittaforma cornaea (microsporidiosis)/ Not well defined	All	Ocular microsporidiosis	Albendazole[2] + fumagillin[5] (eye drops)				There is no known effective therapy for microsporidial infection. **Fumagillin** is used to control microsporidial disease in honey bees, and fumagillin eye drops have been helpful in some HIV-infected patients. **Albendazole** may reduce symptoms. HIV-positive patients may benefit from highly active antiretroviral therapy to improve their own immunity.
	All	Disseminated microsporidiosis	Albendazole[2]				There is no known effective therapy for microsporidial infection. **Albendazole** may reduce symptoms. HIV-positive patients may benefit from highly active antiretroviral therapy to improve their own immunity.
Wuchereria bancrofti (filariasis)/Tropics worldwide		Tropical pulmonary eosinophilia	Diethylcarbamazine[4] (6 mg/kg/day in 3 doses)	21 days	Albendazole + [ivermectin or diethylcarbamazine]	1 dose 1 dose 1 dose	Antihistamines or corticosteroids may be required to decrease allergic reaction to microfilarial disintegration. Alternative therapy suppresses microfilaria but does not kill the adult forms.

ECTOPARASITES

Organism/Distribution	Host	Infection	Drug of Choice	Dosage	Alternative	Dosage	Comments
Lice/Worldwide	All	Pediculosis capitis (head lice), Pediculosis corporis (body lice), Pediculosis pubis (pubic lice)	Malathion (0.5%, topical) or Permethrin (1% topical)	Apply once	Pyrethrin with piperonyl butoxide (topical) or Ivermectin (200 µg/kg PO)	3 times daily on days 1, 2, and 10	If **permethrin** or **pyrethrin** is used, a second application is recommended 1 wk later. Petrolatum for pubic lice in eyelashes.
Sarcoptes scabiei (Scabies)/Worldwide	Immunocompetent	Cutaneous infection	Permethrin (5% topical)	Apply once	Ivermectin (200 µg/ kg PO) or Crotamiton (10% topical)	Once / Once daily × 2 days	**Permethrin** or **ivermectin** treatment may have to be repeated in 10-14 days.
	Immunocompromised	Crusted scabies	Ivermectin (200 µg/ kg PO) ± a topical agent	Once			

1Available from Leiters Park Avenue Pharmacy, San Jose, CA (800-292-6773).
2Approved drug, but considered investigational for this indication.
3Not recommended in pregnancy and in children younger than 8 yr.
4Can be obtained from the CDC Drug Service, telephone 404-639-3670 or 404-639-2888 evenings and weekends.
5Fumagillin is made by Mid-Continent Agrimarketing, Inc., Olathe, Kansas, 800-547-1392.
6Not available commercially. This drug can be compounded as a service by Medical Center Pharmacy, New Haven, CT (203-688-6816) or by Panorama Compounding Pharmacy, 6744 Balboa Blvd, Van Nuys, CA 91406 (800-247-9767).
7Not marketed in the United States.
8Triclabendazole is available from Victoria Pharmacy, Zurich, Switzerland, 41-1-211-24-32.
9Available in limited supply from WHO.
10Not recommended in pregnant or breast-feeding women.
11If quinidine is unavailable, call Eli Lilly (800-821-0538) or the CDC Malaria Hotline (770-488-7788).
Abbreviations are explained in the footnote to Table 1-1.

INFECTIOUS AGENTS AND DRUGS OF CHOICE   1

PARASITE/PROTOZOA TYPES BY CATEGORY

Filaria

> *Brugia malayi*
> *Brugia timori*
> *Loa loa*
> *Mansonella ozzardi*
> *Mansonella perstans*
> *Mansonella streptocerca*
> *Onchocerca volvulus*
> *Wuchereria bancrofti*

Flukes

> *Capillaria philippinensis*
> *Clonorchis sinensis*
> *Fasciola buski*
> *Fasciola hepatica*
> *Heterophyes heterophyes*
> *Metagonimus yokogawai*
> *Metorchis conjunctus*
> *Nanophyetus salmincola*
> *Opisthorchis viverrini*
> *Paragonimus westermani*

Hookworm

> *Ancyclostoma braziliense*
> *Ancyclostoma caninum*
> *Ancyclostoma duodenale*
> *Necator americanus*
> *Uncinaria stenocephala*

Microsporidia

> *Encephalitozoon hellem*
> *Encephalitozoon cuniculi*
> *Encephalitozoon (Septata) intestinalis*
> *Enterocytozoon bieneusi*
> *Pleistophora sp*
> *Trichipleistopora sp*
> *Vittaforma corniaea*

Tapeworms

> *Diphyllabothrium latum*
> *Dipylidium caninum*
> *Hymenolepis nana*
> *Taenia saginata*
> *Taenia sol*

Recommended Empiric Antimicrobial Therapy for Selected Clinical Syndromes

Aaron M. Milstone, MD, Allison Agwu, MD, and Sanjay Jain, MD

RECOMMENDED EMPIRIC ANTIMICROBIAL THERAPY FOR SELECTED CLINICAL SYNDROMES

Syndrome	Host Category	Common Treatable Pathogens	Preferred Treatment	Alternative Treatment	Comments
SYSTEMIC AND INTRAVASCULAR INFECTIONS					
Endocarditis	Native valve (including congenital heart disease)	Streptococci, especially viridans streptococci group, staphylococci, enterococci	[PCN or ampicillin] + vancomycin + gentamicin (if PCN-allergic) Oxacillin/nafcillin + gentamicin		Antimicrobial therapy guided by blood culture results. Consider empiric vancomycin if high prevalence of resistant Gram-positive organisms. AG at synergistic dosage for Gram-positive organisms. Other less common organisms include HACEK group (*Haemophilus parainfluenzae, Haemophilus aphrophilus, Actinobacillus, Cardiobacterium, Eikenella, Kingella*), *Bartonella, Coxiella burnetii, Chlamydia, Brucella, Nocardia, Mycobacterium* spp.
	Prosthetic valve	Coagulase-negative *Staphylococcus, Staphylococcus aureus,* enterococci, viridans streptococci, Gram-negative bacilli, diphtheroids	Vancomycin + gentamicin + rifampin		Surgical consultation. Antimicrobial therapy guided by blood culture results. AG at synergistic dosage for Gram-positive organisms. Other less common organisms include fungi such as *Candida* and *Aspergillus* spp.

	IV drug user	S. aureus (usually MRSA)	Vancomycin + gentamicin	Daptomycin	Daptomycin not approved by the Food and Drug Administration (FDA) for this indication.
Intravascular catheter-related infection (CRI)/ bacteremia	Immunocompetent patient	S. aureus, coagulase-negative staphylococci, less likely enteric Gram-negative rods, Candida spp	Vancomycin + [PCS3 or AG]	Linezolid Synercid*** Daptomycin***	Consider catheter removal, especially if clinical progression or severe illness. Consider Gram-negative coverage, depending on patient risk factors and severity of illness. Add amphotericin B or fluconazole if suspicious of candidemia. Other less common organisms include *Corynebacterium, Bacillus* spp, *Propionibacterium, Enterococcus* spp.
	Immunocompromised patient	S. aureus, coagulase-negative staphylococci, Gram-negative bacilli (especially *Pseudomonas* spp, Enterobacteriaceae), *Corynebacterium* spp	Vancomycin + [Ceftazidime or cefepime or Pip/tazo or AG]	Vancomycin + [Imipenem or meropenem]	Consider catheter removal. Strongly consider adding amphotericin B or fluconazole if suspicious of candidemia.

ANTIMICROBIAL THERAPY FOR SELECTED CLINICAL SYNDROMES

2

Syndrome	Host Category	Common Treatable Pathogens	Preferred Treatment	Alternative Treatment	Comments
Myocarditis	Immunocompetent patient	*Borrelia* spp	Supportive care If Lyme disease suspected, ceftriaxone *or* penicillin IV	If Lyme disease, doxycycline PO if mild/no symptoms and at least 8 yr	Viruses are most common cause of myocarditis (enteroviruses, adenovirus, CMV, influenza virus, parainfluenza virus, mumps virus, HIV). Less common organisms: *Rickettsia* spp, *Treponema pallidum*. Bacteria (especially *S. aureus*, *Neisseria meningitidis*) can cause myocardial abscesses and myocardial dysfunction but rarely cause myocarditis. Role of steroids and IVIg is controversial.
	Immunocompromised patient	*Borrelia* spp and *Toxoplasma*	Same as above for immunocompetent patients		As above. Consider pyrimethamine plus sulfadiazine if toxoplasmosis is suspected.

Pericarditis (purulent)	All	S. aureus, Streptococcus pneumoniae, N. meningitidis, H. influenzae, Enterobacteriaceae, Mycobacterium tuberculosis	Vancomycin + PCS3	Severe PCN allergy: vancomycin + [Aztreonam or FQ]	Broad-spectrum antimicrobial therapy should be initiated empirically for suspected purulent pericarditis. Purulent effusion should be drained as soon as possible. Viral disease likely in nonpurulent pericarditis (enteroviruses). Less common fungal pathogens: other streptococci, anaerobic bacteria, Rickettsia spp, Mycoplasma pneumoniae, Mycoplasma hominis, Ureaplasma urealyticum.
Systemic febrile illness/sepsis	Community-acquired infection, normal host	S. pneumoniae, N. meningitidis, H. influenzae types b, S. aureus, group A Streptococcus, Salmonella	Ceftriaxone	Carbapenem Severe PCN allergy: vancomycin + aztreonam	Consider vancomycin if concern for staphylococcal infection or if CNS involvement is likely. Consider doxycycline in tick-endemic areas or if petechial rash (Ehrlichia, Rickettsia spp). In cases of shock, add vancomycin and consider clindamycin for toxic shock syndrome.

2

ANTIMICROBIAL THERAPY FOR SELECTED CLINICAL SYNDROMES

Syndrome	Host Category	Common Treatable Pathogens	Preferred Treatment	Alternative Treatment	Comments
	Asplenia	*S. pneumoniae, Salmonella, N. meningitidis, H. influenzae* type b, *Capnocytophaga* spp., *Babesia* spp., *Erysipelothrix*	Ceftriaxone	Carbapenem Severe PCN allergy: vancomycin + [Aztreonam or FQ]	Consider vancomycin if concern for staphylococcal infection or if CNS involvement is likely. Consider doxycycline in tick-infested areas or if petechial rash (*Ehrlichia, Rickettsia* spp). Add clindamycin and quinine if *Babesia* is a concern. In cases of shock, add vancomycin and consider clindamycin for toxic shock syndrome.
	GU source	Gram-negative bacilli, enterococci	[Ampicillin + gentamicin] or Ceftriaxone	Pip/tazo or Amp/sulb or FQ	Some experts routinely add AG. Consider resistant organisms and broaden coverage for hosts with indwelling catheters, history of UTI, or other abnormalities of GU tract.
	Hospital-acquired infection	*S. pneumoniae, S. aureus,* other streptococci, Gram-negative bacilli (especially *Pseudomonas aeruginosa*)	Cefepime or Pip/tazo or Imipenem or Meropenem	Severe PCN allergy: vancomycin + [Aztreonam or FQ]	Consider vancomycin if concern for MRSA, shock, or severe illness. Consider amphotericin if suspected fungal etiology. In cases of shock, consider adding an AG.

Intra-abdominal source or biliary source	Enterococci, Enterobacteriaceae, *Bacteroides* spp. Other aerobic and anaerobic Gram-negative bacilli. *Candida* spp less common.	Amp/sulb *or* [Ampicillin + gentamicin + metronidazole] *or* Tic/clav *or* Pip/tazo	Carbapenem Severe PCN allergy: vancomycin + [Aztreonam *or* FQ] + metronidazole	In cases of shock, add an AG (if not already part of the regimen).
Intravenous drug user	*S. aureus*	Oxacillin *or* Vancomycin	Linezolid *or* Synercid *or* Daptomycin	Empiric treatment depends on local antibiotic susceptibility patterns.
Neonate	GBS, *Escherichia coli*, *Listeria*, other enteric Gram-negative bacilli (*Klebsiella*, *Enterobacter*), *S. aureus*	Ampicillin + gentamicin	Ampicillin + cefotaxime	Substitute cefotaxime for gentamicin if meningitis is a possibility or in cases of shock. Consider adding vancomycin or oxacillin if concern for *Staphylococcus* (neonatal intensive care unit patient or community-acquired MRSA). Consider testing for HSV and adding acyclovir if concern for HSV.

2

ANTIMICROBIAL THERAPY FOR SELECTED CLINICAL SYNDROMES

Syndrome	Host Category	Common Treatable Pathogens	Preferred Treatment	Alternative Treatment	Comments
	Hospitalized neonate	GBS, *E. coli*, *Listeria*, other enteric Gram-negative bacilli (*Klebsiella*, *Enterobacter*), *S. aureus*, coagulase-negative *Staphylococcus*, *H. influenzae*, Enterococcus, *Candida* spp	Ampicillin + gentamicin	Ampicillin + cefotaxime	Substitute cefotaxime for gentamicin if meningitis cannot be excluded or depending on local antibiotic susceptibility patterns. Consider vancomycin if concern for *Staphylococcus*. Consider adding amphotericin B for *Candida*. Consider adding acyclovir if concern for HSV.
	Drug-induced neutropenia	Gram-negative bacilli (including *P. aeruginosa*), viridans streptococci, *Staphylococcus* spp, *Candida* spp, other fungi	[Cefepime *or* ceftazidime *or* Pip/tazo] ± AG *or* Imipenem *or* Meropenem	[Imipenem or meropenem] ± AG Severe PCN allergy: [Vancomycin + aztreonam] *or* FQ	Consider vancomycin for central venous line site infection, history of MRSA infection, or hypotension. In case of shock, add vancomycin and an AG. If severe illness or no improvement with antibacterial therapy, add amphotericin B.
Toxic shock syndrome	All	*S. aureus*, GAS	Oxacillin + clindamycin	Vancomycin + clindamycin	Consider IVIg. Seek source. Vancomycin/clindamycin preferred if MRSA prevalence is high.

OCULAR INFECTIONS

Blepharitis	All	Warm compress and eyelid scrub	Unclear etiology; may include *Staphylococcus* spp, seborrhea, meibomian gland dysfunction. Topical antistaphylococcal antimicrobials (e.g., tetracycline, erythromycin, bacitracin) sometimes used to decrease bacterial load on eyelids.
Conjunctivitis (bacterial)	Bacterial: *N. gonorrhoeae*, *C. trachomatis*	[Ceftriaxone or cefotaxime] + [Erythromycin or azithromycin]	[Ceftriaxone or cefotaxime] + sulfonamide	Treat neonate for presumed systemic infection if *N. gonorrhoeae* is suspected: • Oral erythromycin in infants <6 wk old associated with increased risk of pyloric stenosis; risk from azithromycin not well studied. • Sulfonamide can be used beyond immediate neonatal period if intolerant of macrolides. Consider viral disease (HSV) and less common organisms: *Streptococcus* spp, *H. influenzae*, Gram-negative bacilli. Chemical conjunctivitis less common because erythromycin is used as prophylaxis instead of silver nitrate. Consider ophthalmology evaluation. Treat mother and her partner(s) for cases of confirmed STI.

Newborn (ophthalmia neonatorum)

ANTIMICROBIAL THERAPY FOR SELECTED CLINICAL SYNDROMES

2

Syndrome	Host Category	Common Treatable Pathogens	Preferred Treatment	Alternative Treatment	Comments
	Beyond newborn	Bacterial: S. pneumoniae, H. influenzae, Moraxella, ?S. aureus	Polymyxin B + trimethoprim drops	FQ drops	Consider viral disease (adenovirus). Topical therapy not necessary if giving systemic therapy for concomitant OM.
	Sexually active patient and/or associated with genital infection	N. gonorrhoeae, C. trachomatis	Ceftriaxone + doxycycline		Ophthalmic consultation and frequent irrigation if suspected N. gonorrhoeae. Treat partner(s) if confirmed STI.
Dacrocystitis	All	S. pneumoniae, H. influenzae, S. aureus, coagulase-negative staphylococci, Streptococcus pyogenes, P. aeruginosa	Nafcillin/Oxacillin or Cephalexin or Clindamycin	Vancomycin	Consider ophthalmologic consultation to relieve obstruction and to obtain material for culture.
Endophthalmitis	Immunocompetent patient	S. pneumoniae, N. meningitidis, S. aureus, Gram-negative bacilli, coagulase-negative staphylococci, Bacillus spp, Propionibacterium acnes	[Cefotaxime or ceftriaxone] + vancomycin	Vancomycin + FQ	Obtain emergent ophthalmologic evaluation. P. acnes is the most common pathogen following cataract surgery. Blood and vitreal cultures and stains should guide definitive therapy. Intravitreal administration of antibiotics essential in treatment of exogenous (traumatic) endophthalmitis. If history of trauma, consider antipseudomonal coverage.

Immunosuppressed patient	See above bacterial, *Candida* spp, *Aspergillus* spp, *Listeria monocytogenes*, *Nocardia* spp	[Ceftazidime *or* cefepime] + vancomycin + amphotericin B	FQ + voriconazole	Obtain emergent ophthalmologic evaluation. Blood and vitreal cultures and stains should guide definitive therapy.
Keratitis	All	Viral: HSV 1,2; Epstein-Barr virus (EBV), varicella-zoster virus, adenovirus, rubeola virus, rubella virus, mumps virus, measles virus, enteroviruses Bacterial: *S. aureus*, other *Staphylococcus* spp, *S. pneumoniae*, *S. pyogenes*, *C. trachomatis*, *Listeria*, *Moraxella catarrhalis*, Gram-negative bacilli (especially *Pseudomonas*) Fungal: *Aspergillus* sp, *Fusarium* sp, *Candida* sp Protozoal: *Acanthamoeba*, *Hartmanella*	Consider cephalosporin and AG drops pending further evaluation; e.g., cefazolin ophthalmic + AG ophthalmic	FQ ophthalmic	Obtain emergent ophthalmologic evaluation. Cultures and stains to guide therapy. Contact lens wearers at increased risk of *Pseudomonas*.

ANTIMICROBIAL THERAPY FOR SELECTED CLINICAL SYNDROMES 2

Syndrome	Host Category	Common Treatable Pathogens	Preferred Treatment	Alternative Treatment	Comments
Orbital cellulitis	Immunocompetent patient (secondary to sinusitis, trauma, or bacteremia)	Bacterial: *S. pneumoniae, H. influenzae, S. aureus, M. catarrhalis, S. pyogenes* (anaerobes, Gram-negative bacilli)	Amp/sulb *or* [Oxacillin + PCS3] *or* [Clindamycin + PCS3]	Cefuroxime Severe PCN allergy: [Vancomycin or clindamycin] + RFQ *or* Aztreonam	Consider adding vancomycin if concern for MRSA. Recommend ophthalmologic consultation. Evaluate with CT scan for intracranial extension.
	Immunosuppressed patient	See above bacterial, especially *Pseudomonas* spp, other Gram-negative bacilli	Pip/tazo *or* Cefepime	FQ PCN allergy: vancomycin + [Quinolone *or* aztreonam] + metronidazole	Consider adding vancomycin if concern for MRSA. Consider fungi (mucormycosis, *Rhizopus*) and presumptive antifungal therapy.
Preseptal cellulitis	Immunocompetent patient	*Streptococcus* spp, primarily GAS, *S. aureus*, nontypeable *H. influenzae, M. catarrhalis*	Amp/sulb *or* A/C *or* [PCS3 + clindamycin]	Cefuroxime *or* FQ	Consider adding vancomycin, TMP/SMX, or clindamycin if concern for MRSA. If suspected secondary to cutaneous trauma and not suspected to be associated with sinusitis, may choose narrow staphylococcal/streptococcal antibiotic (e.g., clindamycin).

		Organisms	Therapy	Alternative	Comments
Immunosuppressed patient		*Streptococcus* spp, primarily GAS, *S. aureus*, nontypeable *H. influenzae*, *Moraxella*, anaerobes, *Pseudomonas* spp, fungi (*Candida*)	Pip/tazo + vancomycin	[Cefepime + clindamycin] or [Imipenem/meropenem + vancomycin]	Consider adding antifungal.
Stye (hordeolum), external or internal	All	External and internal: *S. aureus*	Warm compress ± dicloxacillin or cephalexin or clindamycin	A/C or TMP/SMX	Internal styes drain spontaneously; external styes usually do not drain spontaneously.
Dental abscess	All	Oral flora: often polymicrobial, including anaerobes	Clindamycin	A/C	Consider surgical drainage.
Parotitis	All	Most common: *S. aureus*. Uncommon: Gram-negative bacilli, oral flora; Chronic: *Mycobacterium*, fungi. Viruses, acute: adenovirus, mumps virus, enteroviruses, influenza virus; chronic: HIV	Oxacillin or Dicloxacillin or Clindamycin or A/C		Cultures guide therapy. For chronic parotitis offer HIV testing.

ANTIMICROBIAL THERAPY FOR SELECTED CLINICAL SYNDROMES

2

Syndrome	Host Category	Common Treatable Pathogens	Preferred Treatment	Alternative Treatment	Comments
GENITOURINARY INFECTIONS					
Cervicitis/ urethritis/ epididymitis (No pelvic inflammatory disease)	All	*C. trachomatis* *N. gonorrhoeae* Uncommon: *Trichomonas vaginalis*, HSV, *Mycoplasma genitalium*, *Ureaplasma urealyticum*	[Azithromycin × 1 dose *or* doxycycline × 7 days] + [Ceftriaxone *or* cefixime *or* ciprofloxacin *or* ofloxacin] × 1 dose	[Erythromycin × 14 days] + [Ceftriaxone *or* cefixime] *or* Spectinomycin* × 1 dose	Treatment for both chlamydial and gonorrheal infections should be given simultaneously due to the high rate of coinfection. Testing for other STIs and HIV should be offered. Sexual partners of patient with confirmed STIs should be examined and treated to avoid reinfection. FQ are no longer recommended for presumptive treatment of gonorrheal infection because of increasing resistance.

Pelvic inflammatory disease (PID)	All	*N. gonorrhoeae, C. trachomatis,* anaerobes (i.e., *Peptostreptococcus, Prevotella* sp, *Clostridia*) Gram-negative organisms: Enterobacteriaceae, *H. influenzae,* streptococci	**Outpatient** [Ceftriaxone IM *or* other PCS3 *or* cefoxitin IM/probenecid PO] + Doxycycline ± metronidazole **Hospitalized patient** [(Cefoxitin *or* cefotetan) + (doxycycline × 14 days)] *or* [Clindamycin IV + gentamicin]	A/C + doxycycline *or* Amp/sulb + doxycycline Penicillin allergy: [(Levofloxacin *or* ofloxacin) ± metronidazole]	For hospitalized patients who improve clinically, parenteral therapy may be replaced after 24 hours. Continuing oral therapy: Doxycycline plus clindamycin to complete 14 days. FQ are no longer recommended for presumptive treatment of gonorrheal infection because of increasing resistence.
UTI	Cystitis	Gram-negative organisms (i.e., *E. coli, Proteus,* Enterobacteriaceae), *Enterococcus* sp, *Staphylococcus saprophyticus* (postpubertal females)	TMP/SMX *or* Cefixime	Nitrofurantoin *or* OCS2 *or* OCS3	For cystitis consider phenazopyridine (Pyridium) for comfort. Note: Urine may turn red.

ANTIMICROBIAL THERAPY FOR SELECTED CLINICAL SYNDROMES

Syndrome	Host Category	Common Treatable Pathogens	Preferred Treatment	Alternative Treatment	Comments
	Pyelonephritis, no urinary tract abnormalities (uncomplicated)	Gram-negative organisms (i.e., *E. coli, Proteus,* Enterobacteriaceae), *Enterococcus*	[Ampicillin + gentamicin] or Ceftriaxone	Cefixime or Ciprofloxacin for severe PCN allergy or resistant organism without other oral treatment options (≥1 year old)	Therapy should be directed by culture results, particularly for those on long-term prophylaxis where the flora may be altered.
	Infants <3 mo	Same as above and group B *Streptococcus*	[Ampicillin + gentamicin] or Ceftriaxone	Cefixime or FQ or AG	Evaluation for urinary tract abnormalities and urinary reflux should be done for all children with UTIs under age of 5 yr, in any boy who gets a UTI, and in older girls with recurrent UTIs.
	Urinary tract abnormalities on prophylaxis	Same as above and resistant Gram-negative organisms	Pip/tazo or Ceftazidime		Pyelonephritis without sepsis may be treated orally on an outpatient basis in selected patients.
	Pregnant patient	Gram-negative organisms (i.e., *E. coli, Proteus*), *Enterococcus* sp, *S. saprophyticus*), group B *Streptococcus*	Nitrofurantoin or OCS2 or OCS3 or TMP/SMX		If TMP/SMX, must be discontinued 2 wk prior to estimated date of delivery due to risk of kernicterus in infant.

Renal abscess	All	S. aureus, Gram-negative organisms (i.e., E. coli, Proteus, Pseudomonas), other Gram-positive organisms (i.e., Enterococcus spp., Streptococcus), anaerobes	Oxacillin + gentamicin + [Metronidazole or clindamycin]	Vancomycin + ceftriaxone	Therapy should be adjusted for abscess culture results as urine and blood cultures may not capture all pathogens. Renal abscess caused by hematogenous source is likely due to S. aureus; abscess secondary to UTI is more likely due to Enterobacteriaceae. Medical management initially, directed by clinical response; however, may need drainage if no resolution or obstruction.
Bacterial vaginosis	Nonpregnant patient	Usually polymicrobial, mostly associated with Gardnerella vaginalis, anaerobic bacteria	Metronidazole intravaginally or PO	Clindamycin vaginal cream or PO	Single-dose metronidazole not as effective as multiday course.
	Pregnant patient		Clindamycin PO or Metronidazole PO or intravaginally		Avoid clindamycin cream in pregnancy.
BONE, JOINT, AND SOFT TISSUE INFECTIONS					
Necrotizing fasciitis	All	S. pyogenes (GAS), Clostridium perfringens and other Clostridium spp, Bacteroides sp, Prevotella sp, Gram-negative organisms, S. aureus	[(Nafcillin or oxacillin) + AG + clindamycin] or [Pip/tazo ± clindamycin] or [Cefepime + clindamycin]	Carbapenem + clindamycin	Antibiotics are adjunctive; early surgical involvement crucial! If S. aureus concern, add vancomycin. Clindamycin may be superior adjunctive antibiotic for GAS due to toxin synthesis inhibition and inoculum effect.

ANTIMICROBIAL THERAPY FOR SELECTED CLINICAL SYNDROMES 2

Syndrome	Host Category	Common Treatable Pathogens	Preferred Treatment	Alternative Treatment	Comments
Osteomyelitis, acute and chronic	All	S. aureus (MSSA/MRSA) GAS and Streptococcus spp, including GBS (neonates) Gram-negative organisms (i.e., Kingella)	Naficillin or Oxacillin or Clindamycin	Vancomycin	Definitive therapy should be guided by biopsy and culture results when available. Biopsy/culture essential before broadening antibiotic coverage for inadequate response to initial empiric therapy. Vancomycin or clindamycin if MRSA prevalent, depending on local susceptibility trends. Rifampin has excellent bone penetration and can be good adjunctive therapy for Gram-positives; it should never be used as monotherapy.
	Osteomyelitis of the foot (result of penetrating injury through sole of shoe)	P. aeruginosa	Ceftazidime or AP pen + AG		Clindamycin alone is not effective treatment for kingella. Initial treatment of penetrating wound to the foot should include antibiotics effective against S. aureus. If osteomyelitis develops, presumptive therapy should include treatment effective against P. aeruginosa.
	Immunocompromised patients and neonates	Candida sp All pathogens listed for normal host, plus Pseudomonas	[Naficillin or oxacillin or clindamycin] + [Ceftazadime or cefepime or AP pen]	Vancomycin + [Ceftazidime or cefepime or AP pen FQ]	Remember: other pathogens, including mycobacteria and fungi, can cause osteomyelitis and should be considered particularly in unusual presentations or lack of clinical response.

Post-spinal fusion infection	All	*Staphylococcus* spp (MSSA/MRSA/MRSE), *Streptococcus* spp, Gram-negative organisms, particularly GI and GU pathogens	Vancomycin + pip/tazo	Although rod removal is usually optimal, it is often difficult or impossible. Deep tissue cultures are essential for directed therapy. Consider adding an AG with or without rifampin.
Pyomyositis	All	*S. aureus* (MSSA/MRSA) *Streptococcus* spp (GAS), anaerobes	Nafcillin or Oxacillin or Cefazolin or Vancomycin or Clindamycin	Early surgical involvement crucial. Therapy should be guided by culture results. With increasing incidence of community-acquired MRSA, low threshold to choose vancomycin or clindamycin. Clindamycin or metronidazole should be part of presumptive therapy when infection is associated with trauma.
Spinal abscess	All	*Staphylococcus aureus* (MSSA/MRSA) *Streptococcus* spp	Oxacillin or Nafcillin or Vancomycin or Clindamycin or Cefazolin	Debridement is an important component of therapy. Therapy should be guided by culture results when available. With increasing incidence of community-acquired MRSA, low threshold to choose vancomycin or clindamycin.

ANTIMICROBIAL THERAPY FOR SELECTED CLINICAL SYNDROMES   2

Syndrome	Host Category	Common Treatable Pathogens	Preferred Treatment	Alternative Treatment	Comments
Arthritis, bacterial	Neonate	S. aureus, GBS, Gram-negative bacilli	(Nafcillin or oxacillin) + (Cefotaxime or gentamicin)	Vancomycin + (Cefotaxime or gentamicin)	Incision and drainage are important components of therapy.
	Child ≤5 yr	S. aureus, group A Streptococcus, S. pneumoniae, K. kingae, Haemophilus spp	(Nafcillin or oxacillin or clindamycin) + cefotaxime	Vancomycin + cefotaxime	Therapy should be guided by Gram-stained smear and culture results when available. Include clindamycin or vancomycin based on local prevalence and susceptibility patterns of MRSA.
	Child >5 yr	S. aureus, Streptococcus spp	Nafcillin or Oxacillin or Clindamycin	Vancomycin	Oral therapy may be appropriate once definite improvement is determined.
	Adolescent	S. aureus, Streptococcus spp, must consider N. gonorrhoeae	[Nafcillin or oxacillin or clindamycin] + ceftriaxone	Vancomycin + (Ceftriaxone or FQ)	In adolescents, ceftriaxone or FQ used when gonorrhea is a consideration.
Diskitis	All	Staphylococcus spp (MSSA/MRSA), Streptococcus spp, K. kingae, Gram-negative bacilli, Mycobacterium (Pott's disease)	Oxacillin or Nafcillin or Clindamycin	Vancomycin	Bed rest is considered essential. Therapy should be directed by clinical progress and recovered pathogen if culture performed. Add Gram-negative coverage if Gram-negative infection suspected.

Folliculitis, furuncles, carbuncles	All	S. aureus (MSSA/MRSA)	Warm compresses, incision, and drainage	Antistaphylococcal agent in more severe infections, i.e., carbuncles: CFZ *or* clindamycin *or* TMP/SMX *or* dicloxacillin	With the increasing incidence of MRSA, clindamycin, TMP/SMX, or vancomycin may be preferred. With recurrent furuncles, boils, consider culturing nares for MRSA and, if positive, for eradication with intranasal mupirocin and/or topical chlorhexidine. Incision, drainage, and culture are important in treatment and determination of definitive antibiotic therapy.
Erysipelas	All	Streptococcus spp, primarily GAS, S. aureus	**Mild** Dicloxacillin or cephalexin	Clindamycin *or* Macrolide	Occasionally, bacteremia may occur; blood cultures should be obtained. TMP/SMX not active against GAS.
			Severe Parenteral penicillin therapy *or* Antistaphylococcal penicillin	Clindamycin *or* Vancomycin	
Cellulitis	Immunocompetent patient	Streptococcus spp, primarily GAS, S. aureus	Cephalexin *or* A/C *or* Clindamycin		Choose non-beta-lactam option if MRSA is common. TMP/SMX not active against GAS.
	Immunocompromised patient, including diabetic individuals	Streptococcus spp, primarily GAS, S. aureus, Pseudomonas, fungi (Candida)	(Clindamycin + ceftazidime) *or* (Pip/tazo + vancomycin)	Vancomycin + AG	For immunocompromised patients, consider presumptive therapy with amphotericin B as well as antibacterials.

ANTIMICROBIAL THERAPY FOR SELECTED CLINICAL SYNDROMES

2

Syndrome	Host Category	Common Treatable Pathogens	Preferred Treatment	Alternative Treatment	Comments
Hidradenitis suppurativa	All	Staphylococcus spp, anaerobes, Pseudomonas, Gram-negative organisms	Clindamycin	Vancomycin	Adjust treatment based on culture results.
Ecthyma gangrenosum	Usually immunocompromised patients but can occur in immunocompetent patients	P. aeruginosa, S. aureus, other Gram-negative organisms, fungal species (Aspergillus, Zygomycetes, Candida spp)	(Ceftazidime + clindamycin) or Cefepime or Pip/tazo	Imipenem or Meropenem or FQ	Sample for culture may be obtained by biopsy or by aspirating sample directly from the cellulitic region. Consider adding amphotericin B, particularly for neutropenic patients.
LOWER RESPIRATORY TRACT INFECTIONS					
Aspiration pneumonia	All	Polymicrobial: oral anaerobes (Bacteroides sp, Fusobacterium), Streptococcus spp, S. aureus, Klebsiella pneumoniae	Clindamycin or BL/BLI	Imipenem or Meropenem	
Lung abscess	All	Polymicrobial: oral anaerobes (Bacteroides sp, Fusobacterium), Streptococcus spp, S. aureus, K. pneumoniae	Clindamycin or BL/BLI	Imipenem or Meropenem	Consider vancomycin for MRSA coverage in severe disease; clindamycin efficacy will depend on local resistance patterns. Consider obtaining needle aspirite for culture

Community-acquired pneumonia	Immunocompetent patient				
	Infant age 4 wk–3 mo	Viruses most common. Bacterial pathogens: S. pneumoniae, C. trachomatis, Bordetella pertussis, S. aureus	**Afebrile, nonseptic** Erythromycin or Azithromycin **Febrile, appears ill** Erythromycin or Azithromycin + cefotaxime	Consider adding vancomycin	Erythromycin may increase the risk of pyloric stenosis in infants <6 wk
	Child age 3 mo–5 yr	Viruses most common, S. pneumoniae, Mycoplasma, Chlamydiophila pneumoniae, GAS, S. aureus (MRSA/MSSA)	**Outpatient** Amoxicillin (high dose) ± azithromycin **Inpatient** Cefotaxime/ceftriaxone + azithromycin	For severe penicillin allergy, consider clindamycin or azithromycin For severe penicillin allergy, [Clindamycin or vancomycin] + azithromycin	Consider including clindamycin or vancomycin if there is pleural effusion, cavitary pneumonia, or more severe illness.
	Child age 5–15 years	Viruses most common, S. pneumoniae, Mycoplasma, C. pneumoniae, GAS, S. aureus (MRSA/MSSA), M. tuberculosis	**Outpatient** Azithromycin ± clindamycin **Inpatient** Ceftriaxone/ cefotaxime + azithromycin	Azithromycin ± clindamycin For severe penicillin allergy, azithromycin + [Clindamycin or vancomycin]	Consider including clindamycin or vancomycin if there is pleural effusion, cavitary pneumonia, or more severe illness.

ANTIMICROBIAL THERAPY FOR SELECTED CLINICAL SYNDROMES   2

Syndrome	Host Category	Common Treatable Pathogens	Preferred Treatment	Alternative Treatment	Comments
Pneumonia	Immunocomprised patient, neutropenia, steroids, immunomodulators, graft-versus-host disease (GVHD)	Same as community-acquired pathogens; additionally, *P. aeruginosa*, other Gram-negative organisms, *Aspergillus, Candida*	[Pip/tazo *or* cefepime] ± AG	Imipenem *or* Meropenem	Send sputum for Gram stain and culture if possible. Therapy should be adjusted for culture data and clinical response. Low threshold for more definitive diagnostic procedures (i.e., bronchoscopy). Consider vancomycin with suspicion for resistant Gram-positive organisms, particularly MRSA. Also consider fungus, pneumocystis, CMV, atypical mycobacteria, and other atypical bacteria, i.e., *Nocardia*.
Cystic fibrosis		*Pseudomonas* sp, *S. aureus*, other Gram-negative organisms, especially *Burkholderia*	[Ceftazidime *or* (tic/clav *or* cefepime] ± AG	[Imipenem *or* meropenem *or* FQ] ± AG	Antimicrobials in conjunction with aggressive pulmonary toilet. Low threshold for adding additional antistaphylococcal coverage, particularly if no improvement. Culture results should be used to guide therapy. Also consider allergic bronchopulmonary aspergillosis, a typical mycobacteria.

HIV	S. pneumoniae, pathogens of community-acquired pneumonia; must also consider pneumocystis, cryptococcosis, histoplasmosis, and tuberculosis based on CD4 count, antibiotic prophylaxis, and past history.	(Ceftriaxone + azithromycin) ± TMP/SMX	Severe penicillin allergy: (Vancomycin + AG) ± TMP/SMX	TMP/SMX for PCP (CD4 <200 or <15%, especially with hypoxia) Induced sputum or BAL should be strongly considered, particularly in patients with CD4 <200 or 15%. Consider Pip/Tazo or cefepime for Pseudomonas if severe immunosuppression, damaged airways, and/or neutropenia.
Neonates (<28 days)	GBS, Streptococcus spp, Listeria, Gram-negative organisms, particularly E. coli, S. aureus, HSV, CMV, enteroviruses	(Ampicillin + gentamicin) ± cefotaxime		For neonates, consider adding vancomycin and acyclovir. Add cefotaxime if meningitis is a possible complication.
Ventilator-associated pneumonia	All	Variable pathogens: S. pneumoniae, Gram-negative bacilli (Pseudomonas, Stenotrophomonas, Acinetobacter, Klebsiella, etc.), S. aureus	Pip/tazo or Cefepime or Imipenem or Meropenem	Clindamycin + AG	Gram-stained smear and culture should help guide therapy. Consider MRSA coverage. Ertapenem does not have antipseudomonal activity.

ANTIMICROBIAL THERAPY FOR SELECTED CLINICAL SYNDROMES

2

Syndrome	Host Category	Common Treatable Pathogens	Preferred Treatment	Alternative Treatment	Comments
Bronchiolitis	All	Respiratory syncytial virus, parainfluenza virus, influenza virus, rhinovirus, human metapneumovirus	Supportive therapy		Infants <2 yr with chronic lung disease, congestive heart disease, and/or prematurity (see AAP guidelines) should receive prophylactic RSV monoclonal antibody.

CENTRAL NERVOUS SYSTEM INFECTIONS

Syndrome	Host Category	Common Treatable Pathogens	Preferred Treatment	Alternative Treatment	Comments
Brain abscess	Previously healthy; complication of sinusitis (beyond neonatal period)	*Streptococcus* spp, Gram-negative enterics, *Eikenella*, anaerobes, *S. pneumoniae, N. meningitidis, S. aureus*	Ceftriaxone + metronidazole	For patient with **severe penicillin allergy,** consider [Chloramphenicol or TMP/SMX] + metronidazole	Consider adding vancomycin (meningitic dose) for resistant *S. aureus* and *S. pneumoniae.* Surgical intervention may be required.
	Immunocompromised patient	Consider *Listeria, Pseudomonas, Nocardia,* anaerobic bacteria, and fungi in addition to pathogens for community-acquired meningitis	(Ceftazidime or cefepime) + vancomycin + metronidazole + ampicillin	For patient with **severe penicillin allergy,** consider aztreonam + vancomycin + metronidazole.	Consider amphotericin B if no response within 1 wk and organism unknown. Consider also *Toxoplasma* in AIDS patients.

Condition	Organism	Therapy	For patient with severe penicillin allergy	Comments
Complication of dental disease	Oral microflora (polymicrobial)	Penicillin (300,000 U/kg/day) + metronidazole	For patient with severe penicillin allergy, consider vancomycin + metronidazole.	Avoid clindamycin because of poor CNS penetration.
Postsurgery (neurosurgery, head trauma, CSF shunt-associated, cochlear implants)	Gram-negative organisms (including *Pseudomonas*) and *S. aureus*	(Ceftazidime or cefepime) + vancomycin	For patient with severe penicillin allergy, consider (Aztreonam or ciprofloxacin) + vancomycin	Add AG if Gram-negative organisms seen on Gram stain.
Neonate	Group B *Streptococcus*, enteric Gram-negative organisms (especially *Citrobacter* and *E. coli*), *Listeria*	Ampicillin + cefotaxime + AG		Attempt should be made to define specific pathogen. *Citrobacter* spp., *Enterobacter sakazakii*, and *Serratia marcescens* cause meningitis associated with brain abscesses.
Encephalitis — Previously healthy and beyond neonatal period	HSV, varicella-zoster virus	Acyclovir		Continue acyclovir until results from HSV PCR are available or alternate organism has been identified. Other etiologies include enteroviruses, arboviruses, including West Nile virus, EBV, cat-scratch disease (*Bartonella henselae*), rabies, Lyme disease (*Borrelia burgdorferi*), TB, malaria, and *Listeria* in immunocompromised patients.

ANTIMICROBIAL THERAPY FOR SELECTED CLINICAL SYNDROMES

2

Syndrome	Host Category	Common Treatable Pathogens	Preferred Treatment	Alternative Treatment	Comments
	Neonates	HSV	Acyclovir (60 mg/kg/day) in divided doses q8 hr		For premature neonates, acyclovir dosage determined according to gestational age. Enteroviruses are most common cause.
Aseptic meningitis		*Borrelia burgdorferi*	Ceftriaxone	Doxycycline	Other causes of aseptic meningitis include viruses: enteroviruses; herpes viruses, lymphocytic choriomeningitis virus, arboviruses; fungi; TB; drugs: NSAIDs, sulfa antibiotics, immune globulins; cancer/systemic inflammatory diseases.
Bacterial meningitis (beyond neonatal period)	Community-acquired infection	*S. pneumoniae, N. meningitidis, H. influenzae* type b (rare in immunized populations)	(Ceftriaxone or cefotaxime) + vancomycin (60 mg/kg/day) divided into 4 daily doses	For patient with severe penicillin allergy, consider chloramphenicol (instead of ceftriaxone or cefotaxime) + vancomycin	Benefit of dexamethasone with first dose (or 15-20 min prior) of antibiotics has been documented only for *H. influenzae* in children. Some experts also use for suspected pneumococcal infection. Prophylaxis of some close contacts is needed for *N. meningitidis* and *H. influenzae* meningitis. See Chapter 8.
	Immunocompromised patient	Consider *Listeria* and *Cryptococcus* in addition to pathogens for community-acquired meningitis.	(Ceftriaxone or Cefotaxime) plus ampicillin plus vancomycin	(Cefepime or meropenem) + TMP/SMX + vancomycin	Consider adding amphotericin B and flucytosine (5-FC) in AIDS patients to treat *Cryptococcus*.

Postsurgery (neurosurgery, head trauma, CSF shunt–associated infection, cochlear implants)	Consider *Pseudomonas* and staphylococci in addition to pathogens for community-acquired meningitis	(Ceftazidime *or* cefepime) + vancomycin	Meropenem + vancomycin
Eosinophilic disease	*Angiostrongylus cantonensis*, *Baylisascaris procyonis*, *Gnathostoma spinigerum*, *Taenia solium*, noninfectious disorders (foreign body)	Identification of causative organism should be made before beginning antimicrobial; corticosteroids are beneficial in some cases	Although justified, examination of stool for ova and parasites may not be useful for all human neurotropic parasites. Neuroimaging may be useful for diagnosis. *A. cantonensis* is most common cause worldwide but not found in mainland United States; *B. procyonis* is found in the United States and associated with exposure to raccoon feces; *G. spinigerum* is found in Southeast Asia in association with consumption of raw fish/poultry. Eosinophils also may be seen in CSF in meningitis due to *Toxoplasma*, *Cyrptococcus*, and coccidioides.
Neonatal	GBS, enteric Gram-negative organisms (especially *E. coli*), *Listeria*	Ampicillin + cefotaxime (+ gentamicin if Gram-negative organisms on Gram-stained smear)	In patients with diagnosis after prolonged hospitalization, consider *S. aureus*, enterococci, resistant enteric Gram-negative organisms, and *Candida*.

ANTIMICROBIAL THERAPY FOR SELECTED CLINICAL SYNDROMES

2

GASTROINTESTINAL INFECTIONS

Syndrome	Host Category	Common Treatable Pathogens	Preferred Treatment	Alternative Treatment	Comments
Intra-abdominal abscess	Community-acquired infection	Enteric Gram-negative organisms, anaerobes, enterococci	Ampicillin + gentamicin + metronidazole	Tic/clav or Pip/tazo or Imipenem or Meropenem For penicillin **allergy,** consider aztreonam + clindamycin	Multiple organisms are usually involved. Surgical drainage may be required.
	Nosocomial infection	Above, + *Pseudomonas*	(Ceftazidime or cefepime) + metronidazole	Pip/tazo or Meropenem For penicillin **allergy,** consider aztreonam + clindamycin.	Surgical drainage may be required.
	Perirectal infection	*S. aureus, S. pyogenes,* enteric Gram-negative organisms and anaerobes	Clindamycin + gentamicin	BL/BLI ± (Clindamycin or vancomyin)	Surgical drainage important.

Hepatic and/or splenic infection	S. aureus, Brucella sp, Bartonella henselae, Gram-negative enterics, anaerobes	Clindamycin + (cefotaxime or ceftriaxone or cefepime or ceftazidime) + metronidazole	Pip/tazo or Imipenem or Meropenem	Entamoeba histolytica can cause liver abscess if intestinal organism migrates through bowel wall to portal circulation. If history and clinical findings suggest cat-scratch disease, azithromycin may shorten the course of illness. Consider CGD.
Retroperitoneal infection	S. aureus, Gram-negative enterics	Clindamycin + (cefotaxime or ceftriaxone or cefepime or ceftazidime)	Vancomycin instead of clindamycin	
Cholecystitis/ cholangitis	Enteric Gram-negative organisms, anaerobes, enterococci	Ampicillin + gentamicin + metronidazole	Tic/clav or Pip/tazo or Imipenem or Meropenem For penicillin **allergy,** consider aztreonam + clindamycin	Drainage of obstructed biliary tract is an important component of therapy for severely ill patients.

2

ANTIMICROBIAL THERAPY FOR SELECTED CLINICAL SYNDROMES

Syndrome	Host Category	Common Treatable Pathogens	Preferred Treatment	Alternative Treatment	Comments
Diarrhea	Antibiotic-associated infection	Perturbation of bowel flora, Clostridium difficile	Stop implicated antibiotic C. difficile-associated: oral metronidazole (use IV drug only if oral drug cannot be administered)	Vancomycin PO or Nitazoxanide	Supportive care to maintain hydration status is important. Antimotility agents should be avoided. Some studies suggest that probiotics such as Lactobacillus are helpful in reducing antibiotic-associated diarrhea.
	Food- or water-borne disease	Bacterial (inflammatory): E. coli, Salmonella, Shigella, Yersinia, Campylobacter; parasitic: Cryptosporidium, Giardia	Antimicrobials are generally not recommended except for certain bacteria (Shigella, Campylobacter) and parasites (Giardia) Presumptive antimicrobial therapy for acute dysentery syndrome (blood and mucus in stool): Cefixime or Azithromycin	Ciprofloxacin or TMP/SMX or Ceftriaxone	Rehydration is the most important component of therapy. Some studies suggest that antimicrobial therapy increases the likelihood of hemolytic uremic syndrome in patients infected with enterohemorrhagic E. coli. Most common causes are not treatable: Toxin-mediated (immediate onset) S. aureus, Bacillus cereus, C. perfringens; viral: norovirus, rotavirus, astrovirus, enteric adenovirus; noninfectious causes (heavy metals, shellfish poisoning).

Immunocompromised patient	In addition to above pathogens, *Listeria*, *Mycobacterium avium-intracellulare*, CMV, *Isospora*, *Cyclospora*, *Microsporidium*	Improve immune status; therapy should be guided by etiologic organism; no clear indication for empiric therapy; see specific organism	Specific laboratory testing and collection containers may be needed. Discuss with laboratory to ensure proper recovery.
Nosocomial infection	*C. difficile*	Stop implicated antibiotic, oral metronidazole (use IV drug only if oral drug cannot be administered).	Vancomycin PO *or* Nitizoxanide	Most common causes are nontreatable: rotavirus, other viruses
Travel-associated infection	Traveler's diarrhea: Enterotoxigenic *E. coli* (ETEC), *Campylobacter*, *Salmonella*, *Shigella*; consider *Vibrio cholerae*, *E. histolytica* depending on epidemiology	Usually self-limited; may consider azithromycin or ciprofloxacin for traveler's diarrhea; see specific organism otherwise		Norovirus has been implicated in outbreaks on cruise ships.
Esophagitis	*C. albicans*, HSV, CMV	Fluconazole	Amphotericin B *or* Caspofungin	Infectious causes should prompt investigation for an immunologic disorder if seen in apparently immunocompetent host. Endoscopy, biopsy, and culture should be undertaken to determine specific pathogen and evaluate for noninfectious causes.
	Almost all cases occur in immunocompromised hosts			

2

ANTIMICROBIAL THERAPY FOR SELECTED CLINICAL SYNDROMES

Syndrome	Host Category	Common Treatable Pathogens	Preferred Treatment	Alternative Treatment	Comments
Necrotizing enterocolitis	Beyond neonatal period Immunocompromised patient: neutropenic host (typhilitis), AIDS, high-dose steroids, severe protein energy malnutrition	Enteric Gram-negative organisms, anaerobes, enterococci; consider *Pseudomonas* in addition in hospitalized patients	(Ceftazidime or cefepime) + metronidazole ± ampicillin	Pip/tazo or Meropenem For penicillin allergy, consider aztreonam + clindamycin	Supportive management. Treat underlying disorder if possible; stop enteral feedings; surgical intervention may be required.
	Neonatal infection	Enteric Gram-negative streptococci, staphylococci, *Candida*	Ampicillin + gentamicin + metronidazole	Ampicillin + cefotaxime + metronidazole	Role of anaerobes is controversial. Adjust antibiotics if pathogen is recovered. Supportive management. Treat underlying disorder if possible; stop enteral feedings; surgical intervention may be required.
Peritonitis	Peritoneal dialysis–associated infection	Coagulase-negative staphylococci, *S. aureus*, Gram-negative organisms, including *Pseudomonas, Candida*	(Ceftriaxone or cefotaxime) + vancomycin		Therapy should be guided by appropriate cultures obtained prior to starting antimicrobials. Catheter removal may be necessary. Intraperitoneal therapy is an alternative to intravenous therapy if the causative agent is known and use of the catheter is to be continued. Vancomycin, cephalosporins, and AGs can be administered by this route.**

Primary infection (spontaneous bacterial peritonitis)	S. pneumoniae, other streptococci, S. aureus, enteric Gram-negative organisms	Ceftriaxone or Cefotaxime	Consider adding vancomycin for resistant S. aureus and S. pneumoniae. Tuberculosis should also be considered in the setting of appropriate epidemiology.
Secondary infection (e.g., bowel perforation)	Enteric Gram-negative organisms, anaerobes, Enterococcus; consider Pseudomonas in addition in hospitalized patients	[(Ampicillin + gentamicin) + (Metronidazole or clindamycin)] or [(Ceftazidime or cefepime) + (Metronidazole or clindamycin)]	Pip/tazo or Meropenem For penicillin allergy, consider aztreonam + clindamycin Surgical management is essential.

Syndrome	Host Category	Common Treatable Pathogens	Preferred Treatment	Alternative Treatment	Comments
ODONTOGENIC INFECTIONS					
Gingivitis	Immunocompetent or neutropenic patient	HSV	Acyclovir for HSV in immunocompromised host		Acyclovir may shorten the duration of symptoms but does not abort them. May be indicated in some healthy hosts with profound disease, hospitalized for, or at risk for, dehydration. Neutropenia and neutrophil defects may be associated with gingivitis. Only normal oral flora are isolated.
Ludwig's angina		Oral microflora (polymicrobial)	Amp/sulb	For penicillin allergy, clindamycin	Surgical drainage essential.
Periodontitis	Immunocompetent or neutropenic patient	Oral microflora (polymicrobial)	A/C or Clindamycin		Neutropenia and neutrophil defects may be associated with gingivitis. Only normal oral flora are isolated.
Stomatitis		HSV, aphthous stomatitis	Acyclovir	Famciclovir or Valacyclovir for adolescents	Acyclovir may be indicated in some healthy hosts with profound disease, hospitalized for, or at risk for, dehydration. Antimicrobials do not shorten the course of aphthous stomatitis.

Thrush	C. albicans	Nystatin topically	Fluconazole or Gentian violet or Clotrimazole	Mucosal candidiasis in >6 months age and in the absence of immunosuppressive or antimicrobial therapy should prompt investigation for immunologic disorder.

UPPER RESPIRATORY TRACT INFECTIONS

Otitis externa

Malignant otitis externa	Generally immunosuppressed patient (AIDS, neutropenia, malignant tumor, or diabetes)	Pseudomonas, Aspergillus	(Ceftazidime or cefepime); consider amphotericin B if spread to soft tissues of face and scalp	Antimicrobials are adjunctive therapy; meticulous debridement and irrigation are essential. Aspergillus infection is associated with high mortality rate.
Swimmer's ear		Pseudomonas, Gram-negative organisms, fungi (Aspergillus niger, Candida)	Local instillation of 2% vinegar or topical otic antibiotic drops (ciprofloxacin or polymyxin-neosporin or TMP-SMX)	Use analgesics for pain. For moderate to severe illness, use wick after removal of excessive debris from ear canal.

ANTIMICROBIAL THERAPY FOR SELECTED CLINICAL SYNDROMES

2

Syndrome	Host Category	Common Treatable Pathogens	Preferred Treatment	Alternative Treatment	Comments
Otitis media					
Acute otitis media (AOM)		S. pneumoniae, M. catarrhalis, H. influenzae non-type b	**Not severe** <2 yr: amoxicillin (high dose); observe if >6 months and diagnosis not certain >2 yr: observe	For penicillin allergy, cefdinir or cefuroxime For severe penicillin allergy, azithromycin If cannot take oral medications, ceftriaxone	Use analgesics when pain present. "Observe" means deferring antimicrobials and then reevaluating at 48–72 hr. Failure to respond in 48–72 hr: if no therapy used initially, start antimicrobial therapy; if amoxicillin used as initial therapy, switch to A/C. Treat for 10 days. Shorter course of 5–7 days okay for healthy children ≥6 yr old.
			Severe (moderate to severe otalgia or fever ≥39°C) A/C (high dose)	Cefuroxime or Cefdinir	Failure to respond in 48–72 hr: ceftriaxone or Consider tympanocentesis and culture.
Chronic suppurative otitis media: See chronic mastoiditis on p. 149.					
Otitis media with effusion		Viruses, prelude/sequela of acute otitis media	Symptomatic treatment		

Parotitis

Acute infection	*S. aureus*, Gram-negative organisms (neonate)	Nafcillin/oxacillin Clindamycin Neonates: vancomycin + (AG or PCS3)	Common causes include viruses: mumps, HIV, EBV, enteroviruses, etc. Surgical drainage and rehydration alone may be curative. Recurrent acute sialadenitis can occur once every few months to years; its pathogenesis is unknown; it usually resolves at adolescence.
Subacute/chronic infection		There is no indication for presumptive therapy without a clear diagnosis	Possible etiologies include mycobacteria, HIV, sarcoidosis, Sjögren's syndrome, tumors.

Infections of Pharynx, Larynx, and Trachea

Epiglottitis	*S. aureus*, *S. pyogenes*, *S. pneumoniae*, *H. influenzae* type b (rare in vaccinated populations)	(Cefotaxime *or* ceftriaxone) + (Clindamycin *or* vancomycin)	Artificial airway should be placed promptly in the operating room under controlled conditions. Frequent suctioning of airway is critical. Effective presumptive antistaphylococcal therapy should be determined based on local susceptibility patterns.
Laryngitis		Symptomatic	Caused by a variety of respiratory viruses.

Syndrome	Host Category	Common Treatable Pathogens	Preferred Treatment	Alternative Treatment	Comments
Lemierre syndrome (jugular vein septic phlebitis)		*Fusobacterium*, oral microflora	Penicillin G	Clindamycin	May require surgical drainage. Some experts also recommend anticoagulation.
Parapharyngeal/ retropharyngeal/ peritonsillar abscess		S. *pyogenes*, other streptococci, S. *aureus*, oral microflora/anaerobes	Amp/sulb *or* [(Ceftriaxone *or* cefotaxime) + clindamycin]		Surgical drainage required. Close observation of the airway as artificial airway may be required.
Pharyngitis, euxudative infection		S. *pyogenes* (GAS), group C and G streptococci, *Arcanobacterium haemolyticum*, *Mycoplasma*	For documented group A streptococcal infection, oral penicillin V. (Amoxicillin is an acceptable alternative.)	For penicillin allergy, Clindamycin *or* Macrolides *or* Cephalosporins	Other potential pathogens include *N. gonorrhoeae*, diphtheria, viruses, including EBV, influenza. For nonstreptococcal pharyngitis, therapy should be determined based on proven or suspected etiology.
		Untreatable: Coxsackievirus, other enteroviruses, HSV			
Vesicular infection			HSV infection: consider acyclovir in immunocompromised host		Acyclovir may be indicated in some healthy hosts with profound disease, hospitalized for, or at risk for, dehydration.

Tracheitis	Normal host; community-acquired infection	Bacterial infection (S. aureus, group A Streptococcus) may complicate viral infection (influenza virus, parainfluenza virus)	Bacterial: Clindamycin, or nafcillin, or oxacillin Viral: Oseltamivir or zanamivir	Vancomycin	Choice of antibacterial should be guided by local MRSA susceptibility patterns. Intubation and suctioning critical for bacterial tracheitis.
	Associated with tracheostomy or intubated trachea/nosocomial	Pseudomonas, other Gram-negative organisms, S. aureus	Cefepime	Pip/tazo or Meropenem For penicillin allergy, consider aztreonam plus clindamycin	Guide therapy based on culture data. Antimicrobials will only treat the acute episode but will not eradicate the organism if device present. Short course of antibiotics (5–7 days) is usually sufficient.
Sinusitis Acute infection	Community-acquired infection	S. pneumoniae, M. catarrhalis, H. influenzae non-type B	**Mild to moderate** Amoxicillin (high dose) **Severe or risk factors for resistance** (day care attendance, recent antimicrobial treatment) A/C (high dose)	For penicillin allergy, cefpodoxime or cefuroxime or cefdinir or azithromycin or RFQ	Failure to respond in 48–72 hours: high-dose A/C. Failure to respond in 48–72 hr: imaging and/or sinus drainage. Alternatively, a trial with IV cefotaxime or ceftriaxone may be used. Treat sinusitis for at least 10–14 days.

ANTIMICROBIAL THERAPY FOR SELECTED CLINICAL SYNDROMES 2

Syndrome	Host Category	Common Treatable Pathogens	Preferred Treatment	Alternative Treatment	Comments
	Immunocompromised patient (neutropenia, diabetes, desferoxamine therapy)	S. aureus, Pseudomonas, Gram-negative organisms, anaerobes, Rhizopus, Mucor, Aspergillus	Cefepime or Pip/tazo + amphotericin B	High-dose liposomal amphotericin B may be more efficacious	Surgical intervention required. Rhizopus, Mucor should be considered in patients on long courses of voriconazole.
	Nosocomial (especially with nasal tubes)	Pseudomonas, Gram-negative organisms, S. aureus, polymicrobial	Cefepime	Pip/tazo or Meropenem For penicillin allergy, consider aztreonam + clindamycin	Remove nasal tube. Guide therapy based on culture data.
Chronic infection		S. pneumoniae, M. catarrhalis, H. influenzae non-type B, S. aureus, anaerobes	A/C (high dose) or Cefuroxime or Cefpodoxime or Cefdinir	[Ceftriaxone or cefotaxime] ± [Clindamycin or vancomycin] or FQ	Consider culture to guide therapy. Continue antibiotic therapy for 14–21 days. Underlying disorders (anatomic defects, allergic rhinitis, cystic fibrosis, immunodeficiency, ciliary dyskinesia) should be ruled out.

Mastoiditis	Acute infection	*S. pneumoniae, S. pyogenes, S. aureus*	Amp/sulb or Clindamycin	For penicillin allergy, cefuroxime	Surgical management required. Definitive therapy should be guided by culture obtained at surgery.
	Chronic (chronic suppurative otitis media)	*Pseudomonas*, Gram-negative organisms, *S. aureus*	Ceftazidime or Cefepime	Ofloxacin otic drops	Daily suctioning of the external canal is an important part of therapy.
Cervical lymphadenitis	Acute infection	*S. aureus, S. pyogenes*; consider GBS in neonates	A/C or Cephalexin or Dicloxacillin or Clindamycin (if MRSA prevalent)	For penicillin allergy, cefdinir or cefuroxime For severe penicillin allergy, vancomycin	Bacteria usually cause unilateral or bilateral lymphadenitis while viruses (EBV, rubella virus, adenovirus) cause bilateral lymphadenitis (lymphadenopathy). Kawasaki disease presents with nonsuppurative, unilateral cervical lymphadenopathy. Surgical drainage may be required in some cases.

AC, amoxicillin/clavulanic acid; AG, aminoglycoside; Amp/sulb, ampicillin/sulbactam; AP pen, antipseudomonal penicillin; BAL, broncho-aveolar lavage; BL/BLI, β-lactam plus β-lactamase inhibitor; CGD, Chronic granulomatous disease; CMV, cytomegalovirus; CNS, central nervous system; CSF, cerebrospinal fluid; FQ, fluoroquinolone; GAS, group A streptococcus; GBS, group B streptococcus; GI, gastrointestinal; GU, genitourinary; HSV, herpes simplex virus; IVIg, intravenous immunoglobulin; MRSA, methicillin-resistant *Staphylococcus aureus*; MRSE, methicillin-resistant *Staphylococcus epidermidis*; MSSA, methicillin-susceptible *Staphylococcus aureus*; NSAIDs, nonsteroidal anti-inflammatory drugs; OM, otitis media; PCN, penicillin; PCR, polymerase chain reaction; PCS3, third-generation parenteral cephalosporin; Pip/tazo, piperacillin/tazobactam; RFQ, respiratory fluroquinolone (levofloxacin, moxifloxacin); STI, sexually trasmitted infection; TB, tuberculosis; Tic/clav, ticarcillin/clavulanic acid; TMP/SMX, trimethoprim/sulfamethoxazole; UTI, urinary tract infection.

*Spectinomycin is unavailable in the United States.

**Perit Dial Int 2005; 25(Suppl 3):S117.

***Pharmacokinetics of synercid and daptomycin have not been studied, and use in children has been limited.

ANTIMICROBIAL THERAPY FOR SELECTED CLINICAL SYNDROMES

2

Drug Dosing in Special Circumstances

Jeffrey L. Wagner, PharmD, and Carlton K.K. Lee, PharmD, MPH

I. GENERAL PEDIATRIC DRUG DOSING

A. BODY MASS CALCULATION

The most common method of individualized pediatric drug dosing is body mass dosing (mg/kg). Conversion from pounds (lb) to metric kilograms (kg):

$$Wt(kg) = \frac{Wt(lb)}{2.2}$$

B. BODY SURFACE AREA CALCULATION

Certain antimicrobial agents (e.g., acyclovir and co-trimoxazole) require body surface area dosing. It has been suggested that drugs that are distributed into extracellular water (ECW) should be dosed by surface area because ECW and total body water are better paralleled by surface area than body weight. The following nomogram or Mosteller formula can be used in children.

1. Nomogram

Surface area is determined by drawing a straight line that connects the patient's height and weight. The intersection of the straight line on the surface area (SA) column reflects the value. If the patient is roughly of average size, SA can be determined by weight alone as indicated in the second column (Fig. 3-1).

2. Alternative Mosteller Formula*

$$BSA(m^2) = \sqrt{\frac{Ht(cm) \times Wt(kg)}{3600}}$$

*Equation from Mosteller RD: Simplified calculation of body surface area. N Engl J Med 1987;317(17):1098.

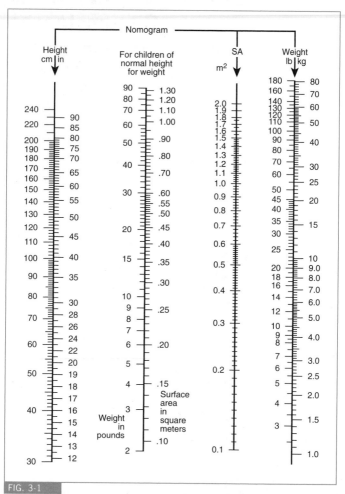

FIG. 3-1

Surface area estimation: pocket calculator versus nomogram. *(Data from Briars Gl, Bailey BJ: Surface area estimation: pocket calculator v nomogram. Arch Dis Child 1994;70:246-247.)*

II. DEVELOPMENTAL DOSING CONSIDERATIONS (DEVELOPMENTAL PHARMACOLOGY)

TABLE 3-1

AGE-DEPENDENT PHYSIOLOGIC VARIABLES INFLUENCING DRUG DISPOSITION IN CHILDREN

Disposition Parameter	Physiologic Variable vs Adult	Age When Adult Level Achieved	Pharmacokinetic Result	Example Drug
ABSORPTION				
Peroral pH	↑ gastric pH (lower acid output)	3 mo	↑ bioavailability of basic drugs ↓ bioavailability of acidic drugs	Penicillin
GI motility	↓ gastric and intestinal motility (gastric emptying time is 6-8 hr at birth)	6-8 mo	Unpredictable bioavailability and prolonged time to peak concentration	
GI contents	↓ bile acids and pancreatic enzymes	~1 yr	↓ bioavailability of fat-soluble drugs	
Intramuscular	↓ vascular perfusion	?		
Percutaneous	↑ absorption	Mo	↑ absorption	Lindane (Kwell) seizures, contraindicated
DISTRIBUTION				
% body water	↑ total body water, ↑ extracellular body water, rapid changes in first year	~12 yr	↑ volume of distribution of water-soluble drugs	Aminoglycosides
% fat	Full-term birth at 12%-16%, ↑ at 5-10 yr of age followed by a ↓	~17 yr		

DRUG DOSING IN SPECIAL CIRCUMSTANCES

TABLE 3-1

AGE-DEPENDENT PHYSIOLOGIC VARIABLES INFLUENCING DRUG DISPOSITION IN CHILDREN—cont'd

Disposition Parameter	Physiologic Variable vs Adult	Age When Adult Level Achieved	Pharmacokinetic Result	Example Drug
Plasma proteins	↓ total protein, albumin, and α-1 acid glycoprotein	Gradual changes over the first year	↑ volume of distribution and free drug concentration of protein-bound drugs	Nafcillin, ampicillin
	↑ unconjugated bilirubin and free fatty acids	Gradual changes over the first year	Potential displacement of bilirubin with highly protein-bound drugs	Sulfamethoxazole, ceftriaxone
Blood-brain barrier	Immature barrier caused by incomplete myelination	?	↑ CNS penetration	Aminoglycosides
METABOLISM				
CYP-450 enzyme				
1A2 isoform	Lower at birth	4 mo; may exceed adult levels before decreasing to adult levels at puberty	Altered drug clearance; maturation dependent	
2C9 isoform*	Lower at birth	6 mo; exceeds adult levels at 3-10 yr before decreasing to adult levels after puberty	Altered drug clearance; maturation dependent	
2C19 isoform*	Lower at birth	~2 yr	Altered drug clearance; maturation dependent	Voriconazole

2D6 isoform*	Lower at birth; 20% of adult at <1 mo	3-5 yr	Altered drug clearance; maturation dependent	
2E1 isoform	Lower at birth	?	Altered drug clearance; maturation dependent	Isoniazid
3A4 isoform*†	Lower at birth; 30%-40% of adult at 1 mo	6 mo; may exceed adult levels at 1-4 mo before decreasing to adult levels after puberty	Altered drug clearance; maturation dependent	Erythromycin, protease inhibitors
Glucuronidation*	Lower at birth	6-24 mo; isoform specific	↓ glucuronide metabolite	Chloramphenicol, zidovudine
Sulphation*	At adult level			
N-acetyltransferase*	Lower	4 yr	Altered drug clearance; maturation and genetic dependence	Sulfamethoxazole, isoniazid
ELIMINATION				
Glomerular filtration	↓ glomerular function	~6 mo	↑ elimination $T_{1/2}$	Aminoglycosides
Tubular secretion	↓ tubular function	~6 mo	↑ elimination $T_{1/2}$	Penicillins, sulfonamides

↑, increased; ↓, decreased; ?, unknown; mo, months; yr, years.

*Pharmacogenomic polymorphisms should be taken under consideration for potential altered net effect.

†Works cooperatively with transporters (e.g., MDR-1 or P-glycoprotein).

Modified from Misap RL, Hill MR, Szefler SL: Special pharmacokinetic considerations in children. In Evans WE (ed): Applied Pharmacokinetics, 3rd ed. Spokane, WA: Applied Therapeutics, 1992; and Blake MJ, Castro L, Leeder SJ, et al.: Ontogeny on drug metabolizing enzymes in the neonate. Seminars in Fetal and Neonatal Medicine 2005;10:123-138.

DRUG DOSING IN SPECIAL CIRCUMSTANCES

3

TABLE 3-2		
NORMAL VALUES OF GLOMERULAR FILTRATION RATE		
Age	GFR (mean) (mL/min/1.73 m²)	Range (mL/min/1.73 m²)
Neonates <34 wk gestational age		
2-8 days	11	11-15
4-28 days	20	15-28
30-90 days	50	40-65
Neonates >34 wk gestational age		
2-8 days	39	17-60
4-28 days	47	26-68
30-90 days	58	30-86
1-6 mo	77	39-114
6-12 mo	103	49-157
12-19 mo	127	62-191
2 yr to adult	127	89-165

From Holliday MA, Barratt TM, Avner ED (eds): Pediatric Nephrology, 3rd ed. Baltimore: Williams & Wilkins, 1994.

III. DRUG DOSING IN RENAL INSUFFICIENCY

Many drugs are excreted by the kidneys and may require dosage adjustments with renal insufficiency. Age-specific normal values of glomerular filtration rates are listed in Table 3-2. See section III.B.3 and Table 3-3 for information on antimicrobials requiring dosage adjustment in renal insufficiency.

A. GLOMERULAR FILTRATION RATE ESTIMATION METHODS

Calculations using either the Cockroft and Gault method or the Jelliffe method are designed for adults and should not be used in pediatrics. The creatinine clearance rate (CrCl) is used clinically as a substitute for actual measuring of the glomerular filtration rate (GFR).

1. URINARY CREATININE METHOD

The urinary creatinine method estimates the GFR.

The CrCl actually measures the theoretical volume of plasma cleared of creatinine in a finite period of time (mL/min). Although creatinine clearance is used to estimate GFR, it usually overestimates GFR (especially when GFR is low) because some creatinine is secreted by the renal tubules. The CrCl is usually inaccurate in children with obstructive uropathy or problems with bladder emptying.

$$\text{Formula* : CrCl} = \frac{Cr_u \times V}{Cr_p} \times \frac{1.73}{BSA}$$

*Equation from Cohen ML, Rifkind D: The Pediatric Abacus: Review of Clinical Formulas and How to Use Them, 1st ed. London: Informa Healthcare; 2002.

where
   CrCl = creatinine clearance (mL/min/1.73 m^2),
   Cr$_u$ = urine creatinine concentration (mg/dL),
   V = volume of urine collected divided by duration of collection
         (mL/min),
   Cr$_p$ = plasma creatinine (mg/dL), may use average of two levels,
   BSA = body surface area (m^2).

2. Schwartz Method
The Schwartz method is used to estimate creatinine clearance without the need for urine collection. Creatinine clearance is used clinically as a substitute for actual measuring of the GFR. Although this method is considered the most widely accepted method for children to date, the Schwartz method is known to overestimate GFR inversely proportional to the level of renal function and in pediatric bone marrow transplant patients.

$$\text{Formula}: \text{CrCl} = \frac{k \times L}{S_{Cr}}$$

where
   CrCl = creatinine clearance (mL/min/1.73 m^2),
   k = constant (see the following list),
   L = body length (cm),
   S$_{cr}$ = serum creatinine concentration (mg/dL).
   Note that k values vary with body size and sex[1-3]:

Age	k value
Preterm infants up to 1 yr	0.33
Full-term infants up to 1 yr	0.45
Children (2-12 yr) and adolescent females (13-21 yr)	0.55
Adolescent males (13-21 yr)	0.70

3. Glomerular Function Determined by Nuclear Medicine Scans
Renal clearance of exogenous radioactive chemicals such as ^{125}I-Iothalamate and ^{54}Cr-EDTA has been used to determine glomerular function.

B. DOSE ADJUSTMENT METHODS FOR ANTIMICROBIAL AGENTS
1. Maintenance Dose
In patients with renal insufficiency, the dose may be adjusted using the following methods:
a. Interval extension (I):
Lengthen the intervals between individual doses, keeping the dose size normal. For this method, the suggested interval is shown in Table 3-3.
b. Dose reduction (D):
Reduce the amount of the individual doses, keeping the interval between the doses normal. This method is particularly recommended for drugs with

which a relatively constant blood level is desired. For this method, the percentage of the usual dose is shown in Table 3-3.

c. Interval extension and dose reduction (DI):
Lengthen the interval and reduce the dose.

d. Interval extension or dose reduction (D, I):
In some instances, either the dose or the interval can be changed.

Note: *These dose adjustments are for infants beyond the neonatal period. These dose modifications are only approximations. Each patient must be monitored closely for signs of drug toxicity, and serum levels must be measured when available. Drug dose and interval should be monitored accordingly.*

2. DIALYSIS

The quantitative effects of hemodialysis (He) and peritoneal dialysis (P) on drug removal are shown. "Y" indicates the need for a supplemental dose with dialysis. "N" indicates no need for adjustment. The designation "No" does not preclude the use of dialysis or hemoperfusion for drug overdose (see Table 3-3).

C. DOSING IN CONTINUOUS RENAL REPLACEMENT THERAPY

The clearance/elimination of certain medications may be affected by continuous renal replacement therapies (CRRT) such as continuous venovenous hemofiltration (CVVH), continuous arteriovenous hemofiltration (CAVH), continuous arteriovenous hemodialysis (CAVHD), continuous venovenous hemodialysis (CVVHD), and continuous venovenous hemodialfiltration (CVVHDF).

1. Factors Influencing Drug Removal with CRRT

a. Drug's physiochemical characteristics favoring removal by convection or diffusion
  i. Low molecular weight
  ii. Low protein binding
  iii. Negative charge (anionic)
  iv. Small volume of distribution
  v. High water solubility/low lipid solubility

b. Technical features of dialysis circuit components and procedure favoring drug removal
  i. Filter properties: Larger membrane pore size
  ii. Increasing blood/dialysate flow rates
  iii. Increasing ultrafiltration rates

2. Optimal Approach to Administering Drugs to Pediatric Patients Receiving CRRT

The optimal approach to administering drugs to pediatric patients receiving CRRT is based on the properties of the drug, specific characteristics of the dialysis system, interactions between the drug and CRRT system that yield the sieving coefficient, and the drug clearance by the CRRT modality chosen.

Text continued on p. 170.

TABLE 3-3

ANTIMICROBIALS REQUIRING ADJUSTMENTS IN RENAL FAILURE[4-6]

Drug	Pharmacokinetics			Adjustments in Renal Failure					Supplemental Dose for Dialysis
	Route of Excretion[a]	Normal $T_{1/2}$ (hr)	Normal Dose Interval	Method		Creatinine Clearance (mL/min)			
					Mild (>50)	Moderate (10-50)	Severe (<10)		
Acyclovir (IV)	Renal	2-4	q8 hr	DI	q8 hr	q12 hr (CrCl 25-50) q24 hr (CrCl 10-25)	50% and q24 hr		Y (He) N (P)
Amantidine	Renal	10-28	q12-24 hr	I	q12-24 hr	q24 hr (CrCl 30-50) q48 hr (CrCl 15-29)	q7 day (CrCl <15)		N (He, P)
Amikacin[b]	Renal	1.5-3	q8-12 hr	I	q8-12 hr	q12-18 hr	q24-48 hr		Y (He, P)
Amoxicillin	Renal	1-3.7	q8-12 hr	I	q8-12 hr	q12 hr (CrCl 10-30)	q24 hr		Y (He, P)
Amoxicillin-clavulanate	Renal	1	q8-12 hr	I	q8-12 hr	q12 hr (CrCl 10-30)	q24 hr		Y (He)
Amphotericin B	Renal 40% up to 7 days	Up to 15 days	qd	D, I	Dosage adjustments are unnecessary with preexisting renal impairment; if decreased renal function is due to amphotericin B, the daily dose can be decreased by 50% or the dose given qod				N (He, P)
Amphotericin B, cholesteryl sulfate		28-29	qd		No guidelines established				N (He)
Amphotericin B, lipid complex	Renal 1%	170	qd		No guidelines established				N (He, P)
Amphotericin B, liposomal	Renal ≤10%	7-153	qd		No guidelines established				
Ampicillin	Renal	1-4	q6 hr	I	q6 hr	q6-12 hr (CrCl 10-30)	q12 hr		Y (He, P)

DRUG DOSING IN SPECIAL CIRCUMSTANCES   3

TABLE 3-3

ANTIMICROBIALS REQUIRING ADJUSTMENTS IN RENAL FAILURE[4-6]—cont'd

	Pharmacokinetics			Adjustments in Renal Failure				
						Creatinine Clearance (mL/min)		
Drug	Route of Excretion[a]	Normal T$_{1/2}$ (hr)	Normal Dose Interval	Method	Mild (>50)	Moderate (10-50)	Severe (<10)	Supplemental Dose for Dialysis
Ampicillin/sulbactam	Renal	1-1.8	q4-6 hr	I	q4-6 hr	q12 hr (CrCl 15-29)	q24 hr (CrCl 5-14)	Y (He, P)
Aztreonam	Renal (hepatic)	1.3-2.2	q6-12 hr	D	100%	50% (CrCl 10-30)	25%	Y (He)
Cefaclor	Renal	0.5-1	q8-12 hr	D	100%	100%	50%	Y (He, P)
Cefadroxil	Renal	1-2	q12 hr	I	q12 hr	q24 hr (CrCl 10-25)	q36 hr	Y (He, P)
Cefazolin	Renal	1.5-2.5	q8 hr	I	q8 hr	q12 hr	q24 hr	Y (He, P)
Cefdinir	Renal	1.1-2.3	q12-24 hr	I	q12-24 hr	7 mg/kg/dose q24 hr or 300 mg q24 hr (CrCl <30)	q24 hr	Y (He)
Cefditoren pivoxil	Renal	1.3-2	q12 hr	DI	100%	200 mg q12 hr (maximum) (CrCl 30-49) 200 mg q24 hr (maximum) (CrCl <30)		?
Cefepime	Renal	1.8-2	q8-12 hr	DI	q12 hr regimens: 100% and q24 hr (CrCl 30-60) q8 hr regimens: 100% and q12 hr (CrCl 30-50)	50% and q24 hr (CrCl 11-29)	25% and q24 hr	Y (He, P)
						100% and q24 hr (CrCl 12-30)	100% and q24-48 hr	

Drug	Route	Half-life (hr)	Dose interval	Method	>50	10–50	<10	Dialysis
Cefixime	Renal (hepatic)	3–4	q12-24 hr	D	100%	75% (CrCl 21-50)	50% (CrCl <20)	N (He, P)
Cefotaxime	Renal	1–3.5	q6-12 hr	D	100%		50% (CrCl <20)	Y (He, P)
Cefotetan	Renal (hepatic)	3.5	q12 hr	I	q12 hr	q24 hr (CrCl 10-30)	q48 hr	Y (He, P)
Cefoxitin	Renal	0.75–1.5	q4-8 hr	I	Normal interval	q8-12 hr (CrCl 30-50) q12-24 hr (CrCl 10-30)	q24-48 hr	Y (He) N (P)
Cefpodoxime proxetil	Renal	2.2	q12 hr	I	q12 hr	q24 hr (CrCl <30)		Y (He) N (P)
Cefprozil	Renal	1.3	q12 hr	D	100%	50% (CrCl <30)		Y (He)
Ceftazidime	Renal	1–2	q8-12 hr	I	q8-12 hr	q12 hr (CrCl 30-50) q24 hr (CrCl 10-30)	q24-48 hr	Y (He, P)
Ceftibuten	Renal	1.5–2.5	q24 hr	D	100%	50% (CrCl 30-49)	25% (CrCl 5-29)	Y (He) N (P)
Ceftizoxime	Renal	1.6	q6-12 hr	I	q8-12 hr	q36-48 hr	q48-72 hr	Y (He, P)
Cefuroxime (IV)	Renal	1.6–2.2	q8-12 hr	I	q8-12 hr	q12 hr (CrCl 10-20)	q24 hr	Y (He) N (P)
Cephalexin	Renal	0.5–1.2	q6 hr	I	q6 hr	q8-12 hr	q12-24 hr	Y (He) N (P)
Cephapirin	Renal	0.6–0.8	q4-6 hr	I	q6 hr	q6-8 hr	q12 hr	Y (He)
Cephradine	Renal	0.7–2	q6-12 hr	D, I	100%	50% or q12-24 hr	25% or q36 hr	Y (He)
Chloroquine hydrochloride/ phosphate	Renal	6–60 days	q24 hr	D	100%	100%	50%	?
Ciprofloxacin (hepatic)	Renal	1.2–5	q8-12 hr	D, I	100%	50%-75% or q18-24 hr (CrCl <30)		Y (He, P)

3

DRUG DOSING IN SPECIAL CIRCUMSTANCES

TABLE 3-3

ANTIMICROBIALS REQUIRING ADJUSTMENTS IN RENAL FAILURE[4-6]—cont'd

Drug	Pharmacokinetics			Adjustments in Renal Failure				
	Route of Excretion[a]	Normal $T_{1/2}$ (hr)	Normal Dose Interval	Method	Creatinine Clearance (mL/min)			Supplemental Dose for Dialysis
					Mild (>50)	Moderate (10-50)	Severe (<10)	
Clarithromycin	Renal/hepatic	3-7	q12 hr	DI	No change	50% and q12-24 hr (CrCl <30)		Y (He) N (P)
Colistimethate sodium	Renal	1.6-4	q6-12 hr	DI	No change	75%-100% and q12 hr (CrCl >20) 50% and q12 hr (CrCl 5-20)	30% and q12-18 hr (CrCl <5)	Y (He)
Co-trimoxazole (sulfamethoxazole/ trimethoprim)	Sulfameth-oxazole: hepatic (renal) Trimethoprim: renal (hepatic)	Sulfamethox-azole: 9-11 Trimethoprim: 8-15	q12 hr	D	No change	50% (CrCl 15-30)	Not recommended (CrCl <15)	
Cycloserine	Renal	10-25	q12 hr	I	100%	q24 hr	q36-48 hr	Y (He)
Daptomycin	Renal	7-11	q24 hr	I	100%	q48 hr (CrCl <30)		Y (He, P)

Drug	Route	$t_{1/2}$	Normal	Method	Adjustment	Dialysis
Didanosine	Renal	1.3-1.5	q12 hr	DI	Patients <60 kg: CrCl 30-59 = 75 mg q12 hr or 150 mg q24 hr (oral solution) or 125 mg once daily (delayed-release capsule) CrCl 10-29 = 100 mg q24 hr or 125 mg once daily (delayed-release capsule) CrCl <10 = 75 mg q24 hr (oral solution) or use alternative formulation (delayed-release capsule) Patients ≥60 kg: CrCl 30-59 = 100 mg q12 hr or 200 mg q24 hr (oral solution) or 200 mg once daily (delayed-release capsule) CrCl 10-29 = 150 mg q24 hr (oral solution) or 125 mg once daily (delayed-release capsule) CrCl <10 = 100 mg q24 hr (oral solution) or 25 mg once daily (delayed-release capsule)	N (He, P)
Doripenem	Renal	1	q8 hr	DI	100% 50% (CrCl 30-50) 50% and q12 hr (CrCl 10-30) No recommendation available	Y (He)
Emtricitabine	Renal	10	q24 hr	D, I	CrCl 30-49 = q48 hr (capsule) or 50% (solution) CrCl 15-29 = q72 hr (capsule) or 33.3% (solution) CrCl <15 = q96 hr (capsule) or 25% (solution)	Y (He)
Ertapenem	Renal (hepatic)	4	q12-24 hr	D	50% (CrCl <30)	Y (He)
Erythromycin	Hepatic (renal)	1.5-2	q6-8 hr	D	100%	50%-75%	N (He, P)
Ethambutol	Renal (hepatic)	2.5-3.6	q24 hr	I	q24-36 hr q48 hr	Y (He) N (P)
Ethionamide	Renal	1.85-3	q8-12 hr	D	50% (CrCl <30)	N (He, P)
Famciclovir	Renal (hepatic)	2-3	500 mg q8 hr	DI	500 mg q12 hr (CrCl 40-59) 500 mg q24 hr (CrCl 20-39) 250 mg q48 hr (CrCl <20)	Y (He)
Fluconazole[c]	Renal	19-25	q24 hr	D	100% 50% (CrCl <50)	Y (He) N (P)

TABLE 3-3

ANTIMICROBIALS REQUIRING ADJUSTMENTS IN RENAL FAILURE[4-6]—cont'd

| | Pharmacokinetics | | | Adjustments in Renal Failure | | | | |
| | | | | | Creatinine Clearance (mL/min) | | | |
Drug	Route of Excretion[a]	Normal $T_{1/2}$ (hr)	Normal Dose Interval	Method	Mild (>50)	Moderate (10-50)	Severe (<10)	Supplemental Dose for Dialysis
Flucytosine[b]	Renal	3-8	q6 hr	I	q6 hr	q12 hr (CrCl 20-40) q24 hr (CrCl 10-20)	q24-48 hr	Y (He, P)
Foscarnet	Renal	3-4.5	q8-12 hr	D		See package insert		Y (He)
Ganciclovir	Renal	2.5-3.6	IV: q12 hr	DI	Induction (IV): 50% and q12 hr (CrCl 50-69)	50% and q24 hr (CrCl 25-49) 25% and q24 hr (CrCl 10-24)	25% post-HD	Y (He) N (P)
					Maintenance (IV): 50% and q24 hr (CrCl 50-69)	25% and CrCl and q24 hr (CrCl 25-49) 12.5% and q24 hr (CrCl 10-24)	12.5% post-HD	
			PO: tid	DI	50%-100% and tid	50% and bid (CrCl 25-49) 50% and qd (CrCl 10-24)	50% post-HD	
Gentamicin[b,c]	Renal	1.5-3	q8-12 hr	I	q12 hr (CrCl 40-60)	q24 hr (CrCl 20-40)	Monitor levels	Y (He, P)
Imipenem/cilastatin	Renal	1-1.4	q6-8 hr	DI	50% and q6 hr (CrCl 41-70)	37% and q8 hr (CrCl 21-40) 25% and q12 hr (CrCl 6-20)	Avoid unless HD (CrCl <5)	Y (He) N (P)

Drug	Route of Elimination	Half-Life (hr)	Interval	Method	GFR >50	GFR 10-50	GFR <10	Dialysis
Isoniazid	Hepatic (renal)	2-4 (slow)[d]; 0.5-1.5 (fast)	q24 hr	D	100%	100%	50%	Y (He); N (P)
Kanamycin	Renal	2-3	q8 hr	DI	60%-90% and q8-12 hr (CrCl 50-80)	30%-70% and q12 hr	20%-30% and q24-48 hr	Y (He, P)
Lamivudine[e]	Renal	1.7-2.5	q12 hr	DI	100%	100% and q24 hr (CrCl 30-49); 66% and q24 hr (CrCl 15-29)	33% and q24 hr (CrCl 5-14); 17% and q24 hr (CrCl < 5)	Y (He)
Levofloxacin	Renal (hepatic)	6-8	q24 hr	DI	500 mg q24 hr regimen: 100%; 750 mg q24 hr regimen: 100%; 250 mg q24 hr regimen:	50% (CrCl 20-49); 100% and q48 hr (CrCl 20-49); 100% (CrCl ≥20)	50% and q48 hr (CrCl ≤19); 66% q48 hr (CrCl ≤19); 100% q48 hr (CrCl ≤19)	N (He, P)
Loracarbef	Renal	0.78-1	q12 hr	D, I	q12 hr	q24 hr or 50%	q72-120 hr	Y (He)
Meropenem	Renal	1-1.4	q8 hr	DI	100% and q8 hr	100% and q12 hr (CrCl 26-50); 50% and q12 hr (CrCl 10-25)	50% and q24 hr	Y (He); N (P)
Methenamine	Renal	4.3	q6-12 hr	D	100%	Avoid use (CrCl <50)		N (He, P)
Metronidazole	Hepatic (renal)	6-12	q6-12 hr	D	100%	100%	50% or q12 hr	Y (He); N (P)

3

DRUG DOSING IN SPECIAL CIRCUMSTANCES

TABLE 3-3

ANTIMICROBIALS REQUIRING ADJUSTMENTS IN RENAL FAILURE[4-6]—cont'd

| | Pharmacokinetics | | | Adjustments in Renal Failure | | | | |
| | | | | | Creatinine Clearance (mL/min) | | | |
Drug	Route of Excretion[a]	Normal $T_{1/2}$ (hr)	Normal Dose Interval	Method	Mild (>50)	Moderate (10-50)	Severe (<10)	Supplemental Dose for Dialysis
Nafcillin	Renal (hepatic)	0.5-1	q4-12 hr	D	100%	100%	Lower range of usual dose or 33%-50% (in patients with both severe renal and hepatic impairment)	N (He, P)
Neomycin	Renal	3	q4-8 hr	I	q6 hr	q12-18 hr	q18-24 hr	Y (He)
Norfloxacin	Hepatic (renal)	3-4	q12 hr	I	q12 hr	q24 hr (CrCl <30)		?
Ofloxacin	Renal	5-7.5	q12 hr	DI	q12 hr	q24 hr (CrCl 20-50)	50% and q24 hr (CrCl <20)	Y (He) N (P)
Oseltamivir	Renal	1-10	q12-24 hr	I	Normal	Treatment: q24 hr (CrCl 10-30) Prophylaxis: q48 hr (CrCl 10-30)	No data No data	?
Oxacillin	Renal (hepatic)	23-45 min	q4-12 hr	D	100%	100%	Use lower range of normal dose	N (He, P)
Penicillin G	Renal (hepatic)	20-50 min	q4-6 hr	I	q4-6 hr	q8-12 hr (CrCl 10-30)	q12-18 hr	Y (He, P)
Penicillin VK (PO)	Renal (hepatic)	30-40 min	q6-8 hr	I	q6 hr	q6 hr	q8 hr	?
Pentamidine	Renal	6.4-9	q24 hr	I	q24 hr	q36 hr (CrCl 10-30)	q48 hr	N (He, P)

Phenazopyridine	Renal (hepatic)	?	tid × 2 days	I		Avoid	Avoid	N/A
Piperacillin	Renal (hepatic)	0.5-1.5	q4-6 hr	I	q4-6 hr	q8 hr (CrCl 20-40)	q12 hr (CrCl <20)	Y (He) N (P)
Piperacillin/ tazobactam	Renal (hepatic)	Piperacillin: 0.5-1.5 Tazobactam: 0.7-1.6	q6-8 hr	DI	100% and q6-8 hr	70% and q6 hr (CrCl 20-40)	70% and q8 hr (CrCl <20)	Y (He) N (P)
Pyrazinamide	Renal	9-23	q12-24 hr	D	100%	100%	50% and q24 hr	Y (He, P)
Rifabutin	Renal (hepatic)	36-45	q12-24 hr	D	100%	50% (CrCl <30)		?
Rifampin	Hepatic (renal)	1.5-5	q12-24 hr	D	100%	50%-100%	50%	N (He) Y (P)
Rimantadine	Renal	19.8-36.5	q12-24 hr	I	q12 hr	q12 hr	q24 hr	N (He)
Stavudine	Renal	0.9-1.6	q12 hr	DI	100% and q12 hr	50% and q12 hr (CrCl 26-50) 50% and q24 hr (CrCl 10-25)		Y (He)
Streptomycin	Renal	2.5	q24 hr	DI	50% and q24 hr (CrCl 50-80)	50% and q24-72 hr	50% and q72-96 hr	Y (He, P)
Sulfamethoxazole	Renal	7-12	q12 hr	D	100%	50% (CrCl 10-30)	25%	Avoid
Sulfisoxazole	Renal	4-8	q6-12 hr	I	q6 hr	q8-12 hr	q12-24 hr	Y (He, P)
Tenofovir	Renal	4-8	q24 hr	I	q24 hr	q48 hr (CrCl 30-49) 2×/wk (CrCl 10-29)	No data	Y (He)
Tetracycline	Renal (hepatic)	8-10	q6 hr	I	q8-12 hr (CrCl 50-80)	q12-24 hr	q24 hr	N (He, P)
Ticarcillin[f]	Renal	0.9-1.3	q4-6 hr	I	q4-6 hr	q8 hr (CrCl 10-30)	q12 hr	Y (He, P)

DRUG DOSING IN SPECIAL CIRCUMSTANCES

3

TABLE 3-3

ANTIMICROBIALS REQUIRING ADJUSTMENTS IN RENAL FAILURE[4-6]—cont'd

| | Pharmacokinetics | | | Adjustments in Renal Failure | | | | |
| | | | | | Creatinine Clearance (mL/min) | | | |
Drug	Route of Excretion[a]	Normal $T_{1/2}$ (hr)	Method	Mild (>50)	Moderate (10-50)	Severe (<10)	Supplemental Dose for Dialysis
Ticarcillin-clavulanate[f]	Renal	Ticarcillin: 0.9-1.3 Clavulanate: 1-1.5	I	q4-6 hr	q8 hr (CrCl 10-30)	q12 hr (q24 hr if comorbid hepatic impairment)	Y (He, P)
Trimethoprim	Renal	8-10	D	100%	50% (CrCl 15-30)	Avoid use (CrCl <15)	Y (He, P)
Tobramycin[b,c]	Renal	1.5-3	I	q8-12 hr	q12-18 hr	q24-48 hr	Y (He, P)
Valacyclovir	Hepatic	2.5-3.6	DI	Herpes zoster: 100% and q8 hr	100% and q12 hr (CrCl 30-49) 100% and q24 hr (CrCl 10-29)	50% and q24 hr	Y (He) N (P)
				Genital herpes (initial): 100% and q12 hr	100% and q24 hr (CrCl 10-29)	50% and q24 hr	
				Genital herpes (recurrent): 100% and q12 hr	100% and q24 hr (CrCl 10-29)	50% and q24 hr	

Drug	Route	Half-life	Method	Dose / Normal	Adjustment	Adjustment	Dialysis
Valganciclovir	Renal	0.4-0.6	DI	Genital herpes (suppressive): 100% and q24 hr	50% and q24 hr or 100% and q48 hr (CrCl 10-29)	Not recommended	
				Induction (IV): 50% and q12 hr (CrCl 40-59)	50% and q24 hr (CrCl 25-39) / 50% and q48 hr (CrCl 10-24)	Not recommended	
				Maintenance (IV): 50% and q24 hr (CrCl 40-59)	50% and q48 hr (CrCl 25-39) / 50% and 2×/wk (CrCl 10-24)	Not recommended	
Vancomycin[b]	Renal	2.2-8	I	q6-12 hr	q18-48 hr	q48-96 hr	Y/N (He)[g], N (P)
Zalcitabine	Renal	1-3	I	q8 hr	q12 hr (CrCl 10-40)	q24 hr	Y (He)

?, unknown; CrCl, creatinine clearance; D, dose reduction; DI, dose reduction and interval extension; D,I, dose reduction or interval extension; GFR, glomerular filtration rate; He, hemodialysis; I, interval extension; N, no; N/A, not applicable; P, peritoneal dialysis; Y, yes.

[a]Route in parentheses indicates secondary route of excretion.
[b]Subsequent doses are best determined by measurement of serum levels and assessment of renal insufficiency.
[c]May add to peritoneal dialysate to obtain adequate serum levels.
[d]Rate of acetylation of isoniazid.
[e]GFR ≥5 mL/min, give full dose as first dose; for GFR <5 mL/min, give 33% of full dose as first dose.
[f]May inactivate aminoglycosides in patients with renal impairment.
[g]If using high-flux hemodialysis (polysulfone polyamide and polyacrylonitrile), give supplemental dose after dialysis.

DRUG DOSING IN SPECIAL CIRCUMSTANCES   3

3. Data Regarding Drug Removal by CRRT Are Currently Limited in Both Children and Adults
4. Antimicrobials Requiring Adjustment with CRRT (Table 3-4)

IV. DRUG DOSING IN HEPATIC INSUFFICIENCY

A. CHILD-PUGH SCORE
The Child-Pugh score (also known as the Child-Turcotte-Pugh score) is used to assess the prognosis of chronic liver disease, mainly cirrhosis (Table 3-5).

B. DRUGS REQUIRING ATTENTION IN HEPATIC INSUFFICIENCY
Drugs that require attention in patients with hepatic insufficiency may need to be dose adjusted, discontinued, or used with caution (Table 3-6).

V. DRUG DOSING IN OBESITY

A. DETERMINING APPROPRIATE DOSAGE REGIMENS FOR ANTIMICROBIALS
The most appropriate dosage regimens for antimicrobials in obese individuals are often unknown. Body mass index (BMI) is the ratio of weight in kilograms to the square of height in meters. BMI is widely used to define overweight and obesity because it correlates well with more accurate measures of body adiposity and is derived from commonly available data—weight and height. BMI between the 85th and 95th percentile for age and sex is considered at risk of overweight, and BMI at or above the 95th percentile is considered overweight or obese. Figures 3.2 and 3.3 illustrate the BMI percentiles for children 2 to 20 years. For infants younger than 2 years old, weight-for-length percentile above the 95th percentile for age is considered at risk of overweight. Figures 3.4 and 3.5 illustrate the weight-for-length percentiles for children from birth to 36 months. Additional growth chart information is found on the Centers for Disease Control and Prevention (CDC) Web site at www.cdc.gov/growthcharts (Figs. 3-2, 3-3, 3-4, and 3-5).

B. IDEAL BODY WEIGHT CHARACTERIZATION IN CHILDREN
Adult methods to estimate ideal body weight are unsuitable for pediatric use. The linear equations given in Table 3-7 were derived from revised growth charts (November 2000) to estimate ideal body weight for age in infants and children. The calculated values of ideal weight generally approximate the 50th percentile, and in no instance fall above or below the 75th or 25th percentile, respectively.

C. ANTIMICROBIAL DOSING IN OBESITY
Table 3-8 summarizes known antimicrobial dosage modifications for obese patients. Required elements include the patient's actual or total body weight (TBW) and determination of his or her ideal body weight (IBW).

Text continued on p. 183.

TABLE 3.4

EMPIRIC DOSING RECOMMENDATIONS OF ANTIMICROBIALS KNOWN TO BE AFFECTED BY CRRT[7-10]

Drug	Usual Dosage	Dosages for CAVH/CVVH and CAVHD/CVVHD	
		<1500 mL/m²/hr	≥1500 mL/m²/hr
Acyclovir	5-10 mg/kg IV q8 hr or 250-500 mg/m² IV q8 hr	3.75-7.5 mg/kg IV q24 hr or 175-350 mg/m² IV q24 hr	5-10 mg/kg IV q24 hr or 250-500 mg/m² IV q24 hr
Amikacin	5-7.5 mg/kg IV q8 hr; monitor levels to optimize safety and efficacy	Required dosages are highly variable; 5-7.5 mg/kg IV once, then measure levels to identify appropriate regimen	Required dosages are highly variable; 5-7.5 mg/kg IV once, then measure levels to identify appropriate regimen
Ampicillin	25-50 mg/kg IV q6 hr CNS infections: 50-100 mg/kg IV q6 hr Maximum: 12 g/24 hr	25-50 mg/kg IV q8-12 hr CNS infections: 50-100 mg/kg IV q8-12 hr	25-50 mg/kg IV q6-8 hr CNS infections: 50-100 mg/kg IV q6-8 hr
Cefepime	50 mg/kg IV q8-12 hr Maximum: 6 g/24 hr	25-50 mg/kg IV q12-18 hr	25-50 mg/kg IV q12 hr
Cefotaxime	25-50 mg/kg IV q6-8 hr CNS infections: 75 mg/kg IV q6 hr Maximum: 12 g/24 hr	25-50 mg/kg IV q8-12 hr CNS infections: 75 mg/kg IV q8-12 hr	25-50 mg/kg IV q8 hr CNS infections: 75 mg/kg IV q8 hr
Cefotetan	20-40 mg/kg IV q12 hr Maximum: 6 g/24 hr	10-20 mg/kg IV q12-24 hr	10-25 mg/kg IV q12 hr
Cefoxitin	20-40 mg/kg IV q6 hr	20-40 mg/kg IV q18 hr	20-40 mg/kg IV q12 hr
Ceftazidime	30-50 mg/kg IV q8 hr	15-35 mg/kg IV q12 hr	15-50 mg/kg IV q12 hr
Ceftriaxone	25-50 mg/kg IV q12 hr Maximum: 4 g/24 hr	25-50 mg/kg IV q12-24 hr Maximum: 4 g/24 hr	25-50 mg/kg IV q12 hr Maximum: 4 g/24 hr
Cefuroxime sodium	25-50 mg/kg IV q8 hr Maximum: 6 g/24 hr	25-50 mg/kg IV q12-18 hr	25-50 mg/kg IV q12 hr

DRUG DOSING IN SPECIAL CIRCUMSTANCES   3

TABLE 3-4

EMPIRIC DOSING RECOMMENDATIONS OF ANTIMICROBIALS KNOWN TO BE AFFECTED BY CRRT[7-10]—cont'd

Drug	Usual Dosage	Dosages for CAVH/CVVH and CAVHD/CVVHD	
		<1500 mL/m²/hr	≥1500 mL/m²/hr
Ciprofloxacin	5-10 mg/kg IV q12 hr **Maximum:** 800 mg/24 hr CF: 10 mg/kg IV q8 hr **Maximum** (CF): 1.2 g/24 hr	2.5-5 mg/kg IV q12 hr **Maximum:** 400 mg/24 hr CF: 5 mg/kg IV q8 hr **Maximum** (CF): 600 mg/24 hr	3.75-7.5 mg/kg IV q12 hr **Maximum:** 600 mg/24 hr CF: 7.5 mg/kg IV q8 hr **Maximum** (CF): 900 mg/24 hr
Fluconazole	6-10 mg/kg IV/PO loading; 3-12 mg/kg IV/PO q24 hr	6-10 mg/kg IV/PO loading, then 3-12 mg/kg IV/PO q24 hr	6-10 mg/kg IV/PO loading, then 6-12 mg/kg IV/PO q24 hr
Flucytosine	25-37.5 mg/kg PO q6 hr	25-37.5 mg/kg PO q12-18 hr	25-37.5 mg/kg PO q8-12 hr
Ganciclovir	Induction: (CrCl >70) 5 mg/kg IV q12 hr, (CrCl 50-69) 2.5 mg/kg IV q12 hr Maintenance: (CrCl >70) 2.5 mg/kg IV q12 hr, (CrCl 50-69) 1.25 mg/kg IV q12 hr	Induction: 1.25-2.5 mg/kg IV q24 hr Maintenance: 0.625-1.25 mg/kg IV q24 hr	Induction: 2.5-3.75 mg/kg IV q24 hr Maintenance: 1.25-2.5 mg/kg IV q24 hr
Gentamicin	2-3 mg/kg IV q8 hr; monitor levels to optimize safety and efficacy	Required dosages are highly variable; 2-3 mg/kg IV once, then measure levels to identify appropriate regimen	Required dosages are highly variable; 2-3 mg/kg IV once, then measure levels to identify appropriate regimen
Imipenem-cilastatin	33 mg/kg IV q8 hr or 25 mg/kg IV q6 hr **Maximum:** 4 g/24 hr	15-20 mg/kg IV q12 hr	20-25 mg/kg IV q8-12 hr

Itraconazole	3-5 mg/kg IV/PO q12-24 hr	3-5 mg/kg IV/PO q12-24 hr; avoid IV in patients with CrCl <30	3-5 mg/kg IV/PO q12-24 hr; **avoid** IV in patients with CrCl <30
Linezolid	10 mg/kg IV/PO q8 hr (<3 mo of age) or q12 hr (≥3 mo of age) **Maximum:** 1200 mg/24 hr	10 mg/kg IV/PO q8 hr (<3 mo of age) or q12 hr (≥3 mo of age) **Maximum:** 1200 mg/24 hr	10 mg/kg IV/PO q8 hr (<3 mo of age) or q12 hr (≥3 mo of age) **Maximum:** 1200 mg/24 hr
Meropenem	20 mg/kg IV q18 hr CNS infection: 40 mg/kg IV q8 hr **Maximum:** 6 g/24 hr	10-20 mg/kg IV q12 hr	20-40 mg/kg IV q12 hr
Metronidazole	5-17 mg/kg IV/PO q8 hr **Maximum:** 4 g/24 hr	5-17 mg/kg IV/PO q8 hr **Maximum:** 4 g/24 hr	5-17 mg/kg IV/PO q8 hr **Maximum:** 4 g/24 hr
Oxacillin	25-33 mg/kg IV q4-6 hr **Maximum:** 12 g/24 hr	25-33 mg/kg IV q6 hr	25-33 mg/kg IV q6 hr
Piperacillin	50-75 mg/kg IV q6 hr CF: 85-150 mg/kg IV q6 hr **Maximum:** 24 g/24 hr	50-75 mg/kg IV q8-12 hr CF: 85-150 mg/kg IV q8-12 hr	50-75 mg/kg IV q6-8 hr CF: 85-150 mg/kg IV q6-8 hr
Piperacillin-tazobactam	100 mg/kg IV q6-8 hr **Maximum:** 18 g/24 hr	70 mg/kg IV q6-8 hr	70-100 mg/kg IV q6-8 hr
Ticarcillin	50-75 mg/kg IV q6 hr CF: 75-150 mg/kg IV q6 hr **Maximum:** 24 g/24 hr	50-75 mg/kg IV q8-12 hr CF: 75-150 mg/kg IV q8-12 hr	50-75 mg/kg IV q6-8 hr CF: 75-150 mg/kg IV q6-8 hr
Ticarcillin-clavulanate	50-75 mg/kg IV q6 hr CF: 75-150 mg/kg IV q6 hr **Maximum:** 24 g/24 hr	50-75 mg/kg IV q8-12 hr CF: 75-150 mg/kg IV q8-12 hr	50-75 mg/kg IV q6-8 hr CF: 75-150 mg/kg IV q6-8 hr

TABLE 3-4

EMPIRIC DOSING RECOMMENDATIONS OF ANTIMICROBIALS KNOWN TO BE AFFECTED BY CRRT[7-10]—cont'd

		Dosages for CAVH/CVVH and CAVHD/CVVHD	
Drug	Usual Dosage	<1500 mL/m²/hr	≥1500 mL/m²/hr
Tobramycin	2-3 mg/kg IV q8 hr; monitor levels to optimize safety and efficacy	Required dosages are highly variable; 2-3 mg/kg IV once, then measure levels to identify appropriate regimen	Required dosages are highly variable; 2-3 mg/kg IV once, then measure levels to identify appropriate regimen
Trimethoprim-sulfamethoxazole	3-5 mg/kg IV/PO q12 hr PCP: 5 mg/kg IV/PO q6 hr	3-5 mg/kg IV/PO q18 hr PCP: 5 mg/kg IV/PO q8 hr	4-5 mg/kg IV/PO q18 hr PCP: 5 mg/kg IV/PO q8 hr
Vancomycin	10-15 mg/kg IV q6-8 hr CNS: 15 mg/kg IV q6 hr Usual maximum: 1 g/dose	Required dosages are highly variable; 10-15 mg/kg IV once, then measure levels to identify appropriate regimen	Required dosages are highly variable; 10-15 mg/kg IV once, then measure levels to identify appropriate regimen

CAVH, continuous arteriovenous hemodyalisis; CAVHD, continuous arteriovenous hemodyalisis; CF, cystic fibrosis; CrCl, creatinine clearance rate; CNS, central nervous syndrome; CRRT, continuous renal replacement therapy; CVVH, continuous venovenous hemofiltration; CVVHD, continuous venovenous hemodyalisis; PCP, pneumocystis pneumonia.
Adapted from Veltri MA, Neu AM, Fivush BA, et al: Drug dosing during intermittent hemodialysis and continuous renal replacement therapy: Special considerations in pediatric patients. Pediatr Drugs 2004;6(1):45-65.

TABLE 3-5

CHILD-PUGH SCORE (ALSO KNOWN AS THE CHILD-TURCOTTE-PUGH SCORE)

Clinical and Biochemical Measurements	Points Scored for Increasing Abnormality		
	1	2	3
Hepatic encephalopathy (grade)	None	Grades I-II	Grades III-IV
Ascites	Absent	Mild (suppressed with medication)	Moderate (refractory)
Total bilirubin (mg/dL)	<2.0	2.0-3.0	>3.0
Serum albumin (g/dL)	>3.5	2.8-3.5	<2.8
INR or prothrombin time (seconds prolonged)	<1.70 or <4	1.71-2.20 or 4-6	>2.20 or >6

INTERPRETATION

Points	Child-Pugh Class	1-Year Survival	2-Year Survival
5-6	A	100%	85%
7-9	B	81%	57%
10-15	C	45%	35%

TABLE 3-6

HEPATIC DOSAGE ADJUSTMENT[6,11,12]

Drug	Use with Caution	Contraindicated	Hepatic Adjustment
Abacavir sulfate	+	Contraindicated in patients with moderate or severe hepatic impairment	Mild dysfunction (Child-Pugh score 5-6): 200 mg twice daily (oral solution is recommended) Moderate to severe dysfunction: use is **contraindicated** by the manufacturer
Albendazole	+		
Amantadine	+		

TABLE 3-6

HEPATIC DOSAGE ADJUSTMENT[6,11,12]—cont'd

Drug	Use with Caution	Contraindicated	Hepatic Adjustment
Amoxicillin with clavulanic acid		Contraindicated in patients with history of amoxicillin/clavulanic acid–associated cholestatic jaundice or hepatic impairment	
Amprenavir	+	Contraindicated in patients with hepatic failure	Adults: Capsules: Child-Pugh score 5-8: 450 mg twice daily. Child-Pugh score 9-12: 300 mg twice daily. Solution: Child-Pugh score 5-8: 513 mg (34 mL) twice daily. Child-Pugh score 9-12: 342 mg (23 mL) twice daily
Anidulafungin (Eraxis)	+		
Atazanavir	+		Adolescents ≥16 years and adults: moderate hepatic impairment (Child-Pugh class B): reduce dose to 300 mg once daily. Severe hepatic impairment (Child-Pugh class C): do not use
Azithromycin	+		

TABLE 3-6

HEPATIC DOSAGE ADJUSTMENT[6,11,12]—cont'd

Drug	Use with Caution	Contraindicated	Hepatic Adjustment
Caspofungin	+		Mild hepatic impairment (Child-Pugh score 5-6): no dosage adjustment necessary Moderate hepatic impairment (Child-Pugh score 7-9): decrease daily dose by 30%
Cefazolin	+		
Cefditoren	+		
Cefoperazone	+		Adults: **Maximum** dose with impaired hepatic function: 4 g/24 hr **Maximum** dose with combined hepatic and renal dysfunction: 1-2 g/24 hr
Cefoxitin	+ (increases alanine amino-transferase [ALT] with high doses)		
Cefuroxime (IV/IM)/ cefuroxime axetil	+ (hepatic impairment: at risk of developing fall in prothrombin activity)		
Chloramphenicol	+		Dose reduction should be based on serum chloramphenicol concentrations
Chloroquine hydrochloride/ phosphate	+		

TABLE 3-6

HEPATIC DOSAGE ADJUSTMENT[6,11,12]—cont'd

Drug	Use with Caution	Contraindicated	Hepatic Adjustment
Clarithromycin	+		
Clindamycin	+		Reduce dosage in patients with severe renal or hepatic impairment
Co-trimoxazole	+		
Darunavir	+		
Delavirdine	+		
Didanosine	+		
Doxycycline	+	Contraindicated in severe hepatic dysfunction	
Efavirenz	+		
Emtricitabine	+		
Erythromycin preparations	+	Contraindicated in patients with hepatic impairment	
Ethambutol hydrochloride	+		
Ethionamide (Trecator-SC)	+	Contraindicated in patients with severe hepatic impairment	
Famciclovir	+		
Fluconazole	+		
Fosamprenavir	+		Adults: Unboosted regimens: mild to moderate hepatic impairment (Child-Pugh score 5-8): reduce dosage to 700 mg twice daily (without concurrent ritonavir) Severe hepatic impairment (Child-Pugh score 9-12): use is not recommended

TABLE 3-6

HEPATIC DOSAGE ADJUSTMENT[6,11,12]—cont'd

Drug	Use with Caution	Contraindicated	Hepatic Adjustment
Gatifloxacin	+		
Griseofulvin	+	Contraindicated in patients with severe liver disease	
Hydroxychloroquine	+		
Indinavir	+		Mild to moderate hepatic impairment: adults: decrease dosage from 800 mg every 8 hr to 600 mg every 8 hr
Iodoquinol	+	Contraindicated in patients with hepatic damage	
Isoniazid	+	Contraindicated in patients with acute liver disease and/or previous history of hepatic damage during isoniazid therapy	
Itraconazole	+		
Ketoconazole	+		
Lamivudine	+		
Linezolid	+		
Lopinavir/ritonavir	+		Plasma levels are increased in patients with hepatic impairment; use with caution
Mefloquine hydrochloride	+		Half-life may be prolonged and plasma levels may be higher

TABLE 3-6

HEPATIC DOSAGE ADJUSTMENT[6,11,12]—cont'd

Drug	Use with Caution	Contraindicated	Hepatic Adjustment
Methenamine mandelate	+		Contraindicated in patients with hepatic insufficiency receiving hippurate salt
Metronidazole	+		50%-67% decrease in dosage
Micafungin	+		
Minocycline	+		
Moxifloxacin	+		Not recommended in patients with severe hepatic insufficiency
Nafcillin	+		Use lower range of usual dose or reduce dose 33%-50%
Nelfinavir	+		
Nevirapine	+		
Nitazoxanide	+		
Ofloxacin			Severe impairment: maximum dose: 400 mg/day
Para-aminosalicylic acid	+		
Paromomycin sulfate	+		
Pentamidine isethionate	+		
Phenazopyridine hydrochloride	+	Contraindicated in patients with liver disease	
Posaconazole	+		
Praziquantel	+		
Pyrantel pamoate	+		
Pyrazinamide	+	Contraindicated in patients with hepatic damage	

TABLE 3-6

HEPATIC DOSAGE ADJUSTMENT[6,11,12]—cont'd

Drug	Use with Caution	Contraindicated	Hepatic Adjustment
Pyrimethamine plus sulfadoxine	+		
Quinidine	+		
Quinine	+		
Quinupristin with dalfopristin	+		Dosage adjustment may be necessary
Ribavirin	+	Contraindicated in patients with autoimmune hepatitis	
Rifabutin	+		
Rifampin	+		
Rifapentine (Priftin)	+		
Rimantadine	+		Severe dysfunction: adults: 100 mg/24 hr
Ritonavir	+		Mild to moderate hepatic impairment: no adjustment recommended; lower ritonavir concentrations have been reported in patients with moderate hepatic impairment Severe hepatic impairment: use with caution
Saquinavir	+	Contraindicated in patients with severe hepatic impairment	
Stavudine	+		
Sulfadiazine	+		
Sulfisoxazole	+		

TABLE 3-6

HEPATIC DOSAGE ADJUSTMENT[6,11,12]—cont'd

Drug	Use with Caution	Contraindicated	Hepatic Adjustment
Suramin	+		Dosage reductions of 50%-75% have been suggested for "severe" hepatic dysfunction; however, specific guidelines have not been published
Tenofovir disoproxil fumarate	+		
Terbinafine	+		Clearance is decreased by ~50% with hepatic cirrhosis; use is not recommended
Tetracycline hydrochloride	+	Contraindicated in patients with liver disease	
Thalidomide	+		
Thiabendazole	+		
Tigecycline	+		Mild-to-moderate hepatic disease: no dosage adjustment required Severe hepatic impairment (Child-Pugh class C): initial dose of 100 mg should be followed with 25 mg every 12 hr
Tinidazole	+		
Tipranavir	+	Contraindicated in moderate and severe hepatic impairment (Child-Pugh classes B and C)	

TABLE 3-6
HEPATIC DOSAGE ADJUSTMENT[6,11,12]—cont'd

Drug	Use with Caution	Contraindicated	Hepatic Adjustment
Trimethoprim	+		
Trimetrexate	+		Although it may be necessary to reduce the dose in patients with liver dysfunction, no specific dosage recommendations exist for treatment initiation with hepatic impairment
Voriconazole	+		Child-Pugh class A or B: use standard loading dose; decrease maintenance dose by 50% Child-Pugh class C: not recommended unless benefit outweighs risk
Zalcitabine	+		
Zidovudine	+		

+, use with caution in the presence of hepatic impairment.

Drug-specific defined adjusted body weight (ABW) is then calculated for determining the obese patient's individualized dosage.

For example, to calculate the gentamicin dosage (2.5 mg/kg/dose IV q8 hr) for an obese 8 year old with a TBW of 40 kg and IBW of 25 kg, the following is recommended:

1. Determine the Adjusted Body Weight (ABW)

$$ABW = 25 \text{ kg} + 0.4 \ (40 \text{ kg} - 25 \text{ kg}) = 31 \text{ kg}$$

2. Calculate Dosage with ABW

Gentamicin: [2.5 mg/kg/dose × 31 kg] IV q8 hr or 77.5 mg IV q8 hr

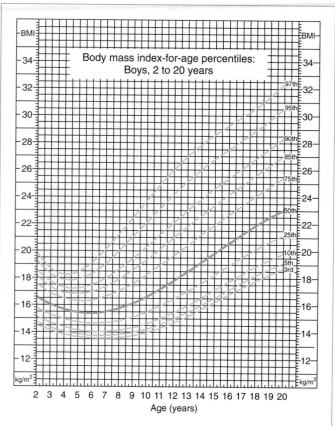

FIG. 3-2

Body mass index for boys 2 to 20 years. *(Developed by the National Center for Health Statistics in collaboration with the National Center for Chronic Disease Prevention and Health Promotion, 2000.)*

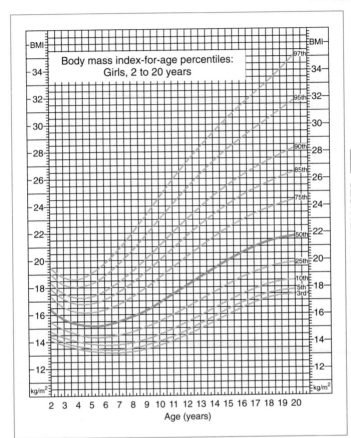

FIG. 3-3

Body mass index for girls 2 to 20 years. *(Developed by the National Center for Health Statistics in collaboration with the National Center for Chronic Disease Prevention and Health Promotion, 2000.)*

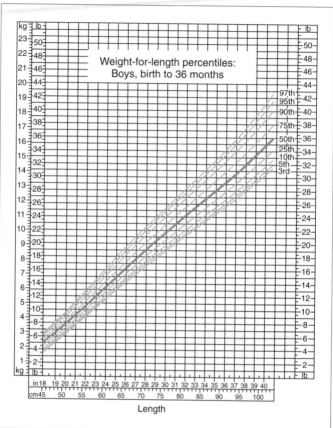

FIG. 3-4

Weight-for-length percentiles for boys, from birth to 36 months. *(Developed by the National Center for Health Statistics in collaboration with the National Center for Chronic Disease Prevention and Health Promotion, 2000.)*

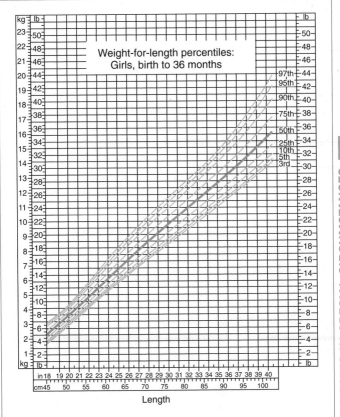

FIG. 3-5

Weight-for-length percentiles for girls, from birth to 36 months. *(Developed by the National Center for Health Statistics in collaboration with the National Center for Chronic Disease Prevention and Health Promotion, 2000.)*

TABLE 3-7

IDEAL WEIGHT

INFANTS AGED 0-24 MO

	0-6 mo	6-12 mo	12-24 mo
Infant boys	$Wt_i = 0.733\ A_{mo} + 3.6$	$Wt_i = 0.433\ A_{mo} + 5.4$	$Wt_i = 0.183\ A_{mo} + 8.4$
Infant girls	$Wt_i = 0.667\ A_{mo} + 3.4$	$Wt_i = 0.400\ A_{mo} + 5.0$	$Wt_i = 0.183\ A_{mo} + 7.6$

CHILDREN AND YOUNG ADULTS AGED 2-20 YEARS

	2-10 yr	10-16 yr	16-20 yr
Boys	$Wt_i = 2.25\ A_{yr} + 8.50$	$Wt_i = 5.00\ A_{yr} + 19.0$	$Wt_i = 2.25\ A_{yr} + 25$
Girls	$Wt_i = 2.38\ A_{yr} + 7.25$	$Wt_i = 3.17\ A_{yr} + 3.33$	$Wt_i = A_{yr} + 38$

A_{mo}, age in months; A_{yr}, age in years; Wt_i, ideal body weight (kg).
From National Center for Health Statistics in collaboration with the National Center for Chronic Disease Prevention and Health Promotion, revised and corrected November 21, 2000.

TABLE 3-8

ANTIMICROBIAL DOSING IN OBESITY[13–15]

Antimicrobial Agent	Recommendations for Weight to Use for Dose Calculation
AMINOGLYCOSIDES	
Amikacin	Initial doses should be based on Vd using ABW with correction factor of 0.4
Gentamicin	(ABW = IBW + 0.4 [TBW − IBW]).
Tobramycin	Final dosage adjustments should be based on serum concentrations.
β-LACTAMS/PENICILLINS	
Ampicillin	No dose adjustment recommended.
Ampicillin-sulbactam	No information on obesity dosing available. Base dose on Vd using ABW with correction factor for H_2O composition of adipose tissue (ABW = IBW + 0.3 [TBW − IBW]).
Nafcillin	Base dose on Vd using ABW with correction factor for H_2O composition of adipose tissue (ABW = IBW + 0.3 [TBW − IBW]).
Penicillin G	No dose adjustment recommended.
Pipercillin-tazobactam	Base dose on diagnosis and CrCl.
Ticarcillin-clavulanate	Base dose on CrCl.

TABLE 3-8

ANTIMICROBIAL DOSING IN OBESITY[13–15]—cont'd

Antimicrobial Agent	Recommendations for Weight to Use for Dose Calculation
β-LACTAMS/CEPHALOSPORINS	
Cefazolin	Use higher end of dosing recommendations.
Cefepime	No information on obesity dosing available. Base dose on Vd using ABW with correction factor for H_2O composition of adipose tissue (ABW = IBW + 0.3 [TBW − IBW]).
Cefotaxime	Base dose on Vd using ABW with correction factor for H_2O composition of adipose tissue (ABW = IBW + 0.3 [TBW − IBW]).
Cefotetan	No dose adjustment recommended.
Ceftazidime	Base dose on CrCl.
Ceftriaxone	No information on obesity dosing available. Base dose on Vd using ABW with correction factor for H_2O composition of adipose tissue (ABW = IBW + 0.3 [TBW − IBW]).
Cefuroxime	Base dose on CrCl.
β-LACTAMS/CARBAPENEMS	
Ertapenem	No dose adjustment recommended.
Meropenem	No dose adjustment recommended.
Imipenem-cilastatin	Base dose on CrCl.
FLUOROQUINOLONES	
Ciprofloxacin	Dose should be based on Vd using ABW with correction factor of 0.45 (ABW = IBW + 0.45 [TBW − IBW])
Levofloxacin	No information on obesity dosing available. Base dose on CrCl.
Moxifloxacin	No dose adjustment recommended.
MACROLIDES	
Azithromycin	No information on obesity dosing available.
Erythromycin	Base dose on IBW.
MISCELLANEOUS	
Acyclovir	Base dose on IBW.
Amphotericin B	Base dose on TBW.
Aztreonam	Use dose at upper end of dosage range for treating serious infections.
Clindamycin	No information on obesity dosing available.
Dalfopristin-quinupristin	Base dose on TBW.
Daptomycin	Base dose on TBW.
Doxycycline	No information on obesity dosing available.

TABLE 3-8

ANTIMICROBIAL DOSING IN OBESITY[13–15]—cont'd

Antimicrobial Agent	Recommendations for Weight to Use for Dose Calculation
Fluconazole	Higher dose is recommended.
Linezolid	No dose adjustment recommended.
Metronidazole	No information on obesity dosing available.
Sulfamethoxazole-trimethoprim	No information on obesity dosing available.
Tigecycline	Traditional dose.
Vancomycin	Base dose on TBW.

ABW, adjusted body weight (kg); CrCl, creatinine clearance (mL/min/1.73 m^2); IBW, ideal body weight (kg); TBW, total or actual body weight (kg); Vd, volume of distribution (L/kg).

VI. ANTIMICROBIAL TISSUE DISTRIBUTION BY KEY ORGAN SYSTEMS

TABLE 3-9

ANTIMICROBIAL TISSUE DISTRIBUTION BY KEY ORGAN SYSTEMS[16,17,18]

Drug	Peak Serum Level (mcg/mL)	CNS	CSF Level Potentially Therapeutic	Bone	Ocular	Bile	Pulmonary	Other
Abacavir sulfate	3	CSF, 18%-33%	No data					
Acyclovir	1.21	CSF, good, 13%-52%	Yes		Aqueous humor, extensive, 37.3%	Liver, good	Lung, significant	Tissues, good (kidney, muscle, spleen, vaginal mucosa, heart tissue)
Albendazole	0.5-1.6	CSF, 43%						Cyst fluid, good, 13%-22%
Amantadine		CSF, 75%						
Amikacin		CSF, 10%-20%; up to 50% with inflamed meninges	No; may consider intrathecal dose of 5-10 mg for potentially therapeutic level		Aqueous humor, poor	Biliary excretion, 10%-60%	Bronchial secretions, 20% Sputum, 24.5%-43%	Body fluids, excellent Blister fluid, 48% Fat and muscle, poor Kidney, excellent Peritoneal fluid, 39% Synovial fluid, excellent Tears, poor

DRUG DOSING IN SPECIAL CIRCUMSTANCES

3

TABLE 3-9

ANTIMICROBIAL TISSUE DISTRIBUTION BY KEY ORGAN SYSTEMS[16,17,18]—cont'd

Drug	Peak Serum Level (mcg/mL)	CNS	CSF Level Potentially Therapeutic	Bone	Ocular	Bile	Pulmonary	Other
Amoxicillin	4-5	CSF, 13%-14%	Yes			Biliary excretion, 100%-3000% Gallbladder and liver, concentrations exceed MIC for most bacteria	Bronchial fluid, 3.8%-7.2% Sputum, 3.8%-7.2% Lung and pleural fluid, concentrations exceed MIC for most bacteria	Middle ear fluid, >2 mcg/mL
Amoxicillin with clavulanic acid	11.6-17/2.1-2.2	CSF, amoxicillin, 5%; clavulanic acid, 0%-8.4%		Bone, adequate		Biliary excretion, 100%-3000%	Mucosa, 200% amoxicillin, 118% clavulanic acid	Peritoneal fluid, 66% clavulanic acid Pus, 27% amoxicillin, 20% clavulanic acid Tonsilar tissue, 23% amoxicillin, 8% clavulanic acid Middle ear effusions, excellent

Drug		CSF		Bone	Aqueous humor	Liver / Biliary	Pleural fluid / Bronchial secretions	Peritoneal fluid / other
Amphotericin B	0.5-3.5	CSF, <2.5%			Aqueous humor, ~67%		Pleural fluid, ~67%	Peritoneal fluid, ~67% Synovial fluid, ~67%
Amphotericin B, cholesteryl sulfate	2.9							
Amphotericin B, lipid complex	1-2.5							
Amphotericin B, liposomal						Liver, 14%-22%	Lung, <1%	Spleen, <6% Heart and kidney, <1%
Ampicillin	47	CSF, 13%-14% with inflamed meninges	Yes	Bone, 4.5%-15.4%	Aqueous humor, adequate	Biliary excretion, 100%-3000% Therapeutic concentrations not obtained with obstructive biliary tract disease	Bronchial secretions, 3.2%-5.2%	Kidney, 50%-80%
Ampicillin with sulbactam	109-150	CSF, 30%		Bone, ampicillin 8%-25%, sulbactam 18%-42%			Bronchial secretions, ampicillin 6%, sulbactam 8%	Peritoneal fluid, ampicillin 92%, sulbactam 96%
Amprenavir	6-9							

DRUG DOSING IN SPECIAL CIRCUMSTANCES

3

TABLE 3-9

ANTIMICROBIAL TISSUE DISTRIBUTION BY KEY ORGAN SYSTEMS[16,17,18]—cont'd

Drug	Peak Serum Level (mcg/mL)	CNS	CSF Level Potentially Therapeutic	Bone	Ocular	Bile	Pulmonary	Other
Anidulafungin	7.2		No					Animal studies with anidulafungin (and other echinocandins) indicate extensive tissue distribution, including brain tissue
Atazanavir	2.3	CSF, low						
Atovaquone plus proguanil (Malarone)	15	CSF, <1%	No					
Azithromycin	0.4-3.6					Biliary excretion, high		Blister fluid, 74% Bronchial secretions, high and persistent Ear, excellent Tissues, excellent

Aztreonam	125	CSF, 3%-52%	+/-	Bone, 20%	Aqueous humor, therapeutic	Biliary excretion, 3%-52% Liver, 50.5%	Bronchial secretions, 10.3%-28.5% Lung, 36.1%-46.3% Pleural fluid, 79.7%	Blister fluid, therapeutic Fat, therapeutic Gallbladder, 26.4% Kidney, 64.4% Small and large intestine, 10.8%-16.9% Pericardial fluid, 34.1%-65.9% Peritoneal fluid, 23.6%-63.5% Muscle, 13.9%-16.4% Skin, 34.3%
Caspofungin	9.9	CSF, 6%	No			Liver, 1600%	Lung, ~100%	Tissues, 90% Kidneys, 300% Heart, 30% Small and large intestine, 100%-200% Spleen, ~100%
Cefaclor	8.4-9.3					Biliary excretion, >60%		
Cefadroxil	16					Biliary excretion, 22%	Pleural fluid and lung, ~50%	Saliva, 9.3%-15.6%
Cefazolin	188	CSF, 1%-4%, minimal	No	Bone, well, especially with inflamed bone		Biliary excretion, 29%-300%	Bronchial secretions, 32%	

3

DRUG DOSING IN SPECIAL CIRCUMSTANCES

TABLE 3-9

ANTIMICROBIAL TISSUE DISTRIBUTION BY KEY ORGAN SYSTEMS[16,17,18]—cont'd

Drug	Peak Serum Level (mcg/mL)	CNS	CSF Level Potentially Therapeutic	Ocular	Bone	Bile	Pulmonary	Other
Cefdinir	1.6						Bronchial mucosa, 27.1%-39%	Maxillary sinus, 65% Skin, 33% Sputum, 1.6%-1.9%
Cefditoren	4					Gallbladder, bile, and liver, high		
Cefepime	193	CSF, 10%	Yes	Aqueous humor, temporarily therapeutic		Bile, therapeutic Gallbladder, therapeutic	Bronchial mucosa, therapeutic	Appendix tissue, therapeutic Blister fluid, therapeutic Peritoneal fluid, therapeutic Sputum, therapeutic Urine, therapeutic
Cefixime	3-5					Biliary excretion, 800%		
Cefoperazone		CSF, 2.3%-4.2%, penetrates inflamed and noninflamed meninges				Bile, ~1000%-2000%		Muscle, 17.1%

Drug			CSF	Aqueous humor	Biliary excretion	Bronchial / Pulmonary	Tissues / Other
Cefotaxime	100	Yes	CSF, 10%	Aqueous humor, 0.16-2.3 mcg/mL	Biliary excretion, 15%-75%	Bronchial mucosa, therapeutic	Tissues, good
Cefotetan	124		CSF, 80%-360%		Biliary excretion, 2%-21%	Bronchial mucosa, therapeutic	
Cefoxitin	110	+/-	CSF, 3%, minimal penetration	Aqueous humor, fair penetration	Biliary excretion, 280%		Peritoneal fluid, 86%
Cefpodoxime proxetil	2.9				Biliary excretion, 115%	Pleural fluid, fluid-to-plasma ratios were 0.24-1.07 Pulmonary tissue, rapid and extensive penetration, 0.53-0.78	Blister fluid, 70% Prostatic fluid, media plasma to prostatic fluid ratio was 0.1
Cefprozil	10.5						Blister fluid, 50%
Ceftazidime	60	Yes	CSF, 20%-40% Intracranial abscess, therapeutic		Biliary excretion, 13%-54%		Peritoneal fluid, 61.6%-75% Tissue fluids, ~50%
Ceftibuten	15					Bronchial secretions, 30% Bronchoalveolar lavage fluid, 81% Lung tissue, 39%	Blister fluid, 85%-132% Nasal secretions, 47% Tracheal secretions, 50%

DRUG DOSING IN SPECIAL CIRCUMSTANCES

3

TABLE 3-9

ANTIMICROBIAL TISSUE DISTRIBUTION BY KEY ORGAN SYSTEMS[16,17,18]—cont'd

Drug	Peak Serum Level (mcg/mL)	CNS	CSF Level Potentially Therapeutic	Bone	Ocular	Bile	Pulmonary	Other
Ceftizoxime	132	CSF, limited, 22.6%		Bone, good		Biliary excretion, 34%-82%	Lung, good	Tissues, good
Ceftriaxone	150	CSF, 8%-16% (bacterial meningitis)	Yes		Aqueous humor, 1.25%	Biliary excretion, 200%-500% Liver, low (increase dose or decrease interval)	Bronchial tissue, good	Blister fluid, excellent Mucus, 25.5%
Cefuroxime (IV/IM)/ cefuroxime axetil	100/4.1	CSF, 17%-88%	Yes	Bone, therapeutic		Biliary excretion, 35%-80%	Bronchial secretions, therapeutic Lung, 33.7%-34.6%	
Cephalexin	18-38			Joints, therapeutic		Biliary excretion, 216%		Sputum, 4%-6%
Cephapirin				Bone, therapeutic				
Cephradine		CSF, does not significantly cross BBB		Bone, penetrates			Bronchial secretions, 16.6%	
Chloramphenicol	11-18	CSF, 45%-89%	Yes			Liver, excellent		

Drug							
Chloroquine hydrochloride/phosphate							Saliva, 53%
Ciprofloxacin	1.6-4.6	CSF, 26%	Inadequate for *Streptococcus* spp	Aqueous humor, fair (23%)	Biliary excretion, 2800%-4500%; Liver, good	Lung, excellent (70%-170%)	Blister fluid, good; Gallbladder, good; Peritoneal, good (95%); Synovial fluid, 93%-647%; Sputum, 22.7%-46.9%
Clarithromycin	2-4	CSF, minimal			Biliary excretion, 7000%	Lung, excellent	Gastric tissue, excellent; Middle ear effusion, good
Clindamycin	2.5-10	CSF, poor even with inflamed meninges	No	Bone, therapeutic	Biliary excretion, 250%-300%	Bronchial secretions, 35%-117%	
Clofazimine					Bile, liver, and gallbladder, excellent		
Cloxacillin	10-15	CSF, poor		Aqueous humor, poor	Bile, good	Pleural fluid, good	Ascites, poor; Saliva, poor; Synovial fluid, good
Colistimethate sodium	5-7.5	CSF, poor	No		Biliary excretion, 0%		

DRUG DOSING IN SPECIAL CIRCUMSTANCES 3

TABLE 3-9

ANTIMICROBIAL TISSUE DISTRIBUTION BY KEY ORGAN SYSTEMS[16,17,18]—cont'd

Drug	Peak Serum Level (mcg/mL)	CNS	CSF Level Potentially Therapeutic	Bone	Ocular	Bile	Pulmonary	Other
Co-trimoxazole		CSF, 40%-50%	Most meningococci resistant			Biliary excretion, 40%-200%		Tissues and fluids, widely distributed
Cycloserine		CSF, 80%-100%						
Dapsone	1.1	CSF, good				Liver, excellent	Lung, good	
Daptomycin	58-99							
Delavirdine	8-30	CSF, very low, 0.4%						Saliva, 6%
Dicloxacillin sodium	10-15			Bone, 15%-72%				Synovial fluid, 70%
Didanosine		CSF, 12%-85%	Yes					
Diethylcarbamazine		CSF, crosses the BBB						
Dirithromycin	0.4						Lung tissue, excellent	Nasal mucosa, excellent Tissue, excellent
Doripenem	23					Bile and gallbladder, excellent		Peritoneal and retroperitoneal fluids and urine, excellent
Doxycycline	1.5-2.1	CSF, 26%	No	Bone, good	Aqueous humor, good	Biliary excretion, 200%-3200%	Bronchial secretions, good (16%) Lung tissue, good	Gynecologic tissues, good

Efavirenz	13 μM	CSF, limited, 0.26%-1.19%	
Emtricitabine	1.8		
Enfuvirtide	5		
Ertapenem	154	CSF, 21% Yes	Biliary excretion, 10%	Blister fluid, 60%
Erythromycin ethylsuccinate and acetylsulfisoxazole		CSF, variable		Lung tissue, good	Middle ear, fair
Erythromycin preparations	0.1-4	CSF, 2%-13% No		Lung tissue, excellent	Middle ear fluid, excellent Sinus secretions, good Sputum, good
Ethambutol hydrochloride	2-6	CSF, 25%-50% No		
Ethionamide		CSF, significant concentrations		
Famciclovir	3-4			
Fluconazole	6.7-14	CSF, 50%-94% (inflamed and normal meninges) Yes		Lung, good	Blister fluid, 200% Saliva, 100%
Flucytosine	30-40	CSF, 60%-100% Yes		Lung, good Aqueous humor, therapeutic

DRUG DOSING IN SPECIAL CIRCUMSTANCES

3

TABLE 3-9

ANTIMICROBIAL TISSUE DISTRIBUTION BY KEY ORGAN SYSTEMS[16,17,18]—cont'd

Drug	Peak Serum Level (mcg/mL)	CNS	CSF Level Potentially Therapeutic	Bone	Ocular	Bile	Pulmonary	Other
Fosamprenavir	6							
Foscarnet	155	CSF, <1%	No					
Fosfomycin	26	CSF, poor		Bone, 3%-28%			Bronchial secretions, 3.5%	
Ganciclovir	8.3	CSF, 24%-68%	Yes		Aqueous humor, poor to good	Liver, 92%	Lung, 99%	
Gentamicin		CSF, 0%-30%	No; may consider intrathecal dose of 5-10 mg for potentially therapeutic level	Bone, limited	Aqueous humor, poor, 4%-9%	Biliary excretion, 10%-60%	Bronchial tree, limited (14%)	Saliva, variable Synovial fluid, good
Griseofulvin								Skin, therapeutic

Imipenem-cilastatin	40	CSF, 8.5%	Yes (concern for seizure potential)	Bone, dry weight bone concentrations 0.4–5.4 mcg/g	Biliary excretion, minimal	Bronchial secretions, 6.7%	Ascitic fluid, exceeds MIC-90 for most organisms that cause peritonitis. Pancreatic secretions, exceeded MIC values for many organisms associated with pancreatic infections. Pericardium, tenfold over the MIC for a majority of pathogens. Peritoneal fluid, ~73%
Indinavir	12.6 µM	CSF, 5%–9%					
Isoniazid	3-5	CSF, 90%	Yes				Saliva, 81%. Synovial fluid, 87.5%–133.3%. Tissues, similar to serum levels

DRUG DOSING IN SPECIAL CIRCUMSTANCES

3

TABLE 3-9

ANTIMICROBIAL TISSUE DISTRIBUTION BY KEY ORGAN SYSTEMS[16,17,18]—cont'd

Drug	Peak Serum Level (mcg/mL)	CNS	CSF Level Potentially Therapeutic	Bone	Ocular	Bile	Pulmonary	Other
Itraconazole	0.3–0.7	CSF, 0%; limited efficacy has been demonstrated in the treatment of cryptococcal and coccidioidal meningitis (penetration into the meninges as opposed to CSF levels)		Bone, excellent		Liver, excellent	Bronchial fluid, excellent	Tissues, excellent (skin, adipose tissue, endometrium, pus) Nail, excellent
Ivermectin	0.05–0.08							
Kanamycin		CSF, 0%–30%	No; may consider intrathecal dose of 5-10 mg for potentially therapeutic level			Biliary excretion, 10%–60%	Pleural fluid, excellent	Ascitic fluid, excellent Synovial fluid, excellent
Ketoconazole		CSF, negligible						Tissues, widely distributed
Lamivudine	2.6	CSF, 6%–11%	No data					

Drug					
Levofloxacin	5.7-8.6	CSF, 30%-50%	Aqueous humor, good	Lung tissue, 200%-500%	Blister fluid, extensive (100%) Tissues, good to excellent (prostate and gynecologic tissues, semen, maxillary sinus mucosa, tonsils, and salivary glands)
Linezolid	15-20	CSF, 60%-70%		Pleural fluid, >4 mcg/mL	Pancreas, 11.0-31.6 mcg/mL
Lopinavir/Ritonavir	9.6/7.8				
Loracarbef	8				Blister fluid, 50% Middle ear fluid, 42%-48% Sinus fluid, 0.16-0.88 mcg/mL Sputum, 0.22-0.37 mcg/mL
Mebendazole		CSF, 8.6 mcg/L			Tissues, detected in liver, kidney, fat, muscle, and spleen
Mefloquine hydrochloride	0.5-1.2	CSF, excellent, >1000 ng/mL			

TABLE 3-9

ANTIMICROBIAL TISSUE DISTRIBUTION BY KEY ORGAN SYSTEMS[1,6,17,18]—cont'd

Drug	Peak Serum Level (mcg/mL)	CNS	CSF Level Potentially Therapeutic	Bone	Ocular	Bile	Pulmonary	Other
Melarsoprol		CSF, low and variable						
Meropenem	49	CSF, ~2%, 0.2-2.8 mcg/mL (20 mg/kg dose); 0.9-6.5 mcg/mL (40 mg/kg dose)	Yes			Biliary excretion, 3%-300%	Bronchial mucosa 4.5 mcg/mL Bronchial secretions, high	Blister, 85% Colon, 2.6 mcg/mL Gynecologic tissue, 1.7-4.2 mcg/mL Muscle, 6.1 mcg/mL Myocardium, 15.5 mcg/mL Peritoneal fluid, 30.2 mcg/mL Skin, 5.3 mcg/mL
Metronidazole	20-25	CSF, 45%-89%				Biliary excretion, 100%	Bronchial secretions, ~100%	Abscesses, significant Saliva, ~100%
Micafungin	5-16		No					
Miconazole		CSF, poor						Tissue, widely distributed
Minocycline	2-3.5	CSF, limited (>doxycycline)		Synovial fluid, limited	Aqueous humor, good, 50%	Biliary excretion, 200%-3200%		Gingival fluid, excellent Saliva/tears, good

Drug	pKa	CSF	Bone	Aqueous humor	Biliary	Bronchial/Lung	Other tissues
Moxifloxacin	4.5	CSF, good penetration				Bronchial mucosa, excellent	Maxillary sinus mucosa, exceeds plasma levels; Saliva, exceeds plasma levels; Blister fluid, 200%
Nafcillin	10-15	CSF, 9%-20% (>oxacillin, cloxacillin, dicloxacillin)	Yes, with high-dose IV therapy		Biliary excretion, >100%		
Nelfinavir	3-4	CSF, undetectable					
Neomycin sulfate							Kidney, good; Inner ear, good; Tissues, good
Nevirapine	2	CSF, present					
Nitazoxanide	3						
Norfloxacin					Bile, good; Gallbladder, good		Blister fluid, good; Prostate, excellent; Tissue, good
Ofloxacin	4.6-6.2	CSF, limited, 50%	Bone, limited, 25%	Aqueous humor, excellent	Bile, excellent; Gallbladder, excellent	Bronchial secretions, good; Lung, excellent	Ascitic fluid, 80%; Blister fluid, good; Middle ear mucosa, excellent; Saliva, limited; Sputum, excellent (71.6%-86%); Tonsils, good

DRUG DOSING IN SPECIAL CIRCUMSTANCES

3

TABLE 3-9

ANTIMICROBIAL TISSUE DISTRIBUTION BY KEY ORGAN SYSTEMS[16,17,18]—cont'd

Drug	Peak Serum Level (mcg/mL)	CNS	CSF Level Potentially Therapeutic	Bone	Ocular	Bile	Pulmonary	Other
Oseltamivir phosphate	0.65/3.5 (carboxylate)						Lung, good to excellent	
Oxacillin	10-15	CSF, poor	Yes, with high-dose IV therapy	Bone, generally not therapeutic	Aqueous humor, poor	Biliary excretion, >20%	Pleural fluid, good	Ascites, poor
Para-aminosalicylic acid		CSF, low concentrations, does not cross the BBB unless meninges are inflamed				Liver, high concentrations	Lung, high concentrations	Kidneys, high concentrations
Penicillin G preparations, aqueous potassium and sodium	20	CSF, 5%-10%, poor, even with inflamed meninges	Yes for penicillin sensitive *Streptococcus pneumoniae*	Bone, sufficient		Biliary excretion, 500%		Fracture hematoma, sufficient Septic joint effusions, sufficient Synovial fluid, variable
Penicillin G preparations, benzathine	0.15							

Drug					
Penicillin G preparations, penicillin G benzathine + penicillin G procaine		CSF, minimal, up to 4.5%, oral probenecid enhances penetration into the CSF resulting in sufficient treponemicidal concentrations (0.018 mcg/mL)			Synovial fluid, good
Penicillin V potassium	5-6	CSF, minimal	Pleural fluid, good		Ascitic fluid, good; Synovial fluid, good; Middle ear concentrations, 2.1-6.3 mcg/mL; Pericardial fluid, good; Saliva, minimal
Pentamidine isethionate				Liver, extensive; Bronchoalveolar lavage fluid, 23.2 ng/mL	Tissues, extensive (spleen, kidney, adrenals)
Piperacillin	400	Not for *Pseudomonas aeruginosa*	CSF, 30%, good with inflamed meninges	Biliary excretion, 3000%-6000%	Adipose tissue, excellent; Gallbladder tissue, excellent; Skeletal muscle, excellent; Sputum, 6%-22%

DRUG DOSING IN SPECIAL CIRCUMSTANCES

3

TABLE 3-9

ANTIMICROBIAL TISSUE DISTRIBUTION BY KEY ORGAN SYSTEMS[16,17,18] —cont'd

Drug	Peak Serum Level (mcg/mL)	CNS	CSF Level Potentially Therapeutic	Bone	Ocular	Bile	Pulmonary	Other
Piperacillin with tazobactam	209	CSF, low, when meninges are not inflamed		Cancellous bone, piperacillin 23%, tazobactam 26% Cortical bone, piperacillin 18%, tazobactam 22%		Biliary excretion, >100%	Lung tissue, 92%	Blister fluid, 35%-42%
Posaconazole (Noxafil)	0.2-1		Yes					
Praziquantel		CSF, 14%-24%						
Pyrazinamide	30-50	CSF, 100%	Yes			Liver, adequate	Lung, adequate	Tissues, adequate penetration
Pyrimethamine plus sulfadoxine		CSF, pyrimethamine, 10%-26.5%						Extravascular fluid, sulfadoxine penetrates well Tissue, sulfadoxine not widely distributed
Quinidine						Liver, high		

Quinine			Red blood cells, 40% Saliva, 25%
Quinupristin with dalfopristin	5		Tissues, good, 83%
Rifabutin			Lung, lung-to-plasma ratio, 6.5:1.0
Rifampin	4-32	Biliary excretion, 10,000% Liver, excellent	Abcesses, 2.4-5.0 mcg/mL Saliva, therapeutic in 2/3 patients Sputum, 1-3 mcg/mL Stomach wall, excellent Ascitic fluid, excellent
		Bone, 3.9%-47.0%	Lung, therapeutic Bronchial mucus, 41.5%
		Yes	CSF, 7%-56%; lower end of range with inflammed meninges or concomitant steroids, ~20% or greater with inflammed meninges
Ribavirin	0.8		Tracheal secretions, >100 × the MIC for RSV after 8 hr of aerosolized therapy
			Red blood cells, may exceed serum level by 50-fold
Rimantadine	0.1-0.4		Nasal mucus, 173%

3

DRUG DOSING IN SPECIAL CIRCUMSTANCES

TABLE 3-9

ANTIMICROBIAL TISSUE DISTRIBUTION BY KEY ORGAN SYSTEMS[16,17,18]—cont'd

Drug	Peak Serum Level (mcg/mL)	CNS	CSF Level Potentially Therapeutic	Bone	Ocular	Bile	Pulmonary	Other
Ritonavir	7.8	CSF, 0.1%-0.5%						
Saquinavir	3.1	CSF, 0.1%-0.2%; combination therapy, <2.5 ng/mL; with NRTI, 167 ng/mL; dual PI, 1094 ng/mL	No					
Stavudine	1.4	CSF, 16%-97%	No					
Stibogluconate (Pentostam)								
Streptomycin sulfate	25-50	CSF, 0%-30%	No; may consider intrathecal dose of 5-10 mg for potentially therapeutic level		Aqueous humor, good (subconjunctival administration)	Bile, 33%	Bronchial secretions, 24% Pleural fluid, 33%	Ascitic fluid, excellent
Sulfadiazine		CSF, 40%-60%						
Sulfisoxazole		CSF, 94 mcg/mL						Lymph, limited Gallbladder, limited
Suramin		CSF, extremely poor						Tissues, 100%

Drug	Serum	CSF	Bone	Bile	Lung/Pleural fluid	Tissues
Tenofovir disoproxil fumarate	0.12					Lymphocytes, extensive
Terbinafine						Tissues, extensive (adipose tissue, skin, nails)
Tetracycline hydrochloride	1.5-2.2	No; Brain, good CSF, 7%	Bone and joints, good	Biliary excretion, 200%-3200%	Bronchial secretions, limited, 10%	Tissues, good (skin, fat) Peridontal tissue, excellent
Thiabendazole		CSF, 1.8 mcg/mL				
Ticarcillin	260	Not for *P. aeruginosa*; CSF, 40%		Bile, good	Pleural fluid, good	Tissues, good
Ticarcillin with clavulanate	330	CSF, ticarcillin, 1.09-34.79 mg/L; clavulanic acid, 0.14-2.69 mg/L	Bone, adequate	Bile, ticarcillin, good; clavulanic acid, 42.8%	Pleural fluid, adequate	Blister fluid, ticarcillin, 58%; clavulanic acid, 77% Lymph fluid, excellent Peritoneal fluid, ticarcillin, 70%; clavulanic acid, 67%
Tigecycline	0.63		Bone, 35% Synovial fluid, 58%	Biliary excretion, 138%	Lung, 8.6-fold higher than serum	Colon, 2.1-fold higher than serum Gallbladder, 38-fold higher than serum

DRUG DOSING IN SPECIAL CIRCUMSTANCES

3

TABLE 3-9

ANTIMICROBIAL TISSUE DISTRIBUTION BY KEY ORGAN SYSTEMS[16,17,18]—cont'd

Drug	Peak Serum Level (mcg/mL)	CNS	CSF Level Potentially Therapeutic	Bone	Ocular	Bile	Pulmonary	Other
Tinidazole					Aqueous humor, 47%	Bile, widely distributed		Skin, similar to plasma tissues, widely distributed (muscle, fat, appendix)
Tipranavir	78-95 μM	CSF, unknown						
Tobramycin		CSF, 0%-30%	No; may consider intrathecal dose of 5-10 mg for potentially therapeutic level	Synovial fluid, excellent, >50%	Aqueous humor, good (subconjunctival injection)	Biliary excretion, 10%-60%	Bronchial secretions, good Interstitial fluid, good	Kidney, good Pericardial fluid, good Peritoneal fluid, excellent, 15%-183% Tears, limited
Trimethoprim	1			Bone, does not penetrate compact bone	Aqueous humor, good although less than plasma	Bile, good although less than plasma	Bronchial secretions, tissue-to-plasma ratio, 2:1	Blister fluid, 76%-141% Saliva, saliva-to-serum ratio, 2:1
Trimetrexate		CSF, poor, 1%-4%					Lung, good	

Valacyclovir	5.6		
Valganciclovir	5.6-9.7		
Vancomycin	20-50	CSF, 7%-14%, increased with meningitis	Need high doses	Biliary excretion, 50%	Pleural fluid, well	Body fluids, well (pericardial, ascitic, synovial, urine, peritoneal)
Vidarabine		CSF, 30%-100%		Liver, good		Tissues, good (kidney, spleen), minimal penetration into skeletal muscle
Voriconazole (VFEND)	3	CSF, 22%-100%	Yes		Pleural fluid, 45.2%-64.5%	
Zalcitabine	0.03	CSF, 9%-37%	Yes			
Zanamivir						Sputum, 47-1336 ng/mL (inhaled); no antiviral activity with systemic administration
Zidovudine	1-2	CSF, 50%-70%	Yes			

+/−, yes in some studies, no others; BBB, blood-brain barrier; CNS, central nervous system; CSF, cerebrospinal fluid; IM, intramuscular; IV, intravenous; MIC, minimum inhibitory concentration; NRTI, nucleoside reverse transcriptase inhibitor; PI, protease inhibitor.

DRUG DOSING IN SPECIAL CIRCUMSTANCES 3

REFERENCES

1. Jacobson P, West N, Hutchinson RJ: Predictive ability of creatinine clearance estimate models in pediatric bone marrow transplant patients. Bone Marrow Transplant 1997;19:481-485.
2. Schwartz GJ, Brion LP, Spitzer A: The use of plasma creatinine concentration for estimating glomerular filtration rate in infants, children, and adolescents. Pediatr Clin North Am 1987;34:571-590.
3. Seikaly MG, Browne R, Gajaj G, et al: Limitations of body length/serum creatinine ratio as an estimate of glomerular filtration in children. Pediatr Nephrol 1996;10:709-711.
4. American Society of Health-System Pharmacists: American Hospital Formulary Service. Bethesda, MD: The Society, 2006.
5. Micromedex Healthcare Series [Intranet database]. Version 133. Greenwood Village, CO: Thomson Micromedex. Copyright 1974-2007.
6. Taketomo C, Hodding JH, Kraus DM: Pediatric Dosage Handbook. 13th ed. Hudson, OH: Lexi-Comp, 2006.
7. Hudson JQ: Drug disposition in patients receiving continuous renal replacement therapies. J Pediatr Pharmacol Ther 2001;6:15-39.
8. Joy MS, Matzke GR, Armstrong DK, et al: A primer on continuous renal replacement therapy for critically ill patients. Ann Pharmacother 1998;32:362-375.
9. Mouser JF, Thompson JB: Drugs removed by renal replacement therapies. J Pediatr Pharmacol Ther 2001;6:79-87.
10. Veltri MA, Neu AM, Fivush BA, et al: Drug dosing during intermittent hemodialysis and continuous renal replacement therapy: Special considerations in pediatric patients. Pediatr Drugs 2004;6(1):45-65.
11. Spray JW, Willett K, Chase D, et al: Dosage adjustment for hepatic dysfunction based on Child-Pugh scores. Am J Health-Syst Pharm 2007;64:690-693.
12. Verbeeck RK, Horsmans Y. Effect of hepatic insufficiency on pharmacokinetics and drug dosing. Pharm World Sci 1998;20(5):183-192.
13. Bearden DT, Rodvold KA: Dosage adjustments for antibacterials in obese patients: Applying clinical pharmacokinetics. Clin Pharmacokinet 2000;38(5):415-426.
14. Erstad BL: Dosing of medications in morbidly obese patients in the intensive care unit setting. Intensive Care Med 2004;30:18-32.
15. Wurtz R, Itokazu G, Rodvold K. Antimicrobial dosing in obese patients. Clin Infect Dis 1997;25(1):112-118.
16. Gilbert DN, Moellering RC, Eliopoulos GM, et al (eds): The Sanford Guide to Antimicrobial Therapy 2007, 37th ed. Sperryville, VA: Antimicrobial Therapy Inc, 2007.
17. Micromedex Healthcare Series (electronic version). Thomson Micromedex, Greenwood Village, CO: Thomson Micromedex, 1974-2007. Available at http://www.thomsonhc.com.
18. Lustar I, McCracken G, Friedland I: Antibiotic pharmacodynamics in cerebrospinal fluid. Clin Inf Dis 1998;27:1117-1129.

Mechanisms of Action and Routes of Administration of Antimicrobial Agents

James D. Dick, PhD

MECHANISMS OF ACTION AND ROUTES OF ADMINISTRATION OF ANTIMICROBIAL AGENTS

Class	Mechanism of Action	Antibacterial	PO	IM	IV	T
ANTIBACTERIAL						
Aminoglycoside	Protein synthesis inhibition	Amikacin		X	X	
		Gentamicin		X	X	X
		Kanamycin		X	X	
		Neomycin				X
		Spectinomycin		X	X	
		Streptomycin		X	X	
		Tobramycin		X	X	
β-Lactam/β-lactamase inhibitor	Cell wall synthesis/β-lactamase inhibitor	Amoxicillin/Clavulanate	X			
		Ampicillin/Sulbactam			X	
		Piperacillin/Tazobactam			X	
		Ticarcillin/Clavulanate			X	
β-Lactam/Carbapenem	Cell wall synthesis	Ertapenem		X	X	
		Imipenem-Cilastatin			X	
		Loracarbef	X			
		Meropenem			X	
β-Lactam/Cephalosporin I	Cell wall synthesis	Cefazolin		X	X	
		Cephalexin	X			

Class	Drug	Mechanism			
β-Lactam/Cephem/Cephalosporin II	Cefaclor	Cell wall synthesis	X	X	
	Cefadroxil		X		
	Cefpodoxime		X		
	Ceprozil		X		
	Ceftibuten		X		
	Cefuroxime		X	X	X
	Cefradine		X		
β-Lactam/Cephalosporin III	Cefixime	Cell wall synthesis	X		
	Cefoperazone			X	X
	Cefotaxime			X	X
	Ceftazidime			X	X
	Ceftibutin		X		
	Ceftizoxime			X	X
	Ceftriaxone			X	X
β-Lactam/Cephalosporin IV	Cefepime	Cell wall synthesis		X	X
β-Lactam/Cephamycin	Cefotetan	Cell wall synthesis		X	X
	Cefoxitin			X	X
β-Lactam/Penicillin	Amoxicillin	Cell wall synthesis	X		
	Ampicillin		X	X	
	Penicillin G		X	X	
	Penicillin V		X	X	

MECHANISMS OF ACTION AND ROUTES OF ADMINISTRATION OF ANTIMICROBIAL AGENTS—cont'd

Class	Mechanism of Action	Antibacterial	PO	IM	IV	T
β-Lactam/Penicillinase stable penicillin	Cell wall synthesis	Dicloxacillin	×			
		Flucloxacillin	×			
		Methicillin		×	×	
		Nafcillin		×	×	
		Oxacillin		×	×	
β-Lactam/Ureidopenicillin	Cell wall synthesis	Mezlocillin		×	×	
		Piperacillin			×	
β-Lactam/Monobactam	Cell wall synthesis	Aztreonam			×	
Fluoroquinolone	Nucleic acid synthesis	Norfloxacin	×			
		Ofloxacin	×	×	×	×
		Ciprofloxacin	×		×	
		Gatifloxacin	×		×	
		Levofloxacin	×		×	
		Moxifloxacin	×		×	
		Pefloxacin	×		×	
		Sparfloxacin	×			
Macrolide	Protein synthesis inhibition	Azithromycin	×		×	
		Clarithromycin	×			
		Dirithromycin	×			
		Erythromycin	×		×	×

Class	Mechanism	Drug			
Sulfonamide	Folate synthesis inhibition	Sulfacetamide	X		
		Sulfadiazine	X		
		Sulfisoxazole	X		
Trimethoprim	Folate synthesis inhibition	Trimethoprim	X		
Trimethoprim/Sulfamethoxazole	Folate synthesis inhibition	Co-Trimoxazole (Trimethoprim-sulfamethoxazole)	X		
Lipopeptide	Membrane disruption	Daptomycin	X		
		Polymyxin B			X
		Colistin		X	X
Tetracycline	Protein synthesis inhibition	Doxycycline	X		
		Minocycline	X		
		Tetracycline	X		
Phenicol	Protein synthesis inhibition	Chloramphenicol	X		
Lincosamide	Protein synthesis inhibition	Clindamycin	X	X	
Steptogramins	Protein synthesis inhibition	Quinupristin/Dalfopristin	X		
Oxazolidinone	Cell wall synthesis	Linezolid	X		
Glycopeptide	Cell wall synthesis	Vancomycin	X		
		Teicoplanin		X	
Fosphomycin	Peptide synthesis inhibition	Fosphomycin	X		
Nitrofuran	Aerobic energy metabolism and synthesis	Furazolidone	X		
		Nitrofurantoin	X		

MECHANISMS OF ACTION AND ROUTES OF ADMINISTRATION OF ANTIMICROBIAL AGENTS—cont'd

Class	Mechanism of Action	Antibacterial	Routes of Administration			
			PO	IM	IV	T
Nitroimidazoles	DNA damage	Metronidazole	×		×	×
Rifamycins	RNA synthesis	Rifampin	×		×	
Pseudomonic acid	Isoleucyl-t RNA synthetase inhibitor	Mupirocin				×
Cyclic peptides	Cell wall synthesis	Bacitracin				×
ANTIMYCOBACTERIAL						
Isonicotinic acid derivative	Cell wall (mycolic acid) synthesis	Isoniazid	×			
		Ethionamide	×			
Rifamycins	RNA sythesis	Rifabutin	×			
		Rifapentine	×			
Ethambutol	Cell wall (arabinogalactan) synthesis	Ethambutol	×			
Salicylic acid	Salicylic acid metabolism	p-Aminosalicylic acid	×			
Pyrazinoic acid	Membrane potential/proton motive force	Pyrazinamide	×			
Basic peptide	Protein synthesis	Capreomycin	×			
Sulfone	Folate synthesis	Dapsone	×			
ANTIFUNGAL						
Polyenes	Membrane disruption (ergosterol)	Amphotericin B			×	×
		Nystatin	×			×
Antimetabolite	Inhibiton of nucleic acid synthesis	5-Fluorocytosine	×			×

Class	Mechanism	Drug		
Imidazoles	Membrane (ergosterol) biosynthesis	Ketoconazole	X	X
		Clotrimazole	X	X
		Miconazole	X	X
Triazoles	Membrane (eryosterol) biosynthesis	Fluconazole	X	X
		Itraconazole	X	X
		Voriconazole	X	X
		Posaconazole	X	
Echinocandin	Cell wall (glucan) synthesis	Caspofungin		X
Griseofulvin	Inhibition of mitosis and microtubules	Griseofulvin		X
ANTIVIRAL				
Antiherpes virus	Inhibition of viral DNA polymerase	Vidarabine	X	X
		Acyclovir	X	X
		Valacyclovir	X	
		Famiciclovir	X	
		Penciclovir	X	
		Valganciclovir	X	
		Gancyclovir	X	X
Pyrophosphate analog	Blocks pyrophosphate exchange on viral DNA polymerase	Foscarnet	X	X

MECHANISMS OF ACTION AND ROUTES OF ADMINISTRATION

4

MECHANISMS OF ACTION AND ROUTES OF ADMINISTRATION OF ANTIMICROBIAL AGENTS—cont'd

Class	Mechanism of Action	Antibacterial	Routes of Administration			
			PO	IM	IV	T
Antiretroviral-nucleoside analogs	Inhibition of reverse transcriptase	Cidofovir			×	×
		Zidovidine	×		×	
		Didanosine	×			
		Zalcitabine	×			
		Lamivudine	×			
		Abacavir	×			
Antiretroviral	Non-nucleoside reverse transcriptase inhibiton	Nevirapine	×			
		Efavirenz	×			
		Delavirdine	×			
Antiretroviral	Nucleotide analog reverse transcriptase inhibitor	Tenofovir	×			
		Saquinavir	×			
		Indinavir	×			
		Ritonavir	×			
	HIV protease inhibitors	Nelfinavir	×			
		Amprenavir	×			
		Lopinavir/ritonavir	×			
		Atazanavir	×			

Class	Mechanism	Drug			
Tricyclic amine	M2 protein ion channel function/hemagglutinin formation	Amantadine	x		
		Rimantadine	x		
Nucleoside analog	Interferes with capping and elongantion of mRNA	Ribovirin	x		x (aerosol)
Neuraminidase inhibitor	Inhibition of infuenza virus neuraminidase activity	Oseltamivir	x		
		Zanamivir			x (inhalation)
Cytidine analog	Selective inhibitor of HIV1 and 2 and HBV	Emtricitabine	x		
ANTIPARASITIC					
Benzimidazoles	Inhibition of tubulin polymerization, cytoskeletal disruption	Mebendazole	x		
		Thiabendazole	x		
Avermectins	Hyperpolarization of susceptible cell membranes	Ivermectin	x		
Piperazine derivative	Alteration of the surface membrane of microfilarae	Diethylcarbamazine	x		
Quinolone derivatives	Nonenzymatic inhibition heme polymerization	Chloroquine	x	x	
		Hydroxychloroquine	x		
8-Aminoquinolones	Inhibition of parasitic mitochondrial enzymes	Primaquine	x		
Cinchona alkaloids	Interferes with hemoglobin digestion, inhibition of nucleic acid and protein synthesis	Quinine	x	x	
Synthetic quinolines	Interferes with hemoglobin metabolism	Mefloquine	x		
Antifolate	Inhibits plasmodial dihydrofolate reductase	Pyrimethamine-Sulfadoxine	x		

MECHANISMS OF ACTION AND ROUTES OF ADMINISTRATION

4

MECHANISMS OF ACTION AND ROUTES OF ADMINISTRATION OF ANTIMICROBIAL AGENTS—cont'd

Class	Antibacterial	Mechanism of Action	PO	IM	IV	T
Combination agent	Atovaquone/proguanil	Inhibition of electron transport, blocking nucleic synthesis Synergystic loss of mitochondrial membrane potential	X			
Acetanilide	Diloxanide furoate	Unknown	X			
Aromatioc diamidine	Pentamidine isethionate	Inhibition of dihydrofolate reductase, glycolysis, and DNA, RNA, and protein synthesis		X	X	X

HBV, hepatitis B virus; HIV, human immunodeficiency virus; IM, intramuscular; IV, intravenous; PO, by mouth; T, topical.

Mechanisms of Drug Resistance

James D. Dick, PhD

I. COMMON MECHANISMS OF MICROBIAL RESISTANCE

TABLE 5-1

COMMON MECHANISMS OF MICROBIAL RESISTANCE

Resistance Category	Antibiotics	Specific Mechanism
Enzymatic modification or nonactivation of the antimicrobial agent	β-Lactams	β-Lactamases
	Aminoglycosides	Aminoglycoside-inactivating (acetylases, phosphorylases, adenylases) enzymes
	Chloramphenicol	Chloramphenicol acetyltransferases
	Macrolides	Macrolide esterases/phosphorylases
	5-Fluorocytosine	Mutation in cytosine deaminase
	Metronidazole	Decrease in activation by pyravate/ferredoxin oxidoreductase system
Alteration of target site	β-Lactams	Structural change in penicillin-binding proteins
	Macrolides	Methylation of rRNA (macrolide, lincosamide, streptogramin B methylase [MLS_B])
	Clindamycin	
	Streptogramins	
	Fluoroquinolones	Structural change (mutation) of DNA gyrase or topoisomerase IV
	Glycopeptides	Modification of the D-alanine terminus of cell wall pentapeptide
	Rifamycins	Mutation on the RNA polymerase β subunit (rpoB)
	Sulfonamides	Structural change in dihydropteroate synthase
	Trimethoprim	Structural change in dihydrofolate reductase
	All antibiotics	Overproduction of antibiotic target

TABLE 5-1

COMMON MECHANISMS OF MICROBIAL RESISTANCE—cont'd

Resistance Category	Antibiotics	Specific Mechanism
Efflux/permeability	Teteracycline	Efflux pumps
	Macrolides (14- to 15-membered ring)	Efflux pumps
	Fluoroquinolones	Efflux pumps
	Carbapenems	Loss of outer membrane proins
	Aminoglycosides	Decreased uptake/accumualtion

II. DISCORDANCE BETWEEN IN VITRO SUSCEPTIBILITY AND IN VIVO EFFICACY

TABLE 5-2

DISCORDANCE BETWEEN IN VITRO SUSCEPTIBILITY AND IN VIVO EFFICACY

Organisms	May Be Susceptible In Vitro	In Vivo
Salmonella	1st- and 2nd-generation cephalosporins	Poor in vivo efficacy
Shigella	Aminoglycosides	
Extended-spectrum β-lactamase (ESBL)-producing Klebsiella sp Eschericha coli Proteus mirabilis	Cephalosporins Aztreonam ± β-lactam/β-lactamase inhibitors	Poor in vivo efficacy
Methicillin-resistant staphylococci	All β-lactam agents, including penicillin, cephalosporins, and carbapenems	Poor in vivo efficacy
Enterococci spp	All cephalosporin, clindamycin, macrolides, trimethoprim–sulfamethoxazole, and aminoglycosides (except high-level gentamicin <500 µg/mL and streptomycin <2000 mg/mL)	Poor in vivo efficacy
Listeria spp	All cephalosporins	Poor in vivo efficacy
Clostridium difficile	All antibiotics except metronidazole and vancomycin	Poor in vivo efficacy

TABLE 5-2

DISCORDANCE BETWEEN IN VITRO SUSCEPTIBILITY AND IN VIVO EFFICACY —cont'd

Organisms	May Be Susceptible In Vitro	In Vivo
Enterobacter spp *Citrobacter* spp *Serratia* spp *Morganella* spp *Providencia* spp	3rd-generation cephalosporins	Initial susceptibility, but rapid emergence of resistance during therapy. Combination therapy usually required.
Pseudomonas aeruginosa	All antimicrobial agents	Emergence of resistance during therapy. Combination therapy usually required.
Staphylococcus spp	Quinolones, vancomycin (VISA)	Emergence of resistance during prolonged therapy
Staphylococci, Streptococci	Erythromycin resistant, clindamycin susceptible	Macrolide resistance can be due to inducible MLS resistance, which can result in clinical failure with clindamycin. Clindamycin susceptibility should be evaluated using the "D" test if erythromycin resistant.
All cerebrospinal fluid (CSF) isolates	All oral antibiotics Clindamycin Teteracyclines Fluoroquinolones 1st- and 2nd-generation cephalosporins	Poor penetration/concentration in CSF. Poor in vivo efficacy.

Therapeutic Drug Monitoring

Michelle C. Caruso, PharmD, and Carlton K.K. Lee, PharmD, MPH

I. GENERAL PRINCIPLES

A. THERAPEUTIC DRUG MONITORING

Therapeutic drug monitoring (TDM) uses serum drug concentrations, pharmacokinetics, and pharmacodynamics to individualize and optimize drug therapy response in patients (Fig. 6-1).

Dosing and frequency of medication administration are governed largely by two principles:

1. **Pharmacokinetics (PK): the effect of the body on the drug disposition (absorption, distribution, metabolism, and excretion). Factors affecting PK are:**
a. Drug's physiochemical characteristics
b. Maturational physiologic changes
c. Concomitant disease states/medical conditions
d. Drug interactions
e. Pharmacogenomics
2. **Pharmacodynamics (PD): the effect of the drug on the body (clinical effects). Factors affecting PD are:**
a. Concomitant disease states/medical conditions
b. Drug interactions
c. Pharmacogenomics

B. THERAPEUTIC SERUM CONCENTRATIONS OR RANGES

1. Main goal is to enhance efficacy and/or prevent toxicity.
2. Therapeutic ranges based on strong correlation and probabilities between serum concentration with desired (efficacy) and undesired (toxicity) drug effects. Some patients may still experience toxic reactions within therapeutic ranges and others may require "supratherapeutic" levels to obtain desired response.

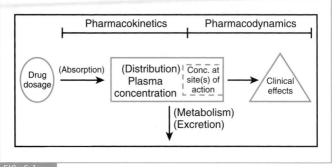

FIG. 6-1

Relationship between pharmacokinetics and pharmacodynamics. *(From McLeod HL, Evans WE: Pediatric pharmacokinetics and therapeutic drug monitoring. Pediatr Rev 1992;13(11):413-421.)*

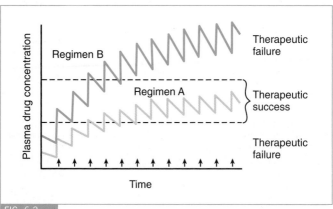

FIG. 6-2

Therapeutic range. Illustrates the concentration time profile following the administration of two different drug regimens, A and B. The dosing intervals are the same for both regimens; however, the dose for regimen B is twice that given in A.

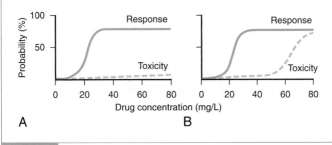

FIG. 6-3

Therapeutic index. Probability of effect (response and toxicity) with drug concentration for two different drugs. Panel A illustrates a hypothetical drug with very little toxicity at concentrations yielding maximum probability of response (wide therapeutic index). Panel B illustrates increasing probability of toxicity as drug concentration increases (narrow therapeutic index). *(From McLeod HL, Evans WE: Pediatric pharmacokinetics and therapeutic drug monitoring. Pediatr Rev 1992;13(11):413-421.)*

3. Serum drug concentration serves as a surrogate site for drug measurement because measurement at the site of action is typically not possible.

C. BENEFITS OF THERAPEUTIC DRUG MONITORING

1. Promotes optimal pharmacologic outcomes for drugs with known "therapeutic concentrations" (Fig. 6-2).
2. Promotes the safe and efficacious use of drugs with a narrow "therapeutic index" (Fig. 6-3).
3. Assists in determining patient status trends and/or changes (physiologic organ system changes, dietary changes, patient compliance issues, and drug interactions).
4. Potential economic impact by decreasing length of hospitalization, fewer hospital admissions, and rational use of serum concentration measurements.

II. ANTIMICROBIALS REQUIRING THERAPEUTIC DRUG MONITORING[1,2]

A. THERAPEUTIC DRUG MONITORING GOALS AND APPROPRIATE TIMES TO SAMPLE SERUM CONCENTRATIONS

TABLE 6-1

THERAPEUTIC DRUG MONITORING GOALS AND APPROPRIATE TIMES TO SAMPLE SERUM CONCENTRATIONS

Drug	When to Draw Peak Levels	When to Draw Trough Levels	Suggested Peak Levels (mg/L)	Suggested Trough Levels (mg/L)	Half-life (hr)[1,2]	Time to Reach Steady State (hr)[3]	Toxicity and Relationship to Serum Concentration
Amikacin	30 min after end of infusion	Within 30 min of next scheduled dose	20-30; 25-30 for CNS, pulmonary, bone, and serious infections; and febrile neutropenic patients	<10	Neonate: 6 ± 2 Infant: 4 ± 1 Child: 2 ± 1 Adolescent: 1.5 ± 1 Adult: 2 ± 1	Neonate: 20-40 Infant: 15-25 Child: 5-12 Adolescent: 5-8 Adult: 8-10	Toxicity risk factors: >5 days of use; dehydration; existing nephro- or ototoxicities; and use of other drugs with similar toxicities. **Nephrotoxicity:** can be associated with high troughs **Ototoxicity (avoid loop diuretics):** —Cochlear: loss of high-frequency tones and related to high peaks; amikacin is most toxic —Vestibular: include nystagmus and ataxia; gentamicin is most toxic

Chloramphenicol	Capsule: 60 min after dose; Suspension: 1.5-3 hr after dose; IV: 0.5-1.5 hr after end of infusion	Immediately before next dose	Meningitis: 15-25; Other infections: 10-20	Meningitis: 5-15; Other infections: 5-10	Neonate (1-2 days of age): 24; Neonate (10-16 days of age): 10; Adult: 1.6-3.3	Neonate: 2-3 days; All others: 12-24	Reversible bone marrow toxicity and anemia: levels > 25 mg/L (Note: rare idiosyncratic, irreversible aplastic anemia has been reported); "Gray baby syndrome" due to immature drug metabolism in neonates (cardiovascular-respiratory collapse): levels >50 mg/L
Flucytosine	60-120 min after an oral dose	Immediately before next dose	Invasive candidiasis: 40-60	≥25	Neonate: 4-34; Infant: 7.4; Adult: 2.5-6	Neonate: 16-136; Infant: 44.4; Adult: 6.4-24	Bone marrow toxicity (anemia, leukopenia, thrombocytopenia): levels >100 mg/L for prolonged periods of time

TABLE 6-1

THERAPEUTIC DRUG MONITORING GOALS AND APPROPRIATE TIMES TO SAMPLE SERUM CONCENTRATIONS—cont'd

Drug	When to Draw Peak Levels	When to Draw Trough Levels	Suggested Peak Levels (mg/L)	Suggested Trough Levels (mg/L)	Half-life (hr)[1,2]	Time to Reach Steady State (hr)[3]	Toxicity and Relationship to Serum Concentration
Gentamicin	30 min after end of infusion	Within 30 min of next scheduled dose	4-10; 8-10 for CNS, pulmonary, bone, and serious infections; and febrile neutropenic patients	<2	Neonate: 6 ± 2 Infant: 4 ± 1 Child: 2 ± 1 Adolescent: 1.5 ± 1 Adult: 2 ± 1	Neonate: 20-40 Infant: 15-25 Child: 5-12 Adolescent: 5-8 Adult: 8-10	Toxicity risk factors: >5 days of use; dehydration; existing nephro- or ototoxicities; and use of other drugs with similar toxicities. **Nephrotoxicity:** can be associated with high troughs **Ototoxicity (avoid loop diuretics):** —Cochlear: loss of high-frequency tones and related to high peaks; amikacin is most toxic —Vestibular: include nystagmus and ataxia; gentamicin is most toxic
Quinidine	N/A	Within 30 min of next scheduled dose	N/A	<8	Child: 2.5-6.7 Adult: 6-8	Child: 10-34 Adult: 24-40	Cardiac arrhythmias (extrasystoles, atrial flutter, ventricular flutter, or fibrillation): may occur with levels ≥5 mg/L

| Tobramycin | 30 min after end of infusion | Within 30 min of next scheduled dose | 4-10; 8-10 for CNS, pulmonary, bone, and serious infections; and febrile neutropenic patients | <2 | Neonate: 6 ± 2
Infant: 4 ± 1
Child: 2 ± 1
Adolescent: 1.5 ± 1
Adult: 2 ± 1 | Neonate: 20-40
Infant: 15-25
Child: 5-12
Adolescent: 5-8
Adult: 8-10 | Toxicity risk factors: >5 days of use; dehydration; existing nephro- or ototoxicities; and use of other drugs with similar toxicities.
Nephrotoxicity: can be associated with high troughs
Ototoxicity (avoid loop diuretics):
—Cochlear: loss of high-frequency tones and related to high peaks; amikacin is most toxic
—Vestibular: include nystagmus and ataxia; gentamicin is most toxic |

TABLE 6-1

THERAPEUTIC DRUG MONITORING GOALS AND APPROPRIATE TIMES TO SAMPLE SERUM CONCENTRATIONS—cont'd

Drug	When to Draw Peak Levels	When to Draw Trough Levels	Suggested Peak Levels (mg/L)	Suggested Trough Levels (mg/L)	Half-life (hr)[1,2]	Time to Reach Steady State (hr)[3]	Toxicity and Relationship to Serum Concentration
Vancomycin	Peak measurement may be recommended for burn patients, clinically nonresponsive by 72 hr, persistent positive cultures, and CNS infections. 60 min after end of 60-min infusion	Within 30 min of next scheduled dose	20-50[4]; peaks >30 have been recommended for CNS infections	5-15[4]; Following troughs have also been suggested: MRSA pneumonia: 15-20; CNS infection: 20; endocarditis: 10-20; bacteremia: 10-15	Premature neonate[5] 30-40 wk and <1.2 kg: 7.8 ± 3 30-42 wk and ≥1.2 kg: 3.8 ± 1.4 >42 wk and >2 kg: 2.1 ± 0.8 Full-term neonate: 6.7 Infant: 4.1 Child: 2.6 ± 0.4 Adult ≥ 16 yr: 7 ± 1.5	Premature neonate[5] 30-40 wk and <1.2 kg: 23-39 30-42 wk and >1.2 kg: 11-19 >42 wk and >2 kg: 6-11 Full-term neonate: 20-34 Infant: 12-21 Child: 8-13 Adult ≥ 16 yr: 21-35	Toxicity risk factors: use with aminoglycoside; preexisting oto- or nephrotoxicity; life-threatening Staphylococcus aureus infection; and >15-21 days of use. Very little new data linking toxicity with serum concentration, which may be attributed to the current improved purified formulation of the drug (versus original "Mississippi Mud" formulation).

CNS, central nervous system; IV, intravenous; MRSA, methicillin-resistant *Staphylococcus aureus.*

[1] Assuming normal renal function

[2] Terminal half-life

[3] These steady-state times are achieved regardless of whether a loading dose is administered.

[4] Data for specific peak and trough levels and efficacy are not well-established. Trough concentration at 4-5 times the MIC has been recommended with higher concentrations; may be needed for sequestered infections or situations of poor vancomycin tissue penetration.

[5] Postconceptual age: the sum of gestational age at birth and chronologic age

III. SPECIAL TOPICS IN ANTIMICROBIAL THERAPEUTIC DRUG MONITORING

A. HIGH-DOSE EXTENDED-INTERVAL DOSING OF AMINOGLYCOSIDES: AMIKACIN, GENTAMICIN, AND TOBRAMYCIN[3,5,6]

1. Also known as once-daily or extended-interval dosing.
2. Designed to enhance efficacy by using concentration-dependent bactericidal properties of aminoglycosides and their post–antibiotic effects (PAE).
3. May reduce nephrotoxicity by decreasing drug accumulation in renal tubular cells.
4. Adult studies have demonstrated equal efficacy and equal or less nephrotoxicity with high-dose extended-interval (HDEI) dosing in select patient populations.
5. Pediatric experience has been limited to patients with cystic fibrosis, pyelonephritis, surgical prophylaxis and treatment, and urinary tract infections; and in the oncology (fever and neutropenia), neonatal intensive care unit (NICU), and pediatric intensive care unit (PICU) populations. A meta-analysis from Contopoulos-Ioannidis et al.[3] comparing HDEI versus traditional multiple daily dosing revealed no differences in clinical and microbiologic failure rates; a statistically significant efficacy benefit for using HDEI with amikacin; no difference in primary nephro- and ototoxicity; and less secondary nephrotoxicity with HDEI. However, gaps remain in knowledge regarding (1) the incidence of ototoxicity, (2) the appropriate dose to use with specific clinical conditions, (3) dosage adjustments in renal insufficiency, and (4) the appropriate method of therapeutic drug monitoring with HDEI.
6. HDEI is not recommended in renal insufficiency (glomerular filtration rate [GFR] < 60 mL/min); unstable renal function; pregnancy; extensive burns (>20% body surface area [BSA]) or trauma; conditions affecting body water such as ascites, extensive edema, and shock; and meningitis.
7. Concerns for using HDEI in children include rapid aminoglycoside clearance, unknown duration of the PAE, safety concerns, and limited clinical and efficacy data.

B. VANCOMYCIN SERUM MONITORING CONTROVERSY

1. Toxicity relationship with serum levels has not been clearly established. Earlier reports of toxicity may be related to the less purified version of vancomycin ("Mississippi Mud").[4,10,11]

a. Nephrotoxicity
    i. High trough or peak levels have NOT caused nephrotoxicity.
    ii. Concomitant use of aminoglycosides or other nephrotoxic drugs, advanced age, or preexisting renal failure can increase risk.
    iii. Usually reversible upon discontinuation.

b. Ototoxicity
  i. High trough or peak levels have *not* caused ototoxicity.
  ii. Concomitant use of aminoglycosides or other ototoxic drugs, pre-existing hearing loss, or kidney dysfunction can increase risk.
  iii. May be reversible upon drug discontinuation.

2. **Monitoring controversy**
a. Lack of evidence supporting relationship between serum vancomycin concentrations and clinical efficacy or toxicity has supported abandoning routine serum concentration monitoring.[10,11]
b. Wide interpatient variability in pharmacokinetics and sites of infection with difficult tissue penetration supports the need for serum concentration monitoring. Patients that should be monitored include those
  i. In intensive care units
  ii. With renal impairment, rapidly changing renal function, and advanced renal failure
  iii. Who are neonates, infants, or children
  iv. With meningitis, pneumonia, or endocarditis
  v. With poor therapeutic response
  vi. Receiving concurrent nephrotoxic medications
c. There is a current trend toward monitoring only trough levels in most patients. Some practitioners initiate serum monitoring only when patients are at risk for nephrotoxicity.

IV. PHARMACOKINETIC MONITORING IN THERAPEUTIC DRUG MONITORING

A. THE ONE-COMPARTMENT FIRST-ORDER ELIMINATION PHARMACOKINETIC MODEL

The one-compartment first-order elimination pharmacokinetic model assumes the following characteristics:

1. Instantaneous distribution and equilibration to all tissues and fluids
2. Drug removal is constant, independent of the dose, and logarithmic over time.

B. BASIC PHARMACOKINETIC TERMS

1. **Bioavailability:** Percentage or fraction of the administered extravascular dose that reaches the patient's bloodstream. Factors influencing bioavailability include the route of administration, drug's dissolution and absorptive characteristics, and precirculation metabolism of drug. General equation:

Amount of drug absorbed or reaching systemic circulation (mg)
$$= S \times F \times dose \ (mg)$$

where S = salt or ester factor and F = bioavailability factor. Both factors are expressed as fractions.

2. **Volume of Distribution (Vd):** A theoretical size of a compartment necessary to account for the total amount of drug in the body if it were present throughout the body at the same concentration found in plasma. General equation:

$$Vd(L) = \frac{\text{Total amount of drug in body (mg)}}{\text{Serum concentration (mg/L)}}$$

a. Usually expressed in liters (L) or liters/kg of body weight (L/kg).
b. Significant changes to just Vd will require a drug dose amount modification with no change in dosage interval. For example, an increase in aminoglycoside volume of distribution due to edema will result in a dose increase in order to maintain the desired serum concentration.
c. Loading doses can be determined when a drug's given volume of distribution and desired serum concentration are known. Loading doses are used to shorten the time to achieve a desired serum concentration. Bioavailability (S and F factors, see earlier) of the medication must be included. General equation:

Loading dose (mg/kg) =

$$\frac{Vd(L/kg) \times [\text{desired serum conc.} - \text{current serum conc.}](mg/L)}{S \times F}$$

3. **Elimination Rate Constant (Kel):** Fraction or percentage of the total amount of drug in the serum removed per unit of time; independent of concentration. General equation:

$$Kel(hr^{-1}) = \frac{Ln[Cp_1 \div Cp_2]}{\Delta t_{1-2}}$$

where
Ln = natural log
Cp_1 = serum concentration at time 1 (mg/L)
Cp_2 = serum concentration at time 2 (mg/L)
  Cp_1 always > Cp_2
Δt_{1-2} = time interval between Cp_1 and Cp_2 (hr)

4. **Elimination Half-Life ($T_{1/2}$):** The time required for a 50% reduction in serum concentration. General equation:

$$T_{1/2}(hr) = \frac{0.693}{Kel(hr^{-1})}$$

a. Significant changes to just the elimination $T_{1/2}$ will require a dosage interval modification without a change in dosage amount. For example, an increase in aminoglycoside elimination $T_{1/2}$ due to renal insufficiency will result in an increase in dosage interval in order to maintain a desired serum trough concentration.

5. **Steady State:** This concept is achieved when the rate of drug administration is equal to the rate of drug removal, and the serum concentration of drug (measured at similar times around any given dose) remains constant. This is also the time when drug accumulation is complete.
   a. Relationship between elimination $T_{1/2}$ and steady state:

No. of Half-lives ($T_{1/2}$)	% Steady State Achieved
1	50
2	75
3	87.5
4	93.75
5	96.88

   b. In clinical practice, steady state is achieved after four to five half-lives.
   c. Any changes in drug dose (amount or interval) will require the same four to five half-lives to reach new steady-state serum concentrations.
   d. Loading doses do not shorten the time to reach steady state.

6. **Clearance (Cl):** The intrinsic ability of the body or its organs of elimination (primarily in liver and kidneys) to remove drug from the blood. Clearance does not represent the amount (mg) of drug removal but describes a theoretical volume of blood being removed (of the drug) per unit time. General equation:

$$Cl(L/hr) = Vd(L) \times Kel(hr^{-1})$$

   a. Usually expressed as a volume per unit time (L/hr)
   b. Significant changes to just clearance will require a dosage interval modification and/or change in dosage amount. For example, increased piperacillin clearance as seen in cystic fibrosis results in higher mg/kg daily dosages; and increased vancomycin clearance as seen in infants results in shorter dosing intervals (e.g., every 6 hours) to prevent subtherapeutic serum levels.

C. SERUM MEASUREMENT METHODS
1. **During steady state**
   a. Maintenance Dose → "Peak" →Trough: Easiest method for calculating elimination rate constant but is not the most efficient method because of the lengthy time interval between the two serum samples.
   b. Trough→ Maintenance Dose → "Peak": Commonly used method of serum level determination. Extrapolating the measured trough as the trough level following the measured peak level is done to facilitate the drug elimination rate constant calculation. Time between serum level measurements is shorter than the preceding method.

2. Non–steady state
a. Useful for preventing toxicity; especially in situations of organ dysfunction.
b. Assessment methods are different from steady-state methods.
c. Non–steady-state levels can be used to predict steady-state levels.

D. CHALLENGES TO TDM
The following issues associated with TDM may result in an improper assessment and incorrect dosing recommendations.
1. Improper serum sampling
a. Measuring pre–steady-state levels but interpreting as steady state
b. Sampling during drug infusion
c. Sampling prior to drug distribution
d. Inappropriately flushing/discarding volume from intravenous (IV) line
2. Improper drug administration
a. Incorrect dose and time of dose
b. Improper site of IV line administration
3. Inaccurate time documentation of serum sampling and/or dose administration
a. Improper serum level assessment
b. Will result in incorrect calculation of key individualized pharmacokinetic parameters (Kel, $T_{1/2}$, and Vd)
4. Drug-drug interactions
a. Inadequate spacing of aminoglycosides and beta-lactam antibiotics can result in falsely lower aminoglycoside serum levels
5. Food and certain electrolytes can reduce absorption of antibiotics
6. Abnormal PK parameter calculations should be explained by a physiologic process (i.e., edema) or improper serum sampling should be considered.

E. ADDITIONAL CONSIDERATIONS IN PHARMACOKINETIC MONITORING
1. Patient age
a. Neonates: reduced renal elimination and protein binding and increased total body water
2. Disease-specific pharmacokinetic parameters and empiric dosages
a. Burns: dynamic renal elimination and body fluid status
b. Cystic fibrosis: pancreatic insufficiency, leaner body mass, hypoalbuminemia, and enhanced drug clearance
c. Oncology: hypoalbuminemia and enhanced drug clearance
d. Renal failure: reduced drug clearance
3. Volume status
a. Fluid overload versus dehydration: increased and decreased volume of distribution of water-soluble drugs, respectively

F. FOR ADDITIONAL ASSISTANCE

Consult a clinical pharmacist who is knowledgeable in pharmacokinetic therapeutic drug monitoring for assistance.

V. PHARMACOKINETIC/PHARMACODYNAMIC (PK/PD) ANTIMICROBIAL RELATIONSHIPS

A. PK/PD RELATIONSHIP CONCEPT

Specific antimicrobial and pathogen PK/PD targets have been developed from in vitro models to enhance efficacy and reduce development of resistance. Most PK/PD indices utilize drug blood concentrations that may differ greatly at the targeted site of action depending on drug protein binding and tissue penetration characteristics. Mechanical factors of the organism, such as biofilm, inoculum effects, and stationary growth phase, may also affect the pharmacodynamic target achievement. Synergistic effects of combination antimicrobial therapy should also be considered.

B. COMMON PK/PD INDICES (Fig. 6-4):

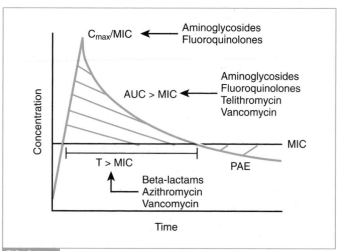

FIG. 6-4

Concentration-versus-time curve with minimum inhibitory concentration superimposed and pharmacokinetic and pharmacodynamic markers. *(Adapted from McKinnon PS, Yu VL: Pharmacologic considerations in antimicrobial therapy, with emphasis on pharmacokinetics and pharmacodynamics: Review for the practicing clinician. Eur J Clin Microbiol Infect Dis 2004;23:271-288.)*

1. **AUC/MIC**: Area under the serum concentration versus time curve (AUC) to minimum inhibitory concentration (MIC) ratio.
a. **MIC**: Used as a surrogate marker for predicting microbiologic activity at the infection site.
2. **C_{max}/MIC**: Maximum serum concentration to MIC ratio.
3. **T > MIC**: Duration of the dosing interval when serum concentrations exceed the MIC.

C. **CONCENTRATION-INDEPENDENT (TIME-DEPENDENT) ANTIMICROBIAL ACTIVITY**
Increasing the dosage of these agents above the MIC of the bacteria will not enhance the bacterial killing rate because the characteristic of killing is not concentration dependent. Time-dependent agents may also have a postantibiotic effect (PAE).

Antimicrobial	Key Predictor of Outcome*
β-Lactams	T > MIC
Macrolides (Azithromycin†)	T > MIC

*Specific outcome predictor numeric value is dependent on specific drug, microbial organism, and in vitro/in vivo/clinical condition.
†Also has a PAE and its AUC/MIC ratio predicts efficacy against *Streptococcus pneumoniae*.

D. **CONCENTRATION-DEPENDENT ANTIMICROBIAL ACTIVITY**
Demonstrates increasing bacterial killing with rising drug concentrations.

Antimicrobial	Key Predictor of Outcome*
Aminoglycosides†	AUC/MIC or C_{max}/MIC
Fluoroquinolones	AUC/MIC or C_{max}/MIC
Glycopeptides (Vancomycin‡)	AUC/MIC
Ketolides (Telithromycin)	AUC/MIC or C_{max}/MIC

*Specific outcome predictor numeric value is dependent on specific drug, microbial organism, and in vitro/in vivo/clinical condition.
†Also has a PAE.
‡Time-dependent activity (T > MIC) has also been suggested.

E. **SELECTED PHARMACOKINETIC AND PHARMACODYNAMIC RELATIONSHIPS OF VARIOUS ANTIMICROBIALS**
1. **Antibacterials** (Tables 6-2, 6-3)
2. **Antimycobacterials** (Table 6-4)
3. **Antifungals** (Table 6-5)

TABLE 6-2

EFFICACY RELATIONSHIPS IN HUMANS

Antibacterial Agent	PK/PD Parameter Associated with Improved Efficacy	Clinical Condition
Aminoglycosides	$C_{max}/MIC > 8:1$ $C_{max}/MIC \geq 10:1$	Gram-negative bacteremia Gram-negative pneumonia
Beta-lactams Cefepime	$T > 4 \times MIC$	Various Gram-negative pneumonia
Fluoroquinolones Ciprofloxacin Levofloxacin/ Gatifloxacin	$AUC/MIC \geq 250$ $AUC/MIC \ 30-40*$	Various Gram-negative infections *Streptococcus pneumoniae* in community-acquired pneumonia and chronic bronchitis
Levofloxacin	$C_{max}/MIC \geq 12:1$	*Streptococcus pneumoniae,* *Staphylococcus aureus, Pseudomonas aeruginosa,* and other Gram-negative infections
Glycopeptides Vancomycin	$AUC/MIC > 125$ $AUC/MIC > 400$	Various *Staphylococcus aureus* infections Methicillin resistant *Staphylococcus aureus* pneumonia

*Reflects free-drug concentration measurements.
AUC/MIC, area under the serum concentration versus time curve to minimum inhibitory concentration ratio; C_{max}/MIC, maximum serum concentration to MIC ratio; $T > MIC$, duration of the dosing interval with serum concentrations exceeds the MIC.
Adapted from McKinnon PS, Davis SL. Pharmacokinetic and pharmacodynamic issues in the treatment of bacterial infectious diseases. Eur J Clin Microbiol Infect Dis 2004;23:271-288.

TABLE 6-3

IN VITRO RESISTANCE RELATIONSHIPS

Antibacterial Agent	PK/PD Parameter Associated with Reduced Resistance	Condition
Fluoroquinolones Levofloxacin	$AUC/MIC \geq 157$	Mouse model evaluating drug exposure and resistant development in *Pseudomonas aeruginosa*
Glycopeptides Vancomycin	$AUC/MIC \geq 382$	Simulated in-vitro PK model using an *agr*-null group II *Staphylococcus aureus* strain.

AUC/MIC, area under the serum concentration versus time curve to minimum inhibitory concentration ratio; PK, pharmacokinetics.
Adapted from Rybak MJ, Pharmacodynamics: Relation to antimicrobial resistance. Am J Med 2006;119(6A):S37-44.

TABLE 6-4

EFFICACY RELATIONSHIPS OF ANTIMYCOBACTERIAL AGENTS

Antimycobacterial Agent	PK/PD Parameter Associated with Improved Efficacy	Condition
Isoniazid	C_{max}/MIC > 15	Mouse model
Rifampin	AUC/MIC ≥ 500 or AUC_{free}/MIC ≥ 75-100	Mouse model and human pharmacokinetic simulations

AUC/MIC, area under the serum concentration versus time curve to minimum inhibitory concentration ratio; C_{max}/MIC, maximum serum concentration to MIC ratio; PD, pharmacodynamic; PK, pharmacokinetic.
Adapted from Nuermberger E, Grosset J. Pharmacokinetic and pharmacodynamic issues in the treatment of mycobacterial infections. Eur J Clin Microbiol Infect Dis 2004;23:243-255.

TABLE 6-5

IN VIVO PHARMACODYNAMIC CHARACTERISTICS OF ANTIFUNGAL DRUG CLASSES IN NEUTROPENIC MOUSE MODELS

Antifungal Class	Candida	Aspergillus
Polyenes (Amphotericins)	C_{max}/MIC*	Unknown
Flucytosine	T > MIC*	N/A†
Triazoles	AUC/MIC*	Unknown
Echinocandins	C_{max}/MIC AUC/MIC	Unknown

*Post-antifungal effects (PAFEs) have been identified for certain drugs within the indicated antifungal drug class and specific Candida strain.
†Not indicated in Aspergillus due to poor activity.
AUC/MIC, area under the serum concentration versus time curve to minimum inhibitory concentration ratio; C_{max}/MIC, maximum serum concentration to MIC ratio; N/A, not applicable; T > MIC, duration of the dosing interval with serum concentrations exceeds the MIC.
Adapted from Groll AH, Kolve H. Antifungal agents: In vitro susceptibility testing, pharmacodynamics, and prospects for combinational therapy. Eur J Clin Microbiol Infect Dis 2004;23:256-270.

VI. DRUG INTERACTIONS

Drug interactions may result in increased drug effects/toxicity, or decreased effects because of a variety of mechanisms. They may include alterations in drug absorption, protein binding, metabolism, and clearance; additive/synergistic drug toxicity; and antagonistic effects on efficacy. Major drug-drug interactions are described in specific antimicrobial drug monographs of the formulary section. The following is a summary of those drug interactions that are considered contraindicated, where the risks associated with concomitant use usually outweigh the benefits. Data demonstrate the specified agents that may interact with each other in a clinically significant manner (Table 6-6).

TABLE 6-6

CONTRAINDICATED DRUG INTERACTIONS FOR ANTIMICROBIAL AGENTS[8,9]

Antimicrobial	Interacting Drug(s)	Toxic Effect
Amprenavir	Alcohol (ethyl), disulfiram, or metronidazole	Propylene glycol toxicity (from amprenavir suspension)
	Amiodarone	Bradycardia, hypotension, cardiogenic shock, heart block, QT prolongation, hepatotoxicity, (Amiodarone toxicity)
	Cisapride	QT prolongation, cardiac arrhythmias
	Ergot derivatives	Vasospasm resulting in peripheral, cardiac and/or cerebral ischemia; ↑ or ↓ in blood pressure or heart rate; seizures; headache
	Pimozide	QT prolongation, ventricular arrhythmias; hypotension; seizures; anticholinergic and extrapyramidal effects
	Quinidine	Tachycardia, hypotension, heart block, ventricular fibrillation, syncope, vascular collapse (quinidine toxicity)
	St. John's wort	Decreased amprenavir efficacy
Atazanavir	Amiodarone	Bradycardia, hypotension, cardiogenic shock, heart block, QT prolongation, hepatotoxicity, (amiodarone toxicity)
	Cisapride	QT prolongation, cardiac arrhythmias
	Ergot derivatives	Vasospasm resulting in peripheral, cardiac and/or cerebral ischemia; ↑ or ↓ in blood pressure or heart rate; seizures; headache
	Pimozide	QT prolongation, ventricular arrhythmias; hypotension; seizures; anticholinergic and extrapyramidal effects
	Quinidine	Tachycardia, hypotension, heart block, ventricular fibrillation, syncope vascular collapse (quinidine toxicity)

Ciprofloxacin	St. John's wort	Decreased atazanavir efficacy
	Tizanidine	Hypotension, bradycardia, drowsiness, lethargy, agitation, vomiting, respiratory depression, coma
Clarithromycin	Cisapride	QT prolongation, cardiac arrhythmias
	Disopyramide	QT prolongation, ventricular arrhythmias, hypotension, heart failure, anticholinergic effects, apnea, cardiac arrest
	Pimozide, thioridazine	QT prolongation, cardiac arrhythmias, hypotension, anticholinergic and extrapyramidal effects, agitation
Clindamycin	Erythromycin	Clindamycin diminishes erythromycin efficacy
Cotrimoxazole	Dofetilide	Decreased excretion of dofetilide (QT prolongation, ventricular arrhythmias, complete heart block)
Delavirdine	Thioridazine	QT prolongation, cardiac arrhythmias, hypotension, anticholinergic and extrapyramidal effects, agitation
Erythromycin	Cisapride	QT prolongation, cardiac arrhythmias
ethylsuccinate and acetylsulfisoxazole	Disopyramide	QT prolongation, ventricular arrhythmias, hypotension, heart failure, anticholinergic effects, apnea, cardiac arrest
	Lincosamide antibiotics (clindamycin, lincomycin)	Decreased erythromycin efficacy
	Pimozide, thioridazine	QT prolongation, cardiac arrhythmias, hypotension, anticholinergic and extrapyramidal effects, agitation

THERAPEUTIC DRUG MONITORING

6

TABLE 6-6

CONTRAINDICATED DRUG INTERACTIONS FOR ANTIMICROBIAL AGENTS[8,9]—cont'd

Antimicrobial	Interacting Drug(s)	Toxic Effect
Erythromycin preparations	Cisapride	QT prolongation, cardiac arrhythmias
	Disopyramide	QT prolongation, ventricular arrhythmias, hypotension, heart failure, anticholinergic effects, apnea, cardiac arrest
	Lincosamide antibiotics (clindamycin, lincomycin)	Decreased erythromycin efficacy
	Pimozide, thioridazine	QT prolongation, cardiac arrhythmias, hypotension, anticholinergic and extrapyramidal effects, agitation
Fosamprenavir	Amiodarone	Bradycardia, hypotension, cardiogenic shock, heart block, QT prolongation, hepatotoxicity, (amiodarone toxicity)
	Cisapride	QT prolongation, cardiac arrhythmias
	Ergot derivatives	Vasospasm resulting in peripheral, cardiac, and/or cerebral ischemia; ↑ or ↓ in blood pressure or heart rate; seizures; headache
	Pimozide	QT prolongation, ventricular arrhythmias; hypotension; seizures; anticholinergic and extrapyramidal effects
	Quinidine	Tachycardia, hypotension, heart block, ventricular fibrillation, syncope, vascular collapse (quinidine toxicity)
	St. John's wort	Decreased fosamprenavir efficacy
Foscarnet	Thioridazine	QT prolongation, cardiac arrhythmias, hypotension, anticholinergic and extrapyramidal effects, agitation

Furazolidone	Alpha-/beta-agonists (indirect-acting)	Hypertension, tachycardia, followed by bradycardia, arrhythmias, seizures, cerebral hemorrhages, ischemia and/or vasoconstriction; psychosis, hyperthermia
	Alpha₁-agonists	Hypertension, headache, tachycardia followed by bradycardia, arrhythmias, seizures, cerebral hemorrhages, ischemia and/or vasoconstriction; psychosis, hyperthermia
	Alpha₂-agonists (ophthalmic)	Hypertension, tachycardia, followed by profound hypotension, bradycardia, cardiac arrhythmias
	Amphetamines, buspirone, dexmethylphenidate, methylphenidate	Hypertension
	Antidepressants (serotonin/norepinephrine reuptake inhibitors); cyclobenzaprine, dextromethorphan, meperidine, selective serotonin reuptake inhibitors, sibutramine	Serotonin syndrome (mental status changes, agitation, myoclonus, hyperreflexia, diaphoresis, dilated pupils, shivering, tremor, diarrhea, fever)
	Atomoxetine, bupropion, mirtazapine	Nausea, vomiting, flushing, dizziness, tremor, myoclonus, rigidity, diaphoresis, hyperthermia, autonomic instability
	Tricyclic antidepressants	Hypertensive crisis, serotonin syndrome (mental status changes, agitation, myoclonus, hyperreflexia, diaphoresis, dilated pupils, shivering, tremor, diarrhea, fever)
Ganciclovir	Imipenem	Seizures
Griseofulvin	Contraceptives (progestins)	Contraceptive failure, breakthrough bleeding

THERAPEUTIC DRUG MONITORING 6

TABLE 6-6

CONTRAINDICATED DRUG INTERACTIONS FOR ANTIMICROBIAL AGENTS[8,9]—cont'd

Antimicrobial	Interacting Drug(s)	Toxic Effect
Imipenem-Cilastatin	Ganciclovir	Seizures
Indinavir	Amiodarone	Bradycardia, hypotension, cardiogenic shock, heart block, QT prolongation, hepatotoxicity (amiodarone toxicity)
	Cisapride	QT prolongation, cardiac arrhythmias
	Ergot derivatives	Vasospasm resulting in peripheral, cardiac and/or cerebral ischemia; ↑ or ↓ in blood pressure or heart rate; seizures; headache
	Pimozide	QT prolongation, ventricular arrhythmias; hypotension; seizures; anticholinergic and extrapyramidal effects
	Quinidine	Tachycardia, hypotension, heart block, ventricular fibrillation, syncope, vascular collapse (quinidine toxicity)
	St. John's wort	Decreased indinavir efficacy
	Thioridazine	QT prolongation, cardiac arrhythmias, hypotension, anticholinergic and extrapyramidal effects, agitation
Isoniazid	Conivaptan	Decreased metabolism of conivaptan, increased drug serum levels
Itraconazole	Dofetilide	Decreased metabolism and renal excretion of dofetilide (QT prolongation, ventricular arrhythmias, complete heart block)
	Pimozide	QT prolongation, ventricular arrhythmias; hypotension; seizures; anticholinergic and extrapyramidal effects
	Ranolazine	Decreased metabolism of ranolazine; dizziness, nausea/vomiting, QT prolongation, diplopia, paresthesia, confusion, syncope

Ketoconazole	Conivaptan	Decreased metabolism of conivaptan, increased drug serum levels
	Dofetilide	Decreased metabolism and renal excretion of dofetilide (QT prolongation, ventricular arrhythmias, complete heart block)
	Pimozide	QT prolongation, ventricular arrhythmias; hypotension; seizures; anticholinergic and extrapyramidal effects
	Ranolazine	Decreased metabolism of ranolazine; dizziness, nausea/vomiting, QT prolongation, diplopia, parethesia, confusion, syncope
	Thioridazine	QT prolongation, cardiac arrhythmias, hypotension, anticholinergic and extrapyramidal effects, agitation
Levofloxacin	Thioridazine	QT prolongation, cardiac arrhythmias, hypotension, anticholinergic and extrapyramidal effects, agitation
Linezolid	Alpha-/beta-agonists (indirect-acting)	Hypertension, tachycardia, followed by bradycardia, arrhythmias, seizures, cerebral hemorrhages, ischemia and/or vasoconstriction; psychosis, hyperthermia
	Alpha₁-agonists	Hypertension, headache, tachycardia, followed by bradycardia, arrhythmias, seizures, cerebral hemorrhages, ischemia and/or vasoconstriction; psychosis, hyperthermia
	Alpha₂-agonists (ophthalmic)	Hypertension, tachycardia followed by profound hypotension, bradycardia, cardiac arrhythmias
	Amphetamines, buspirone, dexmethylphenidate, methylphenidate	Hypertension

TABLE 6-6

CONTRAINDICATED DRUG INTERACTIONS FOR ANTIMICROBIAL AGENTS[8,9]—cont'd

Antimicrobial	Interacting Drug(s)	Toxic Effect
Linezolid—cont.	Antidepressants (serotonin/norepinephrine reuptake inhibitors); cyclobenzaprine, dextromethorphan, meperidine, selective serotonin reuptake inhibitors, sibutramine	Serotonin syndrome (mental status changes, agitation, myoclonus, hyperreflexia, diaphoresis, dilated pupils, shivering, tremor, diarrhea, fever)
	Atomoxetine, bupropion, mirtazapine	Nausea, vomiting, flushing, dizziness, tremor, myoclonus, rigidity, diaphoresis, hyperthermia, autonomic instability
	Tricyclic antidepressants	Hypertensive crisis, serotonin syndrome (mental status changes, agitation, myoclonus, hyperreflexia, diaphoresis, dilated pupils, shivering, tremor, diarrhea, fever)
Lopinavir with ritonavir	Amiodarone	Bradycardia, hypotension, cardiogenic shock, heart block, QT prolongation, hepatotoxicity, (amiodarone toxicity)
	Cisapride	QT prolongation, cardiac arrhythmias
	Disulfiram	Decreased metabolism of ritonavir; decreased metabolism of alcohol contained in Kaletra brand of oral solution with accumulation of acetaldehyde
	Ergot derivatives	Vasospasm resulting in peripheral, cardiac and/or cerebral ischemia; ↑ or ↓ in blood pressure or heart rate; seizures; headache
	Flecainide	Cardiac arrhythmias (ventricular tachydysrhythmias, severe bradycardia, AV block)
	Pimozide	QT prolongation, ventricular arrhythmias; hypotension; seizures; anticholinergic and extrapyramidal effects

	Propafenone	Cardiac arrhythmias, seizures, hypotension, gastrointestinal upset, blurred vision
	Quinidine	Tachycardia, hypotension, heart block, ventricular fibrillation, syncope, vascular collapse (quinidine toxicity)
	St. John's wort	Decreased lopinavir/ritonavir efficacy
	Thioridazine	QT prolongation, cardiac arrhythmias, hypotension, anticholinergic and extrapyramidal effects, agitation
	Voriconazole	Decreased voriconazole efficacy
Metronidazole	Amprenavir	Propylene glycol toxicity (from amprenavir suspension)
Miconazole	Conivaptan	Decreased metabolism of conivaptan, increased drug serum levels
	Dofetilide	Decreased metabolism and renal excretion of dofetilide (QT prolongation, ventricular arrhythmias, complete heart block)
	Pimozide	QT prolongation, ventricular arrhythmias; hypotension; seizures; anticholinergic and extrapyramidal effects
	Ranolazine	Decreased metabolism of ranolazine; dizziness, nausea/vomiting, QT prolongation, diplopia, paresthesia, confusion, syncope
	Thioridazine	QT prolongation, cardiac arrhythmias, hypotension, anticholinergic and extrapyramidal effects, agitation
Moxifloxacin	Thioridazine	QT prolongation, cardiac arrhythmias, hypotension, anticholinergic and extrapyramidal effects, agitation

TABLE 6-6

CONTRAINDICATED DRUG INTERACTIONS FOR ANTIMICROBIAL AGENTS[8,9]—cont'd

Antimicrobial	Interacting Drug(s)	Toxic Effect
Nelfinavir	Amiodarone	Bradycardia, hypotension, cardiogenic shock, heart block, QT prolongation, hepatotoxicity, (amiodarone toxicity)
	Cisapride	QT prolongation, cardiac arrhythmias
	Ergot derivatives	Vasospasm resulting in peripheral, cardiac and/or cerebral ischemia; ↑ or ↓ in blood pressure or heart rate; seizures; headache
	Pimozide	QT prolongation, ventricular arrhythmias; hypotension; seizures; anticholinergic and extrapyramidal effects
	Quinidine	Tachycardia, hypotension, heart block, ventricular fibrillation, syncope, vascular collapse (quinidine toxicity)
	St. John's wort	Decreased nelfinavir efficacy
Norfloxacin	Thioridazine	QT prolongation, cardiac arrhythmias, hypotension, anticholinergic and extrapyramidal effects, agitation
Pentamidine	Thioridazine	QT prolongation, cardiac arrhythmias, hypotension, anticholinergic and extrapyramidal effects, agitation
Polymyxin B sulfate, neomycin sulfate, hydrocortisone	Vaccines (live organisms)	Vaccinial infections
Quinidine gluconate	Protease inhibitors	Tachycardia, hypotension, heart block, ventricular fibrillation, syncope, vascular collapse (quinidine toxicity)
	Thioridazine	QT prolongation, cardiac arrhythmias, hypotension, anticholinergic and extrapyramidal effects, agitation

Ritonavir	Amiodarone	Bradycardia, hypotension, cardiogenic shock, heart block, QT prolongation, hepatotoxicity, (amiodarone toxicity)
	Cisapride	QT prolongation, cardiac arrhythmias
	Disulfiram	Decreased metabolism of ritonavir; decreased metabolism of alcohol contained in Kaletra brand of oral solution with accumulation of acetaldehyde
	Ergot derivatives	Vasospasm resulting in peripheral, cardiac and/or cerebral ischemia; ↑ or ↓ in blood pressure or heart rate; seizures; headache
	Flecainide	Cardiac arrhythmias (ventricular tachydysrhythmias, severe bradycardia, AV block)
	Pimozide	QT prolongation, ventricular arrhythmias; hypotension; seizures; anticholinergic and extrapyramidal effects
	Propafenone	Cardiac arrhythmias, seizures, hypotension, gastrointestinal upset, blurred vision
	Quinidine	Tachycardia, hypotension, heart block, ventricular fibrillation, syncope, vascular collapse (quinidine toxicity)
	St. John's wort	Decreased ritonavir efficacy
	Thioridazine	QT prolongation, cardiac arrhythmias, hypotension, anticholinergic and extrapyramidal effects, agitation
	Voriconazole	Decreased voriconazole efficacy
Saquinavir	Amiodarone	Bradycardia, hypotension, cardiogenic shock, heart block, QT prolongation, hepatotoxicity, (amiodarone toxicity)
	Cisapride	QT prolongation, cardiac arrhythmias
	Ergot derivatives	Vasospasm resulting in peripheral, cardiac, and/or cerebral ischemia; ↑ or ↓ in blood pressure or heart rate; seizures; headache

THERAPEUTIC DRUG MONITORING 6

TABLE 6-6
CONTRAINDICATED DRUG INTERACTIONS FOR ANTIMICROBIAL AGENTS[8,9]—cont'd

Antimicrobial	Interacting Drug(s)	Toxic Effect
Saquinavir—cont.	Pimozide	QT prolongation, ventricular arrhythmias; hypotension; seizures; anticholinergic and extrapyramidal effects
	Quinidine	Tachycardia, hypotension, heart block, ventricular fibrillation, syncope, vascular collapse (quinidine toxicity)
	St. John's wort	Decreased saquinavir efficacy
Terbinafine	Thioridazine	QT prolongation, cardiac arrhythmias, hypotension, anticholinergic and extrapyramidal effects, agitation
Thalidomide	Vaccines (live organisms)	Vaccinial infections
Trimethoprim	Dofetilide	Decreased excretion of dofetilide (QT prolongation, ventricular arrhythmias, complete heart block)
Trimetrexate glucuronate	Vaccines (live organisms)	Vaccinial infections
Voriconazole	Ritonavir	Decreased voriconazole efficacy
	Sirolimus	Decreased metabolism of sirolimus, increases sirolimus drug levels
	Thioridazine	QT prolongation, cardiac arrhythmias, hypotension, anticholinergic and extrapyramidal effects, agitation

REFERENCES

1. Hammett-Stabler CA, Johns T: Laboratory guidelines for monitoring of antimicrobial drugs. Clin Chem 1998;44(5):1129-1140.
2. 2007-2008 Antibiotic Guidelines: Treatment Recommendations for Adult Inpatients. The Johns Hopkins Hospital Antibiotic Management Program. Johns Hopkins Medicine. Published June 2007.
3. Contopoulos-Ioannidis DG, Giotis ND, Baiatsa DV, et al: Extended-interval aminoglycoside administration for children: A meta-analysis. Pediatrics 2004;114(1):e111-e118.
4. Darko W, Medicis JJ, Smith A, Guharoy R, Lehmann DF: Mississippi mud no more: Cost-effectiveness of pharmacokinetic dosage adjustment of vancomycin to prevent nephrotoxicity. Pharmacotherapy 2003;23(5):643-650.
5. Best EJ, Palasanthiran P, Gazaria M: Extended-interval aminoglycoside in children: More guidance is needed. Pediatrics 2005;115(3):827-828.
6. Knoderer CA, Everett JA, Buss WF: Clinical issues surrounding once-daily aminoglycoside dosing in children. Pharmacotherapy 2003;23(1):44-56.
7. Rybak MJ: Pharmacodynamics: Relation to antimicrobial resistance. Am J Med 2006;119(6A):S37-44.
8. Lexi-Comp's Comprehensive Interaction Analysis Program [Intranet database]. Accessed June 13, 2007.
9. Micromedex Healthcare Series [Intranet database]. Version 133. Greenwood Village, CO: Thomson Micromedex. Accessed June 13, 2007.
10. Rodvold KA, Zokufa H, Rotschafer JC: Routine monitoring of serum vancomycin concentrations: Can waiting be justified? Clin Pharm 1987;6:655-658.
11. Edwards DJ: Therapeutic drug monitoring of aminoglycosides and vancomycin: Guidelines and controversies. J Pharm Pract 1991;4:211-214.

6

THERAPEUTIC DRUG MONITORING

Adverse Drug Effects

*Kara L. Murray, PharmD, Susanna Sowell, PharmD,
and Carlton K. K. Lee, PharmD, MPH*

The following tables list common antimicrobial adverse drug reactions with a 1% or higher incidence. These tables are limited to those adverse reactions for which such incidence has been published. Drugs are categorized by organ system. For additional information, see the specific drug's monograph in the formulary chapter or the package insert.

I. BLOOD

Adverse Effect	Medication
Anemia	Amphotericin B (liposomal), atovaquone, botulinum immune globulin intravenous, caspofungin, cidofovir, flucytosine, foscarnet, ganciclovir, linezolid, meropenem, micafungin, palivizumab, pentamidine isethionate, posaconazole, pyrimethamine, quinupristin + dalfopristin, ribavirin, rifabutin, rifapentine, silver sulfadiazine, sulfadiazine, sulfisoxazole, thalidomide, trimethoprim, trimetrexate, valganciclovir, zalcitabine, zidovudine
Eosinophilia	Caspofungin, cefaclor, cefdinir, cefoperazone, ceftibuten, ceftizoxime, ceftriaxone, cefuroxime, daptomycin, dirithromycin, enfuvirtide, micafungin, ticarcillin, vancomycin
Increased prothrombin time	Amphotericin B, caspofungin, clarithromycin, delavirdine, ertapenem, piperacillin + tazobactam
Leukopenia	Albendazole, amphotericin B (liposomal), atovaquone, caspofungin, ceftriaxone, ertapenem, famciclovir, flucytosine, foscarnet, ganciclovir, ivermectin, linezolid, micafungin, pentamidine isethionate, pyrimethamine, ribavirin, rifabutin, rifapentine, ritonavir, silver sulfadiazine, sulfadiazine, sulfisoxazole, suramin, thalidomide, zidovudine

Adverse Effect	Medication
Neutropenia	Atazanavir, atovaquone, caspofungin, cefoperazone, cephapirin, cidofovir, ertapenem, famciclovir, fosamprenavir, ganciclovir, indinavir, lamivudine, linezolid, lopinavir + ritonavir, maraviroc, micafungin, nelfinavir, posaconazole, rifabutin, rifapentine, ritonavir, tenofovir disoproxil fumarate, thalidomide, trimetrexate, vancomycin
Positive Coombs test	Cefepime, cefoperazone, ceftazidime
Thrombocytopenia	Abacavir sulfate, amphotericin b (cholesteryl sulfate), amphotericin B (liposomal), atazanavir, caspofungin, flucytosine, foscarnet, ganciclovir, lamivudine, linezolid, lopinavir + ritonavir, micafungin, pentamidine isethionate, posaconazole, pyrimethamine, rifabutin, rifapentine, sulfadiazine, sulfisoxazole, suramin, trimetrexate, valganciclovir, voriconazole

II. CARDIOVASCULAR

Adverse Effect	Medication
Arrhythmia	Amphotericin B (liposomal), melarsoprol, quinidine
Bradycardia	Amphotericin B (liposomal)
Chest pain	Amphotericin B (liposomal), daptomycin, ertapenem, foscarnet, levofloxacin, ofloxacin, pentamidine isethionate, saquinavir, zidovudine
Flushing	Amphotericin B (conventional), amphotericin B (liposomal), cytomegalovirus immune globulin intravenous, foscarnet, immune globulin intravenous (human), micafungin
Hypotension	Amantadine, amphotericin b (conventional), amphotericin B, (cholesteryl sulfate), amphotericin B (lipid), amphotericin B (liposomal), bacitracin ± polymyxin B sulfate, botulinum immune globulin intravenous, caspofungin, clindamycin, daptomycin, ertapenem, ethionamide, foscarnet, ivermectin, pentamidine isethionate, quinidine, rho (d) immune globulin intravenous (human), thalidomide, vancomycin, voriconazole
Hypertension	Amphotericin B (conventional), amphotericin b (liposomal), botulinum immune globulin intravenous, caspofungin, daptomycin, ertapenem, foscarnet, imiquimod, itraconazole, lopinavir + ritonavir, maraviroc, melarsoprol, micafungin, piperacillin + tazobactam, posaconazole, rho (d) immune globulin intravenous (human), rifapentine, voriconazole
QTc prolongation	Posaconazole, quinidine
Tachycardia	Amphotericin B (cholesteryl sulfate), amphotericin B (liposomal), botulinum immune globulin intravenous, caspofungin, ertapenem, imipenem + cilastatin, immune globulin intravenous (human), ivermectin, rho (d) immune globulin intravenous (human), voriconazole

III. CENTRAL NERVOUS SYSTEM

Adverse Effect	Medication
Anxiety	Abacavir sulfate, amantadine, amphotericin B (liposomal), atovaquone, daptomycin, delavirdine, efavirenz, ertapenem, foscarnet, rimantadine, ritonavir, saquinavir, thalidomide, zidovudine
Ataxia	Amantadine, foscarnet
Chills/Rigors	Amphotericin B (conventional), amphotericin B (cholesteryl sulfate), amphotericin B (lipid), amphotericin B (liposomal), caspofungin, cidofovir, cytomegalovirus immune globulin intravenous (human), foscarnet, halofantrine, hepatitis B immune globulin intravenous (human), iodoquinol, immune globulin intravenous (human), lamivudine, lopinavir + ritonavir, mefloquine hcl, melarsoprol, micafungin, miconazole, rho (d) immune globulin intravenous (human), terconazole, trimetrexate, vancomycin, voriconazole, zanamivir, zidovudine
Confusion	Amantadine, amphotericin B (conventional), Amphotericin b (liposomal), ertapenem, ethambutol HCL, foscarnet, ganciclovir, griseofulvin, melarsoprol, pentamidine isethionate, thalidomide, trimetrexate, valganciclovir, zidovudine
Depression	Abacavir sulfate, amantadine, amphotericin B (liposomal), amprenavir, atazanavir, delavirdine, efavirenz, emtricitabine, fosamprenavir, foscarnet, lamivudine, lopinavir + ritonavir, maraviroc, saquinavir, tenofovir disoproxil fumarate, valacyclovir, zidovudine
Dizziness	Abacavir sulfate, amphotericin B (liposomal), atazanavir, atovaquone, atovaquone + proguanil, caspofungin, cefprozil, ceftibuten, ciprofloxacin, colistimethate sodium, daptomycin, dirithromycin, efavirenz, emtricitabine, ertapenem, foscarnet, fosfomycin, griseofulvin, halofantrine, hepatitis B immune globulin intravenous (human), hydroxychloroquine, imiquimod, indinavir, isoniazid, itraconazole, ivermectin, lamivudine, levofloxacin, lindane, linezolid, maraviroc, metronidazole, micafungin, nifurtimox, norfloxacin, ofloxacin, pentamidine isethionate, phenazopyridine HCl, posaconazole, praziquantel, quinidine, rho (D) immune globulin intravenous (human), rifapentine, rimantadine, ritonavir, sulfadiazine, sulfisoxazole, tenofovir disoproxil fumarate, terbinafine, thalidomide, thiabendazole, tinidazole, valacyclovir, voriconazole, zalcitabine, zanamivir, zidovudine

Adverse Effect	Medication
Fever	Abacavir sulfate, amoxicillin, amphotericin B (conventional), amphotericin B (cholesteryl sulfate), amphotericin B (lipid), atazanavir, atovaquone, caspofungin, cefepime, ceftizoxime, cidofovir, cytomegalovirus immune globulin intravenous (human), daptomycin, delavirdine, diphtheria antitoxin, emtricitabine, ertapenem, foscarnet, ganciclovir, hepatitis B immune globulin intravenous (human), imiquimod, indinavir, iodoquinol, itraconazole, lamivudine, levofloxacin, linezolid, lopinavir + ritonavir, maraviroc, mefloquine HCl, melarsoprol, miconazole, palivizumab, piperacillin + tazobactam, posaconazole, rabies immune globulin intravenous (human), raltegravir, rho (D) immune globulin intravenous (human), ritonavir, sulfadiazine, sulfisoxazole, suramin, tenofovir disoproxil fumarate, terconazole, tetanus immune globulin intravenous (human), thalidomide, trimetrexate, valganciclovir, vancomycin, voriconazole, zalcitabine, zanamivir
Headache	Abacavir sulfate, acyclovir, albendazole, amantadine, amphotericin B (conventional), amphotericin B (cholesteryl sulfate), amphotericin B (lipid), amphotericin B (liposomal), amprenavir, atazanavir, atovaquone, atovaquone + proguanil, azithromycin, caspofungin, cefdinir, cefditoren, cefepime, ceftibuten, cidofovir, ciprofloxacin, clarithromycin, daptomycin, delavirdine, dirithromycin, doripenem, efavirenz, emtricitabine, ertapenem, famciclovir, fluconazole, fosamprenavir, foscarnet, fosfomycin, furazolidone, ganciclovir, griseofulvin, halofantrine, hepatitis B immune globulin intravenous (human), hydroxychloroquine, imiquimod, indinavir, iodoquinol, itraconazole, ketoconazole, lamivudine, levofloxacin, linezolid, lopinavir + ritonavir, loracarbef, mefloquine HCl, melarsoprol, meropenem, metronidazole, micafungin, mupirocin, nevirapine, nifurtimox, nitazoxanide, nitrofurantoin, norfloxacin, ofloxacin, penciclovir, pentamidine isethionate, phenazopyridine, piperacillin + tazobactam, posaconazole, praziquantel, quinidine, quinine, quinupristin + dalfopristin, raltegravir, retapamulin, rho (D) immune globulin intravenous (human), ribavirin, rifabutin, rifapentine, rimantadine, saquinavir, stavudine, sulfadiazine, sulfisoxazole, suramin, tenofovir disoproxil fumarate, terbinafine, thalidomide, thiabendazole, tinidazole, valacyclovir, valganciclovir, varicella-zoster immune globulin intravenous (human), voriconazole, zalcitabine, zanamivir, zidovudine
Increased intracranial pressure	Albendazole

Adverse Effect	Medication
Insomnia	Amantadine, atazanavir, atovaquone, caspofungin, ciprofloxacin, daptomycin, dirithromycin, efavirenz, emtricitabine, enfuvirtide, ertapenem, foscarnet, griseofulvin, lamivudine, levofloxacin, linezolid, lopinavir + ritonavir, maraviroc, ofloxacin, piperacillin + tazobactam, posaconazole, ribavirin, rimantadine, ritonavir, saquinavir, tenofovir disoproxil fumarate, thalidomide, valganciclovir, zidovudine
Malaise	Acyclovir, amantadine, amphotericin B (conventional), amphotericin B (liposomal), foscarnet, halofantrine, hepatitis B immune globulin intravenous (human), imiquimod, indinavir, itraconazole, praziquantel, rho (D) immune globulin intravenous (human), thalidomide, tinidazole, zalcitabine, zanamivir, zidovudine
Neuropathy	Atazanavir, didanosine, emtricitabine, foscarnet, ganciclovir, isoniazid, iodoquinol, lamivudine, maraviroc, melarsoprol, stavudine, suramin, tenofovir disoproxil fumarate, thalidomide, trimetrexate, valganciclovir, zalcitabine
Neurotoxicity	Amikacin, gentamicin, kanamycin, melarsoprol (encephalopathy), streptomycin sulfate, tobramycin
Pain, unspecified	Amphotericin B (lipid), amphotericin B (liposomal), ampicillin, bacitracin ± polymyxin B sulfate, caspofungin, cefazolin, ciclopirox, cidofovir, efavirenz, imiquimod, kanamycin, kunecatechins, levofloxacin, maraviroc, meropenem, miconazole, ofloxacin, penicillin G (benzathine), penicillin G (procaine), piperacillin, piperacillin + tazobactam, podofilox, polymyxin B sulfate + neomycin sulfate + hydrocortisone, quinupristin + dalfopristin, rifapentine, saquinavir, tenofovir disoproxil fumarate, tetanus immune globulin intravenous (human), thalidomide, ticarcillin, varicella-zoster immune globulin intravenous (human)
Seizure	Foscarnet, imipenem + cilastatin, lindane, melarsoprol, thiabendazole, valganciclovir, zalcitabine, zidovudine
Somnolence	Amphotericin B (liposomal), ciprofloxacin, efavirenz, foscarnet, indinavir, loracarbef, micafungin, ofloxacin, posaconazole, rho (D) immune globulin intravenous (human), thalidomide, zidovudine
Weakness	Amphotericin B (liposomal), atovaquone, atovaquone + proguanil, cidofovir, daptomycin, dirithromycin, emtricitabine, ertapenem, ethionamide, foscarnet, fosfomycin, ganciclovir, indinavir, iodoquinol, isoniazid, lopinavir + ritonavir, norfloxacin, posaconazole, quinidine, rabies immune globulin intravenous (human), rimantadine, ritonavir, saquinavir, tenofovir disoproxil fumarate, thalidomide, tinidazole, zidovudine

7

ADVERSE DRUG EFFECTS

IV. SKIN

Adverse Effect	Medication
Alopecia	Albendazole, amphotericin B (liposomal), cidofovir, hydroxychloroquine, imiquimod, selenium sulfide
Angioedema	Hepatitis B immune globulin intravenous (human), tetanus immune globulin intravenous (human), zidovudine
Dermatitis	Amoxicillin, ampicillin, botulinum immune globulin intravenous, butenafine, ketoconazole, lindane, maraviroc, neomycin sulfate + polymyxin B sulfate ± bacitracin, nystatin, palivizumab, penciclovir, polymyxin B sulfate + neomycin sulfate + hydrocortisone, retapamulin, thalidomide, tolnaftate, undecylenic acid
Erythema multiforme	Kunecatechins, loracarbef, silver sulfadiazine
Hives/Rash	Abacavir sulfate, acyclovir, amoxicillin, amoxicillin + clavulanic acid, amphotericin B (cholesteryl sulfate), amphotericin B (lipid), ampicillin, ampicillin + sulbactam, amprenavir, atazanavir, atovaquone, aztreonam, bacitracin ± polymyxin B sulfate, botulinum immune globulin intravenous, caspofungin, cefaclor, cefdinir, cefepime, cefoperazone, cefotaxime, cefpodoxime proxetil, cefprozil, ceftizoxime, ceftriaxone, cidofovir, ciprofloxacin, clarithromycin, clindamycin, clofazimine, daptomycin, delavirdine, dirithromycin, doripenem, efavirenz, emtricitabine, ertapenem, famciclovir, fluconazole, flucytosine, fosamprenavir, foscarnet, fosfomycin, ganciclovir, griseofulvin, hepatitis B immune globulin intravenous (human), hydroxychloroquine, imipenem + cilastatin, imiquimod, indinavir, iodoquinol, itraconazole, kunecatechins, lamivudine, levofloxacin, linezolid, lopinavir + ritonavir, loracarbef, maraviroc, mefloquine HCl, melarsoprol, meropenem, methenamine mandelate, micafungin, miconazole, mupirocin, nafcillin, nelfinavir, neomycin sulfate + polymyxin B sulfate ± bacitracin, nevirapine, nifurtimox, ofloxacin, palivizumab, pentamadine, permethrin, piperacillin, piperacillin + tazobactam, polymyxin B sulfate + neomycin sulfate + hydrocortisone, posaconazole, quinidine, quinupristin + dalfopristin, rho (D) immune globulin intravenous (human), rifabutin, rifapentine, ritonavir, saquinavir, silver sulfadiazine, stavudine, sulfadiazine, sulfamethoxazole + trimethoprim, sulfisoxazole, suramin, tenofovir disoproxil fumarate, terbinafine, thalidomide, thiabendazole, trimethoprim, trimetrexate, undecylenic acid, vancomycin, varicella-zoster immune globulin intravenous (human), voriconazole, zalcitabine, zidovudine

Adverse Effect	Medication
Itching/Pruritis	Acyclovir, amphotericin B (liposomal), atovaquone, atovaquone + proguanil, bacitracin ± polymyxin B sulfate, butenafine, caspofungin, cefepime, cefotaxime, ceftizoxime, ciclopirox, clofazimine, daptomycin, dirithromycin, efavirenz, ertapenem, famciclovir, fosamprenavir, foscarnet, ganciclovir, gentamicin, halofantrine, hydroxychloroquine, imiquimod, indinavir, itraconazole, ivermectin, ketoconazole, kunecatechins, levofloxacin, loracarbef, maraviroc, meropenem, micafungin, miconazole, mupirocin, naftifine, ofloxacin, oxiconazole, permethrin, piperacillin + tazobactam, podofilox, polymyxin B sulfate + neomycin sulfate + hydrocortisone, posaconazole, pyrethrins + piperonyl butoxide, quinupristin + dalfopristin, retapamulin, rho (D) immune globulin intravenous (human), rifapentine, silver sulfadiazine, sulconazole, sulfacetamide sodium, sulfadiazine, sulfisoxazole, terbinafine, thalidomide, tolnaftate, trimetrexate, varicella-zoster immune globulin intravenous (human), voriconazole, zalcitabine, zidovudine
Stevens-Johnson syndrome	Amprenavir, clindamycin, nystatin, sulfacetamide, sulfadiazine, sulfisoxazole, sulfamethoxazole + trimethoprim, thiabendazole, zidovudine
Toxic epidermal necrolysis syndrome	Zidovudine
Phlebitis/ Thrombophlebitis	Amphotericin B (liposomal), ampicillin + sulbactam, aztreonam, caspofungin, cefuroxime, cephapirin, clindamycin, doripenem, ertapenem, erythromycin, imipenem + cilastatin, melarsoprol, meropenem, micafungin, piperacillin, quinupristin + dalfopristin, ticarcillin

V. GASTROINTESTINAL

Adverse Effect	Medication
Abdominal pain	Albendazole, amoxicillin + clavulanic acid, amphotericin B (conventional), amphotericin B (cholesteryl sulfate), amphotericin B (lipid), amphotericin B (liposomal), ampicillin, atazanavir, atovaquone, atovaquone + proguanil, azithromycin, caspofungin, cefdinir, cefditoren, cefixime, cefpodoxime proxetil, cefprozil, ceftibuten, ciprofloxacin, clarithromycin, clindamycin, clofazimine, cloxacillin, daptomycin, delavirdine, dicloxacillin sodium, dirithromycin, efavirenz, emtricitabine, enfuvirtide, ertapenem, erythromycin, ethambutol HCl, famciclovir, fluconazole, flucytosine, fosamprenavir, foscarnet, fosfomycin, furazolidone, ganciclovir, griseofulvin, halofantrine, hydroxychloroquine, indinavir, iodoquinol, isoniazid, itraconazole, ketoconazole, lamivudine, levofloxacin, lopinavir + ritonavir, loracarbef, maraviroc,

Adverse Effect	Medication
Abdominal pain—cont.	mebendazole, mefloquine HCl, micafungin, nevirapine, nifurtimox, nitazoxanide, norfloxacin, nystatin, ofloxacin, oseltamivir phosphate, para-aminosalicylic acid, paromomycin sulfate, phenazopyridine hcl, piperacillin + tazobactam, posaconazole, praziquantel, primaquine phosphate, pyrantel pamoate, pyrimethamine, quinidine, rho (D) immune globulin intravenous (human), rifabutin, rimantadine, ritonavir, saquinavir, selenium sulfide, tenofovir disoproxil fumarate, terbinafine, terconazole, tinidazole, valacyclovir, valganciclovir, voriconazole, zalcitabine, zanamivir, zidovudine
Anorexia	Amantadine, amphotericin B (conventional), amphotericin B (liposomal), atovaquone, atovaquone + proguanil, bacitracin ± polymyxin B sulfate, caspofungin, cidofovir, efavirenz, enfuvirtide, ethambutol HCl, ethionamide, flucytosine, foscarnet, halofantrine, hydroxychloroquine, indinavir, isoniazid, itraconazole, lamivudine, lopinavir + ritonavir, loracarbef, mefloquine HCl, metronidazole, micafungin, miconazole, nifurtimox, ofloxacin, pentamidine isethionate, posaconazole, praziquantel, pyrantel pamoate, pyrazinamide, pyrimethamine, quinidine, ribavirin, rifabutin, rifapentine, rimantadine, ritonavir, saquinavir, sulfadiazine, sulfamethoxazole + trimethoprim, sulfisoxazole, tenofovir disoproxil fumarate, terbinafine, thalidomide, thiabendazole, tinidazole, zalcitabine, zanamivir, zidovudine
Colitis/ Pseudomembranous enterocolitis	Cefotaxime, clindamycin
Constipation	Amantadine, amphotericin B (liposomal), atovaquone, daptomycin, enfuvirtide, ertapenem, foscarnet, levofloxacin, linezolid, maraviroc, meropenem, piperacillin + tazobactam, posaconazole, saquinavir, thalidomide, tinidazole, zidovudine
Diarrhea	Abacavir sulfate, acyclovir, amantadine, amoxicillin + clavulanic acid, amphotericin B (conventional), amphotericin B (cholesteryl sulfate), amphotericin B (lipid), amphotericin B (liposomal), ampicillin, ampicillin + sulbactam, amprenavir, atazanavir, atovaquone, atovaquone + proguanil, azithromycin, aztreonam, bacitracin ± polymyxin B sulfate, botulinum immune globulin intravenous, caspofungin, cefaclor, cefadroxil, cefazolin, cefdinir, cefditoren, cefepime, cefixime, cefoperazone, cefotaxime, cefotetan, cefoxitin, cefpodoxime proxetil, cefprozil, ceftazidime, ceftibuten, ceftriaxone, cephalexin, cephradine, chloroquine phosphate, cidofovir, ciprofloxacin, clarithromycin, clindamycin, clofazimine, cloxacillin, daptomycin, delavirdine, dicloxacillin sodium, dirithromycin, doripenem, efavirenz, emtricitabine, enfuvirtide, ertapenem, ethionamide, famciclovir, fluconazole, flucytosine,

Adverse Effect	Medication
	fosamprenavir, foscarnet, fosfomycin, furazolidone, ganciclovir, griseofulvin, halofantrine, hydroxychloroquine, imipenem + cilastatin, imiquimod, indinavir, iodoquinol, itraconazole, ivermectin, lamivudine, levofloxacin, linezolid, lopinavir + ritonavir, loracarbef, mebendazole, mefloquine HCl, meropenem, metronidazole, micafungin, miconazole, minocycline, moxifloxacin, nelfinavir, neomycin sulfate, nevirapine, nitazoxanide, nystatin, ofloxacin, oxacillin, palivizumab, para-aminosalicylic acid, paromomycin sulfate, penicillin V potassium, pentamidine isethionate, piperacillin, piperacillin + tazobactam, posaconazole, pyrantel pamoate, quinidine, quinine, quinupristin + dalfopristin, raltegravir, retapamulin, rho (D) immune globulin intravenous (human), rifabutin, rifapentine, ritonavir, saquinavir, stavudine, sulfadiazine, sulfisoxazole, tenofovir disoproxil fumarate, terbinafine, tetracycline HCl, thalidomide, thiabendazole, valganciclovir, voriconazole, zalcitabine, zanamivir
Dyspepsia	Amphotericin B (liposomal), atovaquone, cefditoren, cefixime, ceftibuten, ciprofloxacin, clarithromycin, daptomycin, dirithromycin, efavirenz, emtricitabine, ertapenem, foscarnet, imiquimod, indinavir, lamivudine, levofloxacin, lopinavir + ritonavir, maraviroc, methenamine mandelate, micafungin, piperacillin + tazobactam, posaconazole, rifapentine, ritonavir, saquinavir, tenofovir disoproxil fumarate, terbinafine, tinidazole, zidovudine
Nausea	Abacavir sulfate, acyclovir, albendazole, amantadine, amoxicillin + clavulanic acid, amphotericin B (conventional), amphotericin B (cholesteryl sulfate), amphotericin B (lipid), amphotericin B (liposomal), amprenavir, atazanavir, atovaquone, atovaquone + proguanil, azithromycin, aztreonam, bacitracin ± polymyxin B sulfate, caspofungin, cefdinir, cefditoren, cefepime, cefixime, cefotaxime, cefpodoxime proxetil, cefprozil, ceftibuten, chloroquine phosphate, cidofovir, ciprofloxacin, clarithromycin, clindamycin, clofazimine, clotrimazole, cloxacillin, cytomegalovirus immune globulin intravenous (human), daptomycin, delavirdine, dicloxacillin sodium, dirithromycin, doripenem, efavirenz, emtricitabine, enfuvirtide, ertapenem, erythromycin, ethambutol hcl, ethionamide, famciclovir, fluconazole, flucytosine, fosamprenavir, foscarnet, fosfomycin, furazolidone, ganciclovir, griseofulvin, halfantrine, hepatitis B immune globulin intravenous (human), hydroxychloroquine, imipenem + cilastatin, imiquimod, immune globulin intravenous (human), indinavir, iodoquinol, isoniazid, itraconazole, ivermectin, ketoconazole, lamivudine, levofloxacin, linezolid, lopinavir + ritonavir, loracarbef,

Adverse Effect	Medication
Nausea—cont.	mebendazole, mefloquine HCl, meropenem, methenamine mandelate, metronidazole, micafungin, miconazole, minocycline, moxifloxacin, mupirocin, nelfinavir, neomycin sulfate, nevirapine, nifurtimox, nitazoxanide, nitrofurantoin, norfloxacin, nystatin, ofloxacin, oseltamivir phosphate, oxacillin, para-aminosalicylic acid, paromomycin sulfate, penicillin V potassium, pentamidine isethionate, piperacillin + tazobactam, podofilox, posaconazole, praziquantel, primaquine phosphate, pyrantel pamoate, pyrazinamide, quinidine, quinine, quinupristin + dalfopristin, raltegravir, retapamulin, rho (D) immune globulin intravenous (human), ribavirin, rifabutin, rifapentine, rimantadine, ritonavir, saquinavir, stavudine, sulfadiazine, sulfamethoxazole + trimethoprim, sulfisoxazole, suramin, tenofovir disoproxil fumarate, tetracycline HCl, thalidomide, thiabendazole, tinidazole, trimetrexate, valacyclovir, valganciclovir, vancomycin, varicella-zoster immune globulin intravenous (human), voriconazole, zanamivir, zidovudine
Pancreatitis	Enfuvirtide, lamivudine, linezolid, stibogluconate, zidovudine
Vomiting	Abacavir sulfate, acyclovir, albendazole, amoxicillin + clavulanic acid, amphotericin B (conventional), amphotericin B (lipid), amphotericin B (liposomal), ampicillin, amprenavir, atazanavir, atovaquone, atovaquone + proguanil, azithromycin, aztreonam, bacitracin ± polymyxin B sulfate, botulinum immune globulin intravenous, caspofungin, cefdinir, cefditoren, cefepime, cefotaxime, cefpodoxime proxetil, cefprozil, ceftibuten, cidofovir, ciprofloxacin, clarithromycin, clindamycin, clofazimine, clotrimazole, cloxacillin, cytomegalovirus immune globulin intravenous (human), daptomycin, delavirdine, dirithromycin, efavirenz, emtricitabine, ertapenem, erythromycin, ethambutol HCl, ethionamide, famciclovir, fluconazole, flucytosine, foscarnet, fosamprenavir, furazolidone, ganciclovir, griseofulvin, halofantrine, hepatitis B immune globulin intravenous (human), hydroxychloroquine, imipenem + cilastatin, indinavir, iodoquinol, isoniazid, itraconazole, ketoconazole, lamivudine, levofloxacin, linezolid, lopinavir + ritonavir, loracarbef, mebendazole, mefloquine HCl, meropenem, metronidazole, micafungin, miconazole, neomycin sulfate, nifurtimox, nitazoxanide, nystatin, ofloxacin, oseltamivir phosphate, palivizumab, para-aminosalicylic acid, paromomycin sulfate, penicillin V potassium, pentamidine isethionate, piperacillin + tazobactam, podofilox, posaconazole, praziquantel, primaquine phosphate, pyrantel pamoate, pyrazinamide, pyrimethamine, quinidine, quinine, quinupristin + dalfopristin, rho (D) immune globulin intravenous

Adverse Effect	Medication
	(human), rifabutin, rifapentine, rimantadine, ritonavir, saquinavir, selenium sulfide, stavudine, sulfadiazine, sulfamethoxazole + trimethoprim, sulfisoxazole, suramin, tenofovir disoproxil fumarate, thiabendazole, tinidazole, trimetrexate, valacyclovir, valganciclovir, vancomycin, voriconazole, zalcitabine, zanamivir, zidovudine

VI. ENDOCRINE/METABOLIC

Adverse Effect	Medication
Hyperglycemia	Amphotericin B (liposomal), amprenavir, atazanavir, cefditoren, clofazimine, fosamprenavir, lopinavir + ritonavir, quinupristin + dalfopristin, ritonavir, saquinavir, zalcitabine
Hypoglycemia	Atovaquone, pentamidine isethionate, saquinavir, zalcitabine
Hyperkalemia	Amphotericin B (liposomal), daptomycin, dirithromycin, pentamidine isethionate, saquinavir
Hypokalemia	Amphotericin B (conventional), amphotericin B (cholesteryl sulfate), amphotericin B (lipid), amphotericin B (liposomal), caspofungin, daptomycin, foscarnet, itraconazole, micafungin, posaconazole, voriconazole
Hypernatremia	Amphotericin B (liposomal)
Hyponatremia	Amphotericin B (liposomal), atovaquone, botulinum immune globulin intravenous, foscarnet, trimetrexate, zalcitabine
Hyperuricemia	Didanosine, ethambutol HCl, rifapentine, ritonavir
Increased HDL	Efavirenz
Hypercholesterolemia	Amprenavir, atazanavir, efavirenz, imiquimod, lopinavir + ritonavir, ritonavir, saquinavir
Hypertriglyceridemia	Abacavir sulfate, amprenavir, atazanavir, emtricitabine, enfuvirtide, fosamprenavir, itraconazole, lopinavir + ritonavir, ritonavir, saquinavir

HDL, high density lipoprotein.

VII. RENAL/GENITOURINARY

Adverse Effect	Medication
Azotemia	Amphotericin B (conventional)
Hematuria	Amphotericin B (liposomal), caspofungin, cefditoren, rifapentine, sulfadiazine, thalidomide
Interstitial nephritis	Silver sulfadiazine, sulfadiazine
Nephrotoxicity/Renal failure	Acyclovir, amikacin, amphotericin B (cholesteryl sulfate), amphotericin B (lipid), amphotericin B (liposomal), caspofungin, cidofovir, colistimethate sodium, daptomycin, foscarnet, gentamicin, kanamycin, melarsoprol, neomycin sulfate + polymyxin B sulfate ± bacitracin, pentamidine isethionate, rho (D) immune globulin intravenous (human), streptomycin sulfate, sulfadiazine, suramin, tobramycin

7

ADVERSE DRUG EFFECTS

Adverse Effect	Medication
Renal tubular acidosis	Amphotericin B (conventional)
Vaginitis	Amoxicillin + clavulanic acid, cefaclor, cefprozil, ertapenem, fosfomycin, levofloxacin, loracarbef, ofloxacin, tioconazole

VIII. RESPIRATORY

Adverse Effect	Medication
Bronchospasm	Ampicillin + sulbactam, foscarnet, maraviroc
Dyspnea	Amphotericin B (cholesteryl sulfate), amphotericin B (lipid), amphotericin B (liposomal), botulinum immune globulin intravenous, dirithromycin, ertapenem, foscarnet, immune globulin intravenous (human), levofloxacin, pentamidine isethionate, thalidomide, zidovudine
Pulmonary fibrosis	Nitrofurantoin (long-term use)
Stridor	Botulinum immune globulin intravenous, foscarnet
Tachypnea	Amphotericin B (conventional), botulinum immune globulin intravenous

IX. HEPATIC

Adverse Effect	Medication
AST elevation	Abacavir sulfate, amphotericin B (liposomal), amprenavir, atazanavir, ciprofloxacin, isoniazid, ivermectin, lopinavir + ritonavir, maraviroc, nelfinavir, nevirapine, posaconazole, rifabutin, rifapentine, saquinavir, thalidomide, trimetrexate, valacyclovir, voriconazole
ALT elevation	Amphotericin B (liposomal), amprenavir, atazanavir, ceftibuten, ciprofloxacin, isoniazid, ivermectin, lopinavir + ritonavir, maraviroc, nelfinavir, nevirapine, palivizumab, posaconazole, rifabutin, rifapentine, saquinavir, thalidomide, trimetrexate, voriconazole
Alkaline phosphatase elevation	Amphotericin B (liposomal), caspofungin, cefdinir, ceftizoxime, cefuroxime, daptomycin, ertapenem, micafungin, posaconazole, trimetrexate, voriconazole
Hepatitis	Ethionamide, flucytosine, isoniazid, itraconazole, silver sulfadiazine, sulfadiazine, sulfisoxazole, sulfamethoxazole + trimethoprim, zidovudine
Hepatic failure/ Hepatic toxicity	Abacavir sulfate, cefoperazone, melarsoprol, nevirapine, rifampin, stibogluconate
Hyperbilirubinemia/ Jaundice	Amphotericin B (liposomal), atazanavir, caspofungin, ceftibuten, delavirdine, emtricitabine, erythromycin, ethionamide, famciclovir, flucytosine, indinavir, lopinavir + ritonavir, maraviroc, micafungin, posaconazole, quinupristin + dalfopristin, saquinavir, stavudine, sulfadiazine, suramin, thalidomide, trimetrexate, voriconazole, zalcitabine, zidovudine

ALT, alanine aminotransferase; AST, aspartate aminotransferase.

X. OCULAR

Adverse Effect	Medication
Blurred vision	Ivermectin, posaconazole, quinidine, quinine, voriconazole
Photophobia	Levofloxacin, ofloxacin, voriconazole, zidovudine
Visual disturbances	Foscarnet, hydroxychloroquine, iodoquinol, levofloxacin, ofloxacin, terbinafine, voriconazole

XI. MUSCULOSKELETAL

Adverse Effect	Medication
Arthralgia	Abacavir sulfate, amphotericin B (conventional), amphotericin B (liposomal), cytomegalovirus immune globulin intravenous (human), daptomycin, emtricitabine, foscarnet, hepatitis B immune globulin intravenous (human), ivermectin, lamivudine, melarsoprol, pyrazinamide, quinupristin + dalfopristin, rho (D) immune globulin intravenous (human), rifapentine, ritonavir, stibogluconate, thalidomide, valacyclovir, zanamivir, zidovudine
Myalgia	Abacavir sulfate, amphotericin B (conventional), amphotericin B (liposomal), atazanavir, caspofungin, emtricitabine, enfuvirtide, foscarnet, halofantrine, hepatitis B immune globulin intravenous (human), imiquimod, lamivudine, lopinavir + ritonavir, maraviroc, mefloquine HCl, posaconazole, pyrazinamide, quinupristin + dalfopristin, rho (D) immune globulin intravenous (human), rifabutin, ritonavir, stibogluconate, suramin, tenofovir disoproxil fumarate, thalidomide, varicella-zoster immune globulin intravenous (human), zalcitabine, zanamivir, zidovudine
Rhabdomyolysis	Zidovudine

XII. HYPERSENSITIVITY

Adverse Effect	Medication
Anaphylaxis	Amoxicillin, ampicillin, bacitracin + polymyxin B sulfate, diphtheria antitoxin, erythromycin, hepatitis B immune globulin intravenous, neomycin sulfate + polymyxin B sulfate ± bacitracin, penicillin G (benzathine), rho (D) immune globulin intravenous, tetanus immune globulin intravenous, trimetrexate, varicella-zoster immune globulin intravenous, zidovudine
Serum sickness	Diphtheria antitoxin, immune globulin intravenous

XIII. OTHER

Adverse Effect	Medication
Ototoxicity (hearing loss)	Amikacin, gentamicin, streptomycin sulfate, tobramycin
Vestibular toxicity	Amikacin, gentamicin, minocycline, streptomycin sulfate, tobramycin

REFERENCES

1. Kanamycin: Schaumberg, IL: American Pharmaceutical Partners, Inc. August 2003.
2. Nafcillin: Broomfield, CO: Sandoz, Inc. January 2004.
3. Lexi-Comp Online. Available at: http://online.lexi.com/crlonline
4. Micromedex Healthcare Series. Available at: https://www.thomsonhc.com
5. United States Pharmacopeia: Drug Information and Quality Program. Available at: http://www.uspdqi.org/pubs/monographs/index1.html
6. Drug Facts and Comparisons. CliniSphere Version ISBN 1-57439-036-8. St. Louis, MO: Wolters Kluwer Health, Inc. *Updated monthly*

Recommended Antimicrobial Prophylaxis for Selected Infectious Agents and Conditions

Julia A. McMillan, MD, and George K. Siberry, MD, MPH

RECOMMENDED ANTIMICROBIAL PROPHYLAXIS FOR SELECTED INFECTIOUS AGENTS AND CONDITIONS

Exposure	Recommended Empiric Preventive Therapy	Alternative Preventive Therapy	Comments
SITUATIONAL			
Bite, animal	Amoxicillin/clavulanate × 2-3 days	[3rd-generation cephalosporin or TMP-SMX] + clindamycin	Consider need for tetanus and rabies prophylaxis. Longer treatment indicated for immunocompromised patients and wounds that penetrate joints.
Bite, human	Amoxicilline/clavulanate × 2-3 days	[3rd-generation cephalosporin or TMP-SMX] + clindamycin	Consider need for tetanus prophylaxis. Longer treatment indicated for immunocompromised patients and wounds that penetrate joints.
CSF leak	23-valent pneumococcal polysacride vaccine + meningococcal vaccine (conjugate preferred) if ≥2 years old, in addition to conjugated *Haemophilus influenzae* type b and conjugated pneumococcal vaccines routinely recommended for all infants		Some experts recommend penicillin prophylaxis for traumatic CSF leak, but evidence of benefit is lacking.

Endocarditis	**For dental, oral, or upper respiratory tract or esophageal procedures:** Amoxicillin *Penicillin-allergic* Clindamycin *or* Cephalexin *or* Cefadroxil *or* Azithromycin *or* Clarithromycin	Clindamycin *or* Cefazolin IV *or* Ampicillin IV *or* Ceftriaxone	A single antibiotic dose should be administered 30–60 minutes prior to the procedure. Cephalosporins should not be used for people with immediate-type hypersensitivity to penicillin. Efficacy of prophylaxis is not proven for all circumstances. See Wilson, *Circulation* 2007;15:1 for list of conditions and procedures for which prophylaxis is recommended.
	Cardiac surgery with placement of intracardiac or intravascular material 1st generation cephalosporin **High-risk patient (prior cardiac surgery, prior endocarditis):** [Ampicillin IV or IM + gentamicin IV or IM], *then* Amoxicillin PO or Ampicillin IV *Penicillin-allergic:* Vancomycin IV + gentamicin IV or IM	Vancomycin	Administer antibiotic immediately before the procedure; repeat dose during prolonged procedures; continue prophylaxis no more than 48 hr
Immunocompromised host: asplenic states	Penicillin V <5 yr, 125 mg twice daily ≥5 yr, 250 mg twice daily		Age-appropriate immunization against *Streptococcus pneumoniae*, *H. influenzae*, and *Neisseria meningitidis* is recommended in addition to chemoprophylaxis. ≥2 yr: pneumococcal polysaccharide vaccine and meningococcal conjugate vaccine

RECOMMENDED ANTIMICROBIAL PROPHYLAXIS 8

RECOMMENDED ANTIMICROBIAL PROPHYLAXIS FOR SELECTED INFECTIOUS AGENTS AND CONDITIONS—cont'd

Exposure	Recommended Empiric Preventive Therapy	Alternative Preventive Therapy	Comments
Phagocyte function defect	TMP-SMX		Interferon gamma has been shown to prolong infection-free periods for children with chronic granulomatous disease.
Needle stick (hepatitis B, hepatitis C, HIV)	Immediate cleaning with copious soap and water indicated for all needle sticks.		Exposed person should be tested for HIV and hepatitis C at baseline and 4-6 and 12 wk and at 6 mo postexposure. Risk of HIV infection after percutaneous occupational exposure to HIV-infected blood is 0.03%; 0.09% after mucous membrane exposure. Risk after nonoccupational exposure is lower. CDC National Clinician's Postexposure hotline: 888-448-4911
Hepatitis B	No action if exposed person already hepatitis B immune. Source with unknown infection status: Hepatitis B vaccine series for nonimmune contact Source HBsAg+: One dose of hepatitis B immune globulin plus Hepatitis B vaccine series		

HIV	*Known HIV+ source:* 2- to 3-drug regimen for 4 wk depending on volume of exposure and HIV class status of source (see **http://www.cdc.gov/ mmwr/preview/mmwrhtml/rr5409a1.htm** and article by Havens[1]). Postexposure prophylaxis is generally not recommended following needlestick injury from unknown, nonoccupational source.	For healthy infant born to mother with untreated gonococcal infection, administer 1 dose of ceftriaxone IM or IV (25-50 mg/ kg) or cefotaxime IV or IM (100 mg/kg) in addition to prophylactic topical therapy to prevent *Chlamydia trachomatis.*
Ophthalmia neonatorum	Topical: silver nitrate (1%) *or* erythromycin ointment (0.5%) *or* Tetracycline ointment (1%)	
Recurrent otitis media	Amoxicillin *or* sulfisoxazole	
Rheumatic fever	Penicillin G benzathine 1.2 million U q4 wk *or* Penicillin V, 250 mg twice daily *or* Sulfadiazine or sulfisoxazole ≤27 kg: (0.5 g once daily) >27 kg: (1 g once daily) *Penicillin-allergic:* Erythromycin 250 mg twice daily	

RECOMMENDED ANTIMICROBIAL PROPHYLAXIS 8

RECOMMENDED ANTIMICROBIAL PROPHYLAXIS FOR SELECTED INFECTIOUS AGENTS AND CONDITIONS—cont'd

Exposure	Recommended Empiric Preventive Therapy	Alternative Preventive Therapy	Comments
Sexual contact or assault	**Prepubertal victim:** Ceftriaxone × 1 dose (prevention of gonorrhea) + azithromycin (2 g × 1 dose) *or* Erythromycin base or ethylsuccinate × 1 dose (prevention of *C. trachomatis*) + hepatitis B vaccine series (if not immune) + Consideration of metronidazole tid × 7 days (trichomoniasis and bacterial vaginosis) **Adolescent victim:** [Ceftriaxone × 1 dose *or* cefixime (400 mg) (gonorrhea)] + [Azithromycin (1 g × 1 dose) *or* doxycycline bid × 7 days *if not pregnant* (*C. trachomatis*)] + metronidazole (2 g × 1 dose) (trichomoniasis and bacterial vaginosis) + hepatitis B vaccine series if not immune		Chemoprophylaxis of prepubertal, asymptomatic child may not be indicated if follow-up is ensured. Laboratory tests for sexually transmitted infections should be performed prior to chemoprophylaxis. Consider HIV chemoprophylaxis, depending on circumstances of exposure. Consider emergency contraception.
Urinary tract infection	Nitrofurantoin *or* TMP-SMX		Amoxicillin for neonates

PREVENTION OF INFECTION DUE TO SPECIFIC BACTERIAL PATHOGENS

Note: Many of the infections below must be reported to the Health Department. Contact your local Health Department for the list of reportable diseases in your jurisdiction.

Anthrax	Ciprofloxacin or Doxycycline (for those ≥8 yr) for 60 days	If susceptibility testing confirms penicillin susceptibility, therapy can be changed to amoxicillin (80 mg/kg/day or 500 mg 3 times daily divided q8 hr)
Diphtheria	Erythromycin 50 mg/kg/day (max 2 g/day) × 10 days or IM benzathine penicillin G (600,000 U for children <30 kg and 1.2 million U for those ≥30 kg) + DTaP, dT, or Tdap as appropriate for age	Pharyngeal cultures should be obtained from all contacts prior to chemoprophylaxis. Follow-up cultures should also be obtained following therapy and, if positive, a second 10-day course of erythromycin should be given.
Haemophilus influenzae type b	Rifampin 20 mg/kg/day (in 1 dose/day) × 4 days (maximum 600 mg/day)	Prophylaxis is recommended only for household contacts in which there is at least 1 contact <4 yr who is incompletely immunized or an infant <1 yr who has not completed the primary series, or an immunocompromised child of any age or immunization status; and in nursery schools and child care centers with ≥2 cases of invasive disease within 60 days. Index patient should receive prophylaxis only if <2 yr and lives in a household with a susceptible contact and was treated with antibiotic other than ceftriaxone or cefotaxime. Index patient <2 years old should be reimmunized against Hib.

RECOMMENDED ANTIMICROBIAL PROPHYLAXIS

8

RECOMMENDED ANTIMICROBIAL PROPHYLAXIS FOR SELECTED INFECTIOUS AGENTS AND CONDITIONS—cont'd

Exposure	Recommended Empiric Preventive Therapy	Alternative Preventive Therapy	Comments
Mycobacterium avium complex (MAC)	Azithromycin (20 mg/kg by mouth weekly, max 1200 mg) or Clarithromycin (7.5 mg/kg by mouth twice daily, max 500 mg)	Rifabutin, 5 mg/kg/day (max 300 mg) or Azithromycin 5 mg/kg daily (max 250 mg)	Rifabutin should be used ONLY after tuberculosis disease has been excluded. Prophylaxis is recommended for HIV-infected children if ≥6 yr with CD4 T lymphocytes <50/μL, or 2-6 yr with CD4 T lymphocytes <75/μL, or 1-2 yr with CD4 T lymphocytes <500/μL, or <12 mo with CD4 T lymphocytes <750/μL
Mycobacterium tuberculosis	Isoniazid for all exposed contacts with impaired immunity or with age <4 yr Rifampin or rifabutin if contact's isolate is isoniazid-resistant		Tuberculin skin test (TST) should be performed at baseline and 12 wk after contact. If TST is negative at 12 wk and subject is immunocompetent, discontinue isoniazid. If TST is positive or if subject's TST can't be interpreted because of immune impairment, continue isoniazid for 9 mo (4 mo if rifampin or rifabutin is used because of isoniazid resistance).

Neisseria meningitidis	Rifampin
	<1 mo old: 5 mg/kg every 12 hr × 2 days
	≥1 mo old: 10 mg/kg (max 600 mg) every 12 hr × 2 days
	or
	Ceftriaxone
	<15 yr: 125 mg IM × 1 dose
	≥15 yr: 250 mg IM × 1 dose
	or
	Ciprofloxacin
	≥18 yr: 500 mg × 1 dose
	or
	Azithromycin
	<15 yr: 10 mg/kg × 1 dose
	≥15 yr: 500 mg × 1 dose
			Prophylaxis recommended *only* for household contacts *or* those with the following exposure within 7 days of index patient's illness onset:
			  Child care or nursery school contact
			  Direct exposure to patient secretions
			  Mouth-to-mouth resuscitation
			  Frequently slept in the same dwelling
			  Passenger seated next to index patient on an airline flight of >8 hr

Pertussis	Azithromycin <6 mo: 10 mg/kg/day in 1 dose × 5 days ≥6 mo: 10 mg/kg in 1 dose on day 1 (max dose 500 mg); then 5 mg/kg/day (max 250 mg/day) in 1 dose for 4 days *or* Erythromycin Infants and children: 40-50 mg/kg/day (max 2 g/day) in 4 divided doses × 14 days Adolescents and adults: 2 g/day in 4 divided doses × 14 days *or* Clarithromycin: 15 mg/kg/d (max 1 g/day) in 2 divided doses × 7 days	TMP-SMX: (must be ≥2 mo old) TMP (8 mg/kg/day, max 300 mg/day); SMX (40 mg/kg/day, max 1600 mg/day) in 2 divided doses × 14 days	Antibiotic prophylaxis is recommended for all household contacts and other close contacts (including child care) regardless of immunization status. Clarithromycin is not recommended for infants <1 mo; TMP-SMX is not recommended for infants <2 mo. Erythromycin may increase risk of pyloric stenosis for infants <6 wk.

RECOMMENDED ANTIMICROBIAL PROPHYLAXIS 8

RECOMMENDED ANTIMICROBIAL PROPHYLAXIS FOR SELECTED INFECTIOUS AGENTS AND CONDITIONS—cont'd

Exposure	Recommended Empiric Preventive Therapy	Alternative Preventive Therapy	Comments
Tetanus	For clean wound If <3 prior doses of tetanus toxoid, or if history of vaccination is not known, give Td or Tdap. If ≥3 doses of tetanus toxoid is confirmed, dT or Tdap if ≥10 years since last tetanus vaccine. For dirty wound If <3 prior doses of tetanus toxoid or history (depending on age) of vaccination is not known, give DTaP or Td or Tdap *plus* tetanus immune globulin (250 U IM); if ≤3 prior doses, give Td or Tdap if ≥5 years since last tetanus vaccine.	IV immune globulin can be used if tetanus immune globulin is indicated and not available.	If both tetanus toxoid and immune globulin are indicated they should be injected in separate syringes and at different sites.
PREVENTION OF INFECTION DUE TO SPECIFIC VIRAL PATHOGENS			
Cytomegalovirus	Prevention of transmission to transplant recipient: Ganciclovir or valganciclovir	Foscarnet	CMV immune globulin is moderately effective in preventing CMV in seronegative liver and kidney transplant recipients.
Herpes simplex	Prevention of recurrences: Acyclovir *or* famciclovir *or* valacyclovir		Famciclovir and valacyclovir are not recommended for children.

Hepatitis A	Postexposure in nonimmune person Hepatitis A vaccine (if ≥1 yr) Immune globulin alone if <1 yr
Hepatitis B	Postexposure Source with unknown infection status: Hepatitis B vaccine series for nonimmune contact Source HBSAg+: One dose of hepatitis B immune globulin + Hepatitis B vaccine series
HIV	Prevention of maternal-to-child transmission: Zidovudine, Lamivudine, Nevirapine—see perinatal guidelines at **http://www.aidsinfo.nih.gov** Sexual, occupational, or nonoccupational exposure: Known HIV+ source: 2- to 3-drug regimen depending on volume of exposure and HIV class status of source (see **http://www.cdc.gov/mmwr/preview/mmwrhtml/rr5409a1.htm** and Havens[1]) Postexposure prophylaxis is generally not recommended following needlestick injury from unknown, nonoccupational source	Exposed person should be tested for HIV at baseline and 4-6 and at 6 mo postexposure. Risk of HIV infection after percutaneous occupational exposure to HIV-infected blood is 0.03%; 0.09% after mucous membrane exposure. Risk for nonoccupational exposure is lower. CDC National Clinician's Postexposure hotline: 888-448-4911
Influenza	Zanamivir (≥5 yr) or Oseltamivir (≥1 yr)	Rimantadine or amantadine if circulating influenza known to be susceptible; these 2 agents not active against influenza B

RECOMMENDED ANTIMICROBIAL PROPHYLAXIS

8

RECOMMENDED ANTIMICROBIAL PROPHYLAXIS FOR SELECTED INFECTIOUS AGENTS AND CONDITIONS—cont'd

Exposure	Recommended Empiric Preventive Therapy	Alternative Preventive Therapy	Comments
Measles	Measles vaccine (within 72 hr of exposure) or immune globulin		Immune globulin is recommended for high-risk susceptible household contacts (<1 yr, pregnant women, immunocompromised). The usual dose of IVIg used for immunocompromised people who receive it regularly should provide protection against measles as well. IG to prevent measles should be given within 6 days of exposure, usually at 0.25 mL/kg IM, but at 0.5 mL/kg IM for immunocompromised children (max. dose: 15 mL). If IG is given, delay measles vaccine for 5 mo (if 0.25 mL/kg IM) or 6 mo (if 0.5 mL/kg IM) or 8-11 mo (if IVIg given, depending on dose).
Rubella	Intramuscular immune globulin (0.55 mL/kg)	Rubella vaccine	Immune globulin should be offered as a possible means of reducing the likelihood of fetal infection for susceptible, exposed pregnant women who decline termination of pregnancy. Rubella vaccine (for nonpregnant, exposed people) has not been shown to prevent illness, but if given within 72 hr of exposure it may be preventative.

| Varicella | Postexposure: VariZIG or Acyclovir or Varicella immunization | IVIG | VariZIG is available only through a research protocol. It must be administered within 96 hr of exposure. Immunization should be provided within 72 hr of exposure. IVIG can be used (1 dose ≤96 hr after exposure) if VariZIG is not available. |

PREVENTION OF INFECTION DUE TO SPECIFIC FUNGAL PATHOGENS

| Candida | Fluconazole | | Recommended during periods of neutropenia for children undergoing allogeneic stem-cell transplantation. |
| Pneumocystis | Dapsone (≥1 mo) or aerosolized Pentamidine (≥5 yr) or Atovaquone | TMP/SMX | Recommended for HIV-infected or indeterminant infants aged 1-12 mo and for HIV-infected children with following CD_4 T-lymphocyte counts
1-5 yr: <500/µL
6-12 yr: <200/µL
Recommended for children with a variety of immunocompromising conditions |

PREVENTION OF INFECTION DUE TO SPECIFIC PARASITIC PATHOGENS

| Malaria | Travel to areas without reported chloroquine-resistant malaria: Chloroquine | | Prophylaxis should begin 1 wk before travel and continue for 4 wk after exposure has ended. |

RECOMMENDED ANTIMICROBIAL PROPHYLAXIS

8

RECOMMENDED ANTIMICROBIAL PROPHYLAXIS FOR SELECTED INFECTIOUS AGENTS AND CONDITIONS—cont'd

Exposure	Recommended Empiric Preventive Therapy	Alternative Preventive Therapy	Comments
	Travel to areas with chloroquine-resistant malaria: Atovaquone-proguanil daily		Begin prophylaxis 1 day before exposure and for 1 wk after exposure has ended. Contraindicated in pregnancy.
	or Doxycycline (≥8 yr) daily		Begin prophylaxis 1-2 days before exposure and continue 4 wk after exposure has ended. Contraindicated in pregnancy; caution about diarrhea, photosensitivity, and monilial vaginitis
	or Mefloquine weekly		Begin prophylaxis 1 wk before travel and continue 4 wk after exposure has ended. Contraindicated for people with anxiety disorders, psychosis, schizophrenia, and other major psychiatric disturbances and in those with a history of seizures.
Toxoplasmosis	Prevention of 1st episode in HIV-infected people: TMP-SMX: For infants and children: 1-5 yr if CD₄ count <15%; for children ≥6 yr if CD₄ count <100/mm³ Prevention of recurrence in HIV-infected people: [Sulfadiazine + pyrimethamine + leucovorin]	[Dapsone (≥1 mo) + pyrimethamine + leucovorin] *or* Atovaquone *or* [Clindamycin + pyrimethamine + leucovorin]	

CMV, cytomegalovirus; CSF, cerebrospinal fluid; GI, gastrointestinal; GU, genitourinary; IG, immunoglobulin (IM) IM, intramuscular; IV, intravenous; IVIg, intravenous immunoglobulin; max, maximum; PO, by mouth; TMP/SMX, trimethoprim/sulfamethoxazole.

REFERENCE

1. Havens PL; Committee on Pediatric AIDS: Postexposure prophylaxis in children and adolescents for nonoccupational exposure to human immunodeficiency virus. Pediatrics 2003;111:1475-1489.
2. American Academy of Pediatrics: In: Pickering LK, Baker CJ, Long SS, McMillan JA, eds. Red Book 2006 Report of the Committee on Infectious Diseases, 27th ed. Elk Grove Village, IL: American Academy of Pediatrics, 2006.
3. Wilson W, Taubert KA, Gewitz M, et al: Prevention of Infective Endocarditis: Guidelines from the American Heart Association. Circulation 2007;115:1.

RECOMMENDED ANTIMICROBIAL PROPHYLAXIS

Antimicrobial Desensitization Protocols

Kara L. Murray, PharmD, BCPS, and Carlton K. K. Lee, PharmD, MPH

Rapid desensitization is intended for patients who have or who are strongly suspected of having antibiotic-specific immunoglobulin (Ig)E antibodies. Desensitization does not prevent non–IgE-mediated allergic reactions. Patients with antibiotic-induced Stevens-Johnson syndrome or toxic epidermal necrolysis **should not** receive the antibiotic under any circumstances because of the risk of inducing a progressive life-threatening reaction.[1] Discontinue all beta-blockers before desensitization and do not pretreat (unless indicated) with systemic corticosteroids and antihistamines.

Have patient-specific doses of injectable epinephrine, diphenhydramine, and corticosteroid and appropriate resuscitative equipment available at the bedside. For all injectable infusions, rates should be regulated with a syringe pump.

Most protocols are designed for adults. Please note the cumulative desensitization doses of the following protocols may exceed your patient's dosage. Proportional dose reductions are necessary for pediatric patients, as the final cumulative dose should equal the patient's individualized divided dose. For example, if the antibiotic's usual dose is 30 mg/kg/24 hours divided every 12 hours, the final cumulative dose should be 15 mg/kg. Desensitization may be achieved by intermittent intravenous (IV) infusion, continuous IV infusion, or by the oral route. The oral route is less expensive and safer.

I. PENICILLIN

Mild allergic reactions should be treated; if symptoms do not progress, repeat the same dose or drop back one dose before proceeding. At the completion of desensitization, the therapeutic dose of penicillin may be administered.[2] To maintain the desensitized state, continuous penicillin treatment is required. Unless a long-acting preparation is used, oral penicillin should be taken on a twice-daily basis. If penicillin is discontinued for more than 48 hours, the patient is again at risk for anaphylaxis and desensitization should be repeated.[2]

A. INTERMITTENT IV INFUSION[1]

TABLE 9-1

PENICILLIN INTRAVENOUS DESENSITIZATION PROTOCOL WITH DRUG ADDED BY PIGGYBACK INFUSION

Step*	Penicillin (mg/mL)	Amount (mL)	Dose (mg)	Cumulative Dose (mg)
1	0.1	0.1	0.01	0.01
2	0.1	0.2	0.02	0.03
3	0.1	0.4	0.04	0.07
4	0.1	0.8	0.08	0.15
5	0.1	1.6	0.16	0.31
6	1	0.32	0.32	0.63
7	1	0.64	0.64	1.27
8	1	1.2	1.2	2.47
9	10	0.24	2.4	4.87
10	10	0.48	4.8	10
11	10	1	10	20
12	10	2	20	40
13	100	0.4	40	80
14	100	0.8	80	160
15	100	1.6	160	320
16	1000	0.32	320	640
17	1000	0.64	640	1280

Observe patient for 30 min, then give full therapeutic dose by the desired route.

*Interval between doses is 15 min.
From Solensky R: Drug densensitization. Immunol Allergy Clin N Am 2004;24:425-443.

B. CONTINUOUS IV INFUSION[1,2]

TABLE 9-2

PENICILLIN INTRAVENOUS DESENSITIZATION PROTOCOL USING A CONTINUOUS INFUSION PUMP

Step*	Penicillin (mg/mL)	Flow Rate (mL/hr)	Dose (mg)	Cumulative Dose (mg)
1	0.01	6	0.015	0.015
2	0.01	12	0.03	0.045
3	0.01	24	0.06	0.105
4	0.1	5	0.125	0.23
5	0.1	10	0.25	0.48
6	0.1	20	0.5	1
7	0.1	40	1	2

TABLE 9-2

PENICILLIN INTRAVENOUS DESENSITIZATION PROTOCOL USING A CONTINUOUS INFUSION PUMP—cont'd

Step*	Penicillin (mg/mL)	Flow Rate (mL/hr)	Dose (mg)	Cumulative Dose (mg)
8	0.1	80	2	4
9	0.1	160	4	8
10	10	3	7.5	15
11	10	6	15	30
12	10	12	30	60
13	10	25	62.5	123
14	10	50	125	250
15	10	100	250	500
16	10	200	500	1000

Observe patient for 30 min,
then give full therapeutic dose
by the desired route.

*Interval between doses is 15 min.
From Solensky R: Drug densensitization. Immunol Allergy Clin N Am 2004;24:425-443.

C. ORAL[1,2]

TABLE 9-3

PENICILLIN ORAL DESENSITIZATION PROTOCOL

Step*	Penicillin (mg/mL)	Amount (mL)	Dose (mg)	Cumulative Dose (mg)
1	0.5	0.1	0.05	0.05
2	0.5	0.2	0.1	0.15
3	0.5	0.4	0.2	0.35
4	0.5	0.8	0.4	0.75
5	0.5	1.6	0.8	1.55
6	0.5	3.2	1.6	3.15
7	0.5	6.4	3.2	6.35
8	5	1.2	6	12.35
9	5	2.4	12	24.35
10	5	5	25	49.35
11	50	1	50	100
12	50	2	100	200
13	50	4	200	400
14	50	8	400	800

Observe patient for 30 min,
then give full therapeutic
dose by the desired route.

*Interval between doses is 15 min.
From Solensky R: Drug densensitization. Immunol Allergy Clin N Am 2004;24:425-443.

II. CEPHALOSPORINS

Desensitization protocol generally parallels that of penicillin with progressively increasing doses administered in frequent time intervals. Examples of the intermittent IV infusion and continuous IV infusion methods are described in the next sections.

A. INTERMITTENT IV INFUSION[3]

TABLE 9-4

RAPID INTRAVENOUS CEPHALOSPORIN DESENSITIZATION PROTOCOL: GOAL DOSE, 1 G AND 2 G INTRAVENOUSLY

Dose	Goal Dose, 1 g IV		Goal Dose, 2 g IV	
	mg	mg, rounded	mg, rounded	Time
1	0.1	0.1	0.1	15 min
2	0.2	0.2	0.4	15 min
3	0.7	1	1	15 min
4	2.2	2	4	15 min
5	6.9	10	10	15 min
6	21.8	20	40	15 min
7	69	70	140	15 min
8	218.1	200	400	15 min
9	689.7	700	1400	15 min
Cumulative	1008.6	1003.3	1995.5	2 hr, 15 min

Protocol for intravenous desensitization to all cephalosporins with a goal dose of 1 g and 2 g.
From Win PH, Brown H, Zankar A, et al: Rapid intravenous cephalosporin desensitization. J Allergy Clin Immunol 2005;116(1):225-227.

B. CONTINUOUS IV INFUSION[1]

TABLE 9-5

INTRAVENOUS DESENSITIZATION PROTOCOL USING A CONTINUOUS INFUSION PUMP

Step*	mg/mL	Flow Rate (mL/hr)	Dose (mg)	Cumulative Dose (mg)
1	0.01	6	0.015	0.015
2	0.01	12	0.03	0.045
3	0.01	24	0.06	0.105
4	0.1	5	0.125	0.23
5	0.1	10	0.25	0.48
6	0.1	20	0.5	1
7	0.1	40	1	2
8	0.1	80	2	4
9	0.1	160	4	8
10	10	3	7.5	15

TABLE 9-5

INTRAVENOUS DESENSITIZATION PROTOCOL USING A CONTINUOUS INFUSION PUMP—cont'd

Step*	mg/mL	Flow Rate (mL/hr)	Dose (mg)	Cumulative Dose (mg)
11	10	6	15	30
12	10	12	30	60
13	10	25	62.5	123
14	10	50	125	250
15	100	10	250	500
16	100	20	500	1000
17	100	40	1000	2000

*Interval between doses is 15 min.
From Solensky R: Drug densensitization. Immunol Allergy Clin N Am 2004;24:425-443.

III. TRIMETHOPRIM/SULFAMETHOXAZOLE (TMP/SMX) ORAL

Patients with allergic reactions such as serum sickness, vasculitis, hypersensitivity syndrome, pneumonitis, interstitial nephritis, immune-mediated hematologic disorders, drug fever, Stevens-Johnson syndrome, and toxic epidermal necrolysis are **not** candidates for desensitization.

A. PATIENTS WITH A PREVIOUS (DISTANT) REACTION CONSISTENT WITH AN IGE-MEDIATED MECHANISM[1]

TABLE 9-6

EXAMPLE OF GRADED CHALLENGE WITH ORAL TRIMETHOPRIM/SULFAMETHOXAZOLE (TMP/SMX) IN A PATIENT WITH A DISTANT MILD IMMEDIATE-TYPE ALLERGIC REACTION

Step*	TMP/SMX (SMX mg/mL)	Amount (mL)	SMX Dose (mg)
1	4	0.25	1
2	4	1.	4
3	40	0.5	20
4	40	2.	80
5	NA	1 tablet	400

*Interval between doses is 30 min. Dose is expressed as sulfamethaxazole portion of TMP/SMX.
If an allergic reaction occurs, formal desensitization should be performed.
NA, not applicable.
From Solensky R: Drug densensitization. Immunol Allergy Clin N Am 2004;24:425-443.

B. PATIENTS WITH A HISTORY OF TYPICAL DELAYED MACULOPAPULAR REACTION

Cutaneous reactions occur in 40% to 80% of HIV-positive patients compared with 3.3% in non-HIV individuals. Many different TMP/SMX desensitization protocols for HIV are reported in the literature. Here is an example of an oral adult regimen[4] (Tables 9-7, 9-8, and 9-9).

TABLE 9-7

DILUTION FOR TRIMETHOPRIM/SULFAMETHOXAZOLE DESENSITIZATION

Final Concentration of TMP/SMZ	Bottle Assignment	Procedure
200/40 mg per 5 mL	A	Conventional oral TMP/SMZ suspension 5 mL = 200/40 mg
2/0.4 mg per 1 mL	B	1. Add 5 mL of conventional oral TMP/SMZ suspension (from Bottle A) to 95 mL of sterile water. 2. Shake well. Recipe will equal 2/0.4 mg per 1 mL.
0.02/0.004 mg per 1 mL	C	1. Add 1 mL of Bottle B to 99 mL of sterile water. 2. Shake well. Recipe will equal 0.02/0.004 mg per 1 mL.

TABLE 9-8

ADVERSE REACTIONS AND RESPONSE DURING DESENSITIZATION

Type of Reaction	Alteration of Protocol
Mild (rash, fever, nausea)	Diphenhydramine (PO) *or* Ibuprofen (PO)
Urticaria, dyspnea, severe vomiting, and/or hypotension	**Stop** the desensitization **immediately**. Treat with epinephrine and corticosteroids.

TABLE 9-9

DESENSITIZATION PROTOCOL

Hour	Dose of TMP/SMZ	Form/Bottle Number	Suggested Volume
0	0.02/0.004 mg	C	1 mL
1	0.2/0.04 mg	C	10 mL
2	2/0.4 mg	B	1 mL
3	20/4 mg	B	10 mL
4	200/40 mg	A	5 mL
5	800/160 mg	NA	1 single-strength tablet

Drink 180 mL of water after each dose of TMP/SMZ. Subjects tolerating this protocol were prescribed 800/160 mg TMP/SMZ every Monday, Wednesday, and Friday for low-dose *Pneumocystis carinii* prophylaxis.

NA, not applicable.

From Gluckstein D, Ruskin J: Rapid oral desensitization to trimethoprim-sulfamethoxazole (TMP-SMZ): use in prophylaxis for *Pneumocystis carinii* pneumonia in patients with AIDS who were previously intolerant to TMP-SMZ. Clin Infect Dis 1995;20:849-853.

IV. FLUOROQUINOLONE

A. INTRAVENOUS CIPROFLOXACIN DESENSITIZATION PROTOCOL

The following is an example of a successful intravenous ciprofloxacin desensitization protocol from a 29-month-old with a gluteal abscess and chronic osteomyelitis experiencing anaphylaxis[5] (Table 9-10).

B. ORAL CIPROFLOXACIN DESENSITIZATION PROTOCOL

The following is an example of a successful oral ciprofloxacin desensitization protocol from a 15-year-old with cystic fibrosis experiencing urticarial reaction[6] (Table 9-11).

TABLE 9-10

SAMPLE INTRAVENOUS CIPROFLOXACIN DESENSITIZATION PROTOCOL

Dose*	Concentration (mg/mL)	Volume Given (mL)	Absolute Amount (mg)	Cumulative Total Dose (mg)
1	0.000002	5	0.00001	0.00001
2	0.00002	5	0.0001	0.0001
3	0.0002	5	0.001	0.001
4	0.002	5	0.01	0.01
5	0.004	5	0.02	0.03
6	0.008	5	0.04	0.07
7	0.016	5	0.08	0.15
8	0.032	5	0.16	0.31
9	0.064	5	0.32	0.63
10	0.128	5	0.64	1.27
11	0.256	5	1.28	2.55
12	0.512	5	2.56	5.11
13	1.024	5	5.12	10.23
14	2	5	10	20.23
15	2	10	20	40.23
16	2	20	40	80.23
17	2	40	80	160.23

*Administer doses as continuous 15-min infusions, except for the last 3 doses, which are given as 30-min infusions with no intervals between the doses.

From Erdem G, Staat MA, Connelly BL, et al: Anaphylactic reaction to ciprofloxacin in a toddler: Successful desensitization. Pediatr Infect Dis J 1999;18(6):563-564.

9

ANTIMICROBIAL DESENSITIZATION PROTOCOLS

TABLE 9-11

CIPROFLOXACIN ORAL DESENSITIZATION PROTOCOL

Step*	Ciprofloxacin (mg/mL)	Amount (mL)	Dose (mg)	Cumulative Dose (mg)
1	0.1	0.5	0.05	0.05
2	0.1	1	0.1	0.15
3	0.1	2	0.2	0.35
4	0.1	4	0.4	0.75
5	0.1	8	0.8	1.55
6	1	1.6	1.6	3.15
7	1	3.2	3.2	6.35
8	1	6.4	6.4	12.75
9	1	12.8	12.8	25.55
10	10	2.5	25	50.55
11	10	5	50	100.55
12	10	10	100	200.55
13	NA	1 tablet	250	450.55

*Interval between doses is 15 min.
NA, not applicable.
From Lantner RR: Ciprofloxacin desensitization in a patient with cystic fibrosis. J Allergy Clin Immunol 1995;96:1001-1002.

V. VANCOMYCIN

Desensitization should be considered in hypersensitivity reactions, red-man syndrome that does not respond to the usual treatment measures, and vancomycin-induced anaphylaxis.[7] Concomitant use of medications that induce mast-cell degranulation may lead to an unsuccessful desensitization.[7] These medications include ciprofloxacin, barbiturates, narcotic analgesics (fentanyl rarely induces histamine release), atracurium, cisatracurium, succinylcholine, propofol, dextran, and radiocontrast agents.[7] Concurrent use of opioids has produced a synergistic response.[8]

A. RAPID VANCOMYCIN DESENSITIZATION[9] (Table 9-12)

Rapid desensitization is the preferred method that is effective in most patients.

Preparation of vancomycin injections for desensitization:

1. Prepare a standard bag of vancomycin (500 mg in 250 mL NS [NaCl 0.9%] or D5W [dextrose 5% in water]); label as infusion no. 5 (vancomycin 2 mg/mL).

TABLE 9-12

RAPID VANCOMYCIN DESENSITIZATION PROTOCOL

Infusion no.	Dilution	Vancomycin Dose (mg)	Vancomycin Concentration (mg/mL)
1	1:10,000	0.02	0.0002
2	1:1000	0.2	0.002
3	1:100	2	0.02
4	1:10	10	0.2
5	Standard	500	2

From Lerner A, Dwyer JM: Desensitization to vancomycin [letter]. Ann Intern Med 1984;100:157.

2. Draw up 10 mL of the standard vancomycin (2 mg/mL) and place in a 100-mL bag of NS or D5W; label as infusion no. 4 (vancomycin 0.2 mg/mL).
3. Draw up 10 mL from infusion no. 4 (vancomycin 0.2 mg/mL) and place in a 100-mL bag of NS or D5W; label as infusion no. 3 (vancomycin 0.02 mg/mL).
4. Draw up 10 mL from infusion no. 3 (vancomycin 0.02 mg/mL) and place in a 100-mL bag of NS or D5W; label as infusion no. 2 (vancomycin 0.002 mg/mL).
5. Draw up 10 mL from infusion no. 2 (vancomycin 0.002 mg/mL) and place in a 100-mL bag of NS or D5W; label as infusion no. 1 (vancomycin 0.0002 mg/mL).

Infusion Directions:

1. Diphenhydramine and hydrocortisone injections are given 15 min prior to initiation of this desensitization protocol and then every 6 hr throughout the protocol.
2. Initiate infusion rate at 0.5 mL/min (30 mL/hr) and increase by 0.5 mL/min (30 mL/hr) as tolerated every 5 min to a **maximum rate** of 5 mL/min (300 mL/hr). If pruritis, hypotension, rash, or difficulty breathing occurs, stop infusion and reinfuse the previously tolerated infusion at the highest tolerated rate. This step may be repeated up to 3 times for any given concentration.
3. Upon completion of infusion no. 5, immediately administer the required dose of vancomycin in the usual dilution of NS or D5W over 2 hr. Decrease rate if patient becomes symptomatic or, alternatively, increase rate if patient tolerates dose. Administer diphenhydramine orally 60 min prior to each dose.

B. SLOW DESENSITIZATION[10] (Table 9-13)

Use of slow desensitization should be reserved **only** for patients who fail the rapid desensitization protocol.

TABLE 9-13

SLOW VANCOMYCIN DESENSITIZATION PROTOCOL

Premedication: Diphenhydramine 1.25 mg/kg (**max. dose**: 50 mg) IV 15 min prior to protocol initiation, then every 6 hr throughout protocol.

Day	Infusion No.	Dose Provided	Vancomycin Dose (mg)	Concentration (mg/mL)
1	1	0.5 mg in 500 mL	0.5	0.001
2	2	5 mg in 500 mL	5	0.01
3	3	10 mg in 500 mL	10	0.02
4	4	50 mg in 500 mL	50	0.10
5	4	50 mg in 500 mL	50	0.10
6	5	100 mg in 500 mL	100	0.2
7*	6	100 mg in 250 mL × 2	200	0.4
8	7	150 mg in 250 mL × 2	300	0.6
9	8	250 mg in 250 mL × 2	500	1
10	9	500 mg in 250 mL × 2	1000	2
11	9	500 mg in 250 mL × 2	1000	2
12	9	500 mg in 250 mL × 2	1000	2
13	10	1000 mg in 250 mL	1000	4

*Beginning on day 7, doses infused consecutively.
From Lin RY: Desensitization in the management of vancomycin hypersensitivity. Arch Intern Med 1990;150:2197-2198.

Infusion Directions:
1. Infuse each dose over 5 hr. If pruritus, hypotension, rash or difficulty breathing occurs, stop the infusion and reinfuse the previously tolerated infusion.
2. On day 14, administer the required dose of vancomycin in the usual dilution of NS or D5W (e.g., 1000 mg in 250 mL) at a rate of 100 mL/hr. Decrease rate if patient becomes symptomatic or, alternatively, increase rate if patient tolerates dose. Consider oral antihistamine prior to each dose.

VI. AMINOGLYCOSIDES

A. INTRAVENOUS TOBRAMYCIN DESENSITIZATION PROTOCOL
The following is an example of a successful intravenous tobramycin desensitization protocol from a 15-year-old with cystic fibrosis experiencing urticarial reactions to tobramycin and gentamicin.[11]

TABLE 9-14

SAMPLE TOBRAMYCIN DESENSITIZATION PROTOCOL

Dose	Elapsed Time (hr)	Tobramycin (mg)	Cumulative Dose (mg)
1	0	0.001	0.001
2	0.5	0.002	0.003
3	1	0.004	0.007
4	1.5	0.008	0.015
5	2	0.016	0.031
6	2.5	0.032	0.063
7	3	0.064	0.127
8	3.5	0.125	0.255
9	4	0.256	0.511
10	4.5	0.512	1.023
11	5	1	2.023
12	5.5	2	4.023
13	6	4	8.023
14	6.5	8	16.023
15	7	16	32.023
16	7.5	32	64.023
17	8	16	80.023

From Earl HS, Sullivan TJ: Acute desensitization of a patient with cystic fibrosis allergic to both beta-lactam and aminoglycoside antibiotics. J Allergy Clin Immunol 1987;79:477-483.

Directions (Table 9-14):

1. Each tobramycin dose should be diluted in 20 mL of normal saline.
2. Each tobramycin dose should be infused over 20 min and then flushed with 10 mL of normal saline.
3. Subsequent desensitization dosages should be given 10 min following the completion of the prior infusion (time from beginning of infusion to next infusion = 30 min).

B. INHALED TOBRAMYCIN DESENSITIZATION PROTOCOL

The following is an example of a successful inhaled tobramycin desensitization protocol from a 9-year-old with cystic fibrosis experiencing a rash following a course of intravenous gentamicin.[12]

Directions (Table 9-15):

1. Each inhaled tobramycin (TOBI) dose should be diluted in 5 mL of normal saline.
2. Each dose is nebulized on an every 2-hr schedule until the full dose of 300 mg is given.

TABLE 9-15

INHALED TOBRAMYCIN DESENSITIZATION PROTOCOL

Treatment No.	Dose (mg)
1	0.3
2	0.6
3	0.9
4	1.2
5	1.5
6	3
7	6
8	12
9	24
10	48
11	96
12	150
13	200
14	250
15	300

From Spigarelli MG, Hurwitz ME, Nasr SZ: Hypersensitivity to inhaled TOBI following reaction to gentamicin. Pediatr Pulmonol 2002;33:311-314.

REFERENCES

1. Solensky R: Drug desensitization. Immunol Allergy Clin N Am 2004;24:425-443.
2. Sullivan TJ: Drug allergy. In Middleton E, Reed CE, Ellis EF, et al (eds). Allergy: Principles and Practice, 4th edition. St. Louis, Mosby, 1993, pp 1726-1746.
3. Win PH, Brown H, Zankar A, et al: Rapid intravenous cephalosporin desensitization. J Allergy Clin Immunol 2005;116(1):225-227.
4. Gluckstein D, Ruskin J: Rapid oral desensitization to trimethoprim-sulfamethoxazole (TMP-SMZ): Use in prophylaxis for *Pneumocystis carinii* pneumonia in patients with AIDS who were previously intolerant to TMP-SMZ. Clin Infect Dis 1995;20:849-853.
5. Erdem G, Staat MA, Connelly BL, et al: Anaphylactic reaction to ciprofloxacin in a toddler: successful desensitization. Pediatr Infect Dis J 1999;18(6):563-564.
6. Lantner RR: Ciprofloxacin desensitization in a patient with cystic fibrosis. J Allergy Clin Immunol 1995;96:1001-1002.
7. Wazny LD, Daghigh B: Desensitization protocols for vancomycin hypersenstivity. Ann Pharmacother 2001;35(11):1458-1464.
8. Wong JT, Ripple RE, MacLean JA, et al: Vancomycin hypersensitivity: Synergism with narcotics and desensitization by a rapid continuous intravenous protocol. J Allergy Clin Immunol 1994;94(2):189-194.
9. Lerner A, Dwyer JM: Desensitization to vancomycin [letter]. Ann Intern Med 1984;100:157.

10. Lin RY: Desensitization in the management of vancomycin hypersensitivity. Arch Intern Med 1990;150:2197-2198.
11. Earl HS, Sullivan TJ: Acute desensitization of a patient with cystic fibrosis allergic to both beta-lactam and aminoglycoside antibiotics. J Allergy Clin Immunol 1987;79:477-483.
12. Spigarelli MG, Hurwitz ME, Nasr SZ: Hypersensitivity to inhaled TOBI® following reaction to gentamicin. Pediatr Pulmonol 2002;33:311-314.

9

ANTIMICROBIAL DESENSITIZATION PROTOCOLS

Drug Doses

Carlton Lee, PharmD, MPH

10

II. SAMPLE ENTRY

Pregnancy: Refer to explanation of pregnancy categories (on facing page).
Breast: Refer to explanation of breast-feeding categories (on facing page).
Kidney: Indicates need for caution or need for dose adjustment in renal impairment (see also Chapter 3).
Liver: Indicates need for caution or need for dose adjustment in hepatic impairment.

How supplied

CHLOROQUINE HCL/PHOSPHATE ← Generic name

Yes   Yes   1   C

Aralen and others ← Trade name and other names
Amebicide, antimalarial ← Drug category
Tabs: 250, 500 mg as phosphate (150,300 mg base, respectively)
Oral suspension: 16.67 mg/mL as phosphate (10 mg/mL base), 15 mg/mL as phosphate (9 mg/mL base) ← Mortar and pestle: Indicates need for extemporaneous compounding by a pharmacist
Injection: 50 mg/mL as HCl (40 mg/mL base) (5 mL)

Doses expressed in mg of chloroquine base.
Malaria prophylaxis (start 1 wk prior to exposure and continue for 4 wk after leaving endemic area):
  Child: 5 mg/kg/dose PO Q wk; **max. dose:** 300 mg/dose
  Adult: 300 mg/dose PO Q wk
Malaria treatment (chloroquine sensitive strains):
For treatment for malaria, consult with ID specialist or see the latest edition of the AAP Red Book. For IV use, consider safer alternatives such as quinidine or quinine.
  Child: 10 mg/kg/dose (**max. dose:** 600 mg/dose) PO × 1; followed by 5 mg/kg/dose (**max. dose:** 300 mg/dose) 6 hr later and then once daily for 2 days.
  Adult: 600 mg/dose PO × 1; followed by 300 mg/dose 6 hr later and then once daily for 2 days.

Drug dosing

Contraindications: Hypersensitivity to 4-aminoquinoline compounds; and retinal/visual changes.
Warnings/Precautions: **Use with caution** in liver disease, preexisting auditory damage or seizures, G6PD deficiency, psoriasis, porphyria or concomitant hepatotoxic drugs. **Adjust dose in renal failure (see Chapter 3).**
Adverse Effects: ECG abnormalities, prolonged QT interval, pruritis, GI disturbances, skeletal muscle weakness, amnesia, blurred vision, retinal and corneal changes. Headaches, confusion, and hair depigmentation have been reported.
Drug Interactions: Chloroquine is a substrate for CYP 450 2D6 and 3A4 and inhibitor of CYP 450 2D6.
  Antacids, ampicillin, and kaolin may decrease the absorption of chloroquine (allow 4 hr interval between chloroquine). May increase serum cyclosporine levels. Cimetidine may increase effects/toxicity of chloroquine.
Drug Administration: Administer oral doses with meals to reduce GI complications. Mixing tablets with chocolate syrup or placing tablets in capsules may be used to mask bitter taste.
Brief remarks about contraindications, warning/precautions (including therapeutic drug monitoring), adverse effects, drug interactions, and drug administration.

III. EXPLANATION OF BREAST-FEEDING CATEGORIES

See sample entry.
1 Compatible
2 Use with caution
3 Unknown with concerns
X Contraindicated
? Safety not established

IV. EXPLANATION OF PREGNANCY CATEGORIES

A Adequate studies in pregnant women have not demonstrated a risk to the fetus in the first trimester of pregnancy, and there is no evidence of risk in later trimesters.

B Animal studies have not demonstrated a risk to the fetus, but there are no adequate studies in pregnant women; or animal studies have shown an adverse effect, but adequate studies in pregnant women have not demonstrated a risk to the fetus during the first trimester of pregnancy, and there is no evidence of risk in later trimesters.

C Animal studies have shown an adverse effect on the fetus, but there are no adequate studies in humans; or there are no animal reproduction studies and no adequate studies in humans.

D There is evidence of human fetal risk, but the potential benefits from the use of the drug in pregnant women may be acceptable despite its potential risks.

X Studies in animals or humans demonstrate fetal abnormalities or adverse reaction; reports indicate evidence of fetal risk. The risk of use in pregnant women clearly outweighs any possible benefit.

V. DRUG INDEX

Trade Name	Generic Name
1592*	Abacavir sulfate
3TC*	Lamivudine
5-FC*, 5-Fluorocytosine	Flucytosine
A-200	Pyrethrins
ABCD*	Amphotericin B cholesteryl sulfate
Abelcet	Amphotericin B lipid complex
ABLC*	Amphotericin B lipid complex
Acticin	Permethrin
Aczone	Dapsone
Aftate	Tolnaftate
Agenerase	Amprenavir
AK-Poly-Bac Ophthalmic	Bacitracin + polymyxin B
AK-Spore H.C. Otic	Polymyxin B sulfate, neomycin sulfate, and hydrocortisone

*Common abbreviation or other name (not recommended for use when writing a prescription).

Trade Name	Generic Name
AK-Sulf	Sulfacetamide sodium, ophthalmic
AKTob	Tobramycin
AK-Tracin Ophthalmic	Bacitracin
Albenza	Albendazole
Aldara	Imiquimod
Alinia	Nitazoxanide
Altabax	Retapamulin
AmBisome	Amphotericin B, liposomal
Amikin	Amikacin sulfate
Aminosalicylic acid	Para-aminosalicylic acid
Amoxil	Amoxicillin
Amphocin	Amphotericin B
Amphotec	Amphotericin B cholesteryl sulfate
Ancef	Cefazolin
Ancobon	Flucytosine
AntibiOtic	Neomycin/Polymyxin B/Hydrocortisone
Antiminth	Pyrantel pamoate
Antrypol	Suramin
Aptivus	Tipranavir
APV*	Amprenavir
Aralen	Chloroquine HCL/Phosphate
Arestin	Minocycline
Arsobal	Melarsoprol
Arsobal	Suramin
ATV*	Atazanavir
Augmentin, Augmentin ES-600, Augmentin XR	Amoxicillin with clavulanic acid
Avelox, Avelox IV	Moxifloxacin
Axo-Standard [OTC]	Phenazopyridine HCL
Azactam	Aztreonam
Azasite	Azithromycin
AZT*	Zidovudine
BabyBIG	Botulinum immune globulin intravenous, human
Baciguent Topical	Bacitracin
Bactrim	Sulfamethoxazole and trimethoprim
Bactroban, Bactroban Nasal	Mupirocin
Bayer 205	Suramin
Bayer 2502	Nifurtimox
BayHep-B	Hepatitis B immune globulin
BayRab	Rabies immune globulin
BayTet	Tetanus immune globulin
Belganyl	Suramin
Biaxin, Biaxin XL	Clarithromycin

*Common abbreviation or other name (not recommended for use when writing a prescription).

Trade Name	Generic Name
Bicillin C-R, Bicillin C-R 900/300	Penicillin G preparations—Penicillin G benzathine and Penicillin G procaine
Bicillin L-A	Penicillin G preparations—Benzathine
BIG-IV	Botulinum immune globulin intravenous, human
Biltricide	Praziquantel
Biocet	Cephalexin
Bleph 10	Sulfacetamide sodium, ophthalmic
Caldesene	Undecylenic acid
Cancidas	Caspofungin
Carbamazine	Diethylcarbamazine
Ceclor, Ceclor CD	Cefaclor
Cedax	Ceftibuten
Cefadyl	Cephapirin
Cefizox	Ceftizoxime
Cefobid	Cefoperazone
Cefotan	Cefotetan
Ceftin	Cefuroxime axetil (PO)
Cefzil	Cefprozil
Ceptaz (arginine salt)	Ceftazidime
Chibroxin	Norfloxacin
Chloromycetin	Chloramphenicol
Ciloxan ophthalmic	Ciprofloxacin
Cipro, Cipro XR, Ciprodex, Cipro HC Otic	Ciprofloxacin
Claforan	Cefotaxime
Cleocin, Cleocin-T	Clindamycin
Cloxapen	Cloxacillin
Colistin, Colistin Sodium Methanesulfonate	Colistimethate sodium
Coly-Mycin M Parenteral	Colistimethate sodium
Condylox	Podofilox
Copegus	Ribavirin
Cortisporin Otic	Neomycin/Polymyxin B/Hydrocortisone
Cortisporin Otic	Polymyxin B sulfate, neomycin sulfate, and hydrocortisone
Cortisporin TC Otic	Neomycin/Colistin/Hydrocortisone
Co-trimoxazole	Sulfamethoxazole and trimethoprim
Crixivan	Indinavir
Cruex	Clotrimazole
Cruex	Undecylenic acid
Cubicin	Daptomycin
CytoGam	Cytomegalovirus immune globulin
Cytovene	Ganciclovir

Trade Name	Generic Name
d4T*	Stavudine
Daraprim	Pyrimethamine
ddC*	Zalcitabine
Dideoxycytidine	Zalcitabine
ddI*	Didanosine
DDS*	Dapsone
DEC*	Diethylcarbamazine
Denavir	Penciclovir
DesenexMyax	Terbinafine
Diaminodiphenylsulfone	Dapsone
Dideoxyinosine	Didanosine
Diethylcarbamazine citrate	Diethylcarbamazine
Diflucan	Fluconazole
Diiodhydroxyquin	Iodoquinol
Diiodohydroxyquinoline	Iodoquinol
Diquinol	Iodoquinol
DisperMox	Amoxicillin
DLV*	Delavirdine
DMP-266*	Efavirenz
Doribax	Doripenem
DRV*	Darunavir
Duricef	Cefadroxil
Dycill	Dicloxacillin sodium
Dynabac, Dynabac D5-Pak	Dirithromycin
Dynacin	Minocycline
Elimite	Permethrin
Elon Dual Defense Anti-Fungal Formula	Undecylenic acid
Emtriva	Emtricitabine
E-Mycin	Erythromycin preparations
Epivir, Epivir-HBV	Lamivudine
Epzicom	Abacavir sulfate + lamivudine
Eraxis	Anidulafungin
Ery-Ped	Erythromycin preparations
Erythrocin	Erythromycin preparations
Eryzole	Erythromycin ethylsuccinate and acetylsulfisoxazole
Exelderm	Sulconazole
Famvir	Famciclovir
Fansidar	Pyrimethamine + sulfadoxine
f-APV*	Fosamprenavir
Flagyl, Flagyl ER	Metronidazole
Floxin, Floxin Otic	Ofloxacin
Flumadine	Rimantadine
Fortaz	Ceftazidime
Foscavir	Foscarnet
Fourneau 309	Suramin
FTC*	Emtricitabine

*Common abbreviation or other name (not recommended for use when writing a prescription).

Trade Name	Generic Name
Fungizone	Amphotericin B
Fungoid AF	Undecylenic acid
Furadantin	Nitrofurantoin
Furoxone	Furazolidone
Fuzeon	Enfuvirtide
Gamma benzene hexachloride	Lindane
Gantrisin	Sulfisoxazole
Garamycin	Gentamicin
Germanin	Suramin
Goordochom	Undecylenic acid
Grifulvin V	Griseofulvin
Grisactin	Griseofulvin
Griseofulvin Microsize	Griseofulvin
Gris-PEG	Griseofulvin
Gyne-Lotrimin 3	Clotrimazole
Gyne-Lotrimin 7	Clotrimazole
Halfan	Halofantrine
HBIG*	Hepatitis B immune globulin
HepaGam B	Hepatitis B immune globulin
Hetrazan	Diethylcarbamazine
Hiprex	Methenamine preparations
Hivid	Zalcitabine
Humatin	Paromomycin sulfate
IDV*	Indinavir
Imogam Rabies-HT	Rabies Immune globulin
INH*	Isoniazid
Invanz	Ertapenem
Invirase	Saquinavir mesylate
Iostat	Potassium iodide
Isentress	Raltegravir
Kaletra	Lopinavir with ritonavir
Kantrex	Kanamycin
Keflex	Cephalexin
Lamisil, Lamisil AT	Terbinafine
Lampit	Nifurtimox
Lamprene	Clofazimine
Laniazid	Isoniazid
Lariam	Mefloquine HCL
Levaquin, Quixin, Iquix	Levofloxacin
Lexiva	Fosamprenavir
Loprox	Ciclopirox/Ciclopirox olamine
Lorabid	Loracarbef
Lotrimim Ultra	Butenafine
Lotrimin AF	Miconazole
Lotrimin AF	Clotrimazole
LPV/RTV*	Lopinavir with ritonavir
Macrobid	Nitrofurantoin

*Common abbreviation or other name (not recommended for use when writing a prescription).

Trade Name	Generic Name
Macrodantin	Nitrofurantoin
Malarone Pediatric Tablets, Malarone Tablets	Atovaquone + proguanil
Maxipime	Cefepime
Mefoxin	Cefoxitin
Mel B	Melarsoprol
Mel B	Suramin
Melarsen Oxide-BAL	Melarsoprol
Mentax	Butenafine
Mepron	Atovaquone
Merrem	Meropenem
Methenamine mandelate	Methenamine preparations
MetroGel, MetroLotion, MetroCream, MetroGel-Vaginal	Metronidazole
Micatin	Miconazole
Minocin	Minocycline
Mintezol	Thiabendazole
Monistat	Miconazole
Monistat 1	Tioconazole
Monurol	Fosfomycin tromethamine
Moranyl	Suramin
Myambutol	Ethambutol HCL
Mycamine	Micafungin sodium
Mycelex, Mycelex-7	Clotrimazole
Mycifradin	Neomycin sulfate
Mycobutin	Rifabutin
Mycostatin	Nystatin
Nabi-HB	Hepatitis B immune globulin
Naftin Cream, Naftin Gel	Naftifine
Nallpen	Nafcillin
Naphuride	Suramin
Nebcin	Tobramycin
NebuPent	Pentamidine isethionate
Neo-Fradin, Neo-Tabs	Neomycin sulfate
Neosporin GU Irrigant, Neosporin, Neosporin Ophthalmic	Neomycin/Polymyxin B/± Bacitracin
NeuTrexin	Trimetrexate glucuronate
NFV*	Nelfinavir
Nilstat	Nystatin
Nix	Permethrin
Nizoral, Nizoral A-D	Ketoconazole
Noritate	Metronidazole
Noroxin	Norfloxacin
Norvir	Ritonavir
Noxafil	Posaconazole
NVP*	Nevirapine
Nydrazid	Isoniazid
Ocuflox	Ofloxacin

*Common abbreviation or other name (not recommended for use when writing a prescription).

Trade Name	Generic Name
Ocusulf-10	Sulfacetamide sodium, ophthalmic
Omnicef	Cefdinir
Omnipen	Ampicillin
Ovide	Malathion
Oxistat	Oxiconazole
Pamix	Pyrantel pamoate
PAS*	Para-aminosalicylic acid
Paser Granules	Para-aminosalicylic acid
Pathocil	Dicloxacillin sodium
Pediamycin	Erythromycin preparations
Pediazole	Erythromycin ethylsuccinate and acetylsulfisoxazole
PediOtic	Polymyxin B sulfate, neomycin sulfate, and hydrocortisone
Penlac	Ciclopirox/Ciclopirox olamine
Pentam 300	Pentamidine isethionate
Pentavalent antimony	Stibogluconate
Pentostam	Stibogluconate
Periostat	Doxycycline
Pfizerpen	Penicillin G preparations—Aqueous potassium and sodium
Pima	Potassium iodide
Pin-Rid	Pyrantel pamoate
Pin-X	Pyrantel pamoate
Pipracil	Piperacillin
Plaquenil, Quineprox	Hydroxychloroquine
PMPA*	Tenofovir disoproxil fumarate
Podocon-25,	Podophyllin/Podophyllum resin
Podofin	Podophyllin/Podophyllum resin
Polymox	Amoxicillin
Polysporin Ophthalmic, Polysporin Topical	Bacitracin + polymyxin B
Polytrim Ophthalmic Solution	Polymyxin B sulfate and trimethoprim sulfate
Prezista	Darunavir
Priftin	Rifapentine
Primaxin IV, Primaxin IM	Imipenem-Cilastatin
Primsol	Trimethoprim
Principen	Ampicillin
Proloprim	Trimethoprim
Pronto	Pyrethrins
Prostat	Metronidazole
Pyrazinoic acid amide	Pyrazinamide
Pyridium	Phenazopyridine HCL
Qualaquin	Quinine sulfate
Quineprox	Hydroxychloroquine
Raniclor	Cefaclor
Rebetol	Ribavirin

*Common abbreviation or other name (not recommended for use when writing a prescription).

Trade Name	Generic Name
Reese's Pinworm	Pyrantel pamoate
Relenza	Zanamivir
Rescriptor	Delavirdine
Retrovir	Zidovudine
Reyataz	Atazanavir
Ribaspheres	Ribavirin
RID	Pyrethrins
Rifadin	Rifampin
Rimactane	Rifampin
Rocephin	Ceftriaxone
Selsun	Selenium sulfide
Selzentry	Maraviroc
Septra	Sulfamethoxazole and trimethoprim
Seromycin	Cycloserine
Silvadene	Silver sulfadiazine
Sinecatechins	Kunecatechins
Spectazole	Econazole nitrate
Spectracef	Cefditoren pivoxil
Sporanox	Itraconazole
SSD Cream, SSD AF Cream	Silver sulfadiazine
SSKI	Potassium iodide
Stromectol	Ivermectin
Sulfatrim	Sulfamethoxazole and trimethoprim
Sumycin	Tetracycline HCL
Suprax	Cefixime
Sustiva	Efavirenz
Symmetrel	Amantadine hydrochloride
Synagis	Palivizumab
Synercid	Quinupristin with dalfopristin
T-20*	Enfuvirtide
Tamiflu	Oseltamivir phosphate
Tazicef	Ceftazidime
Tazidime	Ceftazidime
TDF*	Tenofovir disoproxil fumarate
Tegopen	Cloxacillin
Terazol 3, Terazol 7	Terconazole
Thalomid	Thalidomide
Thermazene	Silver sulfadiazine
ThyroShield	Potassium iodide
Ticar	Ticarcillin
Timentin	Ticarcillin with clavulanate
Tinactin	Tolnaftate
Tindamax	Tinidazole
Tioconazole 1	Tioconazole
Tisit	Pyrethrins
TMC 114*	Darunavir
TMP*	Trimethoprim

*Common abbreviation or other name (not recommended for use when writing a prescription).

Trade Name	Generic Name
TMP-SMX*	Sulfamethoxazole and trimethoprim
TOBI	Tobramycin
Tobrex	Tobramycin
Totacillin	Ampicillin
TPV*	Tipranavir
Trecator, Trecator-SC	Ethionamide
Trifluorothymidine	Trifluridine
Trimox	Amoxicillin
Trizivir	Abacavir sulfate + zidovudine and lamivudine
Trobicin	Spectinomycin
Tygacil	Tigecycline
Unasyn	Ampicillin with sulbactam
Unipen	Nafcillin
Urex	Methenamine preparations
Vagistat-1	Tioconazole
Valcyte	Valganciclovir
Valtrex	Valacyclovir
Vancocin	Vancomycin
Vantin	Cefpodoxime proxetil
VariZig	Varicella-Zoster immune globulin (human)
Veetids	Penicillin V potassium
Velosef	Cephradine
Veregen	Kunecatechins
Vermox	Mebendazole
Vfend	Voriconazole
Vibramycin	Doxycycline
Videx, Videx EC	Didanosine
Vigamox	Moxifloxacin
Viracept	Nelfinavir
Viramune	Nevirapine
Virazole	Ribavirin
Viread	Tenofovir disoproxil fumarate
Viroptic	Trifluridine
Vistide	Cidofovir
VZIG*	Varicella-zoster immune globulin (human)
Wycillin	Penicillin G preparations—Procaine
Wymox	Amoxicillin
Xolegel	Ketoconazole
Yodoxin	Iodoquinol
Zazole	Terconazole
Zerit	Stavudine
Ziagen	Abacavir sulfate
Zinacef	Cefuroxime (IV, IM)
Zithromax, Zithromax TRI-PAK	Azithromycin

*Common abbreviation or other name (not recommended for use when writing a prescription).

Trade Name	Generic Name
Zolicef	Cefazolin
Zosyn	Piperacillin/Tazobactam
Zovirax	Acyclovir
Z-PAK, Zmax	Azithromycin
Zyvox	Linezolid

FORMULARY

VI. DRUG DOSES

ABACAVIR SULFATE
Ziagen, 1592; In combination with zidovudine and
lamivudine: Trizivir; In combination with lamivudine:
Epzicom

Yes	No	3	C

*Antiviral agent, nucleoside analogue reverse
transcriptase inhibitor*

Tabs: 300 mg
Oral solution: 20 mg/mL (240 mL)
In combination with zidovudine (AZT) and lamivudine (3TC) as Trizivir:
    Tabs: 300 mg abacavir + 300 mg zidovudine + 150 mg lamivudine
In combination with lamivudine (3TC) as Epzicom:
    Tabs: 600 mg abacavir + 300 mg lamivudine

1–3 mo (investigational dose): 8 mg/kg/dose PO BID
≥3 mo–16 yr (see remarks): 8 mg/kg/dose PO BID; **max. dose:** 300 mg BID
Adult: 600 mg/24 hr PO ÷ QD-BID
    Mild hepatic impairment (Child-Pugh score 5 to 6): 200 mg PO BID
Trizivir (see remarks):
    Adolescent and adult (≥40 kg): 1 tablet PO BID
Epzicom (see remarks):
    Adult: 1 tablet PO QD

Contraindications: Hypersensitivity to abacavir or any other components in the
formulation; and moderate/severe hepatic impairment.
Warnings/Precautions: Fatal hypersensitivity reactions (5%) is characterized by
a sign or symptom in 2 or more of the following groups: (1) fever, (2) skin rash, (3)
gastrointestinal, including nausea, vomiting, diarrhea, or abdominal pain, (4)
constitutional, including malaise, fatigue, or achiness, and (5) respiratory, including
cough, dyspnea, and pharyngitis. Discontinue use of drug as soon as hypersensitivity
reaction is suspected and and monitor closely. **Do not** restart medication following
hypersensitivity reaction because more severe life-threatening symptoms will recur.
Adolescent Dosing: Patients in early puberty (Tanner I–II) should be dosed with
pediatric regimens and those in late puberty (Tanner IV) should be dosed with adult
regimens. Adolescents who are at the midst of their growth spurt (Tanner III females
and Tanner IV males) can be dosed by either pediatric or adult regimen with close
monitoring of efficacy and toxicity.
    Use abacavir in combination with other antiretrovirals. Suboptimal virologic
response has been reported with once daily three-drug combination therapy with
lamivudine and tenofovir in therapy-naïve adults.
Use of Combination Products: For Trizivir, **do not** use in patients with creatinine
clearance <50 mL/min or patients with impaired hepatic function. For Epzicom, **do
not** use in patients with creatinine clearance <50 mL/min. No dosing information is
currently available for children with mild hepatic impairment or for adults with
moderate/severe hepatic impairment. There is no current data to support once daily
dosing for adolescents. See http://aidsinfo.nih.gov/guidelines for the latest
information.
Adverse Effects: In addition to hypersensitivity (see Warnings/Precautions), nausea,
vomiting, diarrhea, mild hyperglycemia (more frequent in children), mild triglyceride
elevation, decreased appetite, and insomnia may occur. Lactic acidosis and severe
hepatomegaly with steatosis have also been reported.
Drug Interactions: Ethanol decreases the elimination of abacavir. Abacavir may
increase the clearance of methadone.
Drug Administration: Doses may be administered with food or on an empty stomach.

For explanation of icons, see p. 306.

ACYCLOVIR
Zovirax and various generics
Antiviral

No   Yes   1   B

Capsules: 200 mg
Tabs: 400, 800 mg
Oral suspension: 200 mg/5 mL; may contain parabens
Ointment: 5% (15 g)
Cream: 5% (2 g)
Injection in powder (with sodium): 500, 1000 mg
Injection in solution (with sodium): 50 mg/mL
Contains 4.2 mEq Na/1 g drug

IMMUNOCOMPETENT:
Neonatal (HSV and HSV encephalitis):
   <35 wk postconceptional age: 40 mg/kg/24 hr ÷ Q12 hr IV × 14–21 days
   ≥35 wk postconceptional age: 60 mg/kg/24 hr ÷ Q8 hr IV × 14–21 days
Mucocutaneous HSV (including genital):
Initial infection:
   IV: 15 mg/kg/24 hr or 750 mg/m²/24 hr ÷ Q8 hr × 5–7 days
   PO: 1200 mg/24 hr ÷ Q8 hr × 7–10 days with a **max. dose** in children at 80 mg/kg/24 hr ÷ Q6–8 hr
Recurrence:
   PO: 1200 mg/24 hr ÷ Q8 hr or 1600 mg/24 hr ÷ Q12 hr × 5 days with a **max. dose** in children at 80 mg/kg/24 hr ÷ Q6–8 hr
Chronic suppressive therapy:
   PO: 800–1000 mg/24 hr ÷ 2–5×/24 hr for up to 1 year with a **max. dose** in children at 80 mg/kg/24 hr ÷ Q6–8 hr
Zoster:
   IV: 30 mg/kg/24 hr or 1500 mg/m²/24 hr ÷ Q8 hr × 7–10 days
   PO: 4000 mg/24 hr ÷ 5×/24 hr × 5–7 days for patients ≥12 yr
Varicella:
   IV: 30 mg/kg/24 hr or 1500 mg/m²/24 hr ÷ Q8 hr × 7–10 days
   PO: 80 mg/kg/24 hr ÷ QID × 5 days (begin treatment at earliest signs/symptoms); **max. dose:** 3200 mg/24 hr
Max. dose of oral acyclovir in children = 80 mg/kg/24 hr
IMMUNOCOMPROMISED:
HSV:
   IV: 750–1500 mg/m²/24 hr ÷ Q8 hr × 7–14 days
   PO: 1000 mg/24 hr ÷ 3–5 times/24 hr × 7–14 days
HSV prophylaxis:
   IV: 750 mg/m²/24 hr ÷ Q8 hr during risk period
   PO: 600–1000 mg/24 hr ÷ 3–5 times/24 hr during risk period
Varicella or zoster:
   IV: 1500 mg/m²/24 hr ÷ Q8 hr × 7–10 days
   PO: 250–600 mg/m²/dose 4–5 times/ 24 hr
CMV prophylaxis:
   IV: 1500 mg/m²/24 hr ÷ Q8 hr during risk period
   PO: 800–3200 mg/24 hr ÷ Q6–24 hr during risk period
Max. dose of oral acyclovir in children = 80 mg/kg/24 hr.

ACYCLOVIR *continued*

TOPICAL:
> Apply 0.5 inch ribbon of 5% ointment for 4 inch square surface area 6 times a day × 7 days.

Contraindications: Hypersensitivity to acyclovir or any other of its components. Warnings/Precautions: Use with **caution** in patients with pre-existing neurologic or renal impairment **(adjust dose; see Chapter 3)** or dehydration. **Do not** use topical product on the eye or for the prevention of recurrent HSV infections.
Resistant strains of HSV and VZV have been reported in immunocompromised patients (e.g., advanced HIV infection). See most recent edition of the AAP Red Book for additional information.

Use ideal body weight for obese patients when calculating dosages. Drug is removed by hemodialysis. Peritoneal dialysis and blood exchange transfusion do not appear to appreciably remove the drug. **Dose alteration is necessary in patients with impaired renal function (see Chapter 3).**

Adverse Effects
> Systemic route: May cause renal impairment; has been infrequently associated with headache, vertigo, insomnia, encephalopathy, GI tract irritation, elevated liver function tests, rash, urticaria, arthralgia, fever, and adverse hematologic effects. Inflammation/phlebitis at injection site is common with IV route.
> Topical route: May cause a local pain and irritation.

Drug Interactions: Probenecid decreases acyclovir renal clearance. Acyclovir may increase the concentration of tenofovir, and meperidine and its metabolite (normeperidine).

Drug Administration: Maintain adequate hydration while on therapy.
> IV: Slow (1 hr) IV administration at a concentration ≤ 7 mg/mL are essential to prevent crystallization in renal tubules and risk of phlebitis.
> PO: Doses may be administered with or without food. Shake oral suspension well before each use.

ALBENDAZOLE
Albenza
Anthelmintic, benzimidazole derivative

Yes   Yes   ?   C

Tabs: 200 mg

Hydatid disease (tapeworm, Echinococcus granulosus):
> *<60 kg:* 15 mg/kg/24 hr ÷ BID PO (**max. dose:** 800 mg/24 hr) × 1–6 mo
> *≥60 kg:* 400 mg BID PO × 1–6 mo

Neurocysicercosis (tapeworm, Cysticerus cellulosae; use with concurrent anticonvulsant and corticosteroid therapy):
> *<60 kg:* 15 mg/kg/24 hr ÷ BID PO (**max. dose:** 800 mg/24 hr) × 8–30 days, may be repeated if necessary
> *≥60 kg:* 400 mg BID PO × 8–30 days, may be repeated if necessary

Ancylostoma caninum (Eosinophilic enterocolitis), ascariasis (roundworm), hookworm (Ancylstoma duodenale, Necator americanus), Trichostrongylus: 400 mg PO × 1

Cutaneous larva migrans, Trichuriasis (whipworm or Trichuris trichiura): 400 mg QD PO × 3 days

Visceral larva migrans (toxocariasis): 400 mg QD PO × 5 days

Fluke (Clonorchirs sinensis, Chinese liver fluke): 10 mg/kg/dose PO QD × 7 days

Enterobius vermicularis (pinworm): 400 mg PO × 1, repeat × 1 in 2 wk

Continued

ALBENDAZOLE *continued*

Filariasis (Mansonella perstans), Capillariasis (alternative therapy, mebendazole is drug of choice): 400 mg QD PO × 10 days
Gnathostomiasis (Gnathostoma spinigerum): 400 mg QD PO × 21 days
Trichinosis (Trichinella spiralis): 400 mg BID PO × 8–14 days

> ***Contraindications:*** Hypersensitivity to albendazole or benzimidazole products.
> ***Warnings/Precautions:*** Prior to initiating therapy for neurocysticercosis, assess for retinal lesions to weigh the risk/benefit of potential retinal damage caused by albendazole-induced changes to the existing retinal lesion. Patients treated for neurocysticercosis should receive appropriate steroid and anticonvulsant therapy to minimize cerebral hypertensive episodes. **Should not** be used in pregnancy unless in circumstances where no alternative management is appropriate. Patients **should not** become pregnant at least 1 month following the cessation of therapy. Rare granulocytopenia/pancytopenia resulting in fatalities and hepatotoxicity have been reported; blood counts and LFTs should be monitored with prolonged regimens (prior to each 28-day cycle and every 2 weeks).
>
> Extrahepatic obstruction increases the systemic availability of albendazole sulfoxide (prolonged rate of absorption/conversion and elimination).
> ***Adverse Effects:*** Gastrointestinal disturbances (abdominal pain, nausea and vomiting) and headache are common. Rare but serious effects include acute renal failure, hepatotoxicity with increased LFTs, leukopenia and thrombocytopenia.
> ***Drug Interactions:*** Dexamethasone and praziquantel may increase albendazole sulfoxide levels. Albendazole is an inducer of CYP 450 1A2 and a substrate for 3A4 (major) and 1A2 (minor).
> ***Drug Administration:*** Administer doses with meals.

AMANTADINE HYDROCHLORIDE
Symmetrel and others
Antiviral agent

Yes	Yes	3	C

Capsule: 100 mg
Tabs: 100 mg
Syrup: 50 mg/5 mL (480 mL); may contain parabens

> *Influenza A prophylaxis and treatment (for treatment, it is best to initiate therapy immediately after the onset of symptoms; within 2 days):*
> **1–9 yr:** 5 mg/kg/24 hr PO ÷ QD-BID; **max. dose:** 150 mg/24 hr
> **>9 yr:**
> **<40 kg:** 5 mg/kg/24 hr PO ÷ QD-BID; **max. dose:** 200 mg/24 hr
> **≥40 kg:** 200 mg/24 hr ÷ QD-BID
> ***Alternative dosing for influenza A prophylaxis:***
> **Child >20 kg and adult:** 100 mg/24 hr PO ÷ QD-BID
> ***Prophylaxis (duration of therapy):***
> **Single exposure:** at least 10 days
> **Repeated/uncontrolled exposure:** up to 90 days
> **Use with influenza A vaccine when possible**
> ***Symptomatic treatment (duration of therapy):***
> Continue for 24–48 hr after disappearance of symptoms

AMANTADINE HYDROCHLORIDE *continued*

Contraindications: Hypersensitivity to amantadine or any of its components. **Do not** use in the first trimester of a pregnancy.

Warnings/Precautions: Individuals immunized with live attenuated influenza vaccine should not receive amantadine prophylaxis for 14 days after the vaccine. Chemoprophylaxis does not interfere with immune response to inactivated influenza vaccine. Use with **caution** in patients with liver disease, seizures, renal disease, congestive heart failure, peripheral edema, orthostatic hypotension, history of recurrent eczematoid rash, serious mental illness, and in those receiving CNS stimulants. Neuroleptic malignant syndrome has been reported with abrupt dose reduction or discontinuation (especially if patient is receiving neuroleptics). **Adjust dose in patients with renal insufficiency (see Chapter 3).**

Adverse Effects: May cause dizziness, anxiety, depression, mental status change, rash (livedo reticularis), nausea, orthostatic hypotension, edema, CHF, and urinary retention.

Drug Interactions: Anticholinergic drugs may potentiate the anticholinergic side effect of amantadine. Quinidine, quinine, triamterene and trimethoprim may increase the effects/toxicity of amantadine. Use with CNS stimulants may enhance CNS stimulant effects.

Drug Administration: Administer doses with meals to enhance absorption and decrease GI symptoms and **do not** administer within 4 hr of bedtime to prevent insomnia.

AMINOSALICYLIC ACID

See *Para-Aminosalicylic Acid*

AMIKACIN SULFATE
Amikin
Antibiotic, aminoglycoside

No   Yes   1   C

Injection: 50, 250 mg/mL; may contain sodium bisulfite

 Neonates: See following table.

Postconceptional Age (wk)	Postnatal Age (days)	Dose (mg/kg/dose)	Interval (hr)
≤29*	0–7	18	48
	8–28	15	36
	>28	15	24
30–33	0–7	18	36
	>7	15	24
34–37	0–7	15	24
	>7	15	18–24
≥38	0–7	15	24
	>7	15	12–18

*Or significant asphyxia, PDA, indomethicin use, poor cardiac output, reduced renal function

Continued

For explanation of icons, see p. 306.

AMIKACIN SULFATE *continued*

Infant and child: 15–22.5 mg/kg/24 hr ÷ Q8 hr IV/IM; infants and patients requiring higher doses may receive initial doses of 30 mg/kg/24 hr ÷ Q8 hr IV/IM
Adult: 15 mg/kg/24 hr ÷ Q8–12 hr IV/IM
Initial **max. dose:** 1.5 g/24 hr, then monitor levels

> ***Contraindications:*** Hypersensitivity to amikacin and aminoglycosides.
> ***Warnings/Precautions:*** Use with **caution** in pre-existing renal, vestibular or auditory impairment; concomitant anesthesia or neuromuscular blockers, neurotoxic; concomitant neurotoxic, ototoxic, or nephrotoxic drugs; sulfite sensitivity; and dehydration.
>
> **Adjust dose in renal failure (see Chapter 3).** Rapidly eliminated in patients with cystic fibrosis, burns, and in febrile neutropenic patients. Longer dosing intervals may be necessary for neonates receiving indomethacin for PDAs and for all patients with poor cardiac output.
>
> Therapeutic Levels: Peak, 20–30 mg/L; trough <10 mg/L. Recommended serum sampling time at steady state: trough within 30 min prior to the third consecutive dose and peak 30–60 min after the administration of the third consecutive dose. Peak levels of 25–30 mg/L have been recommended for CNS, pulmonary, bone, life-threatening infections and in febrile neutropenic patients.
>
> ***Adverse Effects:*** May cause ototoxicity, nephrotoxicity, neuromuscular blockade, and rash.
>
> ***Drug Interactions:*** Loop diuretics may potentiate the ototoxicity of all aminoglycoside antibiotics. See Warning/Precautions. Beta-lactam antibiotics may inactivate aminoglycosides in vitro and in vivo in patients with severe renal failure. Degradation depends on beta-lactam concentration, storage time and temperature.
>
> ***Drug Administration:*** IM or IV infusion over 30 min at a concentration ≤10 mg/mL. **Do not** administer beta-lactam antibiotics within 1 hr before or after amikacin dose.

AMOXICILLIN
Amoxil, Trimox, Wymox, Polymox, DisperMox, and others
Antibiotic, aminopenicillin

No   Yes   1   B

Drops: 50 mg/mL (15, 30 mL)
Oral suspension: 125, 250 mg/5 mL (80, 100, 150 mL); and 200, 400 mg/5 mL (50, 75, 100 mL)
Caps: 250, 500 mg
Tablets: 500, 875 mg
Chewable tabs: 125, 200, 250, 400 mg
Tablets for oral suspension (DisperMox): 200, 400 mg; contains phenylalanine

---

Infant ≤3 months: 20–30 mg/kg/24 hr ÷ Q12 hr PO
Child:
  Standard dose: 25–50 mg/kg/24 hr ÷ Q8–12 hr PO
  High dose (resistant S. pneumoniae): 80–90 mg/kg/24 hr ÷ Q12 hr PO
Adult:
  Mild/moderate infections: 250 mg/dose Q8 hr PO OR 500 mg/dose Q12 hr PO
  Severe infections: 500 mg/dose Q8 hr PO OR 875 mg/dose Q12 hr PO
Max. dose: 2–3 g/24 hr
Recurrent otitis media prophylaxis: 20 mg/kg/dose QHS PO
SBE prophylaxis:
  Child: 50 mg/kg/dose × 1 PO 1 hr before procedure; **max. dose:** 2 g/dose

AMOXICILLIN *continued*

Adult: 2 g/dose × 1 PO 1 hr before procedure
Early Lyme disease:
  Child: 50 mg/kg/24 hr ÷ Q8 hr PO × 14–21 days; **max. dose:** 1.5 g/24 hr
  Adult: 500 mg/dose Q8 hr PO × 14–21 days

Contraindications: Hypersensitivity to penicillins.
Warnings/Precautions: Epstein-Barr virus infection, acute lymphocytic leukemia or CMV infections may increase risk for amoxicillin-induced maculopapular rash. Chewable tablets and DisperMox may contain phenylalanine and **should not** be used by phenyketonurics.
  High-dose regimen increasingly useful in respiratory infections, especially acute otitis media and sinusitis, due to increasing incidence of penicillin-resistant pneumococci. **Adjust dose in renal failure (see Chapter 3).**
Adverse Effects: Rash, diarrhea, nausea and vomiting.
Drug Interactions: Use with allopurinol increases risk for rash. Decreases the efficacy of oral contraceptives. Probenecid increases serum amoxicillin levels.
Drug Administration: Doses may be administered with or without food.
DisperMox oral suspension is prepared by swirling/stirring each tablet thoroughly in approximately 10 mL of water only. **Do not** chew or swallow (whole tablets) DisperMox.

AMOXICILLIN WITH CLAVULANIC ACID
Augmentin, Augmentin ES-600, Augmentin XR, and various generic products
Antibiotic, aminopenicillin with beta lactamase inhibitor

Yes   Yes   1   B

Tabs:
  For TID dosing: 250, 500 mg (with 125 mg clavulanate)
  For BID dosing: 875 mg amoxicillin (with 125 mg clavulanate); Augmentin XR: 1 g amoxicillin (with 62.5 mg clavulanate)
Chewable tabs:
  For TID dosing: 125, 250 mg amoxicillin (31.25 and 62.5 mg clavulanate, respectively); contains saccharin
  For BID dosing: 200, 400 mg amoxicillin (28.5 and 57 mg clavulanate, respectively); contains saccharin and aspartame
Oral suspension:
  For TID dosing: 125, 250 mg amoxicillin/5mL (31.25 and 62.5 mg clavulanate/5 mL, respectively) (75, 100, 150 mL); contains saccharin
  For BID dosing: 200, 400 mg amoxicillin/5 mL (28.5 and 57 mg clavulanate/5 mL, respectively) (50, 75, 100 mL); 600 mg amoxicillin/5 mL (Augmentin ES-600; contains 42.9 mg clavulanate/5 mL) (50, 75, 100, 150 mL); contains saccharin and/or aspartame
  Contains 0.63 mEq K$^+$ per 125 mg clavulanate (Augmentin ES-600 contains 0.23 mEq K$^+$ per 42.9 mg clavulanate)

Dosage based on amoxicillin component.
Child <3 mo: 30 mg/kg/24 hr ÷ Q12 hr PO (recommended dosage form is 125 mg/5 mL suspension)
Child ≥3 mo:
  TID dosing (see remarks):
    20–40 mg/kg/24 hr ÷ Q8 hr PO

Continued

AMOXICILLIN WITH CLAVULANIC ACID *continued*

> **BID dosing (see remarks):**
>> 25–45 mg/kg/24 hr ÷ Q12 hr PO
>
> **Augmentin ES-600:**
>> **≥3 mo and <40 kg:** 90 mg/kg/24 hr ÷ Q12 hr PO × 10 days
>
> **Adult:** 250–500 mg/dose Q8 hr PO or 875 mg/dose Q12 hr PO for more severe and respiratory infections
>> **Augmentin XR:**
>>> **≥16 yr and adult:** 2 g Q12 hr PO × 10 days for acute bacterial sinusitis or × 7–10 days for community acquired pneumonia

Contraindications: Hypersensitivity to penicillins and patients with a history of cholestatic jaundice/hepatitic dysfunction associated with amoxicillin-clavulanic acid. Augmentin XR is **contraindicated** in patients with CrCl <30 mL/min.

Warnings/Precautions: For BID dosing, the 875 mg, 1 g tablets, the 200 mg, 400 mg chewable tablets or the 200mg/5mL, 400mg/5mL, 600 mg/5mL suspensions should be used. These BID dosage forms contain phenylalanine and **should not** be used by phenyketonurics. For TID dosing, the 250 mg, 500 mg tablets, the 125 mg, 250 mg chewable tablets or the 125mg/5mL, 250mg/5mL suspensions should be used. The 250 or 500 mg tablets **cannot** be substituted for Augmentin XR. See amoxicillin for additional information.

Higher doses of 80–90 mg/kg/24 hr (amoxicillin component) have been recommended for resistant strains of *S. pneumoniae* in acute otitis media (use BID formulations containing 7:1 ratio of amoxicillin to clavulanic acid or Augmentin ES-600). See amoxicillin.

Adjust dose in renal failure (see Chapter 3).

Adverse Effects: Rash, urticaria, diarrhea (clavulanate increases risk), nausea and vomiting are common. BID dosing schedule is associated with less diarrhea. Rare hepatoxicity has been reported.

Drug Interactions: See amoxicillin.

Drug Administration: May be administered without regard to meals; administering doses prior to meals may enhance absorption and minimize GI side effects. **Do not** administer with high-fat meals; may decrease absorption of clavulanate.

AMPHOTERICIN B
Fungizone, Amphocin
Antifungal, polyene

Yes   Yes   ?   B

Injection: 50 mg vials

IV: See Drug Administration section.
> **Optional test dose:** 0.1 mg/kg/dose IV up to **maximum** 1 mg (followed by remaining initial dose).

Initial dose: 0.5–1 mg/kg/24 hr; if test dose *not* used, infuse first dose over 6 hr and monitor frequently during the first several hours.

Increment: Increase as tolerated by 0.25–0.5 mg/kg/24 hr QD or QOD

Usual maintenance:
> **QD dosing:** 0.5–1 mg/kg/24 hr QD
> **QOD dosing:** 1.5 mg/kg/dose QOD

Max. dose: 1.5 mg/kg/24 hr

Intrathecal: 25–100 mcg Q48–72 hr. Increase to 500 mcg as tolerated.

AMPHOTERICIN B *continued*

Bladder irrigation for urinary tract mycosis: 5–15 mg in 100 mL sterile water for irrigation at 100–300 mL/24 hr. Instill solution into bladder, clamp catheter for 1–2 hr then drain; repeat TID-QID for 2–5 days.

> **Contraindications:** Hypersensitivity to any form of amphotericin B.
> **Warnings/Precautions:** Primarily used for severe, progressive, life-threatening fungal infections. Anaphylaxis has been reported. **Avoid** other nephrotoxic drugs. Monitor renal, hepatic, electrolyte, and hematologic status closely.
> ~66% of plasma concentrations detected in fluids from inflamed pleura, peritoneum, synovium and aqueous humor. Good placenta penetration. Poor CSF (≤4% of serum concentration) and eye penetration. CNS/CSF levels are lower than amphotericin B, liposomal (AmBisome). **(For dosing information in renal failure, see Chapter 3).**
> **Adverse Effects:** Common infusion-related reactions include fever, chills, headache, hypotension, nausea, vomiting; may premedicate with acetaminophen and diphenhydramine 30 min before and 4 hr after infusion. Meperidine useful for chills. Hydrocortisone, 1 mg/kg ampho (**max. dose:** 25 mg) added to bottle may help prevent immediate adverse reactions. Hypercalciuria, hypokalemia, hypomagnesemia, RTA, renal failure (salt loading with 10–15 mL/kg of NS infused prior to each dose may minimize risk), acute hepatic failure, hypotension, and phlebitis may occur.
> **Drug Interactions:** Nephrotoxic drugs such as aminoglycosides, chemotherapeutic agents, and cyclosporine may result in synergistic toxicity. May increase the toxicity of neuromuscular blocking agents and cardiac glycosides due to hypokalemia.
> **Drug Administration:** For IV route, mix with D_5W to concentration 0.1 mg/mL (peripheral administration) or 0.25 mg/mL (central line only). pH >4.2. Infuse over 2–6 hr.

AMPHOTERICIN B CHOLESTERYL SULFATE
Amphotec, ABCD
Antifungal, polyene

Yes · No · ? · B

Injection: 50, 100 mg (vials)
(formulated as a 1:1 molar ratio of amphotericin B complexed to cholesteryl sulfate)

> **IV:** See Drug Administration section.
> Start at 3–4 mg/kg/24 hr QD, dose may be increased to 6 mg/kg/24 hr if necessary. A 10 mL test dose of the diluted solution administered over 15–30 min has been recommended. Doses of 3–6 mg/kg/24 hr have been used to treat invasive *Candida* or *Cryptococcus* infections in patients who have failed to respond to or could not tolerate conventional amphotericin B. Doses as high as 7.5 mg/kg/24 hr have been used to treat invasive fungal infections in BMT patients.

> **Contraindications:** Hypersensitivity to any form of amphotericin B.
> **Warnings/Precautions:** Primarily used for severe, progressive, life-threatening fungal infections. Monitor renal, hepatic, electrolyte, and hematologic status closely.
> In animal models, concentrations in the spleen, kidneys, lungs, heart, and brain are lower than conventional amphotericin B. CNS/CSF levels are lower than amphotericin B, liposomal (AmBisome). Pharmacokinetics in severe renal and hepatic impairment have not been studied.

Continued

AMPHOTERICIN B CHOLESTERYL SULFATE *continued*

Adverse Effects: Common infusion-related reactions including fever, chills, rigors, nausea, vomiting, hypotension, and headache are more frequent with the initial doses; may premedicate with acetaminophen, diphenhydramine and meperidine (see Amphotericin B remarks). Thrombocytopenia, anemia, leukopenia, tachycardia, hypokalemia, hypomagnesemia, hypocalcemia, hyperglycemia, diarrhea, dyspnea, back pain, nephrotoxicity, and increases in serum creatinine, aminotransferases and bilirubin may occur.

Drug Interactions: See amphotericin B.

Drug Administration: Mix with D_5W to concentration 0.16–0.83 mg/mL. Infusion Rate: Give first dose at 1 mg/kg/hr, if well tolerated, infusion time can be gradually shortened to a minimum of 2 hr. **Do not** use an inline filter.

AMPHOTERICIN B LIPID COMPLEX
Abelcet, ABLC
Antifungal, polyene

Yes   No   ?   B

Injection: 5 mg/mL (10, 20 mL)
(formulated as a 1:1 molar ratio of amphotericin B to lipid complex comprised of dimyristoylphosphatidylcholine and dimyristoylphosphatidylglycerol)

IV: See Drug Administration section.
2.5–5 mg/kg/24 hr QD
For visceral leishmaniasis that failed to respond to or replased after treatment with antimony compound, a dosage of 1–3 mg/kg/24 hr QD × 5 days has been used.

Contraindications: Hypersensitivity to any form of amphotericin B.
Warnings/Precautions: Primarily used for severe, progressive, life-threatening fungal infections. Monitor renal, hepatic, electrolyte, and hematologic status closely.

Highest concentrations achieved in spleen, lung, and liver from human autopsy data from one heart transplant patient. CNS/CSF levels are lower than amphotericin B, liposomal (AmBisome). In animal models, concentrations are higher in the liver, spleen, and lungs but the same in the kidneys when compared to conventional amphotericin B. Pharmacokinetics in renal and hepatic impairment have not been studied.

Adverse Effects: Common infusion-related reactions include fever, chills, rigors, nausea, vomiting, hypotension, and headache; may premedicate with acetaminophen, diphenhydramine and meperidine (see amphotericin B remarks). Thrombocytopenia, anemia, leukopenia, hypokalemia, hypomagnesemia, diarrhea, respiratory failure, nephrotoxicity, skin rash, and increases in serum creatinine, liver enzymes and bilirubin may occur.

Drug Interactions: See amphotericin B.

Drug Administration: Mix with D_5W to concentration 1 mg/mL or 2 mg/mL for fluid restricted patients.
Infusion Rate: 2.5 mg/kg/hr; shake the infusion bag every 2 hr if total infusion time exceeds 2 hr. **Do not** use an inline filter.

AMPHOTERICIN B, LIPOSOMAL
AmBisome
Antifungal, polyene

Yes | No | ? | B

Injection: 50 mg (vials); contains sucrose
(formulated in liposomes composed of hydrogenated soy phosphatidylcholine, cholesterol, distearoylphosphatidylglycerol, and alpha-tocopherol)

IV: See Drug Administration section.
Empiric therapy for febrile neutropenia: 3 mg/kg/24 hr QD
Systemic fungal infections: 3–5 mg/kg/24 hr QD; an upper dosage limit of 10 mg/kg/24 hr has been suggested based on pharmacokinetic endpoints and risk for hypokalemia. However, dosages as high as 15 mg/kg/24 hr have been used. Dosages as high as 10 mg/kg/24 hr have been used in patients with aspergillus.
Cryptococcal meningitis in HIV: 6 mg/kg/24 hr QD
Leishmaniasis:
Immunocompetent patient: 3 mg/kg/24 hr on days 1–5, 14, and 21; a repeat course may be necessary if infection does not clear.
Immunocompromised patient: 4 mg/kg/24 hr on days 1–5, 10, 17, 24, 31, and 38; a repeat course may be necessary if infection does not clear.

Contraindications: Hypersensitivity to any form of amphotericin B.
Warnings/Precautions: Primarily used for severe, progressive, life-threatening fungal infections. Monitor renal, hepatic, electrolyte, and hematologic status closely. Safety and effectiveness in neonates have not been established.
When compared to conventional amphotericin B, higher concentrations found in the liver and spleen; and similar concentrations found in the lungs and kidney. CNS/CSF concentrations are higher than other amphotericin B products. Pharmacokinetics in renal and hepatic impairment have not been studied.
Adverse Effects: Common infusion-related reactions include fever, chills, rigors, nausea, vomiting, hypotension, and headache; may premedicate with acetaminophen, diphenhydramine and meperidine (see amphotericin B remarks). Thrombocytopenia, anemia, leukopenia, tachycardia, hypokalemia, hypomagnesemia, hypocalcemia, hyperglycemia, diarrhea, dyspnea, skin rash, low back pain, nephrotoxicity, and increases in serum creatinine, liver enzymes and bilirubin may occur.
Drug Interactions: See amphotericin B.
Drug Administration: Mix with D_5W to concentration 1–2 mg/mL (0.2–0.5 mg/mL may be used for infants and small children).
Infusion Rate: Administer dose over 2 hr; infusion may be reduced to 1 hr if well tolerated. A ≥1 micron inline filter may be used.

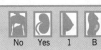

AMPICILLIN
Omnipen, Principen, Totacillin, and others
Antibiotic, aminopenicillin

No | Yes | 1 | B

Oral suspension: 125 mg/5 mL (100, 150, 200 mL), 250 mg/5 mL (100, 200 mL)
Caps: 250, 500 mg
Injection: 250, 500 mg; 1, 2, 10 g
Contains 3 mEq Na/1 g IV drug

Continued

A

FORMULARY

AMPICILLIN *continued*

Neonate (IM/IV):
   <7 days:
     <2 kg: 50–100 mg/kg/24 hr ÷ Q12 hr
     ≥2 kg: 75–150 mg/kg/24 hr ÷ Q8 hr
       Group B streptococcal meningitis: 200–300 mg/kg hr ÷ Q8 hr
   ≥7 days:
     <1.2 kg: 50–100 mg/kg hr ÷ Q12 hr
     1.2–2 kg: 75–150 mg/kg/24 hr ÷ Q8 hr
     >2 kg: 100–200 mg/kg/24 hr ÷ Q6 hr
       Group B streptococcal meningitis: 300 mg/kg/24 hr ÷ Q4–6 hr
Infant/child:
   Mild-moderate infections:
     IM/IV: 100–200 mg/kg/24 hr ÷ Q6 hr
     PO: 50–100 mg/kg/24 hr ÷ Q6 hr; **max. PO dose:** 2–3 g/24 hr
   Severe infections: 200–400 mg/kg/24 hr ÷ Q4–6 hr IM/IV
Adult:
   IM/IV: 500–3000 mg Q4–6 hr
   PO: 250–500 mg Q6 hr
Max. IV/IM dose: 12 g/24 hr
SBE prophylaxis:
   Moderate risk patients:
     Child: 50 mg/kg/dose × 1 IV/IM 30 min before procedure; **max. dose:**
     2 g/dose
     Adult: 2 g/dose × 1 IV/IM 30 min before procedure
   High risk patients with GU and GI procedures: Above doses *plus* gentamicin 1.5
   mg/kg × 1 (**max. dose:** 120 mg) IV within 30 min of starting procedure.

Contraindications: Hypersensitivity to penicillins.
Warnings/Precautions: Epstein-Barr virus infection may increase risk for
maculopapular rash. Use higher doses to treat CNS disease. **Adjust dose in
renal failure (see Chapter 3).**
Adverse Effects: Produces the same side effects as penicillin, with cross-reactivity.
Rash commonly seen at 5–10 days and rash may occur with concurrent EBV
infection or allopurinol use. May cause interstitial nephritis, diarrhea, and
pseudomembranous enterocolitis.
Drug Interactions: Chloroquine reduces ampicillin's absorption. May decrease the
effectiveness of estrogen-containing oral contraceptives.
Drug Administration
   PO: Doses should be administered on an empty stomach; 1–2 hr prior to food.
   IV: Doses may be given via IV push at a concentration ≤100 mg/mL over 3–5
   min or via intermittent IV infusion at ≤30 mg/mL over 15–30 min. IV doses have
   a shorter stability when diluted in dextrose containing solutions.

AMPICILLIN WITH SULBACTAM
Unasyn
*Antibiotic, aminopenicillin with beta-lactamase
inhibitor*

No   Yes   2   B

Injection:
1.5 g = ampicillin 1 g + sulbactam 0.5 g
3 g = ampicillin 2 g + sulbactam 1 g
Contains 5 mEq Na per 1.5 g drug combination

AMPICILLIN WITH SULBACTAM *continued*

Dosage based on ampicillin component.
Infant ≥1 mo:
   Mild/moderate infections: 100–150 mg/kg/24 hr ÷ Q6 hr IM/IV
   Meningitis/severe infections: 200–300 mg/kg/24 hr ÷ Q6 hr IM/IV
Child:
   Mild/moderate infections: 100–200 mg/kg/24 hr ÷ Q6 hr IM/IV
   Meningitis/severe infections: 200–400 mg/kg/24 hr ÷ Q4–6 hr IM/IV
Adult: 1–2 g Q6–8 hr IM/IV
Max. dose: 8 g ampicillin/24 hr

Contraindications: Hypersensitivity to ampicillin, penicillin, or sulbactam products.
   Warnings/Precautions: See ampicillin. Similar spectrum of antibacterial activitiy to ampicillin with the added coverage of beta-lactamase producing organisms. Total sulbactam dose **should not exceed** 4 g/24 hr.
Adjust dose in renal failure (see Chapter 3).
Adverse Effects: See ampicillin.
Drug Interactions: See ampicillin.
Drug Administration
   IV: Dilute medication at a concentration ≤30 mg/mL ampicillin and 15 mg/mL sulbactam. IV solution stability is shorter when diluted in dextrose containing solutions. For slow IV injection give over 10–15 min. For intermittent IV injection give over 15–30 min.
   IM: Administer at concentrations of 250 mg/mL ampicillin and 125 mg sulbactam. Drug may be diluted in sterile water for injection, or 0.5 or 2% lidocaine (assess risk-benefit for using lidocaine as a diluent).

AMPRENAVIR
Agenerase, APV
Antiviral, protease inhibitor

Yes	Yes	3	C

Capsules: 50 mg; each capsule contains 19 mg propylene glycol and 36.3 IU vitamin E (*d*-alpha tocopherol)
Oral solution: 15 mg/mL (240 mL); each 1 mL contains 46 IU vitamin E (*d*-alpha tocopherol) and 550 mg propylene glycol

---

Child 4–12 yr and adolescent 13–16 yr <50 kg:
   Oral solution: 22.5 mg/kg/dose PO BID or 17 mg/kg/dose PO TID up to a **max. dose** of 2800 mg/24 hr
   Capsules: 20 mg/kg/dose PO BID or 15 mg/kg/dose PO TID up to a **max. dose** of 2400 mg/24 hr
Adolescent 13–16 yr ≥50 kg and adult:
   Oral solution: 1400 mg PO BID; switch to capsules as soon as possible to lower the amount of propylene glycol and vitamin E content
   Capsules: 1200 mg PO BID
Capsules in combination with efavirenz and ritonavir:
   Adult: 1200 mg amprenavir PO BID + 600 mg efavirenz PO QD + and 200 mg ritonavir PO BID; only amprenavir boosted with ritonavir should be used in combination with efavirenz
In combination with ritonavir:
   Adult: 600 mg amprenavir PO BID + 100 mg ritonavir PO BID, OR 1200 mg amprenavir PO QD + 200 mg ritonavir PO QD

Continued

FORMULARY

AMPRENAVIR *continued*

 Contraindications: Hypersensitivity to amprenavir or any of its components. Oral solution is **contraindicated** in children <4 yr old, pregnant women, patients with hepatic or renal failure, and patients receiving metronidazole or disulfiram. **Do not** coadminister the following drugs: astemizole, terfenadine, cisapride, midazolam, triazolam, ergot derivatives, lipid lowering agents (e.g., atorvastatin and cervistatin) and pimozide. Concomitant flecainide and propafenone are **contraindicated** when amprenavir is coadministered with ritonavir.

Warnings/Precautions: Drug contains significant amounts of vitamin E and propylene glycol. Therapeutic dosages of the oral solution will provide 1650 mg/kg/24 hr of propylene glycol and 138 IU/kg/24 hr of vitamin E. Use with caution in sulfonamide allergic patients because the drug is a sulfonamide; potential risk for cross-sensitivity reactions is unknown. Oral solutions of amprenavir and ritonavir **should not** be used in combination because of significant of propylene glycol and alcohol, respectively. Oral liquid and capsules are not interchangeable on a mg per mg basis; oral solution is 14% less bioavailable. Noncompliance can quickly promote resistant HIV strains. Many drug interactions, see contraindications and drug interaction sections.

Adolescent Dosing: Patients in early puberty (Tanner I–II) should be dosed with pediatric regimens and those in late puberty (Tanner IV) should be dosed with adult regimens. Adolescents who are at the midst of their growth spurt (Tanner III females and Tanner IV males) can be dosed by either pediatric or adult regimen with close monitoring of efficacy and toxicity.

The following dosage adjustment for adults with hepatic insufficiency have been recommended:

Child-Pugh Score	Dose for Capsules	Dose for Solution
5 to 8	450 mg PO BID	513 mg PO BID
9 to 12	300 mg PO BID	342 mg PO BID

Adverse Effects: Rash, hyperglycemia, hypertriglyceridemia, GI symptoms and discomfort, headache and paresthesia may occur. Severe life-threatening rashes (~1% of patients) have been reported.

Drug Interactions: Amprenavir is a substrate and inhibitor of CYP 450 3A4. Efavirenz, rifampin, rifabutin, anticonvulsants, oral contraceptives and St. John's wort can lower amprenavir levels. Always check the potential for other drug interactions when either initiating therapy or adding new drug onto an existing regimen. See contraindications section.

Drug Administration: Drug may be taken with or without food; avoid administering with high-fat meals. Administer drug 1 hr before or after antacid or didanosine use.

ANIDULAFUNGIN
Eraxis
Antifungal, echinocandin

Yes   No   ?   C

Injection: 50 mg with separate 15 mL vial diluent containing 20% (w/w) dehydrated alcohol in water for injection.

Child: Recommended dosages based on steady-state pharmacokinetic data in immunocompromised children 2–17 yrs. Efficacy data is incomplete.
   To mimic an adult dosage of 50 mg/24 hr: 0.75 mg/kg/dose IV QD
   To mimic an adult dosage of 100 mg/24 hr: 1.5 mg/kg/dose IV QD

ANIDULAFUNGIN *continued*

Adult:
    Candidal infections (excluding esophagitis): 200 mg IV × on day 1, then 100 mg IV QD for at least 14 days after the last positive culture.
    Candidal esophagitis: 100 mg IV × on day 1, then 50 mg IV QD for at least 14 days after the last positive culture.

Contraindications: Hypersensitivity to anidulafungin and any other components in the formulation or other echinocandins.
Warnings/Precautions: Hepatic dysfunction and abnormal or worsening of liver function tests have occurred.
Adverse Effects: Hypokalemia, diarrhea and abnormal liver function tests may occur. Histamine-mediated effects such as rash, urticaria, flushing, pruritus, dyspnea and hypotension are minimized with IV infusion rates <1.1 mg/min.
Drug Interactions: Drug is not metabolized by CYP 450 metabolizing enzymes.
Drug Administration: Dilute dose with either D$_5$W or NS at a concentration ≤0.5 mg/mL. **Do not** infuse dose >1.1 mg/min.

ANTITOXIN, DIPHTERIA

See *Diphtheria Antitoxin*

ATAZANAVIR
Reyataz, ATV
Antiviral, protease inhibitor

                                                          Yes   Yes   3   B

Caps: 100, 150, 200 mg

Adolescent ≥16 yr–adult:
    Antiretroviral-naïve: 400 mg PO QD
    Antiretroviral-experienced: Atazanavir 300 mg PO QD and ritonavir 100 mg PO QD
In combination with efavirenz (must be administered with ritonavir):
    Antiretroviral-naïve adult: Atazanavir 300 mg PO QD, efavirenz 600 mg PO QD, and ritonavir 100 mg PO QD administered with food.
In combination with tenofovir (must be administered with ritonavir):
    Adult: Atazanavir 300 mg PO QD, tenofovir 300 mg PO QD, and ritonavir 100 mg PO QD

Contraindications: Hypersensitivity to atazanavir or any of its components. **Do not** coadminister the following drugs: astemizole, terfenadine, cisapride, midazolam, triazolam, ergot derivatives, lipid lowering agents (e.g., atorvastatin and cervistatin) and pimozide. **Should not** be used in severe hepatic impairment (Child-Pugh class C).
Warnings/Precautions: Many drug interactions, see contraindications and drug interactions sections. Use with indinavir is **not recommended** due to increased risk for hyperbillirubinemia and jaundice. Use with **caution** in mild/moderate hepatic impairment (dose reduction of 300 mg PO QD has been recommended in patients with Child-Pugh class B), pre-exising cardiac conduction disorders, other drugs known to prolong PR interval (e.g., calcium channel blockers, beta-blockers, and digoxin). Many drug interactions, see contraindications and drug interactions sections. Patients with hepatitis B or C infections with elevated transaminases may be at risk for further elevations and hepatic decompensation.

Continued

ATAZANAVIR *continued*

Adverse Effects: Hyperbilirubinemia, jaundice, headache, fever, arthralgia, depression, insomnia, dizziness, GI symptoms, and parasthesias are common. Cardiac PR interval prolongation, AV block, rash (including Stevens-Johnson syndrome), hyperglycemia, serum transaminase elevation, spontaneous bleeding in hemophiliacs, fat redistribution and lipid abnormalities have been reported.

Drug Interactions: Atazanavir is a substrate and inhibitor of CYP 450 3A. Also inhibits the glucuronidation enzyme UGT1A1, and CYP 450 1A2 and 2C9. Antacids, H_2 antagonists, proton pump inhibitors, rifampin, St. John's wort, nevirapine, tenofovir and efavirenz decrease atazanavir levels/effects. Voriconazole and ritonavir may increase atazanavir levels/effects. Always check the potential for other drug interactions when either initiating therapy or adding new drug onto an existing regimen. See contraindications and warnings/precautions sections.

Drug Administration: Doses should be administered with food to enhance absorption. Administer doses 2 hr prior and 1 hr after antacids and buffered formulations of didanosine or other medications. Administer 12 hr apart from H_2 antagonists.

ATOVAQUONE ± PROGUANIL

Mepron; in combination with proguanil: Malarone
Pediatric Tablets, Malarone Tablets
Antiprotozoal, antimalarial agent

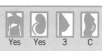

Yes   Yes   3   C

Oral suspension: 750 mg/5 mL (210 mL); contains benzyl alcohol
In combination with proguanil:
    Malarone Pediatric Tablets: 62.5 mg atovaquone and 25 mg proguanil
    Malarone Tablets: 250 mg atovaquone and 100 mg proguanil

Atovaquone:
  Pneumocystis carinii pneumonia (PCP):
    Treatment (21-day course):
      Child: 30–40 mg/kg/24 hr PO ÷ BID with fatty foods; **max. dose:** 1500 mg/24 hr. Infants 3–24 mo may require higher doses of 45 mg/kg/24 hr.
      ≥13 yr and adult: 750 mg/dose PO BID
  Prophylaxis (1st episode and recurrence):
    Child 1–3 mo or >24 mo: 30 mg/kg/24 hr PO QD; **max. dose:** 1500 mg/24 hr
    Child 4–24 mo: 45 mg/kg/24 hr PO QD: **max. dose:** 1500 mg/24 hr
    ≥13 yr and adult: 1500 mg/dose PO QD
  Toxoplasma gondii:
    Child:
      1st episode prophylaxis: Use PCP prophylaxis dosages.
    Adult:
      Treatment: 1500 mg/dose PO BID ± sulfadiazine 1000–1500 mg PO Q6 hr.
      1st episode prophylaxis: 1500 mg/dose PO QD ± pyrimethamine 25 mg PO QD PLUS leucovorin 10 mg PO QD.
      Recurrence prophylaxis: 750 mg/dose PO Q6–12 hr ± pyrimethamine 25 mg PO QD PLUS leucovorin 10 mg PO QD.
  Baesiosis (duration of therapy 7–10 days):
    Child: 40 mg/kg/24 hr PO ÷ BID (**max. dose:** 1500 mg/24 hr) PLUS azithromycin 12 mg/kg/dose PO QD × 7–10 days.
    ≥13 yr and adult: 750 mg/dose PO BID *plus* azithromycin 600 mg PO QD × 7–10 days.

ATOVAQUONE ± PROGUANIL *continued*

Atovaquone with proguanil (Malarone):
Malaria (Chloroquine-resistant P. falciparum):
Treatment (use for a total of 3 days):

Treatment Dosages

Age	Daily Dosage (Atovaquone/Proguanil) ÷ QD–BID PO
Child:	
5–8 kg	125 mg/50 mg
9–10 kg	187.5 mg/75 mg
11–20 kg	250 mg/100 mg
21–30 kg	500 mg/200 mg
31–40 kg	750 mg/300 mg
>40 kg	1000 mg/400 mg
Adult	1000 mg/400 mg

Prophylaxis (initiate therapy 1–2 days before travel, during stay and for 1 wk after leaving):

Prophylaxis Dosages

Age	Daily Dosage (Atovaquone/Proguanil) QD PO
Child:	
11–20 kg	62.5mg/25 mg
21–30 kg	125 mg/50 mg
31–40 kg	187.5 mg/75 mg
>40 kg	250 mg/100 mg
Adult	250 mg/100 mg

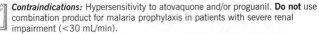

Contraindications: Hypersensitivity to atovaquone and/or proguanil. **Do not** use combination product for malaria prophylaxis in patients with severe renal impairment (<30 mL/min).
Warnings/Precautions: Atovaquone is **not recommended** in the treatment of severe PCP due to the lack of clinical data. Patients with GI disorders or severe vomiting and who cannot tolerate oral therapy should consider alternative IV therapies. Use the combination product with **caution** in severe hepatic impairment.
Adverse Effects: Rash, pruritus, sweating, GI symptoms, LFT elevation, dizziness, headache, insomnia, anxiety, cough and fever are common with both agents. Anemia has been reported with atovaquone and rare anaphylaxis with the combination product.
Drug Interactions
    Atovaquone: Metoclopramide, rifampin, rifabutin and tetracycline may decrease atovaquone levels.
    Proguanil: Inhibitors or substrates to CYP 450 2C19 may potentially decrease the conversion of cycloguanil. May increase anticoagulation effects of warfarin.
Drug Administration
    Atovaquone: Shake oral suspension well before dispensing all doses. Take all doses with high-fat foods to maximize absorption.

Continued

ATOVAQUONE ± PROGUANIL *continued*

Atovaquone/Proguanil: Take all doses with food or milky drink. If vomiting occurs within 1 hr of dosing, repeat dose.

AZITHROMYCIN

Zithromax, Zithromax TRI-PAK, Zithromax Z-PAK,
Zmax (extended-release oral suspension), Azasite
Antibiotic, macrolide

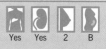

Yes   Yes   2   B

Tablets: 250, 500, 600 mg
   TRI-PAK: 500 mg (3s as unit dose pack)
   Z-PAK: 250 mg (6s as unit dose pack)
Oral suspension: 100 mg/5 mL (15 mL), 200 mg/5 mL (15, 22.5, 30 mL)
Oral powder (Sachet): 1 g (3s, 10s)
Extended-release oral suspension (microspheres):
   Zmax: 2 g reconstituted with 60 mL of water
Injection: 500 mg; contains 9.92 mEq Na/1 g drug
Ophthalmic solution (Azasite): 1% (2.5 mL)

Child:
  Otitis media (≥6 mo):
     5 day regimen: 10 mg/kg PO day 1 (**max. dose:** 500 mg), followed by 5 mg/kg/24 hr PO QD (**max. dose:** 250 mg/24 hr) on days 2–5
     3 day regimen: 10 mg/kg/24 hr PO QD × 3 days (**max. dose:** 500 mg/24 hr)
     1 day regimen: 30 mg/kg/24 hr PO ×1 (**max. dose:** 1500 mg/24 hr)
  Community acquired pneumonia (≥6 mo): Use otitis media 5 day regimen from above
  Pharyngitis/tonsillitis (2–15 yrs): 12 mg/kg/24 hr PO QD × 5 days (**max. dose:** 500 mg/24 hr)
  M. avium complex in HIV (see www.aidsinfo.nih.gov/guidelines for most current recommendations):
     Prophylaxis for first episode: 20 mg/kg/dose PO Q7 days (**max. dose:** 1200 mg/dose); alternatively, 5 mg/kg/24 hr PO QD (**max. dose:** 250 mg/dose) with or without rifabutin.
     Prophylaxis for recurrence: 5 mg/kg/24 hr PO QD (**max. dose:** 250 mg/dose), plus ethambutol 15 mg/kg/24 hr (**max. dose:** 900 mg/24 hr) PO QD with or without rifabutin 5 mg/kg/24 hr (**max. dose:** 300 mg/24 hr).
     Treatment: 10–12 mg/kg/24 hr PO QD (**max. dose:** 500 mg/24 hr) × 1 mo or longer, plus ethambutol 15–25 mg/kg/24 hr (**max. dose:** 1g/24 hr) PO QD with or without rifabutin 10–20 mg/kg/24 hr (**max. dose:** 300 mg/24 hr).
  Anti-inflammatory agent in cystic fibrosis:
     25–39 kg: 250 mg PO every Monday, Wednesday and Friday.
     ≥40 kg: 500 mg PO every Monday, Wednesday and Friday.
Adolescent and adult:
  Pharyngitis, tonsillitis, skin, and soft tissue infection: 500 mg PO day 1, then 250 mg/24 hr PO on days 2–5
  Mild/moderate bacterial COPD exacerbation: Above 5 day dosing regimen OR 500 mg PO QD × 3 days
  Community acquired pneumonia:
     Tablets: 500 mg PO day 1, then 250 mg/24 hr PO on days 2–5
     Extended-release oral suspension (Zmax): Single dose 2 g PO

AZITHROMYCIN *continued*

IV and tablet regimen: 500 mg IV QD × 2 days followed by 500 mg PO QD to complete a 7–10 day regimen (IV and PO)
Sinusitis:
    Tablets: 500 mg PO QD × 3 days
    Extended-release oral suspension (Zmax): Single dose 2 g PO
Uncomplicated chlamydial cervicitis or urethritis: Single 1 g dose PO
Gonococcal cervicitis or urethritis: Single 2 g dose PO
Acute PID (chlamydia): 500 mg IV QD × 1–2 days followed by 250 mg PO QD to complete a 7 day regimen (IV and PO).
M. avium complex in HIV (see www.aidsinfo.nih.gov/guidelines for most recent recommendations):
    Prophylaxis for first episode: 1200 mg PO Q7 days with or without rifabutin 300 mg PO QD
    Prophylaxis for recurrence: 500 mg PO QD, plus ethambutol 15 mg/kg/dose PO QD, with or without rifabutin 300 mg PO QD
    Treatment: 500–600 mg PO QD with ethambutol 15 mg/kg/dose PO QD with or without rifabutin 300 mg PO QD.
Anti-inflammatory agent in cystic fibrosis: Use same dosing in children.
Ophthalmic:
    ≥1 yr and adult: Instill one drop into the affected eye(s) BID, 8–12 hr apart, × 2 days, followed by one drop QD for the next 5 days.

Contraindications: Hypersensitivity to macrolides, ketolides or any other components in the formulation.
Warnings/Precautions: Use with **caution** in impaired hepatic function, GFR <10 mL/min (limited data), and prolonged QT intervals. CNS penetration is poor. Extended-release oral suspension (Zmax) is currently **not approved** in children.
Adverse Effects: Can cause increase in hepatic enzymes, cholestatic jaundice, GI discomfort, and pain at injection site (IV use). Vomiting, diarrhea and nausea have been reported at higher frequency in otitis media with 1 day dosing regimen. Stevens-Johnson syndrome and TEN have been reported rarely. Eye irritation is common with ophthalmic use.
Drug Interactions: Compared to other macrolides, less risk for drug interactions. Nelfinavir may increase azithromycin levels; monitor for liver enzyme abnormalities and hearing impairment. Interaction studies have not been completed for the following medications by which macrolides may increase their effects/toxicity: digoxin, ergotamine, dihydroergotamine, cyclosporine, hexobarbital and phenytoin. Despite not affecting prothrombin time to a single dose of warfarin, careful monitoring of prothrombin time is recommended with warfarin.
Drug Administration
    PO: Oral dosage forms may be administered with or without food but **do not** give simultaneously with aluminum or magnesium containing antacids.
    IV: Dilute dose to 1–2 mg/mL and infuse dose over 60 min (**do not** infuse dose <60 min).
    Ophthalmic drops: Apply finger pressure to lacrimal sac during and for 1–2 min after dose application. **Do not** touch the applicator tip and **do not** wear contact lenses.

For explanation of icons, see p. 306.

AZTREONAM
Azactam
Antibiotic, monobactam

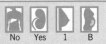

No | Yes | 1 | B

Injection: 0.5, 1, 2 g
Frozen injection: 1 g/50 mL 3.4% dextrose, 2 g/50 mL 1.4% dextrose (iso-osmotic solutions)
Each 1 g drug contains approximately 780 mg L-arginine

Neonate:
30 mg/kg/dose:
   <1.2 kg and 0–4 wk age: Q12 hr IV/IM
   1.2–2 kg and 0–7 days old: Q12 hr IV/IM
   1.2–2 kg and >7 days old: Q8 hr IV/IM
   >2 kg and 0–7 days old: Q8 hr IV/IM
   >2 kg and >7 days old: Q6 hr IV/IM
Child: 90–120 mg/kg/24 hr ÷ Q6–8 hr IV/IM
Cystic fibrosis: 150–200 mg/kg/24 hr ÷ Q6–8 hr IV/IM
Adult:
   Moderate infections: 1–2 g/dose Q8–12 hr IV/IM
   Severe infections: 2 g/dose Q6–8 hr IV/IM
Max. dose: 8 g/24 hr

Contraindications: Hypersensitivity to aztreonam or any other of its components.
Warnings/Precautions: Use with **caution** in arginase deficiency. Low cross-allergenicity between aztreonam and other beta-lactams. Good CNS penetration. **Adjust dose in renal failure (see Chapter 3).**
Adverse Effects: Thrombophlebitis, eosinophilia, leukopenia, neutropenia, thrombocytopenia, liver enzyme elevation, hypotension, seizures, and confusion.
Drug Interactions: Probenecid and furosemide increases aztreonam levels.
Drug Administration: For IV, dose may be administered via IV push (**max. concentration** of 66 mg/mL over 3–5 min) or intermittent infusion (**max. concentration** of 20 mg/mL over 20–60 min). For IM, administer into a large muscle such as the upper outer quadrant of the gluteus maximus or lateral part of the thigh. See package insert for recommended IM concentration.

BACITRACIN ± POLYMYXIN B
AK-Tracin Ophthalmic, Baciguent Topical, and others;
in combination with polymyxin B: AK-Poly-Bac
Ophthalmic, Polysporin Ophthalmic, Polysporin
Topical and others
Antibiotic, topical

No | No | ? | C

BACITRACIN:
   Ophthalmic ointment: 500 units/g (3.5, 3.75 g)
   Topical ointment: 500 units/g (0.9, 15, 30, 120, 454 g)
BACITRACIN IN COMBINATION WITH POLYMYXIN B:
Ophthalmic ointment: 500 units bacitracin + 10,000 units polymyxin B/g (3.5 g)
Topical ointment: 500 units bacitracin + 10,000 units polymyxin B/g (0.9, 15, 30 g)
Topical powder: 500 units bacitracin + 10,000 units polymyxin B/g (10 g)

BACITRACIN ± POLYMYXIN B *continued*

BACITRACIN
Child and adult:
> *Topical:* Apply to affected area 1–5 times/24 hr.
> *Ophthalmic:* Apply 0.25–0.5 inch ribbon into the conjunctival sac of the infected eye(s) Q3–12 hr; frequency depends on severity of infection.

BACITRACIN + POLYMYXIN B
Child and adult:
> *Topical:* Apply ointment or powder to affected area QD–TID
> *Ophthalmic:* Apply 0.25–0.5 inch ribbon into the conjunctival sac of the infected eye(s) Q3–12 hr; frequency depends on severity of infection.

Contraindications: Hypersensitivity to bacitracin and/or polymyxin B or any other components in the formulation.
   Warnings/Precautions: **Do not use** topical ointment for the eyes. Ophthalmic dosage form may retard corneal wound healing. For neomycin containing products, see Neomycin/Polymyxin B/± Bacitracin.
Adverse Effects: Topical dosage form may cause rash, itching, burning, edema, and contact dermatitis. Ophthalmic dosage form may cause temporary blurred vision.
Drug Interactions: None identified.
Drug Administration: For ophthalmic use, **avoid** contact of ointment tube tip with skin or eye and apply dose into the conjuctival sac of the infected eye(s).

BOTULINUM IMMUNE GLOBULIN INTRAVENOUS, HUMAN
BabyBIG, BIG-IV
Immune globulins, botulism

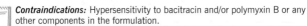
No   Yes   ?   ?

IV preparation in powder for reconstitution: 100 ± 20 mg vial of type A and B immunoglobulins; diluted with 2 mL sterile water for injection (each vial contains 1% albumin, 5% sucrose, 0.02 M sodium phosphate buffer and trace amounts of IgA and IgM).
   Product potency is ≥15 IU/mL anti-type A toxin and ≥4 IU/mL anti-type B toxin activities.

Infant botulism:
> *IV infusion:* 50 mg/kg × 1 as soon as clinical diagnosis is made

Contraindications: Prior history of severe reactions to other human immunoglobulin preparations. May cause anaphylaxis in IgA-deficient patients because product contains trace amounts of IgA.
Warnings/Precautions: Product contains sucrose; minimize risk for renal dysfunction by administering at the minimum concentration available and at the minimum rate of infusion (see later discussion). Like other plasma products, the risk for transmission of unrecognized blood-borne viral agents may occur. Monitor vital signs during drug administration. Product has only been evaluated in children <1 yr old.
Adverse Effects: Anaphylaxis or hypotension may occur; discontinue use and administer supportive care immediately. Chills, muscle cramps, back pain, fever, nausea, vomiting and wheezing may occur; slow rate of infusion or temporarily interrupt the infusion. Erythematous rash, blood pressure changes and other GI disturbances have also been reported.
Drug Interactions: Defer administration of live virus vaccines approximately 5 mo after BIG-IV.

Continued

BOTULINUM IMMUNE GLOBULIN INTRAVENOUS, HUMAN *continued*

Drug Administration: Following initial reconstitution to 50 mg/mL, the solution should be infused within 4 hr. May be further diluted to a minimum concentration of 16.7 mg/mL. Administer with an 18 micron inline or syringe-tip sterile filter is recommended. Use this product only if it is colorless, free of particulate matter, and not turbid.

Initiate infusion at a rate of 25 mg/kg/hr (0.5 mL/kg/hr with a 50 mg/mL solution) for the first 15 min. If tolerated, increase rate to a **maximum** of 50 mg/kg/hr. Discontinue infusion and give epinephrine if anaphylaxis or significant hypotension occurs. Slow infusion rate or temporarily interrupt infusion if minor side effects (i.e., flushing; see preceding discussion) occur.

BUTENAFINE
Mentax, Lotrimin Ultra
Antifungal, benzylamine

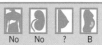

| No | No | ? | B |

Cream: 1% (12, 15, 24, 30 g)

> **≥12 yr:**
> ***Pityriasis versicolor, tinea corporis, tinea, cruris:*** Apply topically to affected areas once daily × 2 weeks
> ***Tinea pedis, interdigital:*** Apply topically to affected areas BID × 7 days, or once daily × 4 weeks

---

Contraindications: Hypersensitivity to butenafine products or any of its components.

Warnings/Precautions: **Use with caution** in patients sensitive to allylamine antifungals. **Avoid** contact with eyes, nose, mouth and mucous membranes. Safety and efficacy studies have not been conducted for children <12 yr.
Adverse Effects: May cause burning/stinging, irritation and itching. Contact dermatitis and exacerbation of fungal infection have been reported.
Drug Interactions: None identified.
Drug Administration: Apply to cover affected areas and immediately surrounding skin avoiding the eyes, nose, mouth and mucous membranes.

CASPOFUNGIN
Cancidas
Antifungal, echinocandin

| Yes | No | ? | C |

Injection: 50, 70 mg; contains sucrose (39 mg in 50 mg vial and 54 mg in 70 mg vial)

> ***Neonate (dosage used in case studies, but pharmacokinetic studies are limited):***
> 1 mg/kg/dose IV QD × 2, then 2 mg/kg/dose IV QD.
> ***Child (pharmacokinetic data in 2–17 yr old with oncological fever and neutropenia, see remarks):***
> 50 mg/m²/dose IV QD; **max. dose:** 50 mg/dose

Adolescent and adult (see remarks):
> **Loading dose:** 70 mg IV × 1
> **Maintenance dose:**
> > **Usual:** 50 mg IV QD. If tolerated and response is inadequate, may increase to 70 mg IV QD.
> > **Hepatic insufficiency (Child-Pugh score 7 to 9):** 35 mg IV QD
> > **Concomitant rifampin:** 70 mg IV QD

CASPOFUNGIN *continued*

 Contraindications: Hypersensitivity to caspofungin or any other components in the formulation.
Warnings/Precautions: **Use with caution** in hepatic impairment and concomitant enzyme inducing drugs. Higher maintenance doses (70 mg QD in adults) may be necessary for concomitant use of enzyme inducers such as carbamazepime, dexamethasone, phenytoin, nevirapine, or efavirenz. In moderate hepatic impairment (Child-Pugh score 7 to 9), decrease dose by 30%.
Adverse Effects: May cause fever, facial swelling, rash, nausea/vomiting, headache, infusion site phlebitis, and LFT elevation.
Drug Interactions: Cyclosporine may cause transient increase in LFTs and caspofungin level elevations. May decrease tacrolimus levels. See preceding Warnings/Precautions section.
Drug Administration: Administer doses by slow IV infusion over 1 hr at a concentration ≤0.47 mg/mL. **Do not** mix or co-infuse with other medications and **avoid** using dextrose-containing diluents (e.g., D_5W).

CEFACLOR
Ceclor, Ceclor CD, Raniclor, and others
Antibiotic, cephalosporin (second generation)

No Yes 1 B

Caps: 250, 500 mg
Extended-release tabs (Ceclor CD): 375, 500 mg
Chewable tabs (Raniclor): 125, 187, 250, 375 mg; contains phenylalanine
Oral suspension: 125 mg/5 mL (75, 150 mL); 187 mg/5 mL (50, 100 mL); 250 mg/5 mL (75, 150 mL); 375 mg/5 mL (50, 100 mL)

 Child >1 mo old (use regular release dosage forms): 20–40 mg/kg/24 hr PO ÷ Q8 hr; **max. dose:** 2 g/24 hr (Q12 hr dosage interval optional in otitis media or pharyngitis)
Adult: 250–500 mg/dose PO Q8 hr; **max. dose:** 4 g/24 hr
  Extended-release tablets: 375–500 mg/dose PO Q12 hr

Contraindications: Hypersensitivity to cephalosporin antibiotics.
Warnings/Precautions: **Use with caution** in patients with penicillin allergy or renal impairment **(adjust dose in renal failure; see Chapter 3).** Extended-release tablets are **not recommended** for children.
Adverse Effects: Elevated liver function tests, bone marrow suppression, and moniliasis. Serum sickness reactions have been reported in patients receiving multiple courses of cefaclor.
Drug Interactions: Probenecid increases cefaclor concentration. May cause positive Coombs' test or false-positive test for urinary glucose.
Drug Administration: Administer all doses on an empty stomach; 1 hr before or 2 hr after meals. **Do not** crush, cut, or chew extended-release tablets.

CEFADROXIL
Duricef and others
Antibiotic, cephalosporin (first generation)

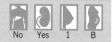

No   Yes   1   B

Suspension: 125, 250, 500 mg/5 mL (50, 75, 100 mL)
Tabs: 1 g
Caps: 500 mg

Infant and child: 30 mg/kg/24 hr PO ÷ Q12 hr (daily dose may be administered QD for group A beta-hemolytic streptococci pharyngitis/tonsillitis); **max. dose:** 2 g/24 hr
   Bacterial endocarditis prophylaxis for dental and upper airway procedure: 50 mg/kg/dose (**max. dose:** 2 g) × 1 PO 1 hr before procedure
Adolescent and adult: 1–2 g/24 hr PO ÷ Q12–24 hr (administer Q12 hr for complicated UTIs); **max. dose:** 2 g/24 hr
   Bacterial endocarditis prophylaxis for dental and upper airway procedure: 2 g × 1 PO 1 hr before procedure

Contraindications: Hypersensitivity to cephalosporin antibiotics.
Warnings/Precautions: **Use with caution** in penicillin allergic patients and renal insufficiency **(adjust dose in renal failure; see Chapter 3).**
Adverse Effects: Rash, nausea, vomiting, and diarrhea are common. Transient neutropenia, and vaginitis have been reported.
Drug Interactions: Probenecid increases serum cefadroxil levels. May cause false-positive urinary reducing substances (Clinitest).
Drug Administration: Doses may be given with or without food.

CEFAZOLIN
Ancef, Zolicef, and others
Antibiotic, cephalosporin (first generation)

Yes   Yes   1   B

Injection: 0.5, 1, 5, 10, 20 g
Frozen injection: 1 g/50 mL 5% dextrose (iso-osmotic solutions)
Contains 2.1 mEq Na/g drug

Neonate IM, IV:
Postnatal age ≤7 days: 40 mg/kg/24 hr ÷ Q12 hr
Postnatal age >7 days:
   ≤2000 g: 40 mg/kg/24 hr ÷ Q12 hr
   >2000 g: 60 mg/kg/24 hr ÷ Q8 hr
Infant >1 mo and child: 50–100 mg/kg/24 hr ÷ Q8 hr IV/IM; **max. dose:** 6 g/24 hr
   Bacterial endocarditis prophylaxis for dental and upper airway procedure: 25 mg/kg/dose (**max. dose:** 1 g) IV/IM 30 min prior to procedure.
Adult: 2–6 g/24 hr ÷ Q6–8 hr IV/IM; **max. dose:** 12 g/24 hr
   Bacterial endocarditis prophylaxis for dental and upper airway procedure: 1 g IV/IM 30 min prior to procedure

Contraindications: Hypersensitivity to cephalosporin antibiotics.
Warnings/Precautions: **Use with caution** in penicillin allergy, patients stabilized on anticoagulants, and hepatic or renal impairment **(adjust dose in renal failure; see Chapter 3).** Does not penetrate well into CSF.
Adverse Effects: GI disturbances are common. Leukopenia, thrombocytopenia, hepatotoxicity, and Stevens-Johnson syndrome have been reported.

C

FORMULARY

CEFAZOLIN *continued*

Drug Interactions: Probenecid increases serum cefazolin levels. May cause transient liver enzyme elevation, false-positive urine reducing substance (Clinitest) and Coombs' test.

Drug Administration
    IV: IV push, infuse over 3–5 min at a concentration ≤100 mg/mL. For intermittent infusion, infuse over 10–60 min at a concentration of 20 mg/mL. Fluid restricted patients have received 138 mg/mL via IV push.
    IM: Dilute with sterile water to 225–330 mg/mL.

CEFDINIR
Omnicef
Antibiotic, cephalosporin (third generation)

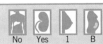

No   Yes   1   B

Caps: 300 mg
Oral suspension: 125 mg/5 mL (60, 100 mL)

---

6 mo–12 yr:
    Otitis media, sinusitis, pharyngitis/tonsillitis: 14 mg/kg/24 hr PO ÷ Q12–24 hr; **max. dose:** 600 mg/24 hr
    Uncomplicated skin infections: 14 mg/kg/24 hr PO ÷ Q12 hr; **max. dose:** 600 mg/24 hr
≥13 yr and adult:
    Bronchitis, sinusitis, pharyngitis/tonsillitis: 600 mg/24 hr PO ÷ Q12–24 hr
    Community acquired pneumonia, uncomplicated skin infections: 600 mg/24 hr PO ÷ Q12 hr

---

Contraindications: Hypersensitivity to cephalosporin antibiotics.
Warnings/Precautions: **Use with caution** in penicillin-allergic patients or in presence of renal impairment **(adjust dose in renal failure; see Chapter 3)**. Good gram-positive cocci activity. Once daily dosing has not been evaluated in pneumonia and skin infections.
Adverse Effects: Diarrhea (especially in children <2 yr), headache and vaginitis are common. Eosinophilia and abnormal liver function tests have been reported with higher than usual doses.
Drug Interactions: Iron-containing vitamins and antacids containing aluminum or magnesium may decrease the drug's absorption. Probenecid increases serum cefdinir levels. May cause false-positive urine reducing substance (Clinitest) and Coombs' test.
Drug Administration: Doses may be taken without regard to food. Administer doses at least 2 hr before or after antacids (containing magnesium or aluminum) or iron supplements.

CEFDITOREN PIVOXIL
Spectracef
Antibiotic, cephalosporin (third generation)

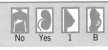

No   Yes   1   B

Tabs: 200 mg

≥12 yr:
    Acute bacterial exacerbation in COPD: 400 mg BID PO × 10 days
    Community acquired pneumonia: 400 mg BID PO × 14 days

Continued

CEFDITOREN PIVOXIL *continued*

≥12 yr
Pharyngitis, tonsillitis, or uncomplicated skin and skin structure infections: 200 mg PO BID PO × 10 days

---

Contraindications: Hypersensitivities to cephalosporins or milk protein (tablet contains sodium caseinate). Carnitine deficiency or inborn errors of metabolism that may result in clinically significant carnitine deficiency (pivulate component causes carnitine renal excretion).
Warnings/Precautions: **Use with caution** in penicillin hypersensitivity. Prolonged use is **not** recommended due to risk for causing carnitine deficiency; 30%–46% transient decrease in carnitine concentrations have been noted in adults treated for community acquired pneumonia for 14 days. **Adjust dose in renal failure (see Chapter 3).**
Adverse Effects: Diarrhea, nausea, headache, abdominal pain, vaginal moniliasis, dyspepsia, and vomiting may occur.
Drug Interactions: Probenecid increases cefditoren levels and antacids (aluminum/magnesium containing) decreases cefditoren absorption.
Drug Administration: Doses may be administered with or without food. Administer doses at least 2 hr before or after antacids (containing magnesium or aluminum) or iron supplements.

CEFEPIME
Maxipime
Antibiotic, cephalosporin (fourth generation)

No Yes 1 B

Injection: 0.5, 1, 2 g
Each 1 g drug contains 725 mg L-arginine

Neonate:
  <14 days: 60 mg/kg/24 hr ÷ Q12 hr IV/IM
  ≥14 days: 100 mg/kg/24 hr ÷ Q12 hr IV/IM. For meningitis or *Pseudomonas* infections, use 150 mg/kg/24 hr ÷ Q8 hr IV/IM
Child ≥2 mo: 100 mg/kg/24 hr ÷ Q12 hr IV/IM
  Meningitis, fever, and neutropenia, or serious infections: 150 mg/kg/24 hr ÷ Q8 hr IV/IM
  Max. dose: 6 g/24 hr
Cystic fibrosis: 150 mg/kg/24 hr ÷ Q8 hr IV/IM, up to a **max. dose** of 6 g/24 hr
Adult: 1–4 g/24 hr ÷ Q12 hr IV/IM
  Severe infections: 6 g/24 hr ÷ Q8 hr IV/IM
  Max. dose: 6 g/24 hr

Contraindications: Hypersensitivity to cephalosporin antibiotics.
Warnings/Precautions: **Use with caution** in patients with penicillin allergy or renal impairment **(adjust dose in renal failure; see Chapter 3)**. Good activity against *P. aeruginosa* and other gram-negative bacterias plus most gram-positives *(S. aureus)*.
Adverse Effects: Rash, GI discomfort, and headache are common. May cause thrombophlebitis and transient increases in liver enzymes.
Drug Interactions: Probenecid increases serum cefepime levels. May cause false-positive urine reducing substance (Clinitest) and Coombs' test. Encephalopathy, myoclonus, seizures, transient leukopenia, neutropenia, agronolocytosis and thrombocytopenia have been reported.
Drug Administration
  IV: For IV push, infuse over 3–5 min at a concentration of 100 mg/mL. For intermittent infusion, infuse over 20–30 min at a concentration ≤40 mg/mL.

C

CEFEPIME *continued*

IM: Dilute with sterile water, D_5W, NS, or lidocaine (0.5 or 1%) to 280 mg/mL. Assess the potential risk/benefit for using lidocaine as a diluent.

CEFIXIME
Suprax
Antibiotic, cephalosporin (third generation)

No Yes 1 B

Tabs: 400 mg
Oral suspension: 100 mg/5 mL (50, 75 mL)

Infant (>6 mo) and child: 8 mg/kg/24 hr ÷ Q12–24 hr PO; **max. dose:** 400 mg/24 hr.
   Acute UTI: 16 mg/kg/24 hr ÷ Q12 hr on day 1, followed by 8 mg/kg/24 hr Q24 hr PO × 13 days. **Max. dose:** 400 mg/24 hr.
   Sexual victimization prophylaxis: 8 mg/kg PO × 1 (**max. dose:** 400 mg) **PLUS** azithromycin 20 mg/kg PO × 1 (**max. dose:** 1 g).
Adolescent and adult: 400 mg/24 hr ÷ Q12–24 hr PO
   Uncomplicated cervical, urethral, or rectal infections due to N. gonorrhoeae: 400 mg × 1 PO.
   Sexual victimization prophylaxis: 400 mg PO × 1, *plus* azithromycin 1 g PO × 1 or doxycycline 100 mg BID PO × 7 days, *plus* metronidazole 2 g PO × 1.

Contraindications: Hypersensitivity to cephalosporin antibiotics.
Warnings/Precautions: Use with caution in patients with penicillin allergy or renal failure (**adjust dose in renal failure; see Chapter 3**). Do not use tablet dosage form for the treatment of otitis media due to reduced bioavailability. Drug is excreted unchanged in urine (50%) and bile (5%–10%).
Adverse Effects: Diarrhea, abdominal pain, nausea, and rash.
Drug Interactions: Probenecid increases serum cefixime levels. May increase carbamazepine serum concentrations. May cause false-positive urine reducing substance (Clinitest), Coombs' test, and nitroprusside test for ketones.
Drug Administration: Doses may be given with or without food.

CEFOPERAZONE
Cefobid
Antibiotic, cephalosporin (third generation)

Yes No 1 B

Injection: 1, 2, 10 g
Contains 1.5 mEq Na/g drug

Infant and child: 100–150 mg/kg/24 hr ÷ Q8–12 hr IV/IM; **max. dose:** 12 g/24 hr
Adult: 2–4 g/24 hr ÷ Q12 hr IV/IM. Doses up to 16 g/24 hr by continuous infusion have been administered to immunocompromised patients without complications (steady-state serum level of 150 mcg/mL).
Maximum doses:
   Usual: 12–16 g/24 hr
   Hepatic disease and/or biliary obstruction: 4 g/24 hr
   Mixed hepatic and renal impairment: 1–2 g/24 hr

Contraindications: Hypersensitivity to cephalosporin antibiotics.
Warnings/Precautions: Use with caution in penicillin-allergic patients or in patients with hepatic failure or biliary obstruction. Bleeding and bruising may occur, especially in patients with vitamin K deficiency. Drug is extensively distributed and excreted in bile. Does not penetrate well into CSF. *Continued*

For explanation of icons, see p. 306.

CEFOPERAZONE *continued*

Adverse Effects: Injection site reaction and phlebitis, and diarrhea are common.
Drug Interactions: May cause disulfiram-like reaction with ethanol, and false-positive urine reducing substance (Clinitest) and Coombs' test.
Drug Administration
    IV: For intermittent infusion, infuse over 15–30 min at a concentration ≤50 mg/mL. For continuous IV infusion, dilute to 2–25 mg/mL.
    IM: Dilute with sterile water or lidocaine 2% (final lidocaine concentration at 0.5%) to 250 or 333 mg/mL. Assess the potential risk/benefit for using lidocaine as a diluent.

CEFOTAXIME
Claforan
Antibiotic, cephalosporin (third generation)

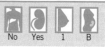
No   Yes   1   B

Injection: 0.5, 1, 2, 10 g
Frozen injection: 1 g/50 mL 3.4% dextrose, 2 g/50 mL 1.4% dextrose (iso-osmotic solutions)
Contains 2.2 mEq Na/g drug

Neonate: IV/IM:
    Postnatal age ≤7 days:
        <2000 g: 100 mg/kg/24 hr ÷ Q12 hr
        ≥2000 g: 100–150 mg/kg/24 hr ÷ Q8–12 hr
    Postnatal age >7 days:
        <1200 g: 100 mg/kg/24 hr ÷ Q12 hr
        1200–2000 g: 150 mg/kg/24 hr ÷ Q8 hr
        >2000 g: 150–200 mg/kg/24 hr ÷ Q6–8 hr
Infant and child (1 mo–12 yr and <50 kg): 100–200 mg/kg/24 hr ÷ Q6–8 hr IV/IM. Higher doses of 150–225 mg/kg/24 hr ÷ Q6–8 hr have been recommended for infections outside the CSF due to penicillin-resistant pneumococci.
    Meningitis: 200 mg/kg/24 hr ÷ Q6 hr IV/IM. Higher doses of 225–300 mg/kg/24 hr ÷ Q6–8 hr, in combination with vancomycin (60 mg/kg/24 hr), have been recommended for meningitis due to penicillin-resistant pneumococci.
    Max. dose: 12 g/24 hr
Child (>12 yr or ≥50 kg) and adult: 1–2 g/dose Q6–8 hr IV/IM
    Severe infection: 2 g/dose Q4–6 hr IV/IM
    Max. dose: 12 g/24 hr
    Uncomplicated gonorrhea: 0.5–1 g × 1 IM

Contraindications: Hypersensitivity to cephalosporin antibiotics.
Warnings/Precautions: Use with caution in penicillin-allergy and renal impairment **(adjust dose in renal failure; see Chapter 3).** Good CNS penetration.
Adverse Effects: Injection site pain and phlebitis, and GI disturbances are common. Stevens-Johnson syndrome, agranulocytosis, and transient elevations in liver function tests have been reported.
Drug Interactions: Probenecid increases serum cefotaxime levels. May cause false-positive urine reducing substance (Clinitest) and Coombs' test, elevated BUN, creatinine, and liver enzymes.

CEFOTAXIME *continued*

Drug Administration
IV: For IV push, infuse over 3–5 min at a concentration ≤100 mg/mL. For intermittent infusion, infuse over 15–30 min at a concentration 20–60 mg/mL. For fluid restricted patients, 150 mg/mL may be administered via IV push over 3–5 min.
IM: Dilute with sterile water to 230–330 mg/mL.

CEFOTETAN
Cefotan
Antibiotic, cephalosporin (second generation)

No   Yes   1   B

Injection: 1, 2, 10 g
Frozen injection: 1 g/50 mL 3.8% dextrose, 2 g/50 mL 2.2% dextrose (iso-osmotic solutions)
Contains 3.5 mEq Na/g drug

Infant and child: 40–80 mg/kg/24 hr ÷ Q12 hr IV/IM
Adolescent and adult: 2–6 g/24 hr ÷ Q12 hr IV/IM
  PID: 2 g Q12 hr IV × 24–48 hr after clinical improvement with doxycycline 100 mg Q12 hr PO/IV × 14 days
Max. dose (all ages): 6 g/24 hr

Contraindications: Hypersensitivity to cephalosporin antibiotics.
Warnings/Precautions: Use with caution in penicillin-allergic patients or in presence of renal impairment (adjust dose in renal failure; see Chapter 3). Has good anaerobic activity but poor CSF penetration.
Adverse Effects: Injection site pain and thrombophlebitis, and diarrhea are common. Hemolytic anemia has been reported.
Drug Interactions: Disulfiram-like reaction may occur when taken with ethanol. May increase effects/toxicities of anticoagulants. May cause false-positive urine reducing substance (Clinitest), and false elevations of serum and urine creatinine (Jaffe method).
Drug Administration
IV: For IV push, infuse over 3–5 min at a concentration 97–180 mg/mL. For intermittent infusion, infuse over 20–60 min at a concentration 10–40 mg/mL.
IM: Dilute with sterile water or lidocaine (0.5 or 1%) to 375 or 472 mg/mL. Assess the potential risk/benefit for using lidocaine as a diluent.

CEFOXITIN
Mefoxin
Antibiotic, cephalosporin (second generation)

No   Yes   1   B

Injection: 1, 2, 10 g
Frozen injection: 1 g/50 mL 4% dextrose, 2 g/50 mL 2.2% dextrose (iso-osmotic solutions)
Contains 2.3 mEq Na/g drug

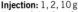
Neonate: 90–100 mg/kg/24 hr ÷ Q8 hr IM/IV
Infant (>3 mo) and child:
  Mild/moderate infections: 80–100 mg/kg/24 hr ÷ Q6–8 hr IM/IV
  Severe infections: 100–160 mg/kg/24 hr ÷ Q4–6 hr IM/IV

Continued

CEFOXITIN *continued*

Adult: 4–12 g/24 hr ÷ Q6–8 hr IM/IV
>**PID:** 2 g IV Q6h × 24–48 hr after clinical improvement with doxycycline 100 mg
>Q12 hr PO/IV × 14 days

Max. dose (all ages): 12 g/24 hr

Contraindications: Hypersensitivity to cephalosporin antibiotics.
Warnings/Precautions: Use with caution in penicillin-allergic patients or in presence of renal impairment **(adjust dose in renal failure; see Chapter 3).** Has good anaerobic activity but poor CSF penetration.
Adverse Effects: Injection site pain, thrombophlebitis, rash, and diarrhea may occur. Immunologic allergic reactions have been reported.
Drug Interactions: Probenecid increases serum cefoxitin levels. May cause false-positive urine reducing substance (Clinitest and other copper reduction method tests), and false elevations of serum and urine creatinine (Jaffe and KDA methods).
Drug Administration
>IV: For IV push, infuse over 3–5 min at a concentration ≤200 mg/mL. For intermittent infusion, infuse over 10–60 min at a concentration ≤40 mg/mL.
>IM: Dilute with sterile water or lidocaine (0.5 or 1%) to 400 mg/mL. Assess the potential risk/benefit for using lidocaine as a diluent.

CEFPODOXIME PROXETIL
Vantin
Antibiotic, cephalosporin (third generation)

No   Yes   1   B

Tabs: 100, 200 mg
Oral suspension: 50, 100 mg/5 mL (50, 75, 100 mL)

---

2 mo–12 yr:
>**Otitis media:** 10 mg/kg/24 hr PO ÷ Q12–24 hr; **max. dose:** 400 mg/24 hr
>**Pharyngitis/tonsillitis:** 10 mg/kg/24 hr PO ÷ Q12 hr; **max. dose:** 200 mg/24 hr
>**Acute maxillary sinusitis:** 10 mg/kg/24 hr PO ÷ Q12 hr; **max. dose:** 400 mg/24 hr

≥13 yr–adult: 200–800 mg/24 hr PO ÷ Q12 hr
>**Uncomplicated gonorrhea:** 200 mg PO × 1

Contraindications: Hypersensitivity to cephalosporin antibiotics.
Warnings/Precautions: Use with caution in penicillin-allergic patients or in presence of renal impairment **(adjust dose in renal failure; see Chapter 3).**
Adverse Effects: May cause diarrhea, nausea, vomiting, and vaginal candidiasis.
Drug Interactions: Probenecid increases serum cefpodoxime levels. High doses of antacids or H_2 blockers may reduce absorption. May cause false-positive Coombs' test.
Drug Administration: Tablets should be administered with food to enhance absorption. Suspension may be administered without regard to food.

CEFPROZIL

Cefzil and others
Antibiotic, cephalosporin (second generation)

No   Yes   1   B

Tabs: 250, 500 mg
Oral suspension: 125 mg/5 mL, 250 mg/5 mL (50, 75, 100 mL) (contains aspartame and phenylalanine)

> *Otitis media:*
>   *6 mo–12 yr:* 30 mg/kg/24 hr PO ÷ Q12 hr
> *Pharyngitis/tonsillitis:*
>   *2–12 yr:* 15 mg/kg/24 hr PO ÷ Q12 hr
> *Acute sinusitis:*
>   *6 mo–12 yr:* 15–30 mg/kg/24 hr PO ÷ Q12–24 hr
> *Uncomplicated skin infections:*
>   *2–12 yr:* 20 mg/kg/24 hr PO Q24 hr
> *Other:*
>   *≥13 yr and adult:* 500–1000 mg/24 hr PO ÷ Q12–24 hr
> **Max. dose** (all ages): 1 g/24 hr

Contraindications: Hypersensitivity to cephalosporin antibiotics.
Warnings/Precautions: **Use with caution** in penicillin-allergic patients or in presence of renal impairment **(adjust dose in renal failure; see Chapter 3).** Oral suspension contains aspartame and phenylalanine and should **not** be used by phenyketonurics.
Adverse Effects: May cause nausea, vomiting, diarrhea, liver enzyme elevations, rash, and vaginitis. Immunological reactions such as erythema muliforme and Stevens-Johnson syndrome have been reported.
Drug Interactions: Probenecid increases serum cefprozil levels. May cause false-positive urine reducing substance (Clinitest and other copper reduction method tests) and Coombs' test.
Drug Administration: Doses may be administered with or without food.

CEFTAZIDIME

Fortaz, Tazidime, Tazicef, Ceptaz (arginine salt)
Antibiotic, cephalosporin (third generation)

    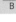

No   Yes   1   B

Injection: 0.5, 1, 2, 6, 10 g
Frozen Injection: 1 g/50 mL 4.4% dextrose, 2 g/50 mL 3.2% dextrose (iso-osmotic solutions)
(Fortaz, Tazicef, Tazidime contains 2.3 mEq Na/g drug)
(Ceptaz contains 349 mg L-arginine/g drug)

> *Neonate: IV/IM:*
> *Postnatal age ≤7 days:*
>   *<2000 kg:* 100 mg/kg/24 hr ÷ Q12 hr
>   *≥2000 kg:* 100–150 mg/kg/24 hr ÷ Q8–12 hr
> *Postnatal age >7 days:*
>   *<1200 g:* 100 mg/kg/24 hr ÷ Q12 hr
>   *≥1200 g:* 150 mg/kg/24 hr ÷ Q8 hr

Continued

CEFTAZIDIME *continued*

Infant and child: 90–150 mg/kg/24 hr ÷ Q8 hr IV/IM; **max. dose:** 6 g/24 hr
    Cystic fibrosis and meningitis: 150 mg/kg/24 hr ÷ Q8 hr IV/IM; **max. dose:**
    6 g/24 hr
Adult: 2–6 g/24 hr ÷ Q8–12 hr IV/IM; **max. dose:** 6 g/24 hr

Contraindications: Hypersensitivity to cephalosporin antibiotics.
Warnings/Precautions: **Use with caution** in penicillin-allergic patients or in
presence of renal impairment **(adjust dose in renal failure; see Chapter 3).**
Good *Pseudomonas* coverage and CSF penetration.
Adverse Effects: May cause diarrhea, phlebitis, injection site pain, rash, and liver
enzyme elevations.
Drug Interactions: Probenecid increases serum ceftazidime levels. May cause
false-positive urine reducing substance (Clinitest and other copper reduction method
tests) and Coombs' test.
Drug Administration
    IV: For IV push, infuse over 3–5 min at a concentration ≤180 mg/mL. For
    intermittent infusion, infuse over 15–30 min at a concentration ≤40 mg/mL.
    IM: Dilute with sterile water or lidocaine (0.5 or 1%) to 280 mg/mL. Assess the
    potential risk/benefit for using lidocaine as a diluent.

CEFTIBUTEN
Cedax
Antibiotic, cephalosporin (third generation)

No   Yes   1   B

Oral suspension: 90 mg/5 mL (30, 60, 90, 120 mL)
Caps: 400 mg

Child:
    Otitis media and pharyngitis/tonsillitis: 9 mg/kg/24 hr PO QD; **max. dose:**
    400 mg/24 hr
    ≥12 yr: 400 mg PO QD; **max. dose:** 400 mg/24 hr

Contraindications: Hypersensitivity to cephalosporin antibiotics.
Warnings/Precautions: **Use with caution** in penicillin-allergic patients or in
presence of renal impairment **(adjust dose in renal failure; see Chapter 3).**
Adverse Effects: May cause GI symptoms, headache, and transient elevations in liver
function tests, eosinophils and BUN.
Drug Interactions: Gastric acid lowering medictions (e.g., ranitidine and omeprazole)
may enhance bioavailability of ceftibuten.
Drug Administration: Oral suspension should be administered 2 hr before or 1 hr
after a meal. Capsules may be administered with or without food.

CEFTIZOXIME
Cefizox
Antibiotic, cephalosporin (third generation)

No   Yes   1   B

Injection: 0.5, 1, 2, 10 g
Frozen injection: 1 g/50 mL 3.8% dextrose, 2 g/50 mL 1.9% dextrose (iso-osmotic
solutions)
Contains 2.6 mEq Na/g drug

CEFTIZOXIME *continued*

Infant >1 mo and <6 mo: 100–200 mg/kg/24 hr ÷ Q6–8 hr IV/IM
Infant ≥6 mo and child: 150–200 mg/kg/24 hr ÷ Q6–8 hr IV/IM; **max. dose:**
12 g/24 hr
Adult: 2–12 g/24 hr ÷ Q8–12 hr IV/IM; **max. dose:** 12 g/24 hr
Uncomplicated gonorrhea: 1 g IM × 1

Contraindications: Hypersensitivity to cephalosporin antibiotics.
Warnings/Precautions: **Use with caution** in penicillin-allergic patients or in
presence of renal impairment **(adjust dose in renal failure; see Chapter 3).**
Good CNS penetration.
Adverse Effects: Injection site pain, pruritus, and rash are common. May cause
transient liver enzyme elevation.
Drug Interactions: Probenecid increases serum ceftizoxime levels. May interfere with
serum and urine creatinine assays (Jaffe method); and cause false-positive urinary
protein and urinary reducing substances (Clinitest, Benedict's solution).
Drug Administration
IV: IV push, infuse over 3–5 min at a concentration of 95 mg/mL. For
intermittent infusion, infuse over 30 min at a concentration of 20 mg/mL.
IM: Dilute with sterile water to 270–280 mg/mL.

CEFTRIAXONE
Rocephin
Antibiotic, cephalosporin (third generation)

Yes   Yes   1   B

Injection: 0.25, 0.5, 1, 2, 10 g
Frozen injection: 1 g/50 mL 3.8% dextrose, 2 g/50 mL 2.4% dextrose (iso-osmotic
solutions)
Intramuscular kit with 1% lidocaine diluent: 0.5, 1 g
Contains 3.6 mEq Na/g drug

Neonate:
Gonococcal ophthalmia or prophylaxis: 25–50 mg/kg/dose IM/IV × 1;
max. dose: 125 mg/dose
Infant and child: 50–75 mg/kg/24 hr ÷ Q12–24 hr IM/IV; **max. dose:** 2 g/24 hr.
Higher doses of 80–100 mg/kg/24 hr ÷ Q12–24 hr (**max. dose:** 2 g/dose and 4 g/24
hr) has been recommended for infections outside the CSF due to penicillin-resistant
pneumococci.
Meningitis (including penicillin resistant pneumococci): 100 mg/kg/24 hr IM/IV
÷ Q12 hr; **max. dose:** 2 g/dose and 4 g/24 hr
Acute otitis media: 50 mg/kg IM × 1; **max. dose:** 1 g
Adult: 1–2 g/dose Q12–24 hr IV/IM; **max. dose:** 2 g/dose and 4 g/24 hr
Uncomplicated gonorrhea or chancroid: 250 mg IM × 1

Contraindications: Hypersensitivity to cephalosporin antibiotics and neonates
with hyperbilirubinemia. **Do not** administer with calcium-containing solutions or
products (mixed or administered simultaneously via different lines) in newborns
because of risk of precipitation of ceftriaxone-calcium salt (see below).
Warnings/Precautions: **Use with caution** in penicillin allergy; patients with
gallbladder, biliary tract, liver, or pancreatic disease; presence of renal impairment; or
in neonates with continuous dosing (risk for hyperbilirubinemia). In neonates,
consider using an alternative third-generation cephalosporin with similar activity.

Continued

CEFTRIAXONE *continued*

Unlike other cephalosporins, ceftriaxone is significantly cleared by the biliary route (35%–45%).

Cases of fatal reactions with calcium-ceftriaxone precipitates in lung and kidneys in term and pre-term neonates have been reported.

Adverse Effects: Rash, injection site pain, diarrhea, and transient increase in liver enzymes are common. May cause reversible cholelithiasis, sludging in gallbladder, and jaundice.

Drug Interactions: High-dose probenecid increases serum ceftriaxone levels. May interfere with serum and urine creatinine assays (Jaffe method); and cause false-positive urinary protein and urinary reducing substances (Clinitest).

Drug Administration

IV: For IV push, infuse over 2–4 min at a concentration ≤40 mg/mL. For intermittent infusion, infuse over 10–30 min at a concentration ≤40 mg/mL.
IM: Dilute drug with either sterile water for injection or 1% lidocaine to a concentration of 250 or 350 mg/mL (250 mg/mL has lower incidence of injection site reactions). Assess the potential risk/benefit for using lidocaine as a diluent.

CEFUROXIME (IV, IM)/CEFUROXIME AXETIL (PO)

IV: Zinacef; PO: Ceftin

Antibiotic, cephalosporin (second generation)

No | Yes | 1 | B

Injection: 0.75, 1.5, 7.5 g
Frozen injection: 750 mg/50 mL 2.8% dextrose, 1.5 g/50 mL water (iso-osmotic solutions)
Injectable dosage forms contain 2.4 mEq Na/g drug
Tabs: 125, 250, 500 mg
Oral suspension: 125, 250 mg/5 mL (50, 100 mL)

IM/IV:
    Neonate: 20–100 mg/kg/24 hr ÷ Q12 hr
    Infant (>3 mo)/child: 75–150 mg/kg/24 hr ÷ Q8 hr
    Adult: 750–1500 mg/dose Q8 hr
    Max. dose: 9 g/24 hr
PO:
    Child (3 mo–12 yr):
        Pharyngitis and tonsillitis:
            Oral suspension: 20 mg/kg/24 hr ÷ Q12 hr; **max. dose:** 500 mg/24 hr
            Tab: 125 mg Q12 hr
        Otitis media, impetigo, and maxillary sinusitis:
            Oral suspension: 30 mg/kg/24 hr ÷ Q12 hr; **max. dose:** 1 g/24 hr
            Tab: 250 mg Q12 hr
        Lyme disease (alternative to doxycycline or amoxicillin):
            Oral suspension: 30 mg/kg/24 hr ÷ Q12 hr; **max. dose:** 500 mg/24 hr × 14–28 days
    Adult: 250–500 mg BID
        Max. dose: 1 g/24 hr

Contraindications: Hypersensitivity to cephalosporin antibiotics.
Warnings/Precautions: **Use with caution** in penicillin-allergic patients or in presence of renal impairment **(adjust dose in renal failure; see Chapter 3). Not recommended for meningitis;** use appropriate third-generation cephalosporin instead. Tablets and suspension are **not** bioequivalent and are **not** substitutable on a mg/mg basis.

CEFUROXIME (IV, IM)/CEFUROXIME AXETIL (PO) *continued*

Adverse Effects: May cause GI discomfort; transient increase in liver enzymes; and thrombophlebitis at the infusion site (IV use).
Drug Interactions: Concurrent use of antacids, H_2 blockers, and proton pump inhibitors may decrease oral absorption. May cause false-positive urine reducing substance (Clinitest and other copper reduction method tests) and Coombs' test; and may interfere with serum and urine creatinine determinations by the alkaline picrate method.
Drug Administration
> IV: For IV push, infuse over 3–5 min at a concentration ≤100 mg/mL. For intermittent infusion, infuse over 15–30 min at a concentration ≤30 mg/mL (137 mg/mL concentration may be used in fluid-restricted patients).
> IM: Dilute with sterile water to 200–220 mg/mL.
> PO: Administer suspension with food. Tablets may be administered with or without food. Avoid crushing tablet because of its bitter taste.

CEPHALEXIN
Keflex, Biocef, and others
Antibiotic, cephalosporin (first generation)

No Yes 1 B

Caps and tabs: 250, 500 mg
Oral suspension: 125 mg/5 mL, 250 mg/5 mL (100, 200 mL)

Infant and child: 25–100 mg/kg/24 hr PO ÷ Q6 hr. Less frequent dosing (Q8–12 hr) can be used for uncomplicated infections. Total daily dose may be divided Q12 hr for streptococcal pharyngitis (>1 yr) and skin or skin structure infections.
> ***Bacterial endocarditis prophylaxis for dental and upper airway procedure:*** 50 mg/kg/dose (**max. dose:** 2 g) × 1 PO 1 hr before procedure
Adult: 1–4 g/24 hr PO ÷ Q6 hr
> ***Bacterial endocarditis prophylaxis for dental and upper airway procedure:*** 2 g × 1 PO 1 hr before procedure
Max. dose: 4 g/24 hr

Contraindications: Hypersensitivity to cephalosporin antibiotics.
Warnings/Precautions: Some cross-reactivity with penicillins. **Use with caution in renal insufficiency (adjust dose in renal failure; see Chapter 3).**
Adverse Effects: May cause GI discomfort and transient elevation of liver enzymes.
Drug Interactions: May increase the effects of metformin. Probenecid increases serum cephalexin levels and concomitant administration with cholestyramine may reduce cephalexin absorption. May cause false-positive urine reducing substance (Clinitest and other copper reduction method tests) and Coombs' test; false elevation of serum theophylline levels (HPLC method); and false urinary protein test.
Drug Administration: Administer doses on an empty stomach; 2 hr prior or 1 hr after meals.

CEPHAPIRIN
Cefadyl
Antibiotic, cephalosporin (first generation)

No Yes 1 B

Injection: 0.5, 1, 2, 4, 20 g
Contains 2.36 mEq Na/g drug

Continued

CEPHAPIRIN *continued*

Child: 40–80 mg/kg/24 hr IV/IM ÷ Q6 hr
Adult: 0.5–1 g/dose IV/IM Q4–6 hr
Max. dose: 12 g/24 hr

Contraindications: Hypersensitivity to cephalosporin antibiotics.
Warnings/Precautions: Use with caution in penicillin-allergic patients or in presence of renal impairment **(adjust dose in renal failure; see Chapter 3).**
Beta-hemolytic streptococci should be treated for at least 10 days.
Adverse Effects: GI disturbances including diarrhea, and thrombophlebitis may occur.
Drug Interactions: May decrease effect of typhoid vaccine.
Drug Administration
    IV: Infuse doses over 3–5 min at concentrations ≤200 mg/mL.
    IM: Dilute drug with sterile water to 500 mg/mL

CEPHRADINE
Velosef and others
Antibiotic, cephalosporin (first generation)

No   Yes   1   B

Oral suspension: 125 mg/5 mL, 250 mg/5 mL (100, 200 mL)
Caps: 250, 500 mg

Infant (≥9 mo) and child: 25–50 mg/kg/24 hr PO ÷ Q6–12 hr
Adult: 1–4 g/24 hr PO ÷ Q6–12 hr
Max. dose: 4 g/24 hr

Contraindications: Hypersensitivity to cephalosporin antibiotics.
Warnings/Precautions: Use with caution in penicillin-allergic patients and renal insufficiency **(adjust dose in renal failure; see Chapter 3).** Does not penetrate well into CSF.
Adverse Effects: GI discomfort and rash are common. May cause transient eosinophilia and neutropenia.
Drug Interactions: Probenecid increases serum cephradine levels. May interfere with serum and urine creatinine assays (Jaffe and KDA methods); theophylline assays (HPLC method); and cause false-positive urinary protein and urinary reducing substances (Clinitest).
Drug Administration: Doses may be given with or without food.

CHLORAMPHENICOL
Chloromycetin and others
Antibiotic

Yes   Yes   3   C

Injection: 1 g
Contains 2.25 mEq Na/g drug

Neonate IV:
Loading dose: 20 mg/kg
Maintenance dose (first dose should be given 12 hr after loading dose):
    ≤7 days: 25 mg/kg/24 hr QD
    >7 days:
        ≤2 kg: 25 mg/kg/24 hr QD
        >2 kg: 50 mg/kg/24 hr ÷ Q12 hr

CHLORAMPHENICOL *continued*

Infant/child/adult: 50–75 mg/kg/24 hr IV ÷ Q6 hr
   Meningitis: 75–100 mg/kg/24 hr IV ÷ Q6 hr
   Max. dose: 4 g/24 hr

   Contraindications: Hypersensitivity to chloramphenicol or any other
components in the formulation.
   ***Warnings/Precautions:* Use with caution** in G6PD deficiency, renal or hepatic
dysfunction, and neonates.
   Dose recommendations are just guidelines for therapy; monitoring of blood levels
is essential in neonates and infants. Follow hematologic status for dose related or
idiosyncratic marrow suppression. "Gray baby" syndrome may be seen with levels
>50 mg/L.
Therapeutic Levels: Peak: 15–25 mg/L for meningitis; 10–20 mg/L for other infections.
Trough: 5–15 mg/L for meningitis; 5–10 mg/L for other infections. Recommended
serum sampling time: trough (IV/PO) within 30 min prior to next dose; peak (IV) 30
min after the end of infusion; peak (PO) 2 hr after oral administration. Time to
achieve steady state: 2–3 days for newborns; 12–24 hr for children and adults.
Note: Higher serum levels may be achieved using the oral, rather than the IV, route.
Adverse Effects: Headache, confusion, neurotoxicity, delirium and depression may
occur.
Drug Interactions: Concomitant use of phenobarbital and rifampin may lower
chloramphenicol serum levels. Phenytoin may increase chloramphenicol serum levels.
Chloramphenicol may increase the effects/toxicity of phenytoin, chlorpropamide,
cyclosporin, tacrolimus and oral anticoagulants; and decrease absorption of vitamin
B_{12}. Chloramphenicol is an inhibitor of CYP 450 2C9.
Drug Administration: For IV push, infuse over 5 min at a concentration ≤100
mg/mL. For intermittent infusion, infuse over 15–30 min at a concentration ≤20
mg/mL. **IM administration is not recommended** since it may be less effective by this
route.

CHLOROQUINE HCL/PHOSPHATE
Aralen and others
Amebicide, antimalarial

Yes   Yes   1   C

Tabs: 250, 500 mg as phosphate (150, 300 mg base, respectively)
Oral suspension: 16.67 mg/mL as phosphate (10 mg/mL base), 15 mg/mL as
phosphate (9 mg/mL base)
Injection: 50 mg/mL as HCl (40 mg/mL base) (5 mL)

Doses expressed in mg of chloroquine base.
***Malaria prophylaxis (start 1 wk prior to exposure and continue for 4 wk after
leaving endemic area):***
   Child: 5 mg/kg/dose PO Q wk; **max. dose:** 300 mg/dose
   Adult: 300 mg/dose PO Q wk
Malaria treatment (chloroquine sensitive strains):
***For treatment for malaria, consult with ID specialist or see the latest edition of the
AAP Red Book. For IV use, consider safer alternatives such as quinidine or quinine.***
   Child: 10 mg/kg/dose (**max. dose:** 600 mg/dose) PO × 1; followed by 5
mg/kg/dose (**max. dose:** 300 mg/dose) 6 hr later and then once daily for 2 days.
   Adult: 600 mg/dose PO × 1; followed by 300 mg/dose 6 hr later and then once
daily for 2 days.

   Contraindications: Hypersensitivity to 4-aminoquinoline compounds; and
retinal/visual changes.   *Continued*

CHLOROQUINE HCL/PHOSPHATE *continued*

Warnings/Precautions: **Use with caution** in liver disease, preexisting auditory damage or seizures, G6PD deficiency, psoriasis, porphyria or concomitant hepatotoxic drugs. **Adjust dose in renal failure (see Chapter 3).**

Adverse Effects: ECG abnormalities, prolonged QT interval, pruritis, GI disturbances, skeletal muscle weakness, amnesia, blurred vision, retinal and corneal changes. Headaches, confusion, and hair depigmentation have been reported.

Drug Interactions: Chloroquine is a substrate for CYP 450 2D6 and 3A4 and inhibitor of CYP 450 2D6.

Antacids, ampicillin, and kaolin may decrease the absorption of chloroquine (allow 4 hr interval between chloroquine). May increase serum cyclosporine levels. Cimetidine may increase effects/toxicity of chloroquine.

Drug Administration: Administer oral doses with meals to reduce GI complications. Mixing tablets with chocolate syrup or placing tablets in capsules may be used to mask bitter taste.

CICLOPIROX/CICLOPIROX OLAMINE
Loprox, Penlac, Ciclopirox olamine
Antifungal, synthetic

| No | No | ? | B |

Shampoo: 1% (120 mL)
Topical gel: 0.77% (30, 45, 100 g)
Topical suspension: 0.77% (30 mL)
Topical nail lacquer solution (Penlac): 8% (3.3, 6.6 mL); contains isopropyl alcohol
Topical cream (Ciclopirox olamine): 0.77, 1% (15, 30, 90 g); contains 1% benzyl alcohol
Topical lotion (Ciclopirox olamine): 0.77, 1% (30, 60 mL); contains 1% benzyl alcohol

---

 (See remarks for Pediatric considerations)
Tinea pedis, tinea cruris, tinea corporis, cutaneous candidasis and tinea versicolor:
    Topical suspension, gel, cream, or lotion: Apply to affected area BID × 4 wk.
Seborrhic dermatitis of scalp:
    Gel: Apply to affected scalp areas BID × 4 wk
    Shampoo: Wet hair and apply 5 mL (up to 10 mL for long hair) to the scalp. Lather, leave on for 3 min, then rinse. Repeat twice weekly for 4 wk with at least 3 days between applications.
Onychomycosis (fingernails or toenails):
    Nail lacquer solution: Apply lacquer once daily (preferably QHS or 8 hr prior to washing) to affected nails, including under nail plate (if free of the nail bed). Daily dose applications should be made over the previous coat and removed with alcohol every 7 days. Also file away loose nail material and trim nails as needed when removing the previous coat. Therapy may last up to 48 wk.

Contraindications: Hypersensitivity to ciclopirox or any other components in the formulation.
Warnings/Precautions: **Not** for ophthalmic, oral, or intravaginal use. Discontinue use of shampoo or nail lacquer form with sensitivity reactions or irritation. **Pediatric studies have not been completed** for the cream and lotion forms (<10 yr old); gel and shampoo forms (<16 yr old); and nail lacquer solution (<12 yr old). Nail lacquer solution is flammable.

CICLOPIROX/CICLOPIROX OLAMINE *continued*

Adverse Effects: Itching, burning and erythemia may occur wth all dosage forms. Nail disorders have been reported with the use of the nail lacquer product. Hair discoloration has been reported with shampoo.
Drug Interactions: None identified.
Drug Administration: **Avoid** contact with eyes and mucous membranes.
Shampoo, gel (seborrhic dermatitis) and nail lacquer: See respective dosage section. Topical suspension, gel, cream, or lotion: Apply to affected areas and surrounding skin. Occlusive dressing should not be used.

CIDOFOVIR
Vistide
Antiviral

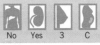

No | Yes | 3 | C

Injection: 75 mg/mL (5 mL); preservative free

Safety and efficacy have not been established in children.
CMV retinitis:
    Induction: 5 mg/kg IV × 1 with probenecid and hydration
    Maintenance: 3 mg/kg IV Q7 days with probenecid and hydration
Adenovirus infection after bone marrow transplant (limited data; see remarks):
    5 mg/kg/dose IV once weekly × 3, followed by 5 mg/kg/dose IV once every 2 wk. Administer oral probenecid 1–1.25 g/m^2/dose (rounded to the nearest 250 mg interval) 3 hr prior to and 1 hr and 8 hr after each dose of cidofovir. Also give IV normal saline at 3 times maintenance fluid 1 hr prior to and 1 hr after cidofovir, followed by 2 times maintenance fluid for an additional 2 hr.

Contraindications: Hypersensitivity to probenecid or sulfa-containing drugs; sCr >1.5 mg/dL, CrCl ≤55 mL/min, urine protein ≥100 mg/dL (2+ proteinuria), direct intraocular injection of cidofovir, and concomitant nephrotoxic drugs.
Warnings/Precautions: Monitor renal function and neutrophil counts during therapy. IV NS prehydration and probenecid must be used to reduce risk of nephrotoxicity. Modify dose in changing renal function. Reduce maintenance dose to 3 mg/kg if sCr increases 0.3–0.4 mg/dL from baseline. Discontinue therapy if sCr increases >0.5 mg/dL from baseline or development of >3+ proteinuria.
Adverse Effects: **Renal impairment is the major dose-limiting toxicity.** May also cause nausea, vomiting, headache, rash, metabolic acidosis, uveitis, decreased intraoccular pressure, and neutropenia.
Drug Interactions: **Nephrotoxic medications** (e.g., aminoglycosides, amphotericin B) increase risk for toxicity and **are contraindicated.** Consider drug interactions of probenecid; increases effects/toxicity of zidovudine.
Drug Administration: IV infusion over 1 hr at a concentration ≤8 mg/mL.

CIPROFLOXACIN
Cipro, Cipro XR, Ciloxan ophthalmic, Ciprodex, Cipro
HC Otic, and others
Antibiotic, quinolone

No | Yes | 1 | C

Tabs: 100, 250, 500, 750 mg
Extended-release tabs (Cipro XR): 500, 1000 mg
Oral suspension: 500 mg/5 mL (100 mL)
Injection: 10 mg/mL (20, 40 mL)

Continued

For explanation of icons, see p. 306.

Premixed injection: 200 mg/100 mL 5% dextrose, 400 mg/100 mL 5% dextrose (iso-osmotic solutions)
Ophthalmic solution: 3.5 mg/mL (2.5, 5, 10 mL)
Ophthalmic ointment: 3.3 mg/g (3.5 g)
Otitic suspension:
    With dexamethasone (Ciprodex): 3 mg/mL ciprofloxacin + 1 mg/mL dexamethasone (7.5 mL); contains benzalkonium chloride
    With hydrocortisone (Cipro HC Otic): 2 mg/mL ciprofloxacin + 10 mg/mL hydrocortisone (10 mL); contains benzyl alcohol

Child:
    PO: 20–30 mg/kg/24 hr ÷ Q12 hr; **max. dose:** 1.5 g/24 hr
    IV: 20–30 mg/kg/24 hr ÷ Q12 hr; **max. dose:** 800 mg/24 hr
    Complicated UTI or pyelonephritis:
        PO: 20–40 mg/kg/24 hr ÷ Q12 hr; **max. dose:** 1.5 g/24 hr
        IV: 18–30 mg/kg/24 hr ÷ Q8 hr; **max. dose:** 1.2 g/24 hr
    Cystic fibrosis:
        PO: 40 mg/kg/24 hr ÷ Q12 hr; **max. dose:** 2 g/24 hr
        IV: 30 mg/kg/24 hr ÷ Q8 hr; **max. dose:** 1.2 g/24 hr
    Anthrax (see remarks):
        Inhalational/systemic/cutaneous: Start with 20–30 mg/kg/24 hr ÷ Q12 hr IV (**max. dose:** 800 mg/24 hr) and convert to oral dosing with clinical improvement at 20–30 mg/kg/24 hr ÷ Q12 hr PO (**max. dose:** 1 g/24 hr). Duration of therapy: 60 days (IV and PO combined)
        Post exposure prophylaxis: 20–30 mg/kg/24 hr ÷ Q12 hr PO × 60 days; **max. dose:** 1 g/24 hr
Adult:
    PO:
        Immediate release: 250–750 mg/dose Q12 hr
        Extended release (Cipro XR):
            Uncomplicated UTI/Cystitis: 500 mg/dose Q24 hr
            Complicated UTI/Uncomplicated pyelonephritis: 1000 mg/dose Q24 hr
        IV: 200–400 mg/dose Q12 hr
        Anthrax (see remarks):
            Inhalational/systemic/cutaneous: Start with 400 mg/dose Q12 hr IV and convert to oral dosing with clinical improvement at 500 mg/dose Q12 hr PO. Duration of therapy: 60 days (IV and PO combined)
            Post exposure prophylaxis: 500 mg/dose Q12 hr PO × 60 days.
Ophthalmic solution: 1–2 drops Q2 hr while awake × 2 days, then 1–2 gtts Q4 hr while awake × 5 days
Ophthalmic ointment: Apply 0.5 inch ribbon TID × 2, then BID × 5 days
Otic:
    Ciprodex:
        Acute otitis media with tympanostomy tubes or acute otitis externa, ≥6 mo and adults: 4 drops to affected ear(s) BID × 7 days
    Cipro HC Otic:
        Otitis externa, >1 yr and adults: 3 drops to affected ear(s) BID × 7 days

Contraindications: Hypersensitivity to ciprofloxacin, fluoroquinolones or any other components in the formulation. Concomitant use with tizanidine may result in excessive sedation and dangerous hypotension. Otic formulation **should not** be used with viral infections of the external ear canal.
Warnings/Precautions: Use with caution in children <18 yr (like other quinolones, tendon rupture can occur during or after therapy, especially with concomitant

CIPROFLOXACIN *continued*

corticosteroid use), alkalinized urine (crystalluria), seizures, excessive sunlight, and renal dysfunction **(adjust dose in renal failure; see Chapter 3). Not recommended** for gonorrhea because of potential resistance. **Do not** use Cipro HC otic suspension with perforated tympanic membranes.

Combinational antimicrobial therapy is recommended for anthrax. For penicillin susceptible strains, consider changing to high-dose amoxicillin (25–35 mg/kg/dose TID PO). See www.bt.cdc.gov for the latest information.

Extended-release tablets is formulated as combination of immediate (~35%) and sustained (~65%) release components.

Adverse Effects

Systemic: GI symptoms, headache, restlessness, and rash are common. Tendinitis, rupture tendon (concomitant corticosteroid use and in elderly), photosensitivity, renal failure, psychosis and seizures have been reported.

Ophthalmic: Burning and discomfort is common. Lid crusting, foreign body sensation and conjunctival hypermia may occur.

Otic: Altered taste sense and otalgia may occur.

Drug Interactions: Inhibits CYP 450 1A2. Ciprofloxacin can increase effects and/or toxicity of caffeine, methotrexate, theophylline, tizanidine, warfarin, and cyclosporine. Probenecid increases serum ciprofloxacin levels

Drug Administration

IV: For intermittent infusion, infuse over 60 min at a concentration ≤2 mg/mL.

PO: All oral dosage forms may be administered with or without food. **Do not** administer antacids, other divalent salts (including dairy products), or sucralfate. Administer ciprofloxacin 2 hr before or 6 hr after taking aforementioned products. **Do not** administer oral suspension through a feeding tube because suspension adheres to tube.

Ophthalmic

Drops: Apply finger pressure to lacrimal sac during and for 1–2 min after dose application.

Ointment: Instill ointment in lower conjunctival sac by **avoiding contact** of ointment tip with eye or skin.

Otic

AOM with tympanostomy tube: Instill drops by having patient lie with affected ear upward. Pump tragus 5 times by pushing inward to facilitate pentration of drops to middle ear and remain in the same position for 1 min.

Otitis external: Patient should lie with the affected ear upward while instilling drops. Remain in this position for 1 min after dosing.

CLARITHROMYCIN
Biaxin, Biaxin XL
Antibiotic, macrolide

| No | Yes | 2 | C |

Film tablets: 250, 500 mg
Extended-release tablets (Biaxin XL): 500 mg
Granules for oral suspension: 125, 250 mg/5 mL (50, 100 mL)

Child:

Acute otitis media, pharyngitis/tonsillitis, pneumonia, acute maxillary sinusitis, or uncomplicated skin infections: 15 mg/kg/24 hr PO ÷ Q12 hr

Bacterial endocarditis prophylaxis: 15 mg/kg **(max. dose:** 500 mg) PO 1 hr before procedure

M. avium complex:

Prophylaxis (1st episode and recurrence): 15 mg/kg/24 hr PO ÷ Q12 hr

Continued

CLARITHROMYCIN *continued*

M. avium complex:
  Treatment: 15 mg/kg/24 hr PO ÷ Q12 hr with other antimycobacterial drugs
 Max. dose: 1 g/24 hr
Adult:
 Pharyngitis/tonsillitis, acute maxillary sinusitis, bronchitis, pneumonia, or uncomplicated skin infections:
  Immediate release: 250–500 mg/dose Q12 hr PO
  Extended release (Biaxin XL): 1000 mg Q24 hr PO (currently not indicated for pharyngitis/tonsillitis or uncomplicated skin infections)
 Bacterial endocarditis prophylaxis: 500 mg PO 1 hr before procedure
 M. avium complex:
  Prophylaxis (1st episode and recurrence): 500 mg/dose Q12 hr PO
  Treatment: 500 mg Q12 hr PO with other antimycobacterial drugs
 H. pylori GI infection: 250 mg Q12 hr to 500 mg Q8 hr PO with omeprazole or ranitidine bismuth; or amoxicillin and omeprazole or lansoprazole.

Contraindications: Hypersensitivity to macrolide antibiotics (e.g., erythromycin). Concomitant cisapride, pimozide, astemizole, terfenadine, ergotamine or dihydroergotamine may result in QT interval prolongation.
Warnings/Precautions: As with other macrolides, clarithromycin has been associated with QT prolongation and ventricular arrhythmias, including ventricular tachycardia and torsades de pointes.
Adjust dose in renal failure (see Chapter 3).
Adverse Effects: Diarrhea, nausea, abnormal taste, dyspepsia, abdominal discomfort (< erythromycin but > azithromycin), and headache. Rare cases of anaphylaxis, Stevens-Johnson syndrome, and toxic epidermal necrolysis have been reported.
Drug Interactions: Substrate and inhibitor of CYP 450 3A4; and inhibitor of CYP 1A2. May increase effects/toxicity of carbamazepine, theophylline, cyclosporine, digoxin, ergot alkaloids, fluconazole, tacrolimus, triazolam and warfarin.
Drug Administration: Extended-release tablets must be administered with food. All other dosage forms may be administered with or without food.

CLINDAMYCIN
Cleocin, Cleocin-T, and others
Antibiotic, lincomycin derivative

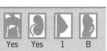

        Yes Yes 1 B

Caps: 75, 150, 300 mg
Oral solution: 75 mg/5 mL (100 mL)
Injection: 150 mg/mL (contains 9.45 mg/mL benzyl alcohol)
Solution, topical (Cleocin-T): 1% (1, 30, 60 mL); may contain 50% isopropyl alcohol
Gel, topical (Cleocin-T): 1% (7.5, 30, 42, 60, 77 g); may contain methylparaben
Lotion, topical (Cleocin-T): 1% (60 mL); may contain methylparaben
Foam, topical: 1% (50 g); contains 58% ethanol
Vaginal cream: 2% (40 g); may contain benzyl alcohol
Vaginal suppository: 100 mg (3s)

Neonate: IV/IM: 5 mg/kg/dose
≤7 days:
 ≤2 kg: Q12 hr
 >2 kg: Q8 hr
>7 days:
 <1.2 kg: Q12 hr
 1.2–2 kg: Q8 hr
 >2 kg: Q6 hr

CLINDAMYCIN *continued*

Child:
> *PO:* 10–30 mg/kg/24 hr ÷ Q6–8 hr
> *IM/IV:* 25–40 mg/kg/24 hr ÷ Q6–8 hr
> ***Bacterial endocarditis prophylaxis:*** 20 mg/kg (**max. dose:** 600 mg) 1 hr before
> procedure with PO route and 30 min prior to procedure with IV route

Adult:
> *PO:* 150–450 mg/dose Q6–8 hr; **max. dose:** 1.8 g/24 hr
> *IM/IV:* 1200–1800 mg/24 hr IM/IV ÷ Q6–12 hr; **max. dose:** 4.8 g/24 hr
> ***Bacterial endocarditis prophylaxis:*** 600 mg 1 hr before procedure with PO route
> and 30 min prior to procedure with IV route

Topical: Apply to affected area BID.

Bacterial vaginosis:
> *Suppositories:* 100 mg/dose QHS × 3 days
> *Vaginal cream (2%):* 1 applicator dose (5 g) QHS for 3 or 7 days in non-pregnant
> patients and for 7 days in pregnant patients in second and third trimester.

> ***Contraindications:*** Hypersensitivity to clindamycin, lincomycin or any other
> components in the formulation.
> ***Warnings/Precautions:*** **Use with caution** in atopic patients. **Not** indicated in
meningitis; CSF penetration is poor. Pseudomembraneous colitis may occur up to
several weeks after cessation of therapy. Capsules may contain FD&C yellow no. 5
(tartrazine); an allergan to susceptible individuals. Dosage reduction may be required
in severe renal or hepatic disease but not necessarily in mild/moderate conditions.
Adverse Effects: Diarrhea, rash, Stevens-Johnson syndrome, granulocytopenia,
thrombocytopenia, or sterile abscess at injection site.
Drug Interactions: Clindamycin may increase the neuromuscular blocking effects of
tubocurarine, pancuronium.
Drug Administration
> IV: For intermittent infusion, infuse over 10–60 min at a rate ≤30 mg/min
> (hypotension, cardiac arrest have been reported with rapid infusions) and at a
> concentration ≤18 mg/mL.
> IM: Use 150 mg/mL injectable solution. **Do not exceed** 600 mg per IM dose.
> PO: All dosage forms may be administered with or without meals. Take capsules
> with a glassful of water. Oral liquid preparation is not palatable; consider use of
> oral capsules as a sprinkle onto applesauce or pudding.

CLOFAZIMINE
Lamprene
Leprostatic agent

No   No   3   C

Caps: 50, 100 mg
Drug is available under an IND held by National Hansen's Disease Programs.
Prescribers must call (225) 578–9861 to obtain drug.

Lepromatous leprosy:
> *Child:* 1 mg/kg/dose (**max. dose:** 100 mg) QD PO with one or more other
> antileprosy drugs

Adult:
> *Dapsone sensitive multibacillary leprosy:* 100 mg QD PO with two other
> antileprosy drugs for at least 2 yr; may decrease to monotherapy when
> negative skin smears are obtained

Continued

CLOFAZIMINE *continued*

>*Dapsone resistant:* 100 mg QD PO with one or more other antileprosy drugs
>× 3 yr followed by clofaximine monotherapy 100 mg QD PO

Erythema nodosum leprosum:
>*Adult:* 100–200 mg QD PO up to 3 mo to facillitate steroid dose reduction or
>elimination, then taper dose to 100 mg as soon as reactive episode is controlled.

Contraindications: Hypersensitivity to clofazimine products.
Warnings/Precautions: Severe GI effects (bowel obstruction, GI hemorrhage,
splenic infarction), some fatal, have been reported rarely. Pink to
brownish-black skin discoloration side effect may take months to years to reverse.
Dosages are generally well tolerated when ≤100 mg/24 hr.
Adverse Effects: Skin discoloration, dry skin, rash, GI disturbances,
conjuctival/corneal pigmentation and abnormal body fluid color. Depression related to
skin discoloration has been reported.
Drug Interactions: Concurrent use with antacids containing aluminum/magnesium
will reduce clofazimine absorption. May reduce phenytoin levels.
Drug Administration: Administer doses with meals.

CLOTRIMAZOLE
Lotrimin AF, Cruex, Gyne-Lotrimin 3, Gyne-Lotrimin 7,
Mycelex, Mycelex-7, and others
Antifungal, imidazole

| No | No | ? | B/C |

Oral troche: 10 mg
Cream, topical (OTC): 1% (12, 15, 24, 30, 45 g); contains benzyl alcohol
Solution, topical (OTC): 1% (10, 30 mL)
Lotion, topical (OTC): 1% (20 mL); contains benzyl alcohol
Vaginal suppository (OTC): 200 mg
Vaginal cream (OTC): 1% (15, 30, 45 g), 2% (21 g)
Combination packs:
>**Mycelex-7 Combination Pack (OTC):** Vaginal suppository 100 mg (7) and
>vaginal cream 1% (7 g)
>**Gyne-Lotrimin 3 Combination Pack (OTC):** Vaginal suppository 200 mg (3) and
>vaginal cream 1% (7 g)

Topical: Apply to skin BID × 4–8 wk
Vaginal candidiasis: (vaginal suppositories)
>100 mg/dose QHS × 7 days, or
>200 mg/dose QHS × 3 days, or
>1 applicator dose (5 g) of 1% vaginal cream QHS × 7–14 days, or
>1 applicator dose of 2% vaginal cream QHS × 3 days

Thrush:
>*>3 yr–adult:* Dissolve slowly (15–30 min) one troche in the mouth 5 times/24 hr
>× 14 days

Contraindications: Hypersensitivity to clotrimazole or any other components in
the formulation.
Warnings/Precautions: **Avoid use** of condoms and diaphragms with vaginal
cream or suppository as latex can be weakened. **Do not** use troches for systemic
infections. Pregnancy code is a "B" for topical and vaginal dosage forms and "C" for
troches.
Adverse Effects: May cause erythema, blistering, or urticaria with topical use. Liver
enzyme elevation, nausea and vomiting may occur with troches.
Drug Interactions: CYP 450 3A substrate and inhibitor; may increase effects/toxicity
of other CYP 450 3A substrates (e.g., ergot derivatives, sirolimus, and tacrolimus).

CLOTRIMAZOLE *continued*

Drug Administration
PO: Troches should be dissolved slowly in the mouth over 15–30 min.
Topical: **Avoid** contact with eyes.
Vaginal: Wash hands before using. Remain lying down for 30 min after application of cream or suppository. Wash applicator after every use. **Do not** use tampons until therapy is completed.

CLOXACILLIN
Tegopen, Cloxapen
Antibiotic, penicillin (penicillinase resistant)

No   No   ?   B

Caps: 250, 500 mg
Oral solution: 125 mg/5 mL (100, 200 mL)
Sodium content:
    250 mg tab = 0.6 mEq
    125 mg suspension = 0.48 mEq

Infant/child: 50–100 mg/kg/24 hr PO ÷ Q6 hr
Adult: 250–500 mg/dose PO Q6 hr
Max. dose: 6 g/24 hr

Contraindications: Hypersensitivity to penicillins.
Warnings/Precautions: **Use with caution** in cephalosporin hypersensitivity. Gastrointestinal disorders such as hypermotility or malabsorption may alter absorption. Not effective against MRSA.
Adverse Effects: May cause nausea, vomiting, diarrhea, rash and fever.
Drug Interactions: May decrease effectiveness of oral contraceptives and increase effects/toxicity of methotrexate and allopurinal. Probenecid increases cloxacillin levels.
Drug Administration: Administer doses on an empty stomach, 1 hr before or 2 hr after meals.

COLISTIMETHATE SODIUM
Coly-Mycin M Parenteral, Colistin, Colistin Sodium
Methanesulfonate
Antibiotic, polypeptide

No   Yes   ?   C

Injection: 150 mg
1 mg pure colistin is equivalent to 30,000 units
Nebulizer solution: 75 mg/3 mL, 150 mg/4 mL (mixed in 0.25% NS, preservative free)
For otic preparation (Cortisporin-TC Otic), see Neomycin/Hydrocortisone Otic Preparations

Dosages are expressed in terms of mg colistin.
Neonate:
    <7 days: 5 mg/kg/24 hr IM ÷ Q12 hr
    ≥7 days: 7.5 mg/kg/24 hr IM ÷ Q8 hr
Child and adult: 2.5–5 mg/kg/24 hr IV/IM ÷ Q6–12 hr; **max. dose:** 7 mg/kg/24 hr ÷ Q8 hr
    Cystic fibrosis: 5–8 mg/kg/24 hr IV ÷ Q8 hr; **max. dose:** 160 mg/dose

Continued

COLISTIMETHATE SODIUM *continued*

Inhalation:
    Cystic fibrosis prophylaxis therapy:
        Use with conventional nebulizer (e.g., PARI LC Plus): 150 mg Q12 hr
        administered in repeated cycles of 28 days on drug followed by 28 days off
        drug.
        Use with eFlow nebulizer: 75 mg Q12 hr administered in repeated cycles of
        28 days on drug followed by 28 days off drug.

Contraindications: Hypersensitivity to colistimethate or any other components
in the formulation.
    Warnings/Precautions: Use with caution in renal impairment **(adjust dose in
renal failure; see Chapter 3)** and with neuromuscular blocking agents. Dose
dependent nephrotoxicity may occur.
    Do not use premixed unit dose vials for inhalation. Premixing colistimethate (a
prodrug) into an aqueous solution and storing it will increase concentrations of the
more active and toxic product, colistin. Inhaled colistin has been shown to cause
massive inflammation in rats and dogs.
Adverse Effects: GI disturbances, rash, and transient neurological symptoms
(circumoral paresthesias, tingling of extremities or tongue). Respiratory distress and
nephrotoxicity have been reported. Bronchospasm may occur with nebulized route,
especially those with CF or asthma.
Drug Interactions: Aminoglycosides, muscle relaxants (e.g., tubocurarine), polymyxin,
succinylcholine, gallamine, decamethonium and sodium citrate may potentiate
neuromuscular blockade. Cephalothin may enhance nephrotoxicity.
Drug Administration
    IV: For intermittent infusion, infuse over 3–5 min at a convenient concentration.
    For continuous infusion, infuse ½ total daily dose over 3–5 min, give remainder
    of dose over 22–23 hr by diluting to a convenient concentration with compatible
    IV fluid (D5, NS and others).
    IM: Dilute to 75 mg/mL concentration with sterile water.
    Inhalation
        Conventional neblizer: If using PARI LC Plus nebulizer, use a DeVilbiss
        Pulmo-Aide compressor. Treatment period is usually over 15 min.
        eFlow nebulizer: Dose may be diluted with NS up to a total volume of 4 mL.
        Treatment period is usually over 10–12 min.

COLISTIN

See *Colistimethate Sodium*

CO-TRIMOXAZOLE

See *Sulfamethoxazole and Trimethoprim*

FORMULARY

CYCLOSERINE
Seromycin
Antituberculosis agent

No   Yes   1   C

Caps: 250 mg

Mycobacterium avium complex and tuberculosis:
  Child: 10–20 mg/kg/24 hr PO ÷ Q12 hr; **max. dose:** 1 g/24 hr
  Adult: 250 mg Q12 hr PO × 14 days, then as tolerated to 250 mg Q6–8 hr; **max. dose:** 1 g/24 hr

Contraindications: Hypersensitivity to cycloserine, epilepsy, depression, anxiety, psychosis, and alcohol abuse.
Warnings/Precautions: **Adjust dose in renal impairment (see Chapter 3).**
Should be given as part of a multi-drug regimen.
Therapeutic Peak Serum Levels: 20–35 mg/L. Recommended serum sampling time at steady state: 2 hr post-dose after 3–4 days of continuous dosing.
Adverse Effects: Confusion, dizziness, headache and somnolence are common. Seizures have been reported.
Drug Interactions: Increases effects/toxicity of phenytoin. Alcohol increases risk of seizures. Ethionamide and isoniazid may increase neurotoxicity.
Drug Administration: Should be given on an empty stomach for maximum absorption.

CYTOMEGALOVIRUS IMMUNE GLOBULIN
CytoGam
Immune globulin, CMV (high titer)

No   Yes   ?   C

Injection: 50 mg/mL (20, 50 mL); each 1 mL contains 50 mg sucrose, 10 mg albumin; 20–30 mEq/L sodium; and trace amounts of IgA and IgM.

CMV prophylaxis following transplant (IV):
  Kidney: 150 mg/kg/dose × 1 within 72 hr prior to transplant, then 100 mg/kg/dose at 2, 4, 6, and 8 wk after transplant, followed by 50 mg/kg/dose at 12 and 16 wk after transplant.
Liver, pancreas, lung, or heart (for CMV negative recipient receiving organ from CMV positive donor; consider concomitant use of ganciclovir) (IV): 150 mg/kg/dose within 72 hr prior to transplant and on 2, 4, 6, and 8 wk after transplant, followed by 100 mg/kg/dose at 12 and 16 wk after transplant.
BMT (IV): 200 mg/kg/dose at 6 and 8 days prior to transplant and on days 1, 7, 14, 21, 28, 42, 56, and 70 after transplant.

Contraindications: History of a prior severe reaction associated with any immunoglobulin preparation; and IgA deficiency.
Warnings/Precautions: **Use with caution** in pre-existing or predisposition to renal insufficiency; formulation contains sucrose. Defer administration of live virus vaccines approximately 3 mo after CMV-IG; revaccination may be necessary if vaccines were administered after CMV-IG.
Adverse Effects: Flushing, shivering, GI disturbances, arthralgia, back pain, cramping, hypotension, wheezing and fever are common and most often infusion related. Anaphylaxis and aseptic meningitis have been reported.
Drug Interactions: Live virus vaccines (e.g., MMR, varicella); see Warnings/Precautions.   *Continued*

CYTOMEGALOVIRUS IMMUNE GLOBULIN *continued*

Drug Administration: Administer via IV infusion at a concentration 16.7–50 mg/mL (not >1:2 dilution) at the following rates:
> Initial dose: 15 mg/kg/hr, if no adverse reaction after 30 min, increase to 30 mg/kg/hr. If no adverse reaction after 30 min, increase to **max. rate** of 60 mg/kg/hr.
> Subsequent doses: 30 mg/kg/hr, if no adverse reaction after 15 min, increase to **max. rate** of 60 mg/kg/hr.

Max. infusion rate: 75 mL/hr of 50 mg/mL concentration or 3750 mg/hr.

DAPSONE
Aczone, Diaminodiphenylsulfone, DDS
Antibiotic, sulfone derivative

No Yes 1 C

Tabs: 25, 100 mg
Oral suspension: 2 mg/mL
Topical gel (Aczone): 5% (30 g)

Pneumocystis carinii prophylaxis:
> ***Child ≥1 mo:*** 2 mg/kg/24 hr PO QD; **max. dose:** 100 mg/24 hr.
> Alternative weekly dosing, 4 mg/kg/dose PO Q7 days; **max. dose:** 200 mg/dose
> ***Adult:*** 100 mg/24 hr PO ÷ QD-BID with pyrimethamine 50 mg PO Q7 days and leucovorin 25 mg PO Q monthly; other combination regimens with pyrimethamine and leucovorin can be used (see http://www.hivatis.org/trtgdlns.html#Opportunistic)

Toxoplasma gondii prophylaxis:
> ***Child ≥1 mo:*** 2 mg/kg/24 hr PO QD; **max. dose:** 25 mg/24 hr with pyrimethamine 1 mg/kg/24 hr PO QD and leucovorin 5 mg PO Q3 days.
> ***Adult:*** 50 mg PO QD with pyrimethamine 50 mg PO Q7 days and leucovorin 25 mg PO Q monthly; other combination regimens with pyrimethamine and leucovorin can be used (see http://www.hivatis.org/trtgdlns.html#Opportunistic)

Leprosy (see www.who.int/lep/disease/disease.htm for latest recommendations including combination regimens such as rifampin ± clofazimine):
> ***Child:*** 1–2 mg/kg/24 hr PO QD; **max. dose:** 100 mg/24 hr
> ***Adult:*** 50–100 mg PO QD

Acne vulgaris:
> ***≥12 yr:*** Apply small amount of topical gel onto clean, acne affected areas BID

> ***Contraindications:*** Hypersensitivity to dapsone products or any other components in the formulation.
> ***Warnings/Precautions:*** Patients with HIV, glutathione deficiency, or G6PD deficiency may be at increased risk for developing methemoglobinemia. Skin discoloration leading to depression and suicide have been reported. Oral suspension may not be absorbed as well as tablets.

Adverse Effects: Hemolytic anemia (dose related), agranulocytosis, methemoglobinemia, aplastic anemia, nausea, vomiting, hyperbilirubinemia, headache, nephrotic syndrome, and hypersensitivity reaction (sulfone syndrome). Cholestatic jaundice, peripheral neuropathy, and suicidal intent have been reported.

Drug Interactions: Didanosine, rifabutin and rifampin decreases dapsone levels. Trimethoprim increases dapsone levels. Pyrimethamine, nitrofurantoin, primaquine and zidovudine increases risk for hematological side effects.

Drug Administration
> PO: Doses may be administered with or without food.
> Topical: Gently wash skin and pat dry prior to use. Apply pea-sized amount in thin layer and rub in completely.

DAPTOMYCIN
Cubicin
Antibiotic, lipopeptide

No   Yes   ?   B

Injection: 250, 500 mg

Adult:
   Complicated skin and skin structure infections: 4 mg/kg/dose IV Q24 hr ×
   7–14 days.
   ***Staphylococcus aureus bacteremia, including those with right-sided
   endocarditis:*** 6 mg/kg/dose IV Q24 hr for a minimum of 2–6 wk.

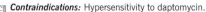

Contraindications: Hypersensitivity to daptomycin.
Warnings/Precautions: **Do not** use for treatment of pneumonia. **Use with
caution** in renal insufficiency **(adjust dose in renal failure; see Chapter 3).**
Concomitant use of HMG-CoA reductase inhibitors (e.g., atorvastatin) increases risk
of myopathy.
   Pediatric pharmacokinetic (PK) data from a single 4 mg/kg dose revealed similar
healthy adult PK profile for adolescents 12 to 17 yr old. Younger children had lower
drug exposures; an inverse linear correlation between plasma clearance and age was
observed (~2-fold increase in clearance for children 2–6 yr old). Additional pediatric
studies are needed.
Adverse Effects: GI disturbances, rash, pruritus, increase in creatine kinase levels,
headache, insomnia, pain, dizziness and dyspnea are common. Jaundice, abnormal
LFTs, rhabdomyolysis and renal failure have been reported.
Drug Interactions: See preceding Warnings/Precautions.
Drug Administration: Dilute drug with NS to a convenient volume and infuse over 30
min.

DARUNAVIR
Prezista, DRV, TMC 114
Antiviral agent, protease inhibitor

Yes   No   3   B

Tabs: 300 mg

≥18 yr and adult: 600 mg PO BID with ritonavir 100 mg PO BID

Contraindications: Hypersensitivity to darunavir or other components of the
formulation. Concomitant administration with drugs that are highly dependent
on CYP 450 3A clearance such as astemizole, cisapride, ergot derivatives,
midazolam, pimozide, terfenadine and triazolam.
Warnings/Precautions: Potential cross-sensitivity with sulfa-allergic patients.
Co-administration with carbamazepine, phenobarbital, phenytoin, rifampin,
lopinavir/ritonavir or saquinavir, and St. John's wort is **not recommended** because of
reducing darunavir levels. Also **not recommended** in combination with lovastatin,
simvastatin and other HMG-CoA reductase inhibitors due to risk for myopathy and
rhabdomyolysis. **Use with caution** in hepatic impairment (primary route of
metabolism; no dose reduction recommendations available), hemophilia type A or B,
and diabetes or hyperglycemia. **Darunavir should always be administered in
combination with ritonavir.**

Continued

DARUNAVIR *continued*

Adverse Effects: GI disturbances, abdominal pain, headache and fatigue are common. Skin rash (including erythema multiforme and Stevens-Johnson syndrome), fever, immune reconstitution syndrome, elevated hepatic transaminases, and lipid abnormalities have been reported.

Drug Interactions: Substrate and inhibitor of CYP 450 3A. Ritonavir boosts darunavir levels and is also a substrate and inhibitor of CYP 450 3A. See preceding Contraindications and Warnings/Precautions sections. Always check the potential for other drug interactions when either initiating therapy or adding new drugs onto an existing regimen.

Drug Administration: Drug is always given in combination with ritonavir. Administer all doses with food.

DELAVIRDINE
Rescriptor, DLV
Antiviral, non-nucleoside reverse transcriptase inhibitor

Yes   No   3   C

Tablets: 100, 200 mg

≥16 yr and adult: 400 mg PO TID
In combination with indinavir:
    Adult: 400 mg delavirdine PO TID and 600 mg indinavir PO TID

Contraindications: Hypersensitivity to delavirdine or any components in the formulation. **Do not** administer with CYP 450 3A substrates with a low therapeutic index (e.g., alprazolam, midazolam, triazolam, cisapride, calcium channel blockers, ergot alkaloid dervatives, amphetamines, cisapride, and sildenafil); increase risk of toxicity of these drugs.

Warnings/Precautions: Use with caution in hepatic disease. Metabolized primarily via CYP 450 3A4 (N-dealkylation and pyridine hydroxylation). CYP 450 2D6, 2C9 and 2C19 may also play a role. Hepatic and renal impairment pharmacokinetics have not been evaluated.

Adverse Effects: Incidence of rash has been reported as high as 50% and occurs within 1–3 wk after initiation of therapy. Dose titration does not significantly reduce the incidence of rash. Other major side effects include headache, fatigue, increased transaminase levels and gastrointestinal complaints. Although less common, hepatic failure has been reported.

Drug Interactions: See Contraindications section for serious interactions. Delavirdine inhibits the CYP450 3A4 and 2C9 drug metabolizing isoenzymes. Antacids, didanosine, H$_2$ antagonists, rifabutin, rifampin, carbamazepine, phenytoin, phenobarbital and saquinavir may decrease delavirdine's efficacy. Ketoconazole, fluoxetine, and clarithromycin may increase delavirdine levels and effects. When administered with protease inhibitors, delavirdine can increase the effects of amprenavir, saquinavir and indinivir. May increase the effects of warfarin. Carefully review the patients' drug profile for other drug interactions each time delavirdine is initiated or when a new drug is added to a regimen containing delavirdine.

Drug Administration: Doses may be administered with or without food. Doses of antacids and didanosine should be administered 1 hr before or 1 hr after taking delavirdine. Only the 100 mg tablets can be dissolved in water (four 100 mg tablets in ≥3 ounces of water) to make a dispersion to be taken immediately; 200 mg tablets **do not** dissolve well in water.

DICLOXACILLIN SODIUM
Dycill, Pathocil, and others
Antibiotic, penicillin (penicillinase-resistant)

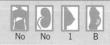

No   No   1   B

Caps: 250, 500 mg; contains 0.6 mEq Na/250 mg

Child (< 40 kg) (see remarks):
　　Mild/moderate infections: 12.5–25 mg/kg/24 hr PO ÷ Q6 hr
　　Severe infections: 50–100 mg/kg/24 hr PO ÷ Q6 hr
Adult (≥40 kg): 125–500 mg/dose PO Q6 hr; **max. dose:** 4 g/24 hr

Contraindications: History of penicillin allergy.
Warnings/Precautions: **Use with caution** in cephalosporin hypersensitivity.
Limited experience in neonates and very young infants. Higher doses (50–100 mg/kg/24 hr) are indicated following IV therapy for osteomyelitis.
Adverse Effects: Nausea, vomiting, and diarrhea are common. Immune hypersensitivity has been reported.
Drug Interactions: May decrease the effects of oral contraceptives and warfarin.
Drug Administration: Administer 1 hr before meals or 2 hr after meals.

DIDANOSINE
Videx, Videx EC, Dideoxyinosine, ddI
Anti-viral agent, nucleoside analogue reverse transcriptase inhibitor

No   Yes   3   B

Tabs (buffered, chewable/dispersable): 25, 50, 100, 150, 200 mg; contains 11.5 mEq sodium, 15.7 mEq magnesium, and phenylalanine per tablet
Capsules (delayed-released, enteric coated beadlets):
　　Videx EC: 125, 200, 250, 400 mg
　　Generic: 200, 250, 400 mg
Oral pediatric powder (10 mg/mL solution reconstituted with antacid solution): 2, 4 g

Neonate and infant:
　　2 wk–4 mo: 100 mg/m²/24 hr ÷ Q12 hr PO
　　>4 mo–8 mo: 200 mg/m²/24 hr ÷ Q12 hr PO
Child >8 mo:
　　Usual dose (in combination with other antiretrovirals): 240 mg/m²/24 hr ÷ Q12 hr PO.
　　Dose range: 180–300 mg/m²/24 hr ÷ Q12 hr; higher dose may required for CNS disease.
Adolescent/adult (see remarks for additional adolescent dosing information):
　　<60 kg:
　　　　Tabs: 250 mg/24 hr ÷ Q12–24 hr PO; Q12 hr dosing interval is preferred for efficacy but Q24 hr dosing may improve compliance.
　　　　Caps (delayed-released, enteric coated beadlets): 250 mg Q24 hr PO
　　≥60 kg:
　　　　Tabs: 400 mg/24 hr ÷ Q12–24 hr PO; Q12 hr dosing interval is preferred for efficacy but Q24 hr dosing may improve compliance.
　　　　Caps (delayed-released, enteric coated beadlets): 400 mg Q24 hr PO
Combination therapy with tenofovir:
　　Adult:
　　　　<60 kg: 200 mg Q24 hr PO using the delayed-released capsule
　　　　≥60 kg: 250 mg Q24 hr PO using the delayed-released capsules

Continued

DIDANOSINE *continued*

Contraindications: Hypersensitivity to didanosine or any other components contained in the formulation.

Warnings/Precautions: Pancreatitis has occurred during therapy in treatment-naïve and -experienced patients regardless of level of immunosuppression. Fatal lactic acidosis has been reported in pregnant women taking didanosine in combination with stavudine.

Use with caution in patients on sodium restriction or with phenylketonuria (buffered tablet contains 11.5 mEq Na/tablet and phenylketonuria). **Reduce dose in renal impairment (see Chapter 3).** Pharmacokinetics in impaired hepatic function is incomplete. Delayed-released capsules should **not** be used for patients <60 kg with GFR <10 mL/min.

Adverse Effects: Headaches, diarrhea, abdominal pain, nausea, vomiting, peripheral neuropathy (dose related), electrolyte abnormalities, hyperuricemia, increased liver enzymes, retinal depigmentation, CNS depression, rash/pruritus, myalgia and pancreatitis (dose related, more in adults when used with tenofovir). Lactic acidosis and severe hepatomegaly with steatosis have been reported.

Drug Interactions: Impairs absorption of drugs requiring an acidic environment and drugs that have impaired absorption in the presence of divalent ions (e.g., ketoconazole and fluoroquinolones, respectively). Didanosine mitochondrial toxicity is enhanced with ribavirin. Use with stavudine or zalcitabine increases risk for lactic acidosis or pancreatitis. Tenofivir may increase didanosine levels.

Drug Administration: Administer all doses on empty stomach (30 min before and 2 hr after a meal). Videx EC should be swallowed intact. Separate dosing when used in combination with the following drugs: 1 hr before or after ddI (indinavir); 2 hr before or after ddI (delavirdine, ritonavir, lopinavir/ritonavir, fluoroquinolones, ketoconazole, itraconazole, tetracyclines, and dapsone). To ensure adequate buffering capacity with the chewable tablet dosage form, administer at least 2 of the appropriate strength tablets (e.g., if the dose is 50 mg, give two 25 mg tablets and not one 50 mg tablet). Consult package insert for additional details.

DIETHYLCARBAMAZINE
Hetrazan, Carbamazine, Diethylcarbamazine citrate, DEC
Anthelmintic

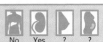

No   Yes   ?   ?

AVAILABLE FROM THE U.S. CENTERS FOR DISEASE CONTROL AND PREVENTION (404-639-3670 Monday-Friday 8:00 am–4:30 pm EST or 404-639-2888 evenings, weekends or holidays)
Tabs: 50 mg

Wuchereria bancrofti, Brugia malayi, or Brugia timori infections:
    Child ≥18 mo and adult (PO): 6 mg/kg/24 hr ÷ TID PO × 12 days; concurrent corticosteroids may be needed to reduce secondary reactions from therapy.
Loa loa (use with caution in heavy infestations as ocular problems or encephalopathy may occur):
    Child ≥18 mo (PO): Start with 1 mg/kg/dose on day 1, then 1 mg/kg/dose TID on day 2, then 1–2 mg/kg/dose TID on day 3, followed by 9 mg/kg/24 hr ÷ TID on days 4–21.
    Adult (PO): Start with 50 mg on day 1, then 50 mg TID on day 2, then 100 mg TID on day 3, followed by 9 mg/kg/24 hr ÷ TID on days 4–21.

DIETHYLCARBAMAZINE *continued*

Onchocerciasis (alternative to ivermectin; therapy should be followed by suramin IV):
    Child ≥18 mo (PO): Start with 0.5 mg/kg/dose TID (**max. dose:** 25 mg/24 hr) × 3 days, then 1 mg/kg/dose TID (**max. dose:** 50 mg/24 hr) for 3–4 additional days, then 1.5 mg/kg/dose TID (**max. dose:** 100 mg/24 hr) for 3–4 additional days, followed by maintenance doses of 2 mg/kg/dose TID × 14–21 days.
    Adult (PO): Start with 25 mg/24 hr QD × 3 days, then 50 mg/24 hr QD for 5 additional days, then 100 mg/24 hr ÷ BID for 3 additional days, followed by maintenance doses of 150 mg/24 hr ÷ TID × 12 days.
Tropical pulmonary eosinophilia (TPE):
    Child ≥18 mo and adult (PO): 6 mg/kg/24 hr ÷ TID PO × 14–21 days.

Contraindications: Hypersensitivity to diethylcarbamazine and its components.
Warnings/Precautions: Dose reductions are indicated in patients with renal insufficiency (>50% drug excreted unchanged in urine), alkaline urine (renal elimination reduced to <10%), or eating a vegetarian diet (alkaline diet). In pregnancy, use of drug is recommended after delivery. Crosses the blood-brain barrier.
Adverse Effects: GI disturbances and drowsiness are common; frequency is proportional with dosage. Headache, lassitude, weakness, general malaise and skin rash have been reported in the treatment of *Wuchereria bancrofti*. Mazzotti reaction, facial edema or pruritus (especially ocular) have been reported in the treatment of onchocerciasis. Giddiness, GI disturbances and malaise have been reported in children treated for ascariasis.
Drug Interactions: None identified.
Drug Administration: Administer doses after meals.
.

DIIODOHYDROXYQUINE

See *Iodoquinol*

DIPHTHERIA ANTITOXIN (EQUINE)
Antitoxin

6.4   No   6.4   No

AVAILABLE FROM THE U.S. CENTERS FOR DISEASE CONTROL AND PREVENTION (404-639-8257 or 770-488-7100)
Injection: 10,000 units

Child and adult:
Diphtheria treatment (in combination with appropriate antibiotic therapy):
    Pharyngeal or laryngeal symptoms of 48 hr duration: 20,000–40,000 units IV/IM × 1
    Nasopharyngeal symptoms: 40,000–60,000 units IV/IM × 1
    Extensive illness of >3 days or in patients with brawny neck swelling: 80,000–120,000 units IV/IM × 1
Diphtheria prophylaxis (in combination with appropriate antibiotic therapy for 7–10 days and active immunization with diphtheria toxoid absorbed): 5,000–10,000 units IM × 1

Continued

DIPHTHERIA ANTITOXIN (EQUINE) *continued*

> ***Serum sensitivity testing (intradermal or scratch skin test and a conjunctival test should be performed):***
>> ***Intradermal skin test:*** Intradermal injection of 0.1 mL of a 1:100 dilution in NS ×1, skin test is read 20 min after injection. Use 0.05 mL of a 1:1000 dilution in NS for patients with allergy history. Administer with NS control test. A positive intradermal skin test reaction consists of an urticarial wheal, with or without pseudopods, surrounded by a zone of erythema.
>> ***Scratch skin test:*** Place one drop of a 1:100 dilution on the skin followed by making a ¼ inch scratch through the drop. Test is read after 20 min. NS control test should be used to facilitate interpretation. A positive scratch skin test reaction consists of an urticarial wheal, with or without pseudopods, surrounded by a zone of erythema.
>> ***Conjunctival test:*** Place 1 drop of a 1:10 dilution into the lower conjunctival sac of one eye. Test is read after 15 min. A NS control test is used in the other eye. Positive conjunctival test reaction consists of itching, burning, redness, and lacrimation; these signs and symptoms can be relieved by placing 1 drop of an ophthalmic solution of epinephrine on the affected eye.
> ***Desensitization:*** Subcutaneous injection of the following dosages and concentrations at 15 min intervals, below. In the event of an immediate sensitivity reaction at any time, apply a tourniquet proximal to the sites of injection and administer epinephrine proximal to the tourniquet. Continue the procedure 1 hr after using the last dose of antitoxin that did not produce a reaction.
>> ***Dose #1:*** 0.05 mL of a 1:20 dilution
>> ***Dose #2:*** 0.1 mL of a 1:10 dilution
>> ***Dose #3:*** 0.3 mL of a 1:10 dilution
>> ***Dose #4:*** 0.1 mL of undiluted diphtheria antitoxin
>> ***Dose #5:*** 0.2 mL of undiluted diphtheria antitoxin
>> ***Dose #6:*** 0.5 mL of undiluted diphtheria antitoxin
>> ***After successfully completing dose #6, the remaining usual dose may be administered IV or IM.***

> ***Contraindications:*** Hypersensitivity to horse serum.
> ***Warnings/Precautions:*** Test for sensitivity to horse serum before administering any doses. **Use with extreme caution** with history of allergic disorders and asthma.
> When the skin or conjunctival test is positive or a doubtful reaction occurs, the risk of administering diphtheria antitoxin should be weighed against the risk of withholding it; if diphtheria antitoxin must be used, desensitization should be performed.
> ***Adverse Effects:*** Dermatological wheal and flare; pain, erythema, urticaria at site of injection; and immediate hypersensitivity reactions may occur. Serum sickness has been reported.
> ***Drug Interactions:*** If being given with diphtheria and tetanus toxoid, administer at separate sites.
> ***Drug Administration:*** Warm drug vial to 90–95° F.
>> IV: Dilute dose to an appropriate volume of NS or D_5W to provide a 1:20 dilution of antitoxin and infuse slowly at a rate not exceeding 1 mL/min.

DIRITHROMYCIN
Dynabac, Dynabac D5-Pak
Antibiotic, macrolide

No   No   ?   C

Tab, enteric coated: 250 mg

≥12 yr:
Mild/moderate COPD exacerbation or bacterial infections: 500 mg PO QD × 5–7 days

Contraindications: Hypersensitivity to dirithromycin, erythromycin, or other macrolide antibiotics.
Warnings/Precautions: Safety data in hepatic impairment (Child's Grade B or greater) is incomplete.
Adverse Effects: GI disturbances and headache are common.
Drug Interactions: Compared to other macrolides, less risk for drug interactions. May increase effects/toxicity of cyclosporin. Interaction studies have not been completed for the following medications by which macrolides may increase their effects/toxicity: digoxin, ergot derivatives, dofetilide, fentanyl, hexobarbital, phenytoin and pimozide.
Drug Administration: Administer with food or within 1 hr after eating to enhance absorption.

DORIPENEM
Doribax
Carbapenem antibiotic

No   Yes   ?   B

Injection: 500 mg

≥18 yr and adult: 500 mg IV Q8 hr with the following recommended duration of therapy:
Complicated intra-abdominal infection: 5–14 days (minimum of 3 days IV with possible switch to appropriate PO therapy).
Complicated UTI and pyelonephritis: 10 days (may be extended up to 14 days in patients with concurrent bacteremia).

Contraindications: Patients sensitive to carbapenems, or with a history of anaphylaxis to beta-lactam antibiotics.
Warnings/Precautions: Use with caution in renal impairment (adjust dose; see Chapter 3). Drug penetrates well into peritoneal and retroperitoneal fluids and tissues.
Adverse Effects: Diarrhea, nausea, headache, rash and phlebitis are common. Dermatologic reactions, including Stevens-Johnson syndrome and TEN, neutropenia, *C. difficile* colitis, anemia, and hypersensitivity reactions have been reported.
Drug Interactions: Probenecid may increase serum doripenem levels. May reduce valproic acid levels.
Drug Administration: Infuse dose over 1 hr at a concentration ≤4.5 mg/mL. Reconstituted IV solutions have short stability times; consult with a pharmacist.

DOXYCYCLINE
Vibramycin, Periostat, and others
Antibiotic, tetracycline derivative

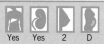

Yes   Yes   2   D

Caps: 20 (Periostat), 50, 75, 100 mg
Tabs: 20 (Periostat), 50, 75, 100 mg
Syrup: 50 mg/5 mL (60 mL)
Oral suspension: 25 mg/5 mL (60 mL)
Injection: 100, 200 mg

Initial:
> **≤45 kg:** 2.2 mg/kg/dose BID PO/IV × 1 day to **max. dose** of 200 mg/24 hr
> **>45 kg:** 100 mg/dose BID PO/IV × 1 day

Maintenance:
> **≤45 kg:** 2.2–4.4 mg/kg/24 hr QD-BID PO/IV
> **>45 kg:** 100–200 mg/24 hr ÷ QD-BID PO/IV

Max. adult dose: 300 mg/24 hr

PID:
> *Inpatient:* 100 mg IV/PO Q12 hr with cefotetan, cefoxitin, or ampicillin/sulbactam. Convert to oral therapy 24 hr after patient improves on IV to complete a 14-day total course (IV and PO).
> *Outpatient:* 100 mg PO Q12 hr × 14 days with ceftriaxone, cefoxitin + probenecid, or other parenteral third-generation cephalosporin ± metronidazole

Anthrax (inhalation/systemic/cutaneous; see remarks): Initiate therapy with IV route and convert to PO route when clinically appropriate. Duration of therapy is 60 days (IV and PO combined):
> **≤8 yr or ≤45 kg:** 2.2 mg/kg/dose BID IV/PO; **max. dose:** 200 mg/24 hr
> **>8 yr and >45 kg:** 100 mg/dose BID IV/PO

Malaria prophylaxis (start 1–2 days prior to exposure and continue for 4 wk after leaving endemic area):
> **>8 yr:** 2 mg/kg/24 hr PO QD; **max. dose:** 100 mg/24 hr
> *Adult:* 100 mg PO QD

Periodontitis:
> *Adult:* 20 mg BID PO × ≤9 mo

Contraindications: Hypersensitivity to doxycycline or tetracycline products.
Warnings/Precautions: Use with caution in hepatic and renal disease and in patients with a history of candidal infections. **Avoid** prolonged exposure to direct sunlight to reduce photosensitivity risk. Generally **not** recommended for use in children <8 yr due to risk for tooth enamel hypoplasia and discoloration. However, the AAP Red Book recommends doxycycline as the drug of choice for rickettsial disease regardless of age.

Doxycycline is approved for the treatment of anthrax (*Bacillus anthracis*) in combination with one or two other antimicrobials. If meningitis is suspected, consider using an alternative agent because of poor CNS penetration. Consider changing to high-dose amoxicillin (25–35 mg/kg/dose TID PO) for penicillin susceptible strains. See www.bt.cdc.gov for the latest information.

Adverse Effects: GI symptoms, photosensitivity, hemolytic anemia, rash and hypersensitivity reactions may occur. Increased intracranial pressure has been reported.

Drug Interactions: Rifampin, barbiturates, phenytoin, and carbamazepine may increase clearance of doxycycline. Doxycycline may enhance the

FORMULARY

DOXYCYCLINE *continued*

hypoprothrombinemic effect of warfarin. See Tetracycline for additional drug/food interactions and comments.
Drug Administration
   IV: Infuse over 1–4 hr at a concentration of 0.1–1 mg/mL.
   PO: Fluid intake should accompany oral administration to reduce risk of esophageal ulceration or irritation. Avoid divalent cations (e.g., antacids, dairy products, iron) for 1 hr before or 2 hr after administration. Doses may be administered with food to decrease GI upset. For periodontitis, take capsules ≥1 hr prior to meals; and take tablets ≥1 hr prior or 2 hr after meals.

ECONAZOLE NITRATE
Spectazole and various generics
Antifungal, imidazole

   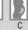

No   No   ?   C

Topical cream: 1% (15, 30, 85 g); contains mineral oil

 Tinea pedis, tinea cruris, tinea corporis, and tinea versicolor (see remarks): Apply to affected areas QD
   Duration of therapy:
      Tinea cruris and tinea corporis: 2 wk
      Tinea pedis: 1 mo
Cutaneous candidiasis: Apply to affected areas BID (morning and evening) × 2 wk

Contraindications: Hypersensitivity to econazole or any other components in the formulation.
Warnings/Precautions: Not for ophthalmic use. If no clinical improvement is seen after the treatment period, consider alternative diagnosis. Clinical and mycological response for tinea versicolor is usually seen after 2 wk of therapy.
Adverse Effects: Burning, itching, stinging and erythema may occur.
Drug Interactions: Econazole, an azole antifungal agent, can inhibit CYP 450 3A4 and may potentially increase the effects of 3A4 substrates (e.g., fentanyl).
Drug Administration: Apply to cover affected areas. **Avoid** contact with eyes.

EFAVIRENZ
Sustiva, DMP-266
Antiviral agent, non-nucleoside reverse transcriptase inhibitor

No   No   3   D

Caps: 50, 100, 200 mg
Tabs: 600 mg
Oral liquid: Available as an investigational agent via Bristol-Myers Squibb (877–372-7397) as an expanded access program of HIV-infected children 3–16 yr.
In combination with emtricitabine and tenofovir as Atripia:
   Tabs: 600 mg efavirenz, 200 mg emtricitabine and 300 mg tenofovir

Continued

EFAVIRENZ *continued*

 Child ≥3 yr and weighing ≥10 kg: Daily PO dose administered QD (see following table)

Body Weight (kg)	Dose (mg)
10–<15	200
15–<20	250
20–<25	300
25–<32.5	350
32.5–<40	400
≥40	600

Adolescent and adult (see remarks): 600 mg/dose PO QD
Atripia:
   Adult (GFRs ≥50 mL/min): 1 tab PO QD on an empty stomach.

Contraindications: Hypersensitivity to efavirenz or any other components in the formulation. **Should not** be used with astemizole, cisapride, triazolam, midazolam, ergot derivatives and voriconazole.

Warnings/Precautions: **Do not** use as a single agent for HIV or added on as a sole agent to a failing regimen. Therapy should always be initiated in combination with at least one other antiretroviral agent to which the patient has not been previously exposed. **Avoid** use in pregnancy; meningomyelocele and Dandy-Walker malformation have been reported in infants.

Adolescent Dosing: Patients in early puberty (Tanner I–II) should be dosed with pediatric regimens and those in late puberty (Tanner IV) should be dosed with adult regimens. Adolescents who are at the midst of their growth spurt (Tanner III females and Tanner IV males) can be dosed by either pediatric or adult regimen with close monitoring of efficacy and toxicity.

   Pharmacokinetics in hepatic or renal impairment have **not** been adequately evaluated.

Adverse Effects: Dizziness, somnolence, insomnia, hallucinations, and euphoria are common side effects. Skin rashes (usually mild-moderate maculopapular eruptions) may occur within the first 2 wk of initiating therapy and usually resolve (with continuing the drug) within 1 mo. Rash is more common in children and more often of greater severity. Discontinue therapy in patients developing severe rash associated with blistering, desquamation, mucosal involvement, or fever. Diarrhea, fever, cough, nausea, vomiting, pancreatitis, and elevations in liver enzymes and serum lipids have been reported.

Drug Interactions: Drug is a substrate and inducer of CYP 450 3A4; and may also inhibit other CYP 450 isoenzymes (2C9, 2C19, and 3A4). Monitor effect/serum levels of drugs metabolized by the aforementioned CYP 450 isoenzymes (e.g., warfarin, rifampin). Increases serum levels of nelfinavir and ritonavir; and decreases levels of indinavir and saquinavir. See preceding Contraindications. May cause false-positive urinary cannabinoid test (CEDIA DAU Multi-Level THC assay).

Drug Administration: Doses should be administered on an empty stomach. **Avoid** high-fat meals (increases absorption). Capsules may be opened and added to liquids or foods, but has a peppery taste; grape jelly may be used to disguise taste. Initiate dosing at bedtime for the first 2–4 wk to reduce central nervous system side effects.

EMTRICITABINE

Emtriva, FTC

Antiviral agent, nucleoside analogue reverse transcriptase inhibitor

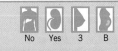

No   Yes   3   B

Caps: 200 mg
Oral solution: 10 mg/mL
In combination with tenofovir as Truvada:
    Tabs: 200 mg emtricitabine and 300 mg tenofovir disoproxil fumarate
In combination with efavirenz and tenofovir as Atripia:
    Tabs: 600 mg efavirenz, 200 mg emtricitabine and 300 mg tenofovir

Child 3 mo–17 yr: 6 mg/kg/24 hr PO QD
    Max. dose: 240 mg/24 hr or 200 mg/24 hr for patients >33 kg using
    capsule dosage form.
≥18 yr–adult:
    Caps: 200 mg PO QD
    Oral solution: 240 mg PO QD
Truvada (GFR ≥30 mL/min and not receiving hemodialysis):
    Adult: 1 tab PO QD with or without food
Atripia (GFR ≥50 mL/min):
    Adult: 1 tab PO QD on an empty stomach

Contraindications: Hypersensitivity to emtricitabine or any of other components
contained in the formulation.
    Warnings/Precautions: Lactic acidosis and severe hepatomegaly with steatosis,
including fatal cases, have been reported. Patients co-infected with HIV and HBV
should be monitored closely for hepatitis several months after stopping treatment
with emtricitabine. **Adjust dosage in renal impairment (see Chapter 3).**
Adverse Effects: Headache, insomnia, diarrhea, nausea, rash and hyperpigmentation
on palms and/or soles (primarily seen in non-Caucasian patients) are common.
Neutropenia, lactic acidosis, and severe hepatomegaly with steatosis have been
reported. Hepatitis exacerbations in patients co-infected with HIV and HBV have
occurred after discontinuing emtricitabine.
Drug Interactions: No major interactions but potential interactions may occur with
drugs that are eliminated via tubular secretion. **Do not** use lamivudine because of
similar resistance profile and no additional additive benefit.
Drug Administration: Doses may be administered with or without food.

ENFUVIRTIDE

Fuzeon, T-20

Antiviral agent, fusion inhibitor

No   No   3   B

Injection: 108 mg; delivers 90 mg/L following reconstitution with 1.1 mL of sterile water
for injection (available in a Convenience Kit containing 60 single-use vials with sterile water
diluent, syringes, and alcohol wipes).

Child 6–16 yr: 2 mg/kg/dose SQ BID; **max. dose:** 90 mg/kg/dose BID
≥16–adult: 90 mg SQ BID

Contraindications: Hypersensitivity to enfuvirtide or any other components in
the formulation.

Continued

ENFUVIRTIDE *continued*

Warnings/Precautions: Currently **not recommended** for antiretroviral-naïve patients due to lack of data. Patients with history of lung disease, low CD4 counts, high initial viral load, IV drug use, or smoking may be at higher risk for bacterial pneumonia. A theoretical production of anti-enfuvirtide antibodies may cross react with HIV-1 gp41 to potentially cause false-positive ELISA test in non-infected HIV individuals. Currently no information on dosing recommendations for patients with GFR <35 mL/min or with hepatic impairment.

Adverse Effects: Local injection site reactions are extremely high (98%) which are usually mild/moderate in severity. Duration of reaction is usually 3–7 days but have been >7 days in about 24% of patients. Hypersensitivity reactions, GI disturbances, fever, chills, rigors, hypotension and elevated liver transaminases have been reported.

Drug Interactions: Unlikely to have significant drug interactions with drug metabolized by CYP 450 enzymes. Currently no interaction has been identified.

Drug Administration: Inject SQ into the upper arm, anterior thigh or abdomen; **avoid** scar tissue, moles, bruises, the naval or a site experiencing an injection site reaction.

ERTAPENEM
Invanz
Antibiotic, carbapenem

No   Yes   ?   B

Injection: 1 g
Contains ~6 mEq Na/g drug

> *3 mo–12 yr:* 15 mg/kg/dose IV/IM Q12 hr; **max. dose:** 1 g/24 hr
> *Adolescent and adult:* 1 g IV/IM Q24 hr
> *Recommended duration of therapy (all ages):*
>   *Complicated intraabdominal infection:* 5–14 days
>   *Complicated skin/subcutaneous tissue infections:* 7–14 days
>   *Diabetic foot infection without osteomyelitis:* Up to 28 days
>   *Community acquired pneumonia, complicated UTI/pyelonephritis:* 10–14 days
>   *Acute pelvic infection:* 3–10 days

Contraindications: Hypersensitivity to ertapenem and other carbapenems (e.g., imipenem, meropenem); and prior anaphylactic reaction to beta-lactams. For IM injection, hypersensitivity to amide-type anesthetics (e.g., lidocaine).

Warnings/Precautions: **Do not** use in meningitis due to poor CSF penetration. **Use with caution** with CNS disorders including seizures. Adjust dosage in renal impairment by decreasing dose by 50% when GFR <30 mL/min. Ertapenem has poor activity against *P. aeruginosa*, *Acinetobacter*, MRSA, and *Enterococcus faecalis*.

Adverse Effects: Diarrhea, infusion complications, nausea, headache, vaginitis, phlebitis/thrombophlebitis, and vomiting are common.
Seizures have been reported primarily in renal insufficiency and/or CNS disorders such as brain lesions or seizures.

Drug Interactions: Probenecid may increase ertapenem levels. May decrease valproic acid levels.

Drug Administration
    IV: For intermittent infusion, infuse over 30 min at a concentration ≤20 mg/mL. **Do not** mix with dextrose-containing solutions. Reconstituted drug is stable for 6 hr at room temperature.
    IM: Reconstitute 1 g vial with 3.2 mL of 1% lidocaine without epinephrine (~280 mg/mL) and use within 1 hr of preparation. Administer by deep IM injection into large muscle mass such as the gluteal muscles or lateral part of thigh.

ERYTHROMYCIN ETHYLSUCCINATE AND ACETYLSULFISOXAZOLE

Pediazole, Eryzole, and others
Antibiotic, macrolide + sulfonamide derivative

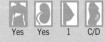

Yes · Yes · 1 · C/D

Oral suspension: 200 mg erythromycin and 600 mg sulfa/5 mL (100, 150, 200, 250 mL)

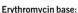

Otitis media: 50 mg/kg/24 hr (as erythromycin) and 150 mg/kg/24 hr (as sulfa) ÷ Q6 hr PO, or give 1.25 mL/kg/24 hr ÷ Q6 hr PO.
Max. dose: 2 g erythromycin, 6 g sulfisoxasole/24 hr

Contraindications: Hypersensitivity to erythromycin or sulfonamides; and liver dysfunction or porphyria.
Warnings/Precautions: **Not** recommended in infants <2 mo old. **Do not** use in renal impairment because dosage adjustments are inconsistent for sulfisoxazole and erythromycin. Pregnancy category changes to "D" if administered near term. See erythromycin and sulfisoxazole for additional information.
Adverse Effects: See erythromycin and sulfisoxazole.
Drug Interactions: See erythromycin and sulfisoxazole.
Drug Administration: May be administered with or without food.

ERYTHROMYCIN PREPARATIONS

Erythrocin, Pediamycin, E-Mycin, Ery-Ped, and others
Antibiotic, macrolide

Yes · Yes · 1 · B

Erythromycin base:
  Tabs: 250, 500 mg
  Delayed-release tabs: 250, 333, 500 mg
  Delayed-release caps: 250 mg
  Topical ointment: 2% (25 g)
  Topical gel: 2% (30, 60 g); contains alcohol 92%
  Topical solution: 1.5%, 2% (60 mL); may contain 44%–66% alcohol
  Topical swab: 2% (60s)
  Ophthalmic ointment: 0.5% (1, 3.5 g)
Erythromycin ethylsuccinate (EES):
  Suspension: 200, 400 mg/5 mL (100, 480 mL)
  Oral drops: 100 mg/2.5 mL (50 mL)
  Chewable tabs: 200 mg
  Tabs: 400 mg
Erythromycin estolate:
  Suspension: 125, 250 mg/5 mL (480 mL)
Erythromycin stearate:
  Tabs: 250 mg
Erythromycin lactobionate:
  Injection: 500, 1000 mg; may contain benzyl alcohol

Oral:
Neonate:
  <1.2 kg: 20 mg/kg/24 hr ÷ Q12 hr PO
  ≥1.2 kg:
    0–7 days: 20 mg/kg/24 hr ÷ Q12 hr PO
    >7 days: 30 mg/kg/24 hr ÷ Q8 hr PO

Continued

ERYTHROMYCIN PREPARATIONS *continued*

Neonate:
> **Chlamydial conjunctivitis and pneumonia:** 50 mg/kg/24 hr ÷ Q6 hr PO ×
> 14 days.
> **Child:** 30–50 mg/kg/24 hr ÷ Q6–8 hr; **max. dose:** 2 g/24 hr
> **Adult:** 1–4 g/24 hr ÷ Q6 hr; **max. dose:** 4 g/24 hr

Parenteral:
> **Child:** 20–50 mg/kg/24 hr ÷ Q6 hr IV
> **Adult:** 15–20 mg/kg/24 hr ÷ Q6 hr IV
> **Max. dose:** 4 g/24 hr

Rheumatic fever prophylaxis: 500 mg/24 hr ÷ Q12 hr PO
Ophthalmic: Apply 0.5 inch ribbon to affected eye BID-QID
Pertussis: Estolate salt: 50 mg/kg/24 hr ÷ Q6 hr PO × 14 days
Preoperative bowel prep: 20 mg/kg/dose PO erythromycin base × 3 doses, with neomycin, 1 day before surgery
Prokinetic agent: 10–20 mg/kg/24 hr PO ÷ TID-QID (QAC or QAC and QHS)

  Contraindications: Hypersensitivity to erythromycin or any other components in the formulation. **Avoid** use with astemizole, cisapride, pimozide or terfenadine.
Warnings/Precautions: Hypertrophic pyloric stenosis in neonates receiving prophylactic therapy for pertussis; and life-threatening episodes of ventricular tachycardia associated with prolonged QTc interval have been reported. **Use with caution** in liver disease. **Adjust dose in renal failure (see Chapter 3).**

Formulations of IV lactobionate dosage form may contain benzyl alcohol. Because of different absorption characteristics, higher oral doses of EES are needed to achieve therapeutic effects. Oral therapy should replace IV as soon as possible.
Adverse Effects: Nausea, vomiting, and abdominal cramps are common. Estolate salt may cause cholestatic jaundice, although hepatotoxicity is uncommon (2% of reported cases). Cardiac dysrhythmia, anaphylaxis and hearing loss have been reported.
Drug Interactions: Inhibits CYP 450 1A2, 3A3/4 isoenzymes. May produce elevated digoxin, theophylline, carbamazapine, clozapine, cyclosporine, and methylprednisolone levels. May produce false-positive urinary catecholamines, 17-hydroxycorticosteroids and 17-ketosteroids.
Drug Administration
PO: Administer doses after meal to reduce GI upset. **Avoid** acid beverages and milk 1 hr before and after dose. Swallow delayed-release or enteric coated dosage forms whole.
IV: For intermittent infusion, infuse over 20–60 min at a concentration 1–2.5 mg/mL (max. 5 mg/mL). For continuous infusion (recommended for decreasing cardiotoxic effects), infuse at a concentration ≤1mg/mL. **Avoid** IM route (pain, necrosis).
Ophthalmic ointment: Instill 0.5–1 cm ointment in lower conjunctival sac by avoiding contact of ointment tip with eye or skin.

ETHAMBUTOL HCL
Myambutol
Antituberculosis drug

No   Yes   1   C

Tabs: 100, 400 mg

  Tuberculosis:
> **Infant, child, adolescent, and adult:** 15–25 mg/kg/dose PO QD or 50 mg/kg/dose PO twice weekly
> **Max. dose:** 2.5 g/24 hr

ETHAMBUTOL HCL *continued*

Nontuberculous mycobacterial infection:
 Child, adolescent, and adult: 15–25 mg/kg/24 hr PO; **max. dose:** 1 g/24 hr
M. avium complex prophylaxis in AIDS (use in combination with other medications):
 Infant, child, adolescent, and adult: 15 mg/kg/dose PO QD; **max. dose:** 900 mg/dose

Contraindications: Hypersensitivity to ethambutol products or any other components in the formulation.
 Do not use in optic neuritis (unless clinically necessary) and in children whose visual acuity cannot be assessed.
Warnings/Precautions: Obtain baseline ophthalmologic studies before beginning therapy and then monthly. Follow visual acuity, visual fields, and (red-green) color vision. **Discontinue** if any visual deterioration occurs. Monitor uric acid, liver function, heme status, and renal function. **Adjust dose with renal failure (see Chapter 3).**
Adverse Effects: Hyperuricemia, nausea, vomiting and mania are common. May cause reversible optic neuritis, especially with larger doses. Thrombocytopenia, neutropenia and peripheral neuropathy have been reported.
Drug Interactions: Coadministration with aluminum hydroxide containing antacids may reduce ethambutol's absorption; space administration by 4 hr.
Drug Administration: Doses may be administered with food; especially with GI symptoms.

ETHIONAMIDE
Trecator, Trecator-SC
Antituberculosis drug

Yes   Yes   ?   C

Tabs: 250 mg

Tuberculosis (as part of combination therapy):
 Infant, child, and adolescent: 15–20 mg/kg/24 hr PO ÷ BID-TID; **max. dose:** 1 g/24 hr
 Adult: 15–20 mg/kg/24 hr (usually 500–750 mg/24 hr) PO ÷ QD-BID; **max. dose:** 1 g/24 hr

 Contraindications: Hypersensitivity to ethionamide or any other components in the formulation; and severe hepatic impairment.
 Warnings/Precautions: May potentiate the adverse effects of other antituberculous drugs (see Drug Interactions). Ophthalmologic examinations should be done before and periodically during therapy. **Use with caution** in diabetes; may cause hypoglycemia. **Avoid** excessive ethanol ingestion because of potential psychotic reaction. Adjust dose in renal insufficiency by administering 50% of normal dose when GFR <10 mL/min.
Adverse Effects: GI disturbances, transient metallic taste, and anorexia are common and may be minimized by dose reduction, drug administration time change, or use of an antiemetic. Orthostatic hypotension, gynecomastia, impotence, acne, hypoglycemia, hypothyroidism, drowsiness and transient increases in bilirubin, SGOT and SGPT have been reported.
Drug Interactions: May increase the effects/toxicity of isoniazid. Seizures have been reported with cycloserine. Increased hepatic side effects may occur with rifampin, pyrazinamide and ethambutol. See Warnings/Precautions.
Drug Administration: Give with meals.

For explanation of icons, see p. 306.

FAMCICLOVIR
Famvir
Antiviral

No   Yes   3   B

Tabs: 125, 250, 500 mg

Adolescent:
  Genital herpes, first episode: 250 mg Q8 hr PO × 7–10 days
  Episodic recurrent genital herpes: 125 mg Q12 hr PO × 3–5 days
  Daily suppressive therapy: 250 mg Q12 hr PO up to 1 yr, then reassess
  HSV recurrence
Adult:
  Herpes zoster: 500 mg Q8 hr PO × 7 days; initiate therapy promptly as soon as
  diagnosis is made (initiation within 48 hr after rash onset is ideal; currently no
  data for starting treatment >72 hr after rash onset).
  Recurrent genital herpes: 1000 mg Q12 hr PO × 1 day; initiate therapy at first
  sign or symptom. Efficacy has not been established when treatment is initiated
  >6 hr after onset of symptoms or lesions.
  Suppression of recurrent genital herpes: 250 mg Q12 hr PO up to 1 yr
  Recurrent mucocutaneous herpes in HIV: 500 mg Q12 hr PO × 7 days

Contraindications: Hypersensitivity to famciclovir, penciclovir, or any other
components in the formulation.
Warnings/Precautions: Drug is converted to its active form (penciclovir). Better
absorption than PO acyclovir. **Reduce dose in renal impairment (see Chapter 3).**
Safety and efficacy in suppression of recurrent genital herpes have not been
established beyond 1 yr.
Adverse Effects: Headache, diarrhea, nausea, and abdominal pain are common.
Erythema multiforme and pruritus have been reported.
Drug Interactions: Concomitant use with probenecid and other drugs eliminated by
active tubular secretion may result in decreased penciclovir (active metabolite)
clearance.
Drug Administration: May be given with or without food.

FLUCONAZOLE
Diflucan and others
Antifungal agent

No   Yes   1   C

Tabs: 50, 100, 150, 200 mg
Injection: 2 mg/mL (100, 200 mL); contains 9 mEq Na/2 mg drug
Oral suspension: 10 mg/mL (35 mL), 40 mg/mL (35 mL)

Neonate:
  Loading dose: 12 mg/kg IV/PO
  Maintenance dose: 6 mg/kg IV/PO with the following dosing intervals (see
  following table)

FLUCONAZOLE *continued*

Postconceptional Age (wk)	Postnatal Age (days)	Dosing Interval (hr) and Time (hr) to Start First Maintenance Dose After Load
≤29	0–14	72
	>14	48
30–36	0–14	48
	>14	24
37–44	0–7	48
	>7	24
≥45	>0	24

Child (IV/PO):

Indication	Loading Dose	Maintenance Dose to Begin 24 hr After Loading Dose
Oropharyngeal candidiasis	6 mg/kg	3 mg/kg
Esophageal candidiasis	12 mg/kg	6 mg/kg
Invasive systemic candidiasis and cryptococcal meningitis	12 mg/kg	6–12 mg/kg
Suppressive therapy for HIV infected with cryptococcal meningitis	6 mg/kg	6 mg/kg

Max. dose: 12 mg/kg/24 hr
Adult:
    Oropharyngeal and esophageal candidiasis: Loading dose of 200 mg PO/IV followed by 100 mg QD 24 hr after; doses up to **max. dose** of 400 mg/24 hr should be used for esophageal candidiasis
    Systemic candidiasis and cryptococcal meningitis: Loading dose of 400 mg PO/IV, followed by 200–800 mg QD 24 hr later
    Bone marrow transplant prophylaxis: 400 mg PO/IV Q24 hr
    Suppressive therapy in for HIV infected with cryptococcal meningitis: 200 mg QD PO/IV Q24 hr
    Vaginal candidiasis: 150 mg PO × 1

    Contraindications: Concomitant administration of fluconazole with cisapride is **contraindicated**; arrhythmias may occur. Hypersensitivity to fluconazole or any other components in the formulation.
Warnings/Precautions: **Use with caution** in patients with proarrhythmic conditions and impaired renal function. **Adjust dose in renal failure (see Chapter 3).** Pediatric to adult dose equivalency: every 3 mg/kg pediatric dosage is equal to 100 mg adult dosage.
Adverse Effects: May cause nausea, headache, rash, vomiting, abdominal pain, hepatitis, liver enzyme elevation, cholestasis, and diarrhea. Neutropenia, agranulocytosis, and thrombocytopenia have been reported.
Drug Interactions: Inhibits CYP 450 2C9/10 and CYP 450 3A3/4 (weak inhibitor). May increase effects, toxicity, or levels of cyclosporine, midazolam, phenytoin, rifabutin, tacrolimus, theophylline, warfarin, oral hypoglycemics, and AZT. Rifampin increases fluconazole metabolism.

Continued

FLUCONAZOLE *continued*

Drug Administration
IV: For intermittent infusion, infuse over 1–2 hr (**not to exceed** 200 mg/hr) at a concentration of 2 mg/mL. Administer doses ≥6 mg/kg/24 hr over 2 hr.
PO: Doses may be given with or without food.

FLUCYTOSINE
Ancobon, 5-FC, 5-Fluorocytosine
Antifungal agent

| No | Yes | 3 | C |

Caps: 250, 500 mg
Oral liquid: 10 mg/mL

 Neonate: 80–160 mg/kg/24 hr ÷ Q6 hr PO
Child and adult: 50–150 mg/kg/24 hr ÷ Q6 hr PO

Contraindications: Hypersensitivity to flucytosine or any other components in the formulation. Use is **contraindicated** in the first trimester of pregnancy.
Warnings/Precautions: Use extreme **caution** in renal impairment **(adjust dose in renal failure; see Chapter 3)**. Monitor CBC, BUN, serum creatinine, alkaline phosphatase, AST, and ALT.
Therapeutic Levels: 25–100 mg/L. Recommended serum sampling time at steady state: Obtain peak level 2–4 hr after oral dose following 4 days of continuous dosing. Peak levels of 40–60 mg/L have been recommended for systemic candidiasis. Maintain trough levels above 25 mg/L. Prolonged levels above 100 mg/L can increase risk for bone marrow suppression. Bone marrow suppression in immunosuppressed patients can be irreversible and fatal.
Adverse Effects: Nausea, vomiting, diarrhea, rash, and CNS disturbance are common. Cardiotoxicity, anemia, leukopenia, and thrombocytopenia have been reported.
Drug Interactions: Amphotericin may increase efficacy and toxicity (enterocolitis, myelosuppression); **use with caution.** Cytarabine may decrease flucytosine activity. Flucytosine interferes with creatinine assay tests using the dry-slide enzymatic method (Kodak Ektachem analyzer).
Drug Administration: Administer dose with food over a 15 min period to decrease nausea and vomiting.

FOSAMPRENAVIR
Lexiva, f-APV
Antiretroviral, protease inhibitor

| Yes | No | 3 | C |

Oral suspension: 50 mg/mL equivalent to 43 mg/mL amprenavir (225 mL)
Tabs: 700 mg; equivalent to 600 mg of amprenavir

 Doses based on mg of fosamprenavir (see Warnings/Precautions).
Child:
    Antiretroviral-naïve:
        2–5 yr: 30 mg/kg/dose PO BID; **max. dose:** 1400 mg BID
        ≥6 yr:
            Regimens without ritonavir: 30 mg/kg/dose PO BID; **max. dose:** 1400 mg BID

FOSAMPRENAVIR *continued*

> > ***Regimens containing ritonavir:*** 18 mg/kg/dose PO BID (**max. dose:** 700 mg BID) with 3 mg/kg/dose ritonavir PO BID (**max. dose:** 100 mg BID)
> ***Therapy-experienced:***
> > **≥6 yr:**
> > > ***Regimens without ritonavir, ≥47 kg:*** 1400 mg (as tablets) PO BID
> > > ***Regimens with ritonavir:*** 18 mg/kg/dose PO BID (**max. dose:** 700 mg BID) with 3 mg/kg/dose ritonavir PO BID (**max. dose:** 100 mg BID). Fosamprenavir tablets may be used for patients ≥39 kg and ritonavir capsules for ≥33 kg.

Adolescent and adult:
> ***Antiretroviral-naïve:***
> > ***Regimens without ritonavir:*** 1400 mg PO BID
> > ***Regimens containing ritonavir:***
> > > ***Once daily regimen:*** 1400 mg fosamprenavir PO QD with 200 mg ritonavir PO QD
> > > ***Twice daily regimen:*** 700 mg fosamprenavir PO BID with 100 mg ritonavir PO BID

> ***Protease inhibitor-experienced:*** 700 mg fosamprenavir PO BID with 100 mg ritonavir PO BID; once daily regimen is not recommended for these patients
Adult:
> ***In combination with efavirenz (should be boosted with ritonavir):***
> > ***Once daily regimen:*** 1400 mg fosamprenavir PO QD with 300 mg ritonavir PO QD and 600 mg efavirenz PO QD
> > ***Twice daily regimen:*** 700 mg fosamprenavir PO BID with 100 mg ritonavir PO BID and 600 mg efavirenz PO QD

Contraindications: Hypersensitivity to fosamprenavir or amprenavir and any of its components. **Do not** use with agents highly dependent on cytochrome P450 3A4 for clearance (e.g., astemizole, terfenadine, cisapride, midazolam, triazolam, ergot derivatives, lipid lowering agents such as atorvastatin and cervistatin, pimozide and triazolam); and antiarrhythmic agents (e.g., flecainide and propafenone).

Warnings/Precautions: **Use with caution** with sulfonamide allergy, hepatic impairment (should **not** be used in severe hepatic disease), and hemophilia (reports of spontaneous bleeding). Patients with hepatitis B or C or marked elevations in transaminases prior to therapy may develop transaminase elevations.

Dosing in hepatic impairment for unboosted regimens (no data available for regimens containing ritonavir):

> *Mild/Moderate impairment (Child-Pugh score 5–8):* 700 mg PO BID
> *Severe impairment (Child-Pugh score 9–12):* Use **not** recommended.

Fosamprenavir is a prodrug of amprenavir and is rapidly hydrolyzed to amprenavir in the GI tract.

For children 2–5 yr, data is currently insufficient to recommend once-daily dosing and dosing for therapy-experienced patients. Adolescent Dosing: patients in early puberty (Tanner I–II) should be dosed with pediatric regimens and those in late puberty (Tanner IV) should be dosed with adult regimens. Adolescents who are at the midst of their growth spurt (Tanner III females and Tanner IV males) can be dosed by either pediatric or adult regimen with close monitoring of efficacy and toxicity.

Adverse Effects: GI disturbances, perioral paresthesias, headache, rash and lipid abnormalities are common. Life-threatening rash (e.g., Stevens-Johnson syndrome), fat redistribution, neutropenia, hyperglycemia, hemolytic anemia and elevations in serum transaminases and creatinine kinase have been reported.

Drug Interactions: Amprenavir is a substrate and inhibitor of CYP 450 3A4. Efavirenz, rifampin, rifabutin, anticonvulsants, oral contraceptives and St. John's wort can lower amprenavir levels. Always check the potential for other drug interactions

Continued

FOSAMPRENAVIR *continued*

when either initiating therapy or adding new drug onto an existing regimen. See Contraindications section.
Drug Administration: Doses may be administered with or without food. Administer doses 1 hr before or after any antacids or buffered medications (e.g., didanosine).

FOSCARNET
Foscavir
Antiviral agent

| No | Yes | 3 | C |

Injection: 24 mg/mL (250, 500 mL)

> ***Adolescent and adult, IV:***
> ***CMV retinitis:***
>   ***Induction:*** 180 mg/kg/24 hr ÷ Q8 hr × 14–21 days
>   ***Maintenance:*** 90–120 mg/kg/24 hr QD
> ***Acyclovir-resistant herpes simplex:*** 40 mg/kg/dose Q8 hr or 40–60 mg/kg/dose Q12 hr for up to 3 wk or until lesions heal

Contraindications: Hypersensitivity to foscarnet or any other components in the formulation.
Warnings/Precautions: **Use with caution** in patients with renal insufficiency. Discontinue use in adults if serum Cr ≥2.9 mg/dL. **Adjust dose in renal failure (see Chapter 3).** Monitoring renal function and plasma minerals and electrolytes (especially calcium and those with neurologic and cardiac conditions) is recommended. Adequate fluid hydration should be maintained during therapy to reduce nephrotoxicity risk.
Adverse Effects: GI disturbances, anemia, headache and fever are common. May cause peripheral neuropathy, seizures, hallucinations, increased LFTs, hypertension, chest pain, ECG abnormalities, coughing, dyspnea, bronchospasm, and renal failure (adequate hydration and avoiding nephrotoxic medications may reduce risk). Hypocalcemia (increased risk if given with pentamidine), hypokalemia, and hypomagnesemia may also occur.
Drug Interactions: Nephrotoxic medications (e.g., amphotericin, aminoglycosides) increase risk of nephrotoxicity. Ciprofloxacin may increase risk for seizures.
Drug Administration: For intermittent infusion, infuse at a rate **not exceeding** 60 mg/kg/dose over 1 hr or 120 mg/kg/dose over 2 hr at a concentration of ≤12 mg/mL for peripheral line administration or ≤24 mg/mL for central line administration.

FOSFOMYCIN TROMETHAMINE
Monurol
Antibacterial, phosphonic acid derivative

| No | No | ? | B |

Oral powder for solution: 3 g single dose sachet

> ***Uncomplicated UTI (acute cystitis):*** 3 g PO × 1.

Contraindications: Hypersensitivity to fosfomycin or any other components in the formulation.

FOSFOMYCIN TROMETHAMINE *continued*

Warnings/Precautions: Multiple daily doses over 2–3 days do **not** offer any advantage over a single dose regimen and can increase incidence of adverse events.
Adverse Effects: GI disturbances, headache, vaginitis and rhinitis are common. Although rare, angioedema, aplastic anemia, jaundice, hepatic necrosis and toxic megacolon have been reported.
Drug Interactions: Drugs which increase GI motility (e.g., metoclopramide and erythromycin) may lower serum concentrations by decreasing fosfomycin's absorption.
Drug Administration: All doses should be dissolved in 3–4 ounces of water (not hot water) and administered immediately. Doses may be given with or without food.

FURAZOLIDONE
Furoxone
Antiprotozoal, antibacterial agent

No   No   ?   C

Tabs: 100 mg
Oral liquid: 50 mg/15 mL (60, 473 mL); may contain methyl- and propyl-parbens)

Child:
Bacterial diarrhea or cholera:
    ≥1 mo: 1.25 mg/kg/dose PO QID × 5–7 days
Giardiasis:
    ≥1 mo: 1.25–2 mg/kg/dose PO QID × 7–10 days; alternative dosage by age as follows (PO QID × 7–10 days):
        1 mo–<1 yr: 8.3–16.7 mg (2.5–5 mL oral liquid)
        1–4 yr: 16.7–25 mg (5–7.5 mL oral liquid)
        ≥5 yr: 25–50 mg (7.5–15 mL oral liquid)
    Max. dose: 8.8 mg/kg/24 hr
Adult:
    Bacterial diarrhea or cholera: 100 mg PO QID × 5–7 days; some recommend shorter courses of 2–5 days
    Giardiasis: 100 mg PO QID × 7–10 days
    H. pylori GI infection with metronidazole resistance: Furazolidone 200 mg PO BID and clarithromycin 500 mg PO BID × 1 wk followed by omeprazole 20 mg PO QD-BID × 4 wk

---

Contraindications: Hypersensitivity to furazolidone or any other components in the formulation. Infants <1 mo because of possible hemolytic anemia. MAO inhibitors, foods containing tyramine, tricyclic antidepressants, and sympathomimetics (e.g., epinephrine, phenylephrine, amphetamines) may result in hypertensive crisis. Alcohol use during and within 4 days of drug use may cause disulfiram-like reaction.
Warnings/Precautions: **Use with caution** with sedating medications (e.g., antihistamines, opioids and tranquilizers) and patients with G6PD deficiency.
Adverse Effects: GI disturbances, discoloration of urine (dark yellow to brown) and headache are common. Hypersensitivity reactions (e.g., hypotension, angioedema, fever, arthralgia, urticaria) and leukopenia have been reported.
Drug Interactions: See Contraindications.
Drug Administration: Doses may be administered with food to reduce GI irritation.

For explanation of icons, see p. 306.

GANCICLOVIR
Cytovene
Antiviral agent

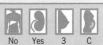

No   Yes   3   C

Injection: 500 mg; contains 4 mEq Na per 1 g drug
Caps: 250, 500 mg
Oral solution: 25, 100 mg/mL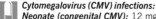

Cytomegalovirus (CMV) infections:
  Neonate (congenital CMV): 12 mg/kg/24 hr ÷ Q12 hr IV × 6 wk
  Child >3 mo and adult:
      Induction therapy (duration 14–21 days): 10 mg/kg/24 hr ÷ Q12 hr IV
      IV maintenance therapy: 5 mg/kg/dose QD IV or 6 mg/kg/dose QD IV for 5 days/wk
  Oral maintenance therapy following induction:
      6 mo–16 yr: 30 mg/kg/dose PO Q8 hr with food
      Adult: 1000 mg PO TID with food
Prevention of CMV in transplant recipients:
  Child and adult:
      Induction therapy (duration 7–14 days): 10 mg/kg/24 hr ÷ Q12 hr IV
      IV maintenance therapy: 5 mg/kg/dose QD IV or 6 mg/kg/dose QD IV for 5 days/wk for 100–120 days post-transplant
      Oral maintenance therapy: See oral doses from CMV maintenance therapy following induction.
Prevention of CMV in HIV-infected individuals (see www.hivatis.org for latest recommendations):
  Infant and child:
      First episode prophylaxis: 30 mg/kg/dose PO Q8 hr with food; consider valganciclovir
      Recurrence prophylaxis: 5 mg/kg/dose IV QD
  Adolescent and adult:
      First episode prophylaxis: 1000 mg PO TID with food
      Recurrence prophylaxis: 5–6 mg/kg/dose IV QD for 5–7 days/wk; or 1000 mg PO TID

Contraindications: Hypersensitivity to ganciclovir/acyclovir products or any of its components; or severe neutropenia (ANC <500/microliter) or severe thrombocytopenia (platelets <25,000/microliter). Any ocular surgery contraindication (infection or severe thrombocytopenia) for the intravitreal implant dosage form.
Warnings/Precautions: Limited experience with use in children <12 yr old. Use with extreme caution. **Reduce dose in renal failure (see Chapter 3).** May impair male and female fertility. Oral absorption is poor; consider the more bioavailable pro-drug, valganciclovir.
Adverse Effects: Neutropenia, thrombocytopenia, anemia, fever and phlebitis are common. Drug reactions alleviated with dose reduction or temporary interruption. With intravitreal implant use, decreased visual acuity may occur 2–4 wk postimplant.
Drug Interactions: Immunosuppressive agents may increase hematologic toxicities. Amphotericin B and cyclosporine and tacrolimus increase risk for nephrotoxicity. May increase the risk for seizures with imipenem/cilastatin and increase didanosine and zidovudine levels. Probenecid, didanosine and zidovudine may decrease ganciclovir levels.
Drug Administration: Use proper procedures for handling and disposal; drug is potentially carcinogenic and mutagenic.

GANCICLOVIR *continued*

IV: For intermittent infusion, infuse ≥1 hr at a concentration ≤10 mg/mL. IM and SC administration are **contraindicated** because of high pH (pH = 11).
PO: Administer doses with food. **Do not** open or crush capsule dosage forms.
Avoid direct contact with open or crushed capsules with the skin or mucous membranes.

GENTAMICIN
Garamycin and many others
Antibiotic, aminoglycoside

No   Yes   1   C

Injection: 10 mg/mL (2 mL), 40 mg/mL (2, 20 mL); some products may contain sodium metabisulfite
Premixed injection in NS: 40 mg (50 mL), 60 mg (50, 100 mL), 70 mg (50 mL), 80 mg (50, 100 mL), 90 mg (100 mL), 100 mg (50, 100 mL), 120 mg (50, 100 mL)
Ophthalmic ointment: 0.3% (3.5 g)
Ophthalmic drops: 0.3% (1, 5, 15 mL)
Topical ointment: 0.1% (15, 30 g)
Topical cream: 0.1% (15, 30 g)

 Parenteral (IM or IV):
Neonate/infant (see following table):

Postconceptional Age (wk)	Postnatal Age (days)	Dose (mg/kg/dose)	Interval (hr)
≤29*	0–7	5	48
	8–28	4	36
	>28	4	24
30–33	0–7	4.5	36
	>7	4	24
34–37	0–7	4	24
	>7	4	18–24
≥38	0–7	4	24
	>7	4	12–18

*Or significant asphyxia, PDA, indomethicin use, poor cardiac output, reduced renal function

    Child: 7.5 mg/kg/24 hr ÷ Q8 hr
    Adult: 3–6 mg/kg/24 hr ÷ Q8 hr
Cystic fibrosis: 7.5–10.5 mg/kg/24 hr ÷ Q8 hr
Intrathecal/intraventricular (use preservative-free product only):
    Newborn: 1 mg QD
    >3 mo: 1–2 mg QD
    Adult: 4–8 mg QD
Ophthalmic ointment: apply Q8–12 hr
Ophthalmic drops: 1–2 drops Q2–4 hr

Contraindications: Hypersensitivity to aminoglycosides or any other components in the formulation.

Continued

GENTAMICIN *continued*

Warnings/Precautions: **Use with caution** in combination with neurotoxic, ototoxic, or nephrotoxic drugs; anesthetics or neuromuscular blocking agents; pre-existing renal, vestibular or auditory impairment; and in patients with neuromuscular disorders. Eliminated more quickly in patients with cystic fibrosis, neutropenia, and burns. **Adjust dose in renal failure (see Chapter 3).** Monitor peak and trough levels.

Therapeutic Peak Levels:
  6–10 mg/L general
  8–10 mg/L in pulmonary infections, neutropenia, osteomyelitis, and severe sepsis

Therapeutic Trough Levels: <2 mg/L. Recommended serum sampling time at steady state: trough within 30 min prior to the 3rd consecutive dose and peak 30–60 min after the administration of the 3rd consecutive dose.

Adverse Effects: May cause nephrotoxicity, ototoxicity, and neuromuscular blockade.
Drug Interactions: Ototoxicity may be potentiated with the use of loop diuretics. See Warnings/Precautions section.
Drug Administration

IV: Infuse over 30–60 min at a concentration ≤10 mg/mL. Administer beta-lactam antibiotics at least 1 hr before or after gentamicin.
IM: Use either undiluted commercial products of 10 or 40 mg/mL.
Intrathecal/intraventricular: Use the preservative-free 10 mg/mL product.
Ophthalmic:
  Drops: Apply finger pressure to lacrimal sac during and for 1–2 min after dose application.
  Ointment: Instill ointment in lower conjunctival sac by **avoiding** contact of ointment tip with eye or skin.

GENTIAN VIOLET
Various generic products
Antifungal agent

No	No	?	C

Topical solution: 1%, 2% (30 mL); contains 10% ethyl alcohol

Topical:
  Child and adult: Apply to lesions BID-TID × 3 days. A 0.25 or 0.5% solution is as effective and may be less irritating than 1%–2% solutions.

Contraindications: Hypersensitivity to gentian violet or any other components in the formulation; porphyria; and use on ulcerative lesions or open wounds.
Warnings/Precautions: Drug stains the skin and clothing purple. Discontinue use if irritation or sensitization occurs.
Adverse Effects: Pruritus, skin irritation, skin ulcer, and skin staining (permanent with granulation tissue) are common.
Drug Interactions: None identified.
Drug Administration: For topical administration, apply to lesion with cotton and **avoid** application to ulcerative lesions. **Avoid** contact with eyes, skin and clothing.

FORMULARY

GRISEOFULVIN

Grifulvin V, Griseofulvin Microsize, Grisactin,
Gris-PEG, and others
Antifungal agent

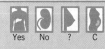

Yes No ? C

Microsize:
    Tabs (Grifulvin V): 500 mg
    Oral suspension (Grifulvin V, Griseofulvin Microsize): 125 mg/5 mL (120 mL);
    contains 0.2% alcohol, parabens and propylene glycol
Ultramicrosize (250 mg ultramicrosize is approximately 500 mg microsize):
    Tabs (Gris-PEG): 125, 250 mg

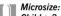

Microsize:
Child >2 yr: 10–20 mg/kg/24 hr PO ÷ QD-BID; give with milk, eggs, fatty
foods. Some have recommended a higher dose of 20–25 mg/kg/24 hr PO for
tinea capitis to improve efficacy due to relative resistance of the organism.
    Adult: 500–1000 mg/24 hr PO ÷ QD-BID
    Max. dose: 1 g/24 hr
Ultramicrosize:
    Child >2 yr: 10–15 mg/kg/24 hr PO ÷ QD-BID
    Adult: 330–750 mg/24 hr PO ÷ QD-BID
    Max. dose: 750 mg/24 hr

Contraindications: Hypersensitivity to griseofulvin products or any other
components in the formulation; porphyria and hepatic disease; and pregnancy
or intention to become pregnant within 1 mo after stopping therapy.
Warnings/Precautions: Monitor hematologic, renal, and hepatic function. Possible
cross-reactivity in penicillin-allergic patients. Usual treatment period is 8 wk for tinea
capitis and 4–6 mo for tinea unguium.
Adverse Effects: Rash, urticaria, erythema and multiforme-like drug reactions are
common. Leukopenia, rash, headache, paresthesias, GI disturbances, and
photosensitivity have been reported.
Drug Interactions: May reduce effectiveness or decrease level of oral contraceptives,
warfarin and cyclosporine; and potentiate the effects of alcohol (flushing and
tachycardia). Induces CYP 450 1A2 isoenzyme. Phenobarbital may enhance
clearance of griseofulvin.
Drug Administration: Administer with fatty meals to increase the drug's absorption.

HALOFANTRINE

Halfan
Antimalarial agent

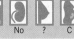

No No ? C

Tabs: 250 mg; orphan drug
Oral suspension: 100 mg/5 mL; contact GlaxoSmithKline (www.gsk.com) for
availability

*Mild to moderate acute malaria caused by susceptible strains of Plasmodium
falciparum and Plasmodium vivax:*
    <40 kg: 8 mg/kg/dose PO Q6 hr × 3 doses; second course of therapy is
    recommended 1 wk later.

Continued

For explanation of icons, see p. 306.

HALOFANTRINE *continued*

> *Alternative dosing by age (administer dose Q6 hr × 3 PO with recommended second course 1 wk later):*
> > *1–2 yr (10–12 kg):* 100 mg
> > *2–5 yr (13–18 kg):* 150 mg
> > *5–8 yr (19–25 kg):* 200 mg
> > *8–10 yr (26–31 kg):* 250 mg
> > *10–12 yr (32–40 kg):* 375 mg
>
> ≥*40 kg:* 500 mg PO Q6 hr × 3 doses; second course of therapy is recommended 1 wk later.

> *Contraindications:* Hypersensitivity to halofantrine and known family history of congenital prolonged QTc intervals.
> *Warnings/Precautions:* **Avoid** use with other drugs that may prolong cardiac QTc interval. Consult with ID specialist or see the latest edition of the AAP Red Book.
> *Adverse Effects:* GI disturbances, cough, headache and pruritis are common. Prolongation of QTc intervals have occurred with use of higher than recommended doses and with interacting medications. Joint pain, loss of appetite and rash have been reported.
> *Drug Interactions:* Use with aurothioglucose may increase risk for blood dyscrasias. Drugs with QTc interval prolongation effects (e.g., bepridil, cisapride, levomethadyl, mefloquine, mesoridazine, pimozide, posaconazole, thioridazine and ziprasidone) and inhibitors of the hepatic CYP 450 3A4 isoenzyme may increase the risk of this effect.
> *Drug Administration:* Take on an empty stomach, 1 hr before or 2 hr after meals.

HEPATITIS B IMMUNE GLOBULIN
BayHep-B, Nabi-HB, HepaGam B, HBIG
Hyperimmune globulin, hepatitis B

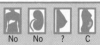

No   No   ?   C

Injection:
> **BayHep-B:** contains ≥217 IU/mL and 0.21–0.32 M glycine
> > Syringe: 0.5 mL
> > Vials: 1, 5 mL
>
> **Nabi-HB:** contains >312 IU/mL and 0.15 M glycine
> > Vials: 1, 5 mL
>
> **HepGam B:** contains >312 IU/mL and 10% maltose and 0.03% polysorbate 80
> > Vials: 1, 5 mL

Contains 4–18% protein (of which not less than 80% is IgG) and trace amounts of IgA

> *Prophylaxis of newborns (along with hepatitis B vaccine series initiated within 12 hr after birth):*
> > *HBsAg-positive mothers:* 0.5 mL IM × 1 within 12 hr after birth
> > *Unknown maternal HBsAG status:* 0.5 mL IM × 1 within 7 days after birth (pending results of materal HBsAg status)
>
> *Postexposure prophylaxis (within 24 hr of needlestick, ocular or mucosal exposure; or within 14 days of sexual exposure):*
> > *<1 yr with <2 hepatitis B vaccine doses administered:* 0.5 mL IM × 1 with completed hepatits B vaccine series
> > ≥*1 yr and adult:* 0.06 mL/kg/dose IM × 1 with completed hepatitis B vaccine series; a second HBIG dose may be given 1 mo later for individuals refusing hepatitis B vaccine or are known non-responders to the vaccine.

HEPATITIS B IMMUNE GLOBULIN *continued*

Contraindications: Anaphylactic or severe systemic reactions to parenteral human globulin products and IgA deficiency.
Warnings/Precautions: **IM administration only**; IV administration may result in serious reactions. Defer administration of live virus vaccines approximately 3 mo after HBIG; revaccination may be necessary if vaccines were administered after HBIG. See AAP Red Book for additional information.

Use of HepaGam product may falsely elevate glucose levels with the glucose dehydrogenase pyrroloquinequinone (GDH-PDQ) method.
Adverse Effects: Injection site pain and erythema, GI disturbances, myalgia, headache and malaise are common and generally mild. Mild leukopenia and elevations in alkaline phosphate, AST/SGOT and serum creatinine have been reported.
Drug Interactions: Live virus vaccines (e.g., MMR, varicella); see Warnings/Precautions.
Drug Administration:. Preferred IM injection sites include the anterolateral aspect of the upper thigh and deltoid muscle. If the buttock is used, use the upper, outer quadrant and avoid the central region.

HYDROXYCHLOROQUINE
Plaquenil, Quineprox
Antimalarial, antirheumatic agent

Yes   Yes   1   C

Tabs: 200 mg (155 mg base)
Oral suspension: 25 mg/mL (19.375 mg/mL base)

Doses expressed in mg of hydroxychloroquine base.
Malaria prophylaxis (start 1 wk prior to exposure and continue for 4 wk after leaving endemic area):
Child: 5 mg/kg/dose PO once weekly; **max. dose:** 310 mg
Adult: 310 mg PO once weekly
Malaria treatment (acute uncomplicated cases): For treatment of malaria, consult with ID specialist or see the latest edition of the AAP Red Book.
Child: 10 mg/kg/dose (**max. dose:** 620 mg) PO × 1 followed by 5 mg/kg/dose (**max. dose:** 310 mg) 6 hr later. Then 5 mg/kg/dose (**max. dose:** 310 mg) Q24 hr × 2 doses starting 24 hr after the first dose.
Adult: 620 mg PO × 1 followed by 310 mg 6 hr later. Then 310 mg Q24 hr × 2 doses starting 24 hr after the first dose.

Contraindications: Hypersensitivity to hydroxychloroquine and 4-aminoquinoline; retinal or visual field changes from prior use; individuals with psoriasis or porphyria; and longer term use in children.
Warnings/Precautions: **Use with caution** in liver disease, G6PD deficiency, concomitant hepatic toxic drugs, renal impairment, and metabolic acidosis or hematologic disorders.
Adverse Effects: May cause headaches, skeletal muscle myopathy, GI disturbances, skin and mucosal pigmentation, agranulcytosis, and visual disturbances.
Drug Interactions: May increase digoxin serum levels. Use with aurothioglucose may increase risk of blood dyscrasias.
Drug Administration: Administer doses with food or milk to reduce GI symptoms.

For explanation of icons, see p. 306.

IMIPENEM-CILASTATIN
Primaxin IV, Primaxin IM
Antibiotic, carbapenem

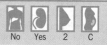

No   Yes   2   C

Injection:
  Primaxin IV: 250, 500 mg; contains 3.2 mEq Na/ g drug
  Primaxin IM: 500, 750 mg; contains 2.8 mEq Na/ g drug
Each 1 mg drug contains 1 mg imipenem and 1 mg cilastatin

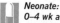

  Neonate:
  0–4 wk and <1.2 kg: 50 mg/kg/24 hr ÷ Q12 hr IV
  <1 wk and ≥1.2 kg: 50 mg/kg/24 hr ÷ Q12 hr IV
  ≥1 wk and ≥1.2 kg: 75 mg/kg/24 hr ÷ Q8 hr IV
Child (4 wk–3 mo): 100 mg/kg/24 hr ÷ Q6 hr IV
Child (>3 mo): 60–100 mg/kg/24 hr ÷ Q6 hr IV; **max. dose:** 4 g/24 hr
  Cystic fibrosis: 90 mg/kg/24 hr ÷ Q6 hr IV; **max. dose:** 4 g/24 hr
Adult:
  IV: 250–1000 mg/dose Q6–8 hr; **max. dose:** 4 g/24 hr or 50 mg/kg/24 hr, whichever is less.
  IM: 500–750 mg/dose Q12 hr

Contraindications: Hypersensitivity to imipenem or cilastatin or any other components in the formulation. Amide local anesthetics hypersensitivity and severe shock or heart block with the IM preparation containing lidocaine.
Warnings/Precautions: Higher risk for seizures may occur with CNS infections, concomitant use with ganciclovir, higher doses and renal impairment. **Use with caution** in penicillin, cephalosporin, and other beta-lactam allergic patients and renal insufficiency **(adjust dose in renal failure; see Chapter 3).** CSF penetration is variable but best with inflamed meninges.
Adverse Effects: Injection site pain, GI disturbances, thrombophlebitis, pruritus, urticaria, dizziness, hypotension, elevated LFTs and blood dyscrasias may occur. See Warnings/Precautions. Nausea may be due to the rapid rate of drug infusion; slowing infusion rate may reduce severity. Nausea and vomiting may be more common at doses exceeding 2 g/24 hr.
Drug Interactions: **Do not administer** with probenecid (increases imipenem/cilastatin levels) and ganciclovir (increases seizure risk).
Drug Administration
  IV: For intermittent IV infusion, infuse over 30–60 min at a concentration ≤5 mg/mL.
  IM: Dilute with 1% lidocaine without epinephrine to a concentration of 250 mg/mL and use within 1 hr of preparation. Assess the potential risk/benefit for using lidocaine as a diluent.

IMIQUIMOD
Aldara
Immunomodulator, topical

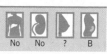

No   No   ?   B

Topical cream: 5% (250 mg single dose packets in a box of 12 packets); contains benzyl alcohol and parabens.

IMIQUIMOD *continued*

Condyloma acuminatum:
    ≥12 yr and adult: Apply to affected areas at bedtime 3 times a wk (avoid consecutive day dosing) for up to a **maximum** of 16 wk. Leave application on for 6–10 hr.

Contraindications: Hypersensitivity to imiquimod or any other components in the formulation.
Warnings/Precautions: May exacerbate inflammatory conditions of the skin.
Use with caution with pre-existing autoimmune conditions. Delay use of imiquimod until genital/perianal tissue is healed from any previous drug or surgical treatment.
Avoid excessive sunlight exposure including sunlamps.
Adverse Effects: Erythema is common; a rest period of several days may be taken to relieve patient discomfort or severe local skin reaction. Skin ulceration/peeling and edema may occur.
Drug Interactions: None identified.
Drug Administration: Apply a thin layer to affected areas; rub area until cream is no longer visable. **Avoid** contact with eyes, lips, and nostrils and **do not** use occlusive dressings. Wash hands before and after administration.

IMMUNE GLOBULIN
Immune globulins

| 6.4 | No | 6.2 | Yes |

IM preparations:
    GamaSTAN S/D: 150–180 mg/mL (2, 10 mL); contains 0.21–0.32 M glycine
IV preparations in solution:
    Flebogamma 5% (50 mg/mL); contains 50 mg/mL sorbitol and ≤6 mg/mL polyethylene glycol
    Gamunex: 10% (100 mg/mL); contains 0.16–0.24 M glycine
    Gammagard liquid: 10% (100 mg/mL)
    Octagam: 5% (50 mg/mL); contains 100 mg/mL maltose
IV preparations in powder for reconstitution:
    Carimune NF: 1, 3, 6, 12 g (contains1.67 g sucrose and <20 mg NaCl per 1 g Ig); dilute to 3, 6, 9 or 12%
    Polygam S/D: 2.5, 5, 10 g (contains 3 mg/mL albumin, 22.5 mg/mL glycine, 20 mg/mL glucose, 2 mg/mL polyethylene glycol, 1 mcg/mL tri-n-butyl phosphate, 1 mcg/mL octoxynol 9, and 100 mcg/mL polysorbate 80); dilute to 5% or 10%

Intramuscular (IM) preparation:
Hepatitis A, prophylaxis:
    Pre-exposure to endemic areas:
        ≤3 mo length of stay: 0.02 mL/kg/dose IM × 1
        >3 mo length of stay: 0.06 mL/kg/dose IM every 4–6 mo
    Post-exposure prophylaxis: 0.02 mL/kg/dose IM × 1 administered within 14 days of exposure
Measles, post-exposure prophylaxis (administered within 6 days of exposure):
    Immunocompetent: 0.25 mL/kg/dose IM × 1; **max. dose:** 15 mL
    Immunodeficient: 0.5 mL/kg/dose IM × 1; **max. dose:** 15 mL
Rubella, post-exposure prophylaxis: 0.55 mL/kg/dose IM × 1 administered within 72 hr of exposure.
Intravenous (IV) preparation:
    Replacement therapy for antibody-deficient disorders: 400–600 mg/kg/dose IV every mo; adjust dosing to maintain trough IgG level of at least 500 mg/dL.

Continued

For explanation of icons, see p. 306.

IMMUNE GLOBULIN *continued*

Idiopathic thrombocytopenia: 400–1000 mg/kg/dose IV QD × 2–5 days, then repeat dose every 3–6 wk based on clinical response and platelet count. May use Rh (D) immunoglobulin in Rh-positive patients.

Kawasaki disease: 2 g/kg/dose IV × 1 administered over 10–12 hr and initiated within the first 10 days of symptoms. Repeat dose of 2 g/kg ×1 may be considered if signs and symptoms persist.

Pediatric HIV:

Hypogammaglobulinemia (<250 mg/dL), recurrent serious bacterial infections (>2 in 1 yr), failure to form antibodies to common antigens, or measles propylaxis: 400 mg/kg/dose IV every 28 days

HIV-associated thromobocytopenia: 500–1000 mg/kg/dose IV QD × 3–5 days

Contraindications: History of severe systemic allergic reaction to human immunoglobulin products. Select IgA deficiency; may cause **anaphylaxis** due to varied amounts of IgA in preparation. Some IV products are IgA depleted; consult a pharmacist. IV or intradermal use and severe thrombocytopenia or any coagulation disorder with the IM preparation.

Warnings/Precautions: These products are derived from human plasma and may contain infectious viruses. Risk for viral infections are reduced by screening donors and testing and/or inactivating certain viruses.

Intravenous preparations containing sucrose **should not be infused** at a rate such that the amount of sucrose exceeds 3 mg/kg/min to decrease risk of renal dysfunction including acute renal failure.

Adverse Effects: Flushing, chills, fever, headache, and hypotension are common. Aseptic meningitis, acute renal failure (IV forms containing sucrose, see above), acute lung injury with pulmonary edema 1–6 hr after IV infusion, and hepatitis have been reported.

Hypersensitivity reaction may occur when IV form is administered rapidly (see Drug Administration). Injection site reaction is common with IM form.

Drug Interactions

IM: Delay live virus vaccines (e.g., MMR and varicella) for at least 3 mo for hepatitis A prophylaxis; for at least 5 mo for immunocompetent measles prophylaxis; and for at least 6 mo for immunodeficient measles prophylaxis.

IV: Delay live virus vaccines after IVIG administration (see latest edition of the AAP Red Book for details).

Drug Administration

IM: **Use IM product only**. Anterolateral aspects of the upper thigh and deltoid muscle of the upper arm are preferred injection sites. **Do not** use the gluteal region routinely because of risk of sciatic nerve injury. Limit single injection volume to 1–3 mL for infants and small children; and 5 mL for large children and adolescents.

IV: Use IV products only. Refer to specific product's package insert. If infusion-related adverse reactions occur, stop infusion until side effects subside and may restart at a rate previously tolerated.

IMMUNE GLOBULIN, BOTULINUM

See *Botulinum Immune Globulin Intravenous*

IMMUNE GLOBULIN, CYTOMEGALOVIRUS

See *Cytomegalovirus Immune Globulin*

IMMUNE GLOBULIN, HEPATITIS B

See *Hepatitis B Immune Globulin*

IMMUNE GLOBULIN, RABIES

See *Rabies Immune Globulin*

IMMUNE GLOBULIN, TETANUS

See *Tetanus Immune Globulin*

IMMUNE GLOBULIN, VARICELLA-ZOSTER

See *Varicella-Zoster Immune Globulin (Human)*

INDINAVIR
Crixivan, IDV
Antiviral agent, protease inhibitor

Yes   No   3   C

Caps: 100, 200, 333, 400 mg

Child (investigational dose): 500 mg/m^2/dose PO Q8 hr; **max. dose:** 800 mg/dose. This dose has resulted in higher AUC and lower trough levels when compared to adults.

Adolescent and adult:
    Usual dose: 800 mg PO Q8 hr
    Needle stick prophylaxis: 800 mg/dose PO TID × 28 days. Use in combination with zidovudine (AZT) 200 mg/dose PO TID or 300 mg/dose PO BID, and lamivudine 150 mg/dose PO BID × 28 days.

Adult:
    In combination with ritonavir: 800 mg PO Q8 hr with 200 mg ritonavir PO BID
    In combination with efavirenz: 1000 mg PO Q8 hr with 600 mg efavirenz PO QD
    In combination with delavirdine: 600 mg PO Q8 hr with 400 mg delavirdine PO TID
    In combination with itraconazole or ketoconazole; or dosing in mild/moderate hepatic impairment: 600 mg PO Q8 hr
    In combination with rifabutin: 1000 mg PO Q8 hr and decrease standard rifabutin dose by 50%

For explanation of icons, see p. 306.

Continued

INDINAVIR *continued*

Contraindications: Hypersensitivity to indinavir or any other components in the formulation. Concomitant use with astemizole, terfenadine, cisapride, ergot alkaloid derivatives, pimozide, triazolam, and/or midazolam.

Warnings/Precautions: **Should not** be used in neonates due to risk for hyperbilirubinemia/kernicterus, and in pregnancy. Reduce dose in mild-moderate hepatic impairment.

Adolescent Dosing: Patients in early puberty (Tanner I–II) should be dosed with pediatric regimens and those in late puberty (Tanner IV) should be dosed with adult regimens. Adolescents who are at the midst of their growth spurt (Tanner III females and Tanner IV males) can be dosed by either pediatric or adult regimen with close monitoring of efficacy and toxicity.

Adverse Effects: GI discomfort, headache, metallic taste, hyperbilirubinemia, dizziness and lipid abnormalities are common. Nephrolithiasis, hyperglycemia, hepatitis, spontaneous bleeding in hemophiliacs, tubulointerstitial nephritis, immune reconstitution syndrome and body fat redistribution have been reported.

Drug Interactions: Like other protease inhibitors, indinavir inhibits the cytochrome P4503A4 isoenzyme to increase the effects or toxicities of many drugs. Rifampin, rifabutin, efavirenz, and nevirapine can decrease indinavir levels; whereas ketoconazole, itraconazole can increase levels. See the above Contraindications. **Carefully review the patient's medication profile for potential interactions!**

Drug Administration: Administer doses on an empty stomach (1 hr before or 2 hr after meals) with adequate hydration (48 ounces/24 hr in adults). If didanosine is included in the regimen, space 1 hr apart on an empty stomach. Capsules are sensitive to moisture and should be stored with a desiccant. **Noncompliance can quickly promote resistant HIV strains.**

IODOQUINOL
Yodoxin, Diquinol, Diiodhydroxyquin,
Diiodohydroxyquinoline
Intestinal amebicide, topical
antibacterial/antifungal

Yes   No   3   C

Powder: 25 g
Tabs: 210, 650 mg
Contains approximately 64% iodine.

Amebiasis, balantidiasis, and dientamoeba fragilis:
  Child: 30–40 mg/kg/24 hr PO ÷ TID × 20 days; **max. dose:** 1.95 g/24 hr. Use 40 mg/kg/24 hr for balantidiasis.
  Adult: 650 mg PO TID × 20 days

Contraindications: Hypersensitivity to iodine and 8-hydroxyquinolones and hepatic impairment.
  Warnings/Precautions: **Use with caution** in thyroid disease, neurologic disorders. **Avoid** long-term use because of risk for optic neuritis, optic atrophy and peripherial neuropathy. **Should not** be used to treat nonspecific diarrhea.

Adverse Effects: Pruritus, urticaria, GI disturbances, headache, fever and shivering are common. Dose-related neurologic and ocular toxicities are the most serious adverse effect; see Warnings/Precautions.

Drug Interactions: May increase iodine levels and interfere with thyroid function tests (may persist up to 6 mo after stopping therapy).

Drug Administration: Take doses after meals. Tablets may be crushed and mixed with applesauce or chocolate syrup for better palatability.

ISONIAZID
INH, Nydrazid, Laniazid, and others
Antituberculous agent

Yes   Yes   1   C

Tabs: 100, 300 mg
Syrup: 50 mg/5 mL (473 mL)
Injection: 100 mg/mL (10 mL); contains 0.25% chlorobutanol

See most recent edition of the AAP Red Book for details and length of therapy.
Prophylaxis:
    Infant and child: 10 mg/kg (**max. dose:** 300 mg) PO QD. After 1 mo of daily therapy and in cases where daily compliance cannot be assured, may change to 20–40 mg/kg (**max. dose:** 900 mg) per dose PO, given twice weekly.
    Adult: 300 mg PO QD
Treatment:
    Infant and child:
        10–15 mg/kg (**max. dose:** 300 mg) PO QD or 20–30 mg/kg (**max. dose:** 900 mg) per dose twice weekly with rifampin for uncomplicated pulmonary tuberculosis in compliant patients. Additional drugs are necessary in complicated disease.
    Adult:
        5 mg/kg (**max. dose:** 300 mg) PO QD or 15 mg/kg (**max. dose:** 900 mg) per dose twice weekly with rifampin. Additional drugs are necessary in complicated disease.
For INH-resistant TB: Discuss with local health dept., or consult ID specialist.

Contraindications: Acute liver disease and previous isoniazid-associated hepatitis.
Warnings/Precautions: **Use with caution** in chronic liver disease and renal impairment **(adjust dose; see Chapter 3). Should not be used alone for treatment. Avoid** daily alcohol use to reduce risk for isoniazid-induced hepatitis. Follow LFTs monthly. Supplemental pyridoxine (1–2 mg/kg/24 hr) is recommended.
Adverse Effects: Peripheral neuropathy, optic neuritis, seizures, encephalopathy and psychosis may occur. Hepatic side effects may occur with higher doses, especially in combination with rifampin. Drug-induced hepatitis risk also increases with age. Agranulocytosis, anemia, thrombocytopenia, and SLE have been reported. Oral liquid dosage form may cause diarrhea.
Drug Interactions: Inhibits CYP 450 1A2, 2C9, 2C19, and 3A3/4 microsomal enzymes; decrease dose of carbamazepine, diazepam, valproic acid and phenytoin. Aluminum salts may decrease absorption. Prednisone may decrease isoniazid's effects. Also a substrate and inducer of CYP 450 2E1 and may potentiate acetaminophen heptatotoxicity. May cause false-positive urine glucose test.
Drug Administration
    PO: Administer 1 hr prior to and 2 hr after meals.
    IM: May be given IM (same as oral doses) when oral therapy is not possible.

ITRACONAZOLE
Sporanox
Antifungal agent, triazole

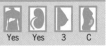

| Yes | Yes | 3 | C |

Caps: 100 mg
Oral solution: 10 mg/mL (150 mL); contains saccharin and sorbitol

Child (limited data): 3–5 mg/kg/24 hr PO ÷ QD-BID; dosages as high as 5–10 mg/kg/24 hr have been used for aspergillus prophylaxis in chronic granulomatous disease. Population pharmacokinetic data in pediatric cystic fibrosis and bone marrow transplant patients suggest an oral liquid dosage of 10 mg/kg/24 hr PO ÷ BID or oral capsule dosage of 20 mg/kg/24 hr ÷ BID to be more reliable for achieving trough plasma concentrations between 500–2000 ng/mL.

Prophylaxis for recurrence of opportunistic disease in HIV:
    Cryptococcus neoformans: 2–5 mg/kg/dose PO Q12–24 hr
    Histoplasma capsulatum or Coccidioides immitis: 2–5 mg/kg/dose PO Q12–48 hr

Adult:
    Blastomycosis and nonmeningeal histoplasmosis:
        PO: 200 mg QD up to a **max. dose** of 400 mg/24 hr ÷ BID (**max. dose:** 200 mg/dose)
        IV: 400 mg/24 hr ÷ BID × 2 days, followed by 200 mg QD; switch to oral therapy as soon as possible.
    Aspergillosis and severe infections:
        PO: 600 mg/24 hr ÷ TID × 3–4 days, followed by 200–400 mg/24 hr ÷ BID; **max. dose:** 600 mg/24 hr ÷ TID
        IV: 400 mg/24 hr ÷ BID × 2 days, followed by 200 mg QD; switch to oral therapy as soon as possible.
    Empiric therapy in febrile, neutropenic patients: 400 mg/24 hr IV ÷ BID × 2 days, followed by 200 mg QD for up to 14 days; continue with the oral solution at 200 mg PO BID until resolution.

Contraindications: Coadministration of cisapride, dofetilide, pimozide, quinidine, triazolam, lovastatin, simvastatin, ergot derivatives and oral midazolam is **contraindicated**. History of itraconazole hypersensitivity.
Warnings/Precautions: Use with caution in hepatic impairment, hypersensitivity to other azole antifungals and with active/prior congestive heart failure. Oral solution and capsule dosage form should **not** be used interchangeably; oral solution is more bioavailable. Achlorhydria reduces absorption of the drug. Only the oral solution has been demonstrated effective for oral and/or esophageal candidiasis.

IV dosage form **should not** be used in patients with GFR <30 mL/min because the hydoxypropyl-beta-cyclodextrin excipient has reduced clearance in patients with renal failure.

Steady-state trough serum concentrations of >250 ng/mL itraconazole and >1000 ng/mL hydroxyitraconazole (metabolite) have been recommended. Recommended serum sampling time at steady state: trough level after 2 wk after continuous dosing.
Adverse Effects: May cause GI symptoms, headaches, rash, liver enzyme elevation, hepatitis, and hypokalemia. Congestive heart failure, Stevens-Johnson syndrome and anaphylaxis have been reported.
Drug Interactions: Like ketoconazole, it inhibits the activity of the cytochrome P450 3A4 drug metabolizing isoenzyme. See Contraindications section.

ITRACONAZOLE *continued*

Grapefruit juice decreases itraconazole oral absorption whereas cola beverage increases oral absorption. See remarks in ketoconazole for additional drug interaction information.

Drug Administration

PO: Administer oral solution on an empty stomach, but administer capsules with food. **Avoid** grapefruit juice.

IV: For intermittent infusion, infuse over 1 hr at a concentration of 3.33 mg/mL. Dilute IV form with NS (not compatible with D_5W or LR).

IVERMECTIN
Stromectol
Antihelmintic

No   No   1   C

Tabs: 3, 6 mg

 Cutaneous larva migrans, or strongyloidiasis: 0.2 mg/kg/dose PO QD × 1–2 days; dosing by body weight (see following table):
Scabies: 0.2 mg/kg/dose PO × 1; dosing by body weight (see following table):

CUTANEOUS LARVA MIGRANS, SCABIES, STRONGYLOIDIASIS

Weight (kg)	Oral Dose
15–24	3 mg
25–35	6 mg
36–50	9 mg
51–65	12 mg
66–79	15 mg
≥80	0.2 mg/kg

Onchocerciasis: 0.15 mg/kg PO × 1; dosing by body weight (see following table):

ONCHOCERCIASIS

Weight (kg)	Single Oral Dose
15–25	3 mg
26–44	6 mg
45–64	9 mg
65–84	12 mg
≥85	0.15 mg/kg

Dose may be repeated every 6–12 mo until asymptomatic.

Contraindications: Hypersensitivity to ivermectin or any other components in the formulation.
Warnings/Precautions: Rare fatal encephalopathy may occur in onchocerciasis with a concurrent heavy Loa loa infection.

Continued

IVERMECTIN *continued*

Adverse Effects: Reactions experienced in strongyloidiasis include diarrhea, nausea, vomiting, pruritus, rash, dizziness, and drowsiness. Adverse reactions experienced in onchocerciasis include cutaneous or systemic allergic/inflammatory reactions of varying severity (Mazzotti reaction), and ophthalmological reactions. Specific reactions may include arthralgia/synovitis, lymph node enlargement and tenderness, pruritus, edema, fever, orthostatic hypotension, and tachycardia. Therapy for postural hypotension may include oral hydration, recumbency, IV normal saline, and/or IV steroids. Antihistamines and/or aspirin have been used for most mild to moderate cases.
Drug Interactions: None identified.
Drug Administration: Take doses on an empty stomach with water.

KANAMYCIN
Kantrex and others
Antibiotic, aminoglycoside

No	Yes	1	D

Caps: 500 mg
Injection: 37.5, 250, 333, 500 mg/mL; may contain sulfites

 Neonate IV/IM administration (see following table):

Birth Weight (kg)	<7 Days	≥7 Days
<2 kg	15 mg/kg/24 hr ÷ Q12 hr	22.5 mg/kg/24 hr ÷ Q8 hr
≥2 kg	20 mg/kg/24 hr ÷ Q12 hr	30 mg/kg/24 hr ÷ Q8 hr

Infant and child: IM/IV: 15–30 mg/kg/24 hr ÷ Q8–12 hr
Adult: IV/IM: 15 mg/kg/24 hr ÷ Q8–12 hr
PO administration for GI bacterial overgrowth: 150–250 mg/kg/24 hr ÷ Q6 hr; **max. dose:** 4 g/24 hr

---

 Contraindications: Hypersensitivity to kanamycin or other aminoglycosides or any other components in the formulation. For oral route, patients with intestinal obstructions.
Warnings/Precautions: **Use with caution** in neuromuscular disorders (e.g., infant botulism, myasthenia gravis), anesthesia and muscle-relaxant medication use and hypermagnesemia (may result in respiratory arrest). Renal toxicity and ototoxicity may occur. **Reduce dosage frequency with renal impairment (see Chapter 3).** Poorly absorbed orally, PO used to treat GI bacterial overgrowth.
Therapeutic Levels: peak: 15–30 mg/L; trough: <5–10 mg/L. Recommended serum sampling time at steady-state: trough within 30 min prior to the 3rd consecutive dose and peak 30–60 min after the administration of the 3rd consecutive dose.
Adverse Effects
  IM/IV: Nephrotoxicity is common. Ototoxicity may occur with the following predisposing factors and may be irreversible: pre-existing renal impairment, high serum drug levels, prolonged use of drug, pre-existing hearing loss, and prior exposure to ototoxic drugs.
  PO: GI disturbances are common. Prolonged use with oral route has induced intestinal malabsorption.

KANAMYCIN *continued*

Drug Interactions: Other ototoxic and nephrotoxic medications may increase risk of toxicities. Loop diuretics (e.g., furosemide) may increase risk for ototoxicity and should be **avoided**. Anesthesia and muscle-relaxant medications may result in neuromuscular blockade with respiratory paralysis.
Drug Administration: IV: For intermittent IV infusion, infuse over 30–60 min at a concentration 2.5–5 mg/mL.

KETOCONAZOLE
Nizoral, Nizoral A-D, Xolegel, and others
Antifungal agent, imidazole

No   No   1   C

Tabs: 200 mg
Oral suspension: 100 mg/5 mL
Cream: 2% (15, 30, 60 g); contains sulfites
Gel (Xolegel): 2% (15 g); contains 34% alcohol
Shampoo: 1% [Nizoral A-D, OTC] (120, 210 mL), 2% (120 mL)

Oral:
Child ≥2 yr: 3.3–6.6 mg/kg/24 hr QD
Adult: 200–400 mg/24 hr QD
Max. dose: 800 mg/24 hr ÷ BID
Topical: 1–2 applications/24 hr
Shampoo: Twice weekly for 4 wk with at least 3 days between applications; intermittently as needed to maintain control
Suppressive therapy against mucocutaneous candidiasis in HIV:
Child: 5–10 mg/kg/24 hr ÷ QD-BID PO; **max. dose:** 800 mg/24 hr ÷ BID
Adolescent and adult: 200 mg/dose QD PO

Contraindications: Hypersensitivity to ketoconazole products or any other components in the formulation. Cardiac arrhythmias may occur when used with cisapride, terfinadine, quinidine, and pimozide; and excessive sedation and prolonged hypnotic effects with triazolam. Concomitant administration of ketoconazole with any of these drugs is **contraindicated**.
Warnings/Precautions: Achlorhydria or drugs that decrease gastric acidity will decrease oral absorption. Monitor LFTs in long-term use.
Adverse Effects
  PO: Nausea, vomiting, rash, headache, pruritus, and fever are common. Gynecomastia and hepatotoxiciy have been reported.
  Topical: Pruritus and stinging may occur.
Drug Interactions: Inhibits CYP 450 3A4. May increase levels/effects of phenytoin, digoxin, cyclosporine, corticosteroids, nevirapine, protease inhibitors, and warfarin. Phenobarbital, rifampin, isoniazid, H_2 blockers, antacids, and omeprazole can decrease levels of ketoconazole. See Contraindications.
Drug Administration
  PO: Administer doses with food or acidic beverages and 2 hr prior to antacids to increase absorption.
  Shampoo: Wet hair and scalp with water, apply sufficient amount to scalp and gently massage for about 1 min. Rinse hair thoroughly, reapply shampoo and leave on the scalp for an additional 3 min; then rinse.
  Topical: Apply sufficient amount and rub gently into affected and surrounding area.

KUNECATECHINS
Veregen, Sinecatechins
Keratolytic, sinecatechins

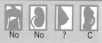

No   No   ?   C

Ointment: 15% (15 g); approximately 2.5% of the product contains caffeine, theobromine and gallic acid

---

Condyloma acuminatum:
Adult: Apply a 0.5 cm strand of ointment TID to each external genital and perianal wart. Continue therapy until complete clearance of warts but no longer than 16 wk.

Contraindications: Hypersensitivity to any component of the product.
Warnings/Precautions: For external use only; not for intra-anal, ophthalmic or intravaginal use. Ointment may weaken condoms and vaginal diaphragms.
Avoid use on open wounds and exposure of treated areas to sunlight and ultraviolet (UV) light. Has not been evaluated for treatment of urethral, intra-vaginal, cervical, rectal or intra-anal human papilloma viral disease.
Adverse Effects: Burning sensation, edema, erythema, skin induration pruritus, vesicular rash and superficial skin ulcer are common.
Drug Interactions: None identified.
Drug Administration: Ointment may stain clothing or bedding. Use fingers to apply ointment to affected area and ensure complete coverage by applying a thin layer of ointment. Wash hands well before and after each application.

LAMIVUDINE
Epivir, Epivir-HBV, 3TC
Antiviral agent, nucleoside analogue reverse transcriptase inhibitor

No   Yes   3   C

Tabs: 100 mg (Epivir-HBV), 150, 300 mg
Oral solution: 5 mg/mL (Epivir-HBV), 10 mg/mL; contains propylene glycol
In combination with zidovudine (AZT) as Combivir:
   Tabs: 150 mg lamivudine + 300 mg zidovudine
In combination with abacavir as Epzicom:
   Tabs: 300 mg lamivudine + 600 mg abacavir
In combination with abacavir and zidovudine (AZT) as Trizivir:
   Tabs: 150 mg lamivudine + 300 mg abacavir + 300 mg zidovudine

---

HIV:
Neonate (<30 days): 2 mg/kg/dose PO BID
Child (3 mo–16 yr): 4 mg/kg/dose PO BID; **max. dose:** 150 mg/dose
   Adolescent (≥16 yr) and adult:
      <50 kg: 4 mg/kg/dose PO BID; **max. dose:** 150 mg/dose
      ≥50 kg: 300 mg/24 hr PO ÷ QD–BID
      Needle stick prophylaxis: 150 mg/dose PO BID × 28 days. Use in combination with zidovudine (AZT) 200 mg/dose PO TID or 300 mg/dose PO BID, and indinavir 800 mg/dose PO TID × 28 days.
Combivir:
   ≥12 yr–adult: 1 tablet PO BID
Epizcom:
   Adult: 1 tablet PO QD
Trizivir:
   Adolescent (≥40 kg)–adult: 1 tablet PO BID

LAMIVUDINE *continued*

Chronic hepatitis B (see remarks):
    2–17 yr: 3 mg/kg/dose PO QD up to a **max. dose** of 100 mg/dose
    Adult: 100 mg/dose PO QD

Contraindications: Hypersensitivity to lamivudine or any other component contained in the formulation.
    Warnings/Precautions: Lactic acidosis, severe hepatomegaly with steatosis, post-treatment exacerbations of hepatitis B and ALT elevations, pancreatitis, and emergence of resistant viral strains have been reported. **Use with caution** in renal impairment; **adjust dose in renal impairment (see Chapter 3)**. For use of any of the combination products (Combivir, Epizcom, and Trizivir), **do not use** in patients with creatinine clearance of <50 mL/min.
Chronic hepatitis B: Use Epivir-HBV product for this indication. Safety and effectiveness beyond 1 yr have **not** been determined. Patients with both HIV and hepatitis B should use the higher HIV doses along with an appropriate combination regimen. Rapid emergence of HIV resistance is likely to occur in HBV patients with unrecognized or untreated HIV infection.
Adverse Effects: Headache, fatigue, nausea, decreased appetite, diarrhea, skin rash, and abdominal pain are common. Pancreatitis (primarily in advanced disease), peripheral neuropathy, anemia, neutropenia, liver enzyme elevation, and fat redistribution may occur. See Warnings/Precautions for other serious side effects.
Drug Interactions: Concomitant use with cotrimoxazole (TMP/SMX) may result in increased lamivudine levels. Should **not** be used in combination with zalcitabine or emtricitabine because it may inhibit intracellular phosphorylation of one another or share similar resistance profiles (no additive benefit), respectively.
Drug Administration: Doses may be administered with or without food.

LEVOFLOXACIN
Levaquin, Quixin, Iquix
Antibiotic, quinolone

| No | Yes | 3 | C |

Tabs: 250, 500, 750 mg
Oral solution: 25 mg/mL (480 mL)
Injection: 25 mg/mL (20, 30 mL)
Prediluted injection in D$_5$W: 250 mg/50 mL, 500 mg/100 mL, 750 mg/150 mL
Ophthalmic drops:
    Quixin: 0.5% (2.5, 5 mL)
    Iquix: 1.5% (5 mL)

Child:
    Recurrent or persistent acute otitis media (6 mo–<5 yr): 10 mg/kg/dose PO Q12 hr ×10 days; **max. dose:** 500 mg/24 hr
    Community acquired pneumonia (10 days of therapy; see remarks) and data from a single-dose pharmacokinetic study to provide similar drug exposures associated with clinical efficacy and safety as seen in adults:
        6 mo–<5 yr: 10 mg/kg/dose PO/IV Q12 hr; **max. dose** 500 mg/24 hr
        5–12 yr: 10 mg/kg/dose PO/IV Q24 hr; **max. dose** 500 mg/24 hr
Adult:
    Community acquired pneumonia: 500 mg PO/IV Q24 hr × 7–14 days; OR 750 mg PO/IV Q24 hr × 5 days
    Complicated UTI/acute pyelonephritis: 250 PO/IV Q24 hr × 10 days; OR 750 mg PO/IV Q24 hr × 5 days
    Uncomplicated UTI: 250 mg PO/IV Q24 hr × 3 days

Continued

LEVOFLOXACIN *continued*

Uncomplicated skin/skin structure infection: 500 mg PO/IV Q24 hr × 7–10 days
Acute bacterial sinusitis: 500 mg PO/IV Q24 hr × 10–14 days; OR 750 mg PO/IV Q24 hr × 5 days
Inhalational anthrax (post-exposure): 500 mg PO/IV Q24 hr × 60 days.
Conjunctivitis:
≥1 yr and adult: Instill 1–2 drops of the 0.5% solution to affected eye(s) Q2 hr up to 8 times/24 hr while awake for the first 2 days, then Q4 hr up to 4 times/24 hr while awake for the next 5 days.
Corneal ulcer:
≥6 yr and adult: Instill 1–2 drops of the 1.5% solution to affected eye(s) Q30 min–2 hr while awake and 4 and 6 hr after retiring for the first 3 days, then Q1–4 hr while awake.

Contraindications: Hypersensitivity to levofloxacin and to other quinolones.
Warnings/Precautions: **Avoid** in patients with history of QTc prolongation or taking QTc prolonging drugs, and excessive sunlight exposure. **Use with caution** in diabetes, seizures, children <18 yr and renal impairment (adjust dose in renal failure; see Chapter 3). **Not** recommended for gonorrhea because of potential resistance.

Levofloxacin was well tolerated with equal efficacy in a comparative study to standard-of-care antibiotics in children 0.5 to 16 yr with community acquired pneumonia. Long-term safety trials are underway in children treated for pneumonia and otitis media.
Adverse Effects: May cause GI disturbances, headache, and blurred vision with the ophthalmic solution. Like other quinolones, tendon rupture can occur during or after therapy.
Drug Interactions: Antacids containing aluminum, magnesium and/or calcium, sucralfate, metal cations (e.g., zinc, iron copper and magnesium), and didanosine may decrease levofloxacin oral absorption. May enhance the effects of warfarin. Use with corticosteroids may increase risk of tendon rupture and use with nonsteroidal anti-inflammatory drugs may increase risk of CNS stimulation and seizures. May cause false-positive opiate immunoassay urine screening tests.
Drug Administration
IV: Infuse IV over 1–1.5 hr at a concentration ≤5 mg/mL. **Avoid** IV push or rapid infusion because of risk of hypotension.
PO: **Do not** administer antacids or other divalent salts with or within 2 hr of oral levofloxacin dose; otherwise may be administered with or without food.
Ophthalmic Drops: Apply finger pressure to lacrimal sac during and for 1–2 min after dose application.

LINDANE
Various brands, Gamma benzene hexachloride
Scabicidal agent, pediculocide

No   No   3   B

Shampoo: 1% (30,60, 473 mL)
Lotion: 1% (30, 60, 473 mL)

Scabies: Apply thin layer of lotion to skin. Bathe and rinse off medication in adults after 8–12 hr; children 6–8 hr. May repeat × 1 in 7 days PRN.
Pediculosis capitis: Apply 15–30 mL of shampoo, lather for 4–5 min, rinse hair and comb with fine comb to remove nits. May repeat × 1 in 7 days PRN.
Pediculosis pubis: May use lotion or shampoo (applied locally).

FORMULARY

LINDANE *continued*

Contraindications: Premature infants and seizure disorders.
Warnings/Precautions: Lindane is considered second-line therapy due to side effect risk. Lindane is systemically absorbed. Risk of toxic effects is greater in young children; use other agents (permethrin) in infants, young children, and during pregnancy.

For scabies, change clothing and bedsheets after starting treatment and treat family members. For pediculosis pubis, treat sexual contacts. Itching may occur after the successful killing of scabies and is not necessarily an indication for retreatment with lindane.
Adverse Effects: May cause a rash; rarely may cause seizures or aplastic anemia.
Drug Interactions: Use with caution with drugs that lower seizure threshold (e.g., antipsychotics, antidepressants, theophylline, cyclosporine).
Drug Administration: Avoid contact with face, eyes, urethral meatus, damaged skin, open cuts, extensive excoriations or mucous membranes. Use of rubber gloves for administration is recommended, especially when applying to more than one person.
Do not wash skin with any lotion, cream or oil; certain ingredients may enhance lindane systemic absorption. **Do not** use any covering (e.g., plastic lining or clothing) over the applied lindane that does not breathe.

LINEZOLID
Zyvox
Antibiotic, oxazolidinone

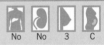

| No | No | 3 | C |

Tabs: 400, 600 mg; contains ~0.45 mEq Na per 200 mg drug
Oral suspension: 100 mg/5 mL (150 mL); contains phenylalanine, sodium benzoate, and 0.8 mEq Na per 200 mg drug
Injection premixed: 200 mg in 100 mL, 400 mg in 200 mL, 600 mg in 300 mL; contains 1.7 mEq Na per 200 mg drug

Neonate <7 days: 10 mg/kg/dose IV/PO Q12 hr; if response is sub-optimal, increase dose to 10 mg/kg/dose Q8 hr
Neonate ≥7 days–11 yr:
    Pneumonia, bacteremia, complicated skin/skin structure infections, Vancomycin-resistant E. faecium (VRE): 10 mg/kg/dose IV/PO Q8 hr. Duration of therapy: 10–14 days, except for VRE (14–28 days).
    Uncomplicated skin/skin structure infections:
        <5 yr: 10 mg/kg/dose PO Q8 hr × 10–14 days
        5–11 yr: 10 mg/kg/dose PO Q12 hr × 10–14 days
≥12 yr and adult:
    MRSA infections: 600 mg Q12 hr IV/PO
    Vancomycin-resistant E. faecium: 600 mg Q12 hr IV/PO × 14–28 days
    Community acquired and nosocomial pneumonia; and bacteremia: 600 mg Q12 hr IV/PO × 10–14 days
    Uncomplicated skin infections:
        ≥12 yr and adolescent: 600 mg Q12 hr PO × 10–14 days
        Adult: 400 mg Q12 hr PO × 10–14 days

Contraindications: Hypersensitivity to linezolid or any other components in the formulation.
Warnings/Precautions: Avoid use with SSRIs (e.g., fluoxetine, paroxetine), tricyclic antidepressants, venlafaxine, and trazodone; may cause serotonin syndrome. **Use caution** when using adrenergic (epinephrine, pseudoephedrine) agents or

Continued

LINEZOLID *continued*

consuming large amounts of foods and beverages containing tyramine; may increase blood pressure. Dosing information in severe hepatic failure and renal impairment with multidoses have not been completed.

Adverse Effects: Diarrhea, headache, and nausea are common. Anemia, leukopenia, pancytopenia, thrombocytopenia may occur in patients who are at risk for myelosuppression and who receive regimens >2 wk. Complete blood count monitoring is recommended in these individuals. Pseudomembranous colitis and neuropathy (peripheral and optic) has also been reported.

Drug Interactions: Reversible inhibitor of monoamine oxidase; see Warnings/Precautions section.

Drug Administration: Protect all dosage forms from light and moisture.
IV: Infuse over 30–120 min at the ready to use concentration of 2 mg/mL. **Do not** further dilute or mix/infuse with other medications.
PO: Oral suspension product must be gently mixed by inverting the bottle 3–5 times prior to each use (**do not shake**). All oral doses may be administered with or without food.

LOPINAVIR WITH RITONAVIR
Kaletra, LPV/RTV
Antiviral, protease inhibitor combination

Yes   No   3   C

Tabs: 200 mg lopinavir and 50 mg ritonavir
Oral solution: 80 mg lopinavir and 20 mg ritonavir/1 mL; contains 42.4% alcohol and saccharin (160 mL)

Neonate and infant <6 mo (investigational dose from ACTG P1030): 300 mg/m^2 lopinavir and 75 mg/m^2 ritonavir BID PO
6 mo–12 yr (administer all doses with food and see remarks):
Not in combination with nevirapine, efavirenz, or amprenavir: 230 mg/m^2/dose lopinavir and 57.5 mg/m^2/dose ritonavir BID PO up to a **maximum** of 400 mg lopinavir and 100 mg ritonavir/dose; OR use the following doses by weight (see following table):

Weight (kg)	Dose (Lopinavir and Ritonavir) BID PO
7–<15	12 mg/kg/dose and 2 mg/kg/dose
15–40	10 mg/kg/dose and 2.5 mg/kg/dose
>40	400 mg and 100 mg

In combination with nevirapine, efavirenz, or amprenavir: 300 mg/m^2/dose lopinavir and 75 mg/m^2/dose ritonavir BID PO up to a **maximum** of 533 mg lopinavir and 133 mg ritonavir/dose; OR use the following doses by weight (see following table):

Weight (kg)	Dose (Lopinavir and Ritonavir) BID PO
7–<15	13 mg/kg/dose and 3.25 mg/kg/dose
15–50	11 mg/kg/dose and 2.75 mg/kg/dose
>50	600 mg and 150 mg

LOPINAVIR WITH RITONAVIR *continued*

≥12 yr and adult (administer all doses with food):
  Not in combination with nevirapine, efavirenz, or amprenavir: 400 mg lopinavir and 100 mg ritonavir BID PO
  In combination with nevirapine, efavirenz, amprenavir, or nelfinavir: 600 mg lopinavir and 150 mg ritonavir BID PO
Adult:
  Treatment naïve and Not in combination with nevirapine, efavirenz, or amprenavir: 800 mg lopinavir and 200 mg ritonavir QD PO
  In combination with saquinavir hard gel caps (Inverase): 400 mg lopinavir and 100 mg ritonavir BID PO

Contraindications: Hypersensitivity to lopinavir, ritonavir, or any other components in the formulation. **Do not** administer with astemizole, cisapride, flecainide, propafenone, ergot alkaloids, pimozide, midazolam, terfenadine, and triazolam; may result in serious/life-threatening events.

Warnings/Precautions: **Use with caution** in hepatic impairment (no dose adjustment information currently available), history of pancreatitis, diabetes, and hemophilia. Fatal cardiogenic shock has been reported in an infant receiving a 10-fold accidental overdose.

BSA dosing in children provides similar AUC as seen in adults but with lower trough levels; some clinicians may initiate therapy with higher LPV/RTV doses in PI-experienced pediatric patients who may have reduced PI susceptibility. Adolescent Dosing: Patients in early puberty (Tanner I–II) should be dosed with pediatric regimens and those in late puberty (Tanner IV) should be dosed with adult regimens. Those who are at the midst of their growth spurt (Tanner III females and Tanner IV males) can be dosed by either pediatric or adult regimen with close monitoring of efficacy and toxicity.

Adverse Effects: May cause diarrhea, headache, asthenia, nausea, vomiting, increase in serum lipids, and rash (in combination with other antiretroviral agents).

Drug Interactions: Ritonavir is combined with lopinavir as an adjuvant for boosting lopinavir levels and not for its antiretroviral properties. Lopinavir/ritonavir is metabolized by CYP P450 3A and also inhibits the same enzyme. Efavirenz, amprenevir and nevirapine induces metabolism of lopinavir; higher doses of lopinavir/ritonavir are necessary. Carbamazepine, dexamethasone, phenobarbital, phenytoin, rifampin, and St. John's wort may decrease lopinavir levels.

Lopinavir/ritonavir may increase effects or toxicity of atorvastatin, cerivastatin, clarithromycin, rifabutin, lidocaine, quinidine, amiodarone, cyclosporine, tacrolimus, rapamycin, calcium channel blockers, ketoconazole, itraconazole, and metronidazole. Lopinavir can decrease the effectiveness of methadone, atovaquone, and birth control pills containing ethinyl estradiol (use alternative methods). Always check the potential for other drug interactions when either initiating therapy or adding new drugs onto an existing regimen.

Drug Administration: Administer oral solution with food for better absorption. Tablets should be taken whole with or without food. If didanosine is included in the regimen, administer didanosine 1 hr prior to or 2 hr after lopinavir/ritonavir. High-fat meal increases absorption (especially with liquid dosage form).

LORACARBEF
Lorabid
Antibiotic, carbacephem

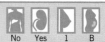

No Yes 1 B

Oral suspension: 100 mg/5 mL, 200 mg/5 mL (100 mL)
Caps: 200, 400 mg

Infant and child (6 mo–12 yr):
Acute otitis media, sinusitis: 30 mg/kg/24 hr ÷ Q12 hr PO × 10 days
Pharyngitis/tonsillitis, impetigo, skin/soft tissue infection: 15 mg/kg/24 hr ÷ Q12 hr PO × 7–10 days
≥13 yr and adult:
Uncomplicated cystitis: 200 mg PO Q24 hr × 7 days
Pharyngitis/tonsillitis, skin/soft tissue infection: 200 mg PO Q12 hr × 7–10 days
Sinusitis: 400 mg PO Q12 hr × 10 days
Pneumonia, uncomplicated pyelonephritis: 400 mg PO Q12 hr × 14 days
Bronchitis: 200–400 mg PO Q12 hr × 7 days

Contraindications: Hypersensitivity to loracarbef products and cephalosporin antibiotics.
Warnings/Precautions: Use with caution in penicillin-allergic patients and history of colitis. **Adjust dose in renal impairment (see Chapter 3).** Use suspension for acute otitis media because of higher peak plasma levels.
Adverse Effects: GI disturbances, rash and headache are common. Serum sickness has been reported.
Drug Interactions: Probenecid increases loracarbef serum levels.
Drug Administration: Administer on an empty stomach 1 hr before or 2 hr after meals.

MALARONE

See *Atovaquone ± Proguanil*

MALATHION
Ovide
Pediculicide, organophosphate

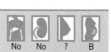

No No ? B

Lotion: 0.5% (59 mL); contains 79% isopropyl alcohol, terpineol, dipentene and pine needle oil

Pediculosis capitis:
≥6 yr and adult: Sprinkle sufficient amounts of lotion onto dry hair and rub gently until the scalp is fully wet (pay special attention to the back of head and neck). Allow the hair to dry naturally; **do not** use hair dryer. After 8–12 hr, wash the hair with a nonmedicated shampoo, rinse and use a fine-toothed comb to remove dead lice and eggs. If lice are still present, a second dose may be administered in 7–9 days.

Contraindications: Neonates and infants; and hypersensitivity to any malathion or any other ingredient in the vehicle.

MALATHION *continued*

Warnings/Precautions: Use only under the direct supervision of an adult. If skin irritation occurs, discontinue use until resolution; then reapply lotion and discontinue use if irritation reoccurs.

Adverse Effects: Contact hypersensitivity reaction and skin and scalp irritation are common.

Drug Internations: None identified.

Drug Administration: **For external use only.** Launder bedding and clothing. **Avoid contact with eyes;** flush eyes immediately with water if accidental exposure. **Do not expose lotion and wet hair to open flame or electric heat, including hair dryers,** because it contains flammable ingredients.

MARAVIROC
Selzentry
Antiviral agent, CCR5 co-receptor antagonist

Yes   No   3   B

Tabs: 150, 300 mg

> **≥17 and adult:**
> *In combination with strong CYP 450 3A inhibitors (with or without CYP 450 3A inducers) including protease inhibitors (except tipranavir/ritonavir, delavirdine):* 150 mg PO BID
> *In combination with weak or non-CYP 450 3A inducers or inhibitors (including tipranavir/ritonavir, nevirapine, all nucleoside reverse transcriptase inhibitors and enfuvirtide):* 300 mg PO BID
> *In combination with CYP 450 3A inducers (without a strong CYP 450 3A inhibitor; including efavirenz):* 600 mg PO BID

Contraindications: Have not been determined.

Warnings/Precautions: Immediately evaluate patients with signs or symptoms of hepatitis or allergic reactions following the use of maraviroc. A systemic allergic reaction (pruritic rash, eosinophilia or elevated IgE) has occurred prior to the development of hepatotoxicity.

Use caution with pre-existing liver dysfunction, hepatitis B or C, or in patients with increased risk of cardiovascular events (more cardiovascular events including myocardial ischemia/infarction were observed in patients receiving the medication). Pharmacokinetics, safety and efficacy have not been evaluated in renal and hepatic impairment.

Adverse Effects: Rash, abdominal pain, cough, pyrexia, upper respiratory infections, musculoskeletal symptoms and dizziness are common. Myocardial infarction/ischemia, cholestatic jaundice, liver cirrhosis and hepatotoxicity (including failure) have been reported.

Drug Interactions: Maraviroc is a substrate of CYP 450 3A isoenzyme and PGP transporter. Drug levels are likely to be altered by inhibitors and inducers of the aforementioned systems. Efavirenz decreases maraviroc levels, whereas lopinavir/ritonavir increases maraviroc levels.

Drug Administration: May be taken with or without food.

For explanation of icons, see p. 306.

MEBENDAZOLE
Vermox and others
Anthelmintic

Yes | No | 1 | C

Chewable tabs: 100 mg (may be swallowed whole or chewed; boxes of 12s)

Child (>2 yr) and adult:
Pinworms (Entererobius): 100 mg PO × 1, repeat in 2 wk if not cured
Hookworms, roundworms (Ascaris), and whipworm (Trichuris): 100 mg PO BID × 3 days. Repeat in 3–4 wk if not cured. Alternatively, may administer 500 mg PO ×1.
Capillariasis: 200 mg PO BID × 20 days
Visceral larva migrans (Toxocariasis): 100–200 mg PO BID × 5 days
Trichinellosis (Trichinella spiralis): 200–400 mg PO TID × 3 days, then 400–500 mg PO TID × 10 days; use with steroids for severe symptoms
Ancylostoma caninum (Eosinophilic enterocolitis): 100 mg PO BID × 3 days.
See latest edition of the AAP Red Book for additional information.

Contraindications: Hypersensitivity to mebendazole products.
Warnings/Precautions: Ineffective in hydatid disease. Experience in children <2 yr and in pregnancy is limited. Family may need to be treated as a group.
Adverse Effects: Rash, GI disturbances and headache are common. May cause diarrhea and abdominal cramping in cases of massive infection. Liver function test elevations and hepatitis have been reported with prolonged courses; monitor hepatic function with prolonged therapy.
Drug Interactions: Therapeutic effect may be decreased if administered to patients receiving carbamazepine or phenytoin.
Drug Administration: Administer doses with food. Tablets may be crushed and mixed with food, swallowed whole, or chewed.

MEFLOQUINE HCL
Lariam and others
Antimalarial

Yes | No | ? | C

Tabs: 250 mg (228 mg base)

Doses expressed in mg mefloquine HCl salt.
Malaria prophylaxis (start 1 wk prior to exposure and continue for 4 wk after leaving endemic area):
    Child (PO, administered Q weekly):
        <10 kg: 5 mg/kg
        10–19 kg: 62.5 mg (¼ tablet)
        20–30 kg: 125 mg (½ tablet)
        31–45 kg: 187.5 mg (¾ tablet)
        >45 kg: 250 mg (1 tablet)
    Adult: 250 mg PO Q weekly
Malaria treatment:
    <45 kg: 15 mg/kg ×1 PO followed by 10 mg/kg × 1 PO 8–12 hr later
    Adult: 750 mg × 1 PO followed by 500 mg × 1 PO 12 hr later
See latest edition of the AAP Red Book for additional information.

MEFLOQUINE HCL *continued*

Contraindications: Active or recent history of depression, anxiety disorders, psychosis or schizophrenia, seizures, or hypersensitivity to mefloquine, quinine or quinidine.

Warnings/Precautions: **Use with caution** in cardiac dysrhythmias and neurologic disease. May cause psychiatric symptoms, ranging from anxiety, paranoia, and depression to hallucinations and psychotic behavior. ECG abnormalities may occur when used in combination with quinine, quinidine, chloroquine, halofantrine, and beta blockers. If any of the aforementioned antimalarial drugs is used in the initial treatment of severe malaria, initiate mefloquine at least 12 hr after the last dose of any of these drugs. Monitor liver enzymes and ocular exams for therapies longer than 1 yr.

Adverse Effects: GI disturbances, dizziness, somnolence, extrasystole and bradycardia are common. May cause headache, syncope, seizures, ocular abnormalities, GI symptoms, leukopenia, and thrombocytopenia. See Warnings/Precautions section.

Drug Interactions: May reduce valproic acid levels. See Warnings/Precautions section.

Drug Administration: **Do not** take on an empty stomach. Administer with at least 240 mL (8 oz) water. Treatment failures in children may be related to vomiting of administered dose. If vomiting occurs less than 30 min after the dose, administer a second full dose. If vomiting occurs 30–60 min after the dose, administer an additional half-dose. If vomiting continues, monitor patient closely and consider alternative therapy.

MELARSOPROL
Arsobal, Mel B, Melarsen Oxide-BAL
Antiprotozoal agent, trypanosomicidal agent

Yes   Yes   ?   ?

AVAILABLE FROM THE U.S. CENTERS FOR DISEASE CONTROL AND PREVENTION (404-639-3670 Monday-Friday 8:00 am–4:30 pm EST or 404-639-2888 evenings, weekends or holidays)
Injection: 180 mg/5 mL; contains propylene glycol

African trypanosomiasis:
Child: Total dose of 18–25 mg/kg IV administered over a 1 mo period as follows. Start at 0.36 mg/kg/24 hr QD, gradually increasing to a **maximum** of 3.6 mg/kg/24 hr at intervals of 1–5 days for a total of 9 or 10 doses.
Adult: 3.6 mg/kg/dose IV QD × 3 days; **max. dose:** 180–200 mg/24 hr. This regimen can be repeated 3–4 times with a 1 wk interval between treatment courses.

Contraindications: Hypersensitivity to melarsoprol.
Warnings/Precautions: **Use with caution** in G6PD deficiency, renal (primary renal excretion; no dosing recommendation available) or hepatic insufficiency and leprosy. Use during febrile episodes have been associated with a reactive arsenical encephalopathy; use during infuenza epidemics is considered **contraindicated.** Crosses the blood-brain barrier; CSF concentration is ~50-fold lower than serum.

Adverse Effects: Jarissch-Herxheimer-like reaction, peripheral neuropathy, phlebitis, reactive arsenical encephalopathy, and local swelling at injection site are common. Hepatic dysfunction, hypertension, arrhythmias, myocardial damage, allergic reactions, exfoliative dermatitis and renal dysfunction have been reported.

Continued

MELARSOPROL *continued*

Drug Interactions: None identified.
Drug Administration: Have patient in the supine, fasting state during and several hr after dose. Administer dose by slow IV injection. Drug is incompatible with water. To reduce incidence of reactive encephalopathy, prednisolone 1 mg/kg/dose PO QD (**max. dose:** 40 mg) starting the day before the first dose and continued through the second course. Taper prednisolone over 3 days after the second course. Reinitiate the same initial dose on the day prior to the third course and discontinue over 3 days.

MEROPENEM
Merrem
Carbapenem antibiotic

No   Yes   ?   B

Injection: 0.5, 1 g
Contains 3.92 mEq Na/g drug

Neonate: 20 mg/kg/dose IV using the following dosage intervals:
   <7 days old: Q12 hr
   ≥7 days old:
      1.2 –2 kg: Q12 hr
      >2 kg: Q8 hr
Infant >3 mo and child:
   Skin and subcutaneous tissue infections: 30 mg/kg/24 IV ÷ Q8 hr; **max. dose:** 1.5 g/24 hr
   Intra-abdominal and mild/moderate infections: 60 mg/kg/24 hr IV ÷ Q8 hr; **max. dose:** 3 g/24 hr
   Meningitis and severe infections: 120 mg/kg/24 hr IV ÷ Q8 hr; **max. dose:** 6 g/24 hr
Adult:
   Skin and subcutaneous tissue infections: 1.5 g/24 hr IV ÷ Q8 hr
   Intra-abdominal and mild/moderate infections: 3 g/24 hr IV ÷ Q8 hr
   Meningitis and severe infections: 6 g/24 hr IV ÷ Q8 hr

Contraindications: Patients sensitive to carbapenems, or with a history of anaphylaxis to beta-lactam antibiotics.
   Warnings/Precautions: Use with caution in meningitis and CNS disorders (may cause seizures) and renal impairment **(adjust dose; see Chapter 3).** Drug penetrates well into the CSF.
Adverse Effects: Diarrhea, nausea, headache and injection site inflammation are common. Dermatological reactions, including Stevens-Johnson syndrome and TEN, neutropenia, leukopenia, hepatic enzyme and bilirubin elevation, and angioedema have been reported. Thrombocytopenia has been reported in patients with renal dysfunction.
Drug Interactions: Probenecid may increase serum meropenem levels. May reduce valproic acid levels.
Drug Administration: For IV push, infuse over 3–5 min at a concentration of 50 mg/mL. For intermittent infusion, infuse over 15–30 min at a concentration ≤50 mg/mL. Reconstituted IV solutions have short stability times; consult with a pharmacist.

FORMULARY

METHENAMINE PREPARATIONS
Hiprex, Urex, and Methenamine mandelate
NOTE: Many methenamine combination products
are also available.
Urinary germicide

Yes   Yes   2   C

Methenamine hippurate (Hiprex, Urex):
 Tabs: 1 g (Hiprex contains tartrazine)
Methenamine mandelate:
 Tabs: 0.5, 1 g
 Enteric coated tabs: 0.5, 1 g
 Oral suspension: 0.5 g/5 mL (480 mL)

Methenamine hippurate:
 Child (6–12 yr): 500–1000 mg/dose PO BID. Alternatively, 25–50 mg/kg/24
 hr PO ÷ Q12 hr has been recommended.
  >12 yr–adult: 1000 mg/dose PO BID
Methenamine mandelate:
 Child (6–12 yr): 500 mg/dose PO QID. Alternatively, 50–75 mg/kg/24 hr PO ÷
 Q6 hr has been recommended.
 Adult: 1000 mg/dose PO QID

Contraindications: Renal insufficiency and severe hepatic impairment; severe
dehydration; hyperphosphatemia; and hypersensitivity to any components in
the formulation. Concurrent sulfonamide use; may form an insoluable
precipitate. Use as a single agent for acute infections with parenchymal involvement.
Warnings/Precautions: Methenamine is hydrolyzed by acidic urine to form
bactericidal formaldehyde and ammonia. *Proteus* or *Pseudomonas* (urea-splitting
organisms) may be resistant to methenamine by inhibiting the release of
formaldehyde; acidification of urine is essential.
 Use only after eradication of urinary tract infection by other appropriate
antimicrobial agents. Large doses have caused bladder irritation, painful and frequent
micturition, proteinuria and gross hematuria. **Use with caution** in gout (may cause
urate crystals in urine) and pre-existing liver disease (worsen by increased ammonia
production).
Adverse Effects: Nausea, upset stomach, dysuria and rash are common. GI
disturbances may be transient or severe enough to discontinue therapy or reduce the
dosage. Headache, dyspnea, bladder irritation and pruritus have been reported.
Drug Interactions: Urinary alkalinizers and sulfonamides may decrease
methenamine's effects. May falsely increase urinary levels of
17-hydroxycorticosteroids, catecholamines and vanillylmandelic acid; and falsely
decrease urinary tests for 5-hydroxyindoleacetic acid and certain pregnancy tests.
Drug Administration: Take with food to minimize GI upset. Acidification of the urine
with ascorbic acid or cranberry juice is recommended to enhance the drug's effect.
Avoid excessive intake of alkalinizing foods and medications such as milk products,
bicarbonate, acetazolamide.

For explanation of icons, see p. 306.

METRONIDAZOLE
Flagyl, Flagyl ER, Protostat, MetroGel, MetroLotion,
MetroCream, Noritate, MetroGel-Vaginal, and others
Antibiotic, antiprotozoal

Yes   Yes   3   B

Tabs: 250, 500 mg
Tabs, extended release (Flagyl ER): 750 mg
Caps: 375 mg
Oral suspension: 20 mg/mL ☑ or 50 mg/mL ☑
Injection: 500 mg; contains 830 mg mannitol/g drug
Ready to use injection: 5 mg/mL (100 mL); contains 28 mEq Na/g drug
Gel, topical (MetroGel): 0.75% (28, 45 g)
Lotion (MetroLotion): 0.75% (60 mL); contains benzyl alcohol
Cream, topical:
    MetroCream: 0.75% (45 g); contains benzyl alcohol
    Noritate: 1% (30 g)
Gel, vaginal (MetroGel-Vaginal): 0.75% (70 g with 5 applicators)

Amebiasis:
    Child: 35–50 mg/kg/24 hr PO ÷ TID × 10 days
    Adult: 500–750 mg/dose PO TID × 10 days
Anaerobic infection:
    Neonate: PO/IV:
      <7 days:
        <1.2 kg: 7.5 mg/kg/dose Q48 hr
        1.2–2 kg: 7.5 mg/kg/dose Q24 hr
        ≥2 kg: 15 mg/kg/24 hr ÷ Q12 hr
      ≥7 days:
        <1.2 kg: 7.5 mg/kg Q24 hr
        1.2–2 kg: 15 mg/kg/24 hr ÷ Q12 hr
        ≥2 kg: 30 mg/kg/24 hr ÷ Q12 hr
    Infant/child/adult:
      IV/PO: 30 mg/kg/24 hr ÷ Q6 hr
      Max. dose: 4 g/24 hr
Other parasitic infections:
    Infant/child: 15–30 mg/kg/24 hr PO ÷ Q8 hr
    Adult: 250 mg PO Q8 hr or 2 g PO × 1
Bacterial vaginosis:
    Adolescent and adult:
      PO: 500 mg BID × 7 days or 2 g × 1dose
      Vaginal: 5 g (1 applicator-ful) BID × 5 days
Giardiasis:
    Child: 15 mg/kg/24 hr PO ÷ TID × 5 days; **max. dose:** 750 mg/24 hr
    Adult: 250 mg PO TID × 5 days
Trichomoniasis (treat sexual contacts):
    Child: 15 mg/kg/24 hr PO ÷ TID × 7 days
    Adolescent/adult: 2 g PO × 1 or 250 mg PO TID or 375 mg PO BID × 7 days
C. difficile infection (IV may be less efficacious):
    Child: 30 mg/kg/24 hr ÷ Q6 hr PO/IV x 10 days
    Adult: 250–500 mg TID-QID PO × 10–14 days, or 500 mg Q8 hr IV × 10–14 days
H. pylori infection (use in combination amoxicillin and bismuth subsalicylate):
    Child: 15–20 mg/kg/24 hr ÷ BID PO × 4 wk
    Adult: 250–500 mg TID PO × 14 days

METRONIDAZOLE *continued*

Inflammatory bowel disease (as alternative to sulfasalazine):
    Adult: 400 mg BID PO
Topical use: Apply and rub a thin film to affected areas at the following frequencies specific to product concentration.
    0.75% cream: BID
    1% cream: QD

> ***Contraindications:*** **Avoid** use in first-trimester of pregnancy. Hypersensitivity to metronidazole or any other components in the formulation.
> ***Warnings/Precautions:*** **Use with caution** in patients with CNS disease, blood dyscrasias, and severe liver or renal disease (GFR <10 mL/min; **see Chapter 3).** Patients should **not** ingest alcohol for 24–48 hr after dose (disulfiram-type reaction). For intravenous use in all ages, some references recommend a 15 mg/kg loading dose. If using single 2 g dose in a breastfeeding mother, discontinue breastfeeding for 12–24 hr to allow excretion of the drug.
> ***Adverse Effects:*** Nausea, vomiting, diarrhea, ataxia, dizziness, headache, worsening of candidiasis, metallic taste and peripheral neuropathy are common. May discolor urine. Leukopenia, thrombocytopenia and ototoxicity have been reported.
> ***Drug Interactions:*** May increase levels or toxicity of phenytoin, lithium, and warfarin. Phenobarbital and rifampin may increase metronidazole metabolism. Alcohol may cause disulfiram-like reactions.
> ***Drug Administration***
>   PO: Give on an empty stomach but may be given with food if GI upset occurs. **Do not** crush extended-release tablets.
>   IV: For intermittent infusion, infuse over 60 min at a concentration of 5–8 mg/mL.
>   Intravaginal: Use vaginal gel product only and **do not** apply to the eye.
>   Topical: Treated areas should be cleansed before drug application.

MICAFUNGIN SODIUM
Mycamine
Antifungal, echinocandin

Yes   Yes   ?   C

Injection: 50, 100 mg; contains lactose

> ***Premature infant >1000 g (based on single-dose pharmacokinetic and safety trial in 18 neonates, 26 ± 2.4 wk gestation):*** 5 mg/kg and 7 mg/kg doses are suggested to provide similar AUC drug exposure of adults receiving daily doses of 100 mg and 150 mg. Dosages ranging from 0.75–3 mg/kg were well tolerated in this study.
> ***Esophageal candidiasis:***
>   ***<50 kg:*** 3 mg/kg/dose IV QD; **max. dose:** 150 mg/dose
>   ***≥50 kg:*** 150 mg IV QD; mean duration for successful therapy was 15 days (range: 10–30 days).
> ***Invasive candidiasis:***
>   ***<40 kg:*** 2–3 mg/kg/dose IV QD; **max. dose:** 150 mg/24 hr
>   ***≥40 kg:*** 100–150 mg IV QD
> ***Candida prophylaxis in hematopoietic stem cell transplant:***
>   ***<50 kg:*** 1–2 mg/kg/dose IV QD; **max. dose:** 50 mg/dose
>   ***≥50 kg:*** 50 mg IV QD; mean duration 19 days (range: 6–51 days)
> ***Invasive aspergilosis (doses under investigation):***
>   ***<50 kg:*** 3–4 mg/kg/dose IV QD
>   ***≥50 kg:*** 150 mg IV QD

Continued

MICANFUNGIN SODIUM *continued*

Contraindications: Hypersensitivity to micafungin or to any component of the product.

Warnings/Precautions: Prior hypersensitivity to other echinocandins (anidulafungin, casopofungin) increases risk. Serious reactions such as anaphylactoid reactions and anaphylaxis with shock have been reported.

Use with caution in hepatic and renal impairment. No dosing adjustments are required based on race or gender, or in patients with severe renal dysfunction or mild to moderate hepatic function impairment. Effect of severe hepatic function impairment on micafungin pharmacokinetics has not been evaluated.

Adverse Effects: GI disturbances, phlebitis, rash, hyperbilirubinemia, liver function test elevation, headache, fever and rigor are common. Anemia, leukopenia, neutropenia, thrombocytopenia and hemolysis have been reported.

Drug Interactions: Micafungin is CYP 450 3A isoenzyme substrate and weak inhibitor. May increase the effects/toxicity of nifedipine and sirolimus.

Drug Administration: IV: Flush line with NS prior to IV administration. Infuse over 1 hr at a concentration of 0.5–1.5 mg/mL in NS or D_5W.

MICONAZOLE
Monistat and others; Topical products: Micatin, Lotrimin AF, and others
Antifungal, imidazole

No   No   ?   C

Cream (OTC): 2% (15, 30, 90 g)
Lotion (OTC): 2% (30, 60 mL)
Ointment (OTC): 2% (28.4 g)
Solution (OTC): 2% with alcohol (7.39, 29.57 mL)
Gel (OTC): 2% with alcohol (24 g)
Topical solution (OTC): 2% with alcohol (7.4, 29.6 mL)
Powder (OTC): 2% (70, 90 g)
Spray, liquid (OTC): 2% (105 mL); contains alcohol
Spray, powder (OTC): 2% (85, 90, 100 g); contains alcohol
Vaginal cream (OTC): 2% (15, 25, 45 g)
Vaginal suppository (OTC): 100 mg (7s), 200 mg (3s)
Vaginal combination packs:
  Monistat 1 (Rx): 1200 mg suppository (1) and 2% cream (9 g)
  M-Zole 3, Monistat 3, Vagistat-3 (OTC): 200 mg suppository (3s) and 2% cream (9 g)
  Monistat 7, M-Zole 7 (OTC): 100 mg suppository (7s) and 2% cream (9 g)

Topical: Apply BID × 2–4 wk
Vaginal: 1 applicator full of cream or 100 mg suppository QHS × 7 days or 200 mg suppository QHS × 3 days
Monistat 1: 1200 mg suppository ×1 at bedtime or during the day.

Contraindications: Hypersensitivity to miconazole or any other components in the formulation.

Warnings/Precautions: Use with caution in hypersensitivity to other imidazole antifungal agents (e.g., clotrimazole, ketoconazole). Vegetable oil base in vaginal suppositories may interact with latex products (e.g., condoms and diaphragms); consider switching to the vaginal cream. **Avoid** contact with the eyes.

MICONAZOLE *continued*

Adverse Effects: Pruritis, rash, burning, phlebitis, headaches, and pelvic cramps.
Drug Interactions: Drug is a substrate and inhibitor of the CYP 450 3A3/4 isoenzymes. Vaginal use with concomittant warfarin use has also been reported to increase warfarin's effect.
Drug Administration
Topical: Apply sparingly to cleansed and dry affected area. For intertriginous areas, rub cream gently into the skin.
Vaginal: Wash hands prior to use. Gently insert suppository or applicator full of cream high into the vagina at bedtime. Remain lying down for 30 min after administration. Wash applicator with soap and water after each use.

MINOCYCLINE
Minocin, Dynacin, Arestin, and others
Antibiotic, tetracycline derivative

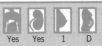

Yes   Yes   1   D

Tabs: 50, 75, 100 mg
Caps: 50, 75, 100 mg
Extended-release tabs: 45, 90, 135 mg
Caps (pellet filled): 50, 100 mg
Sustained-release microspheres (Arestin): 1 mg (12s)
Oral suspension: 50 mg/5 mL (60 mL); contains 5% alcohol

General infections:
Child (8–12 yr): 4 mg/kg/dose × 1 PO, then 2 mg/kg/dose Q12 hr PO; **max. dose:** 200 mg/24 hr
Adolescent and adult: 200 mg/dose × 1 PO, then 100 mg Q12 hr PO
Chlamydia trachomatis/Ureaplasma urealyticum:
Adolescent and adult: 100 mg PO Q12 hr × 7 days
Acne (≥12 yr–adult):
Immediate-release dosage forms: 50–100 mg PO QD-BID
Extended-release tabs:
45–59 kg: 45 mg PO QD
60–90 kg: 90 mg PO QD
91–136 kg: 135 mg PO QD

Contraindications: Hypersensitivity to minocycline, tetracyclines or any other components in the formulation.
Warnings/Precautions: **Not** recommended for children <8 yr and during the last half of pregnancy due to risk of permanent tooth discoloration. **Use with caution** in renal failure, lower dosage may be necessary.
Adverse Effects: High incidence of vestibular dysfunction (30%–90%). Nausea, vomiting, allergy, increased intracranial pressure (leading to headaches, papilledema and blurred vision), photophobia and injury to developing teeth may occur. Hepatitis, including autoimmune hepatitis, and liver failure have been reported.
Drug Interactions: Use with isotretinoin or vitamin A are **not** recommended because of added risk for increased intracranial pressure. May decrease the efficacy of live attenuated oral typhoid vaccine. May increase the effects/toxicity of warfarin. The absorption of the following elements and the absorption of minocycline may be reduced with concomitant administration: aluminum, iron, calcium, magnesium, and zinc.

Continued

MINOCYCLINE *continued*

Drug Administration: Administer tablets and pellet-filled capsules 1 hr before or 2 hr after meals. Capsule and extended-release tablets may be administered with or without food. **Do not** give with dairy products

MOXIFLOXACIN
Avelox, Avelox IV, Vigamox
Antibiotic, quinolone

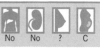

No   No   ?   C

Tabs: 400 mg
Injection, premixed ready to use bags: 400 mg in 0.8% saline (250 mL)
Ophthalmic solution (Vigamox): 0.5% (3 mL)

Adult: 400 mg PO/IV QD
Bacterial conjunctivitis:
  ≥1 yr–adult: Instill 1 drop to affected eye(s) TID × 7 days

Contraindications: Hypersensitivity to moxifloxacin, quinolones or any of the components in the formulation.
Warnings/Precautions
IV/PO: **Avoid** use in patients with QT interval prolongation (including taking other medications with the same effect), bradycardia, myocardial ischemia, or uncorrected hypokalemia. Use with corticosteroids may increase risk for tendon rupture. **Use with caution** in seizures. No dosing adjustment is necessary in renal impairment and mild/moderate hepatic insufficiency (Child Pugh Classes A and B). Has **not** been studied in patients with severe hepatic impairment (Child Pugh Class C).
Ophthalmic: **Avoid** wearing contact lens during active infection. Topical use only; **do not** inject this product.
Adverse Effects
IV/PO: GI disturbances, dizziness and headaches are common. Torsades de pointes, Stevens-Johnson syndrome, severe immune hypersensitivity reaction, tendon rupture and peripheral neuropathy have been reported.
Ophthalmic: Conjunctivitis, decreased visual acuity, dry eyes, keratitis, ocular discomfort, subconjunctival hemorrhage and tearing are common.
Drug Interactions: Use of Class IA (e.g., quinidine, procainamide) and Class III (e.g., amiodarone, sotalol) antiarrhythmics should be **avoided**. Antacids and iron, when administered close together, reduces the absorption of moxifloxacin.
Drug Administration
PO: May be taken with or without food. If patient is to receive antacids containing aluminum or magnesium, sucralfate, iron, multivitamins with zinc, or buffered didanosine, administer dose at least 4 hr before or 8 hr after.
IV: For intermittent IV infusion, infuse over 60 min with the pre-mixed concentration of 1.6 mg/mL.
Ophthalmic Drops: Apply finger pressure to lacrimal sac during and for 1–2 min after dose application.

MUPIROCIN

Bactroban, Bactroban Nasal, and others
Topical antibiotic

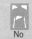

No   No   ?   B

Ointment: 2% (15, 22, 30 g); contains polyethylene glycol
Cream: 2% (15, 30 g); contains benzyl alcohol
Nasal ointment: 2% (1 g), as calcium salt

Topical:
   ≥3 mo–adult: Apply small amount TID to affected area × 5–14 days.
   Ointment may be used in infants ≥2 mo.
   Intranasal: Apply small amount intranasally 2–4 times/24 hr for 5–14 days.

Contraindications: Hypersensitivity to mupirocin products.
Warnings/Precautions: Cream is **not** intended for use in lesions >10 cm in length or 100 cm² in surface area. **Do not** use topical ointment preparation on open wounds due to concerns about systemic absorption of polyethylene glycol.
If clinical response is **not** apparent in 3–5 days with topical use, reevaluate infection.
Intranasal administration may be used to eliminate carriage of *S. aureus*, including MRSA.
Adverse Effects
   Topical: May cause minor local irritation and dry skin.
   Intranasal: Nasal stinging, taste disorder, headache, rhinitis and pharyngitis may occur.
Drug Interactions: None identified.
Drug Administration: **Avoid** contact with eyes.
   Topical: May cover treated areas with gauze dressings.
   Intranasal: Press nostrils together and release repeatedly for 1 min to improve drug distribution in the nares. Discard tube after use **(do not reuse)**.

NAFCILLIN

Unipen, Nallpen, and others
Antibiotic, penicillin (penicillinase resistant)

Yes   Yes   2   B

Caps: 250 mg
Injection: 1, 2, 10 g; contains 2.9 mEq Na/g drug
Injection, premixed in iso-osmotic dextrose: 1 g in 50 mL, 2 g in 100 mL

Neonate: IM/IV:
   ≤7 days:
      <2 kg: 50 mg/kg/24 hr ÷ Q12 hr
      ≥2 kg: 75 mg/kg/24 hr ÷ Q8 hr
   >7 days:
      <1.2 kg: 50 mg/kg/24 hr ÷ Q12 hr
      1.2–2 kg: 75 mg/kg/24 hr ÷ Q8 hr
      ≥2 kg: 100 mg/kg/24 hr ÷ Q6 hr
Infant and child:
   PO: 50–100 mg/kg/24 hr ÷ Q6 hr
   IM/IV:
      Mild to moderate infections: 50–100 mg/kg/24 hr ÷ Q6 hr
      Severe infections: 100–200 mg/kg/24 hr ÷ Q4–6 hr
      Max. dose: 12 g/24 hr

Continued

NAFCILLIN *continued*

Adult:
  PO: 250–1000 mg Q4–6 hr
  IV: 500–2000 mg Q4–6 hr
  IM: 500 mg Q4–6 hr
  Max. dose: 12 g/24 hr

Contraindications: Hypersensitivity to nafcillin, penicillins, or any other components in the formulation.
Solutions containing dextrose may be **contraindicated** in patients with known allergy to corn or corn products.
Warnings/Precautions: Allergic cross-sensitivity with penicillin. **Oral route not recommended** due to unpredictable absorption. CSF penetration is poor unless meninges are inflammed. **Use with caution** in patients with combined renal and hepatic impairment (reduce dose by 33%–50%) and cephalosporin hypersensitivity.
Adverse Effects: High incidence of phlebitis with IV dosing. May cause rash and bone marrow suppression. Acute interstitial nephritis is rare. Hypokalemia has been reported.
Drug Interactions: Nafcillin may increase elimination of cyclosporine and warfarin. Probenecid increases serum nafcillin levels. May cause false-positive urinary and serum proteins.
Drug Administration
  PO: Give on an empty stomach with water; 1 hr before or 2 hr after meals.
  IV: IV push, infuse over 5–10 min at a concentration ≤66.7 mg/mL. For intermittent infusion, infuse over 15–60 min at a concentration ≤40 mg/mL (100 mg/mL for fluid restricted patients).
  IM: Dilute with sterile water or NS to 250 mg/mL and immediately administer by deep intragluteal injection.

NAFTIFINE
Naftin Cream, Naftin Gel
Antifungal, allylamine derivative

No	No	?	B

Cream: 1% (15, 30, 60 g); contains benzyl alcohol
Gel: 1% (20, 40, 60 g); contains alcohol 52% (v/v)

Adult:
Tinea (reevaluate if no clinical effect after 4 wk):
  Cream: Gently massage into affected and surrounding skin areas QD
  Gel: Gently massage into affected and surrounding skin areas BID (morning and evening).

Contraindications: Hypersensitivity to naftifine products and to any of its components.
Warnings/Precautions: Discontinue use if excessive irritation or hypersensitivity develops. Safety and efficacy in children have not been established.
Adverse Effects: Burning/stinging, itching, local irritation, dryness and erythema are common.
Drug Interactions: None identified.
Drug Administration: **Avoid** occlusive dressings unless otherwise directed. **Avoid** contact with eyes, nose, mouth and other mucous membranes. Wash hands after application.

NELFINAVIR
Viracept, NFV
Antiviral, protease inhibitor

Yes   No   3   B

Powder, oral: 200 mg/ level teaspoonful or 50 mg/ level scoop (50 mg/g powder); contains 11.2 mg phenylalanine/g powder
Tabs: 250, 625 mg

≤6 wk (from preliminary pharmacokinetic studies): 40 mg/kg/dose PO BID was well tolerated but one-third of patients did not meet the AUC target. Higher doses are currently being studied. Administer with high-fat meals to assure absorption.
Infant–<2 yr: Effective dose not established. 30–35 mg/kg/dose PO TID (**max. dose:** 750 mg/dose) has been suggested.
2–13 yr: 45–55 mg/kg/dose PO BID (**max. dose:** 1250 mg/dose); or 25–35 mg/kg/dose PO TID (**max. dose:** 750 mg/dose)
Adolescent and adult: 1250 mg PO BID or 750 mg PO TID

Contraindications: Hypersensitivity to nelfinavir or any other components in the formulation. Do **not** coadminister with midazolam, triazolam, lovastatin, simvastatin, ergot derviatives, amiodarone, quinidine, St. John's wort or pimozide.
Warnings/Precautions: Avoid use of oral powder dosage form in patients with phenylketouria since it contains phenylalanine. All dosage forms contain ethyl methanesulfonate (EMS), an impurity formed during the manufacturing process. EMS is a potential human carcinogen. Pediatric and pregnant women **should not initiate** regimens containing nelfinavir. However, pediatric and pregnant women who are stable on nelfinavir should remain on therapy as the benefit-risk ratio remains favorable. **Noncompliance can quickly promote resistant HIV strains. Use with caution** in hepatic impairment; dosing in hepatic impairment has not been studied. Many drug-drug interactions exist; see Drug Interactions section.
Adolescent Dosing: Patients in early puberty (Tanner I–II) should be dosed with pediatric regimens and those in late puberty (Tanner IV) should be dosed with adult regimens. Adolescents who are at the midst of their growth spurt (Tanner III females and Tanner IV males) can be dosed by either pediatric or adult regimen with close monitoring of efficacy and toxicity.
Adverse Effects: Diarrhea and lipodystrophy are common. Asthenia, abdominal pain, rash, hyperglycemia, and exacerbation of chronic liver disease may occur. Spontaneous bleeding episodes in hemophiliacs have been reported.
Drug Interactions: Nelfinavir is a substrate and inhibitor of CYP 450 3A3/4; and substrate for CYP 450 2C19. Rifampin, rifabutin, nevirapine, azithromycin, phenobarbital, phenytoin, and carbamazepine can decrease nelfinavir levels. Nelfinavir can increase the effects/toxicity of rifabutin, tacrolimus, sirolimus, sildenafil and hepatically metabolized benzodiazepines (e.g., midazolam); it can decrease effects/levels of efavirenz, delavirdine, phenytoin, zidovudine, methadone and oral contraceptive effectiveness (use alternative methods). When used in combination with other protease inhibitors (PI), nelfinavir and other PI levels may increase. See Contraindications section. Always check the potential for other drug interactions when either initiating therapy or adding new drugs onto an existing regimen.
Drug Administration: Administer all doses with food; **avoid** mixing with acidic foods or juice. If didanosine is part of the antiviral regimen, nelfinavir should be administered at least 2 hr prior or 1 hr after didanosine. Oral powder dosage form may be mixed with water, milk, pudding, or formula (up to 6 hr).

NEOMYCIN SULFATE

Mycifradin, Neo-Fradin, Neo-Tabs, and others
Antibiotic, aminoglycoside; ammonium detoxicant

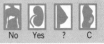

No   Yes   ?   C

Tabs (Neo-Tabs): 500 mg
Oral solution (Mycifradin, Neo-Fradin): 125 mg/5 mL; contains parabens

Diarrhea:
Preterm and newborn: 50 mg/kg/24 hr ÷ Q6 hr PO
Hepatic encephalopathy:
    Infant and child: 50–100 mg/kg/24 hr ÷ Q6–8 hr PO × 5–6 days. **Max. dose:** 12 g/24 hr
    Adult: 4–12 g/24 hr ÷ Q4–6 hr PO × 5–6 days
Bowel prep:
    Child: 90 mg/kg/24 hr PO ÷ Q4 hr × 2–3 days
    Adult: 1 g Q1 hr PO × 4 doses, then 1 g Q4 hr PO × 5 doses. (Many other regimens exist.)

Contraindications: Ulcerative bowel disease or intestinal obstruction. Hypersensitivity to neomycin or aminoglycosides.
    Warnings/Precautions: Use with caution in renal, hearing or vestibular impairment; and neuromuscular disorders. Monitor for nephrotoxicity and ototoxicity. Oral absorption is limited, but levels may accumulate. Consider dosage reduction in the presence of renal failure.
Adverse Effects: GI disturbances are common. May cause itching, redness, edema, colitis, candidiasis, or poor wound healing if applied topically. Prevalence of neomycin hypersensitivity has increased.
Drug Interactions: May potentiate oral anticoagulants and decrease the absorption of penicillin V, vitamin B_{12}, digoxin and methotrexate. Increase in adverse effects of other neurotoxic, ototoxic, or nephrotoxic drugs.
Drug Administration: Specific information not identified.

NEOMYCIN/HYDROCORTISONE OTIC PREPARATIONS

NEOMYCIN/POLYMYXIN B/HYDROCORTISONE:
Cortisporin Otic, AntibiOtic, and others
NEOMYCIN/COLISTIN/HYDROCORTISONE:
Cortisporin TC Otic
Steroid and antibiotic, otic suspension

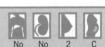

No   No   2   C

Otic suspension:
    Neomycin/Polymyxin B/Hydrocortisone: Each ml contains 3.5 mg neomycin base, 10,000 units polymyxin base and 10 mg (1%) hydrocortisone; may contain metasulfites and propylene glycol (7.5, 10 mL)
    Neomycin/Colistin/Hydrocortisone: Each one mL contains 3 mg colistin sulfate, 3.3 mg neomycin sulfate, 10 mg (1%) hydrocortisone acetate, and 0.5 mg thonzonium bromide; contains 0.002% thimerosal. (7.5 mL) See Colistimethate Sodium for intravenous colistin.

Otitis externa:
Neomycin/Polymyxin B/Hydrocortisone:
    Child: Instill 3 drops in affected ear(s) TID-QID up to a **maximum** of 10 days

NEOMYCIN/HYDROCORTISONE OTIC PREPARATIONS *continued*

Adult: Instill 4 drops in affected ear(s) TID-QID up to a **maximum** of 10 days
Neomycin/Colistin/Hydrocortisone:
Child: Instill 4 drops in affected ear(s) TID-QID up to a **maximum** of 10 days
Adult: Instill 5 drops in affected ear(s) TID-QID up to a **maximum** of 10 days

Contraindications: Hypersensitivity to any of the specific product's components in the formulation. Cutaneous viral infections.
Warnings/Precautions: **Use with caution** with sulfite allergy, perforated tympanic membrane, and chronic otitis media.
Adverse Effects: Allergic skin reactions, stinging and burning in the ear and ototoxicity have been reported. Prevalence of neomycin hypersensitivity has increased
Drug Interactions: None identified.
Drug Administration: Clean and dry the external auditory cannal with a sterile cotton applicator prior to dose. Patient should lie with the affected ear upward when instilling drops. Remain in this position for 5 min after dosing. Alternatively, a cotton wick saturated with suspension may be inserted into the ear canal. Wick should be remoistened every 4 hr and the wick should be replaced once every 24 hr.

NEOMYCIN/POLYMYXIN B/ ± BACITRACIN

Neosporin GU Irrigant, Neosporin, Neosporin
Ophthalmic, and others
Topical antibiotic

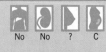

No   No   ?   C

Solution, genitourinary irrigant: 40 mg neomycin sulfate, 200,000 U polymyxin B/ mL (1, 20 mL); multidose vial contains methylparabens
In combination with bacitracin:
Ointment, topical (Neosporin) (OTC): 3.5 mg neomycin sulfate, 400 U bacitracin, 5000 U polymyxin B/g (0.9, 14, 28 g)
Ointment, ophthalmic (Neosporin Ophthalmic): 3.5 mg neomycin sulfate, 400 U bacitracin, 10,000 U polymyxin B/g (3.5 g)

Topical: Apply to minor wounds and burns QD-TID
Ophthalmic: Apply small amount to conjunctiva Q3–4 hr × 7–10 days, depending on the severity of infection.
Bladder irrigation:
Adult: Mix 1 ml in 1000 ml NS and administer via a 3-way catheter at a rate adjusted to the patient's urine output. Do not exceed 10 days of continuous use.

Contraindications: Hypersensitivity to neomycin and polymyxin B or any of its components. **Avoid** use of bladder irrigant in patients with defects in the bladder mucosa or wall.
Warnings/Precautions: **Do not** use for extended periods. May cause superinfection, delayed healing.
Adverse Effects: Ophthalmic preparation may cause stinging and sensitivity to bright light. Prevalence of neomycin hypersensitivity has increased.
Drug Administration
Topical: Apply a thin layer to the cleaned affected area. May be covered with a sterile bandage.
Ophthalmic: Instill ointment in lower conjunctival sac by avoiding contact of ointment applicator tip with eye or skin. **Avoid** contamination with the tube.

Continued

NEOMYCIN/POLYMYXIN B/± BACITRACIN *continued*

Bladder irrigation: **Do not** inject irrigant solution. Connect the container to the inflow lumen of the 3-way catheter. Connect the outflow lumen via a sterile disposable plastic tube to a disposable plastic collection bag. Continuously rinse the bladder; **do not** interrupt the inflow or rinse solution for more than a few minutes.

NEVIRAPINE
Viramune, NVP
Antiviral, non-nucleoside reverse transcriptase inhibitor

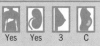

Yes   Yes   3   C

Tabs: 200 mg
Oral suspension: 10 mg/mL (240 mL); contains parabens

Neonate–2 mo: Start with 5 mg/kg/dose or 120 mg/m^2/dose QD PO × 14 days, followed by 120 mg/m^2/dose Q12 hr PO × 14 days, then 200 mg/m^2/dose Q12 hr PO

Child:

 Body surface area dosing used in the majority of clinical trials: Start with 120 mg/m^2/dose (**max. dose:** 200 mg/dose) QD PO × 14 days; if no rash or other side effects, increase dose to 120 mg/m^2/dose Q12 hr PO. Usual maintenance dose: 120–200 mg/m^2/dose Q12 hr PO; **max. dose:** 200 mg/dose Q12 hr. Children <8 yo may require higher dosages (200 mg/m^2/dose Q12 hr).

Alternative FDA approved dosing by body weight:

 2 mo–<8 yr: Start with 4 mg/kg/dose (**max. dose:** 200 mg/dose) QD PO × 14 days; if no rash or other side effects, increase dose to 7 mg/kg/dose (**max. dose:** 200 mg/dose) Q12 hr PO.

 ≥8 yr: Start with 4 mg/kg/dose (**max. dose:** 200 mg/dose) QD PO × 14 days; if no rash or other side effects, increase dose to 4 mg/kg/dose (**max. dose:** 200 mg/dose) Q12 hr PO.

Adolescent–adult: Start with 200 mg/dose QD PO × 14 days; if no rash or other side effects, increase to 200 mg/dose Q12 hr.

Prevention of vertical transmission during high-risk situations:

 Intrapartum at onset of labor: 200 mg PO × 1

 Newborn at 48–72 hr of life: 2 mg/kg/dose PO × 1. If mother did not receive intrapartum dose or received dose <1 hr before delivery, give 2 mg/kg/dose PO immediately after birth followed by second dose 48–72 hr of life.

Contraindications: Hypersensitivity to nevirapine or any of its components.
Warnings/Precautions: **Use with caution** in patients with hepatic or renal dysfunction. **Discontinue therapy** if a severe rash or a rash with fever, blistering, oral lesions, conjunctivitis or muscle aches occur.

 Life-threatening hepatotoxicity has been reported primarily during the first 12 wk of therapy. Patients with increased serum transaminase or a history of hepatitis B or C infection prior to nevirapine are at greater risk for hepatotoxicity. Women, including pregnant women, with CD$_4$ counts >250 cells/mm^3 or men with CD$_4$ counts >400 cells/mm^3 are at risk for hepatotoxicity. Monitor liver function tests and CBCs. Adolescent Dosing: Patients in early puberty (Tanner I–II) should be dosed with pediatric regimens and those in late puberty (Tanner IV) should be dosed with adult regimens. Adolescents who are at the midst of their growth spurt (Tanner III females and Tanner IV males) can be dosed by either pediatric or adult regimen with close monitoring of efficacy and toxicity. Non-compliance can quickly promote resistant HIV strains.

NEVIRAPINE *continued*

Adverse Effects: Skin rash (may be life-threatening, including Stevens-Johnson syndrome; permanently discontinue and never restart), fever, abnormal liver function tests, headache, and nausea are common. Hypersensitivity reactions have been reported. Permanently discontinue and do not restart nevirapine if symptomatic hepatitis, severe transaminase elevations, or hypersensitivity reactions occur. See Warnings/Precautions.

Drug Interactions: Induces the CYP 450 3A4 and 2B6 drug metabolizing isoenzymes and causes an autoinduction of its own metabolism within the first 2–4 wk of therapy and has the potential to interact with many drugs. Drug can decrease levels of itraconazole, ketoconazole, methadone, indinavir, ritonavir, saquinavir, and oral/other hormonal contraceptives. Rifampin and rifabutin can lower serum levels of nevirapine. Cimetidine, clarithromycin, erythromycin, ketoconazole can increase serum levels of nevirapine and are **not** recommended for use. **Carefully review the patients' drug profile for other drug interactions each time nevirapine is initiated or when a new drug is added to a regimen containing nevirapine.**

Drug Administration: Doses can be administered with food and concurrently with didanosine. If therapy is interrupted >7 days, restart therapy with initial once-daily dosing for 14 days followed by BID dosing.

NIFURTIMOX
Lampit, Bayer 2502
Antiprotozoal agent

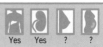

Yes   Yes   ?   ?

AVAILABLE FROM THE U.S. CENTERS FOR DISEASE CONTROL AND PREVENTION (404-639-3670 Monday-Friday 8:00 am–4:30 pm EST or 404-639-2888 evenings, weekends or holidays)
Tabs: 30, 120 mg

Trypanosomiasis:
    Child (duration of treatment: 90 days acute infection and 120 days for chronic infection):
        ≤10 yr: 15–20 mg/kg/24 hr PO ÷ TID-QID after meals
        11–16 yr: 12.5–15 mg/kg/24 hr PO ÷ TID-QID after meals
    Adolescent–adult (acute and chronic infections): 8–10 mg/kg/24 hr PO ÷ TID-QID after meals × 90–120 days

---

Contraindications: Hypersensitivity to nifurtimox.
Warnings/Precautions: **Use with caution** in hepatic and renal impairment; drug is metabolized by the liver and excreted by the kidneys (no dosing recommendations available). Risk-benefit should be considered with seizures or other neurologic disorders, G6PD deficiency, and pulmonary disease.
Adverse Effects: Anorexia, GI discomfort, rash, cutaneous reactions and arthralgias are common. Leukopenia, pancytopenia, hemolytic anemia, abnormal LFTs, pulmonary infiltrates, CNS toxicity and impotence have been reported.
Drug Interactions: None identified.
Drug Administration: May be taken with meals to minimize GI irritation. Tablets may be crushed and mixed with food.

NITAZOXANIDE
Alinia
Antiprotozoal agent

Yes　Yes　?　B

Oral suspension: 100 mg/5 mL (60 mL)
Tabs: 500 mg

 Diarrhea caused by Giardia lamblia or Cryptosporidium parvum (administer all doses with food):
    1–3 yr: 100 mg (5 mL) oral suspension Q12 hr PO × 3 days
    4–11 yr: 200 mg (10 mL) oral suspension Q12 PO × 3 days
    ≥12 yr: 500 mg tablet Q12 hr PO × 3 days

Contraindications: Hypersensitivity to nitazoxanide or any other components in the formulation.
Warnings/Precautions: **Use with caution** in hepatic or renal dysfunction; studies have **not** been completed. Has **not** been shown to be superior to placebo for the treatment of diarrhea caused by *Cryptosporidium parvum* in immunocompromised patients, including HIV. Has **not** been studied for *Giardia lamblia* in HIV or immunocompromised patients. Tablets and oral suspension are **not** bioequivalent; suspension is 70% bioavailable to the tablet.
Adverse Effects: Abdominal pain, diarrhea, headache, nausea and vomiting are common.
Drug Interactions: Drug's metabolite, tizoxanide, is highly protein bound (>99.9%); **use caution** when used with other highly protein bound drugs.
Drug Administration: Administer all doses with food; drug was administered with food in clinical trials.

NITROFURANTOIN
Furadantin, Macrodantin, Macrobid, and others
Antibiotic

No　Yes　1　B

Caps (macrocrystals; Macrodantin): 25, 50, 100 mg
Caps (dual release; Macrobid): 100 mg (25 mg macrocrystal/75 mg monohydrate)
Oral suspension (Furadantin): 25 mg/5 mL (470 mL); contains parabens and saccharin

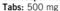 *Child (>1 mo):*
    Treatment: 5–7 mg/kg/24 hr ÷ Q6 hr PO; **max. dose:** 400 mg/24 hr
    UTI prophylaxis: 1–2 mg/kg/dose QHS PO; **max. dose:** 100 mg/24 hr
≥12 yr and adult:
    (Macrocrystals): 50–100 mg/dose Q6 hr PO
    (Dual release): 100 mg/dose Q12 hr PO
    UTI prophylaxis (macrocrystals): 50–100 mg/dose PO QHS

Contraindications: Hypersensitivity to nitrofurantoin, severe renal disease, infants <1 mo of age, GFR <60 mL/min (reduced drug distribution in the urine), and pregnant women at term.
Warnings/Precautions: **Use with caution** in G6PD deficiency, anemia, lung disease and peripheral neuropathy.
Adverse Effects: GI disturbances and loss of appetite are common. Hypersensitivity reactions, cholestatic jaundice, headache, hepatotoxicity, polyneuropathy, and hemolytic anemia may occur.

NITROFURANTOIN *continued*

Drug Interactions: Anticholinergic drugs and high-dose probenecid may increase nitrofurantoin's effects/toxicity. Magnesium salts may decrease the absorption of nitrofurantoin. Causes false-positive urine glucose with Clinitest.
Drug Administration: Give with food or milk.

NORFLOXACIN
Noroxin, Chibroxin
Antibiotic, quinolone

No   Yes   3   C

Tabs: 400 mg
Ophthalmic drops (Chibroxin): 3 mg/mL (5 mL)

   Child:
   UTI (limited data in children 5 mo–19 yr): 9–14 mg/kg/24 hr PO ÷ Q12 hr; **max. dose:** 800 mg/24 hr. For UTI prophylaxis, give 2–6 mg/kg/24 hr.
Adult:
   UTI: 400 mg PO Q12 hr (× 7–10 days for uncomplicated cases and × 10–21 days for complicated cases)
   Prostatitis: 400 mg PO Q12 hr × 28 days
   N. gonorrheae (uncomplicated): 800 mg PO × 1
Ophthalmic
   ≥1 yr–adult: 1–2 drops QID × ≤7 days. May give up to Q2 hr for severe infections during the first day of therapy.

Contraindications: Hypersensitivity to norfloxacin or other quinolones. History of tendinitis or tendon rupture associated with quinolone use.
   Warnings/Precautions: Use with caution in children <18 yr, seizures, proarrhythmic conditions, diabetes, patients receiving Class Ia or Class III antiarrhythmics and impaired renal function **(adjust dose in renal failure, see Chapter 3).** Like other quinolones, there is concern regarding development of arthropathy. Use with corticosteroids may increase risk for tendon rupture. Does **not** adequately treat chlamydia co-infections. UTI dosing can be used for BK virus nephropathy in immunocompromised patients.
Adverse Effects
   PO: GI disturbances, headache and dizziness are common. QTc prolongation, peripheral neuropathy, myasthenia gravis exacerbation and tendon rupture have been reported.
   Ophthalmic dosage form may cause local burning or discomfort, photophobia and bitter taste.
Drug Interactions: Inhibits CYP 450 1A2. May increase serum cyclosporine and theophylline levels; and prolong PT in patients on warfarin. Probenecid may increase norfloxacin's effects/toxicity. Nitrofurantoin may decrease norfloxacin's antibacterial effects.
Drug Administration
   PO: Administer oral doses on an empty stomach. If administering with iron, zinc, aluminum or magnesium containing products, sulcralfate or buffered didanosine, administer dose 2 hr before or after.
   Ophthalmic drops: Apply finger pressure to lacrimal sac during and for 1–2 min after dose application.

FORMULARY

For explanation of icons, see p. 306.

NYSTATIN
Mycostatin, Nilstat, and others
Antifungal agent

No No 1 C

Tabs: 500,000 U
Troches/pastilles: 200,000 U
Oral suspension: 100,000 U/mL (5, 60, 480 mL)
Cream/ointment: 100,000 U/g (15, 30 g)
Topical powder: 100,000 U/g (15, 30 g)
Vaginal tabs: 100,000 U (15s)

Oral:
> *Preterm infant:* 0.5 mL (50,000 U) to each side of mouth QID
> *Term infant:* 1 mL (100,000 U) to each side of mouth QID

Child/adult:
> *Suspension:* 4–6 mL (400,000–600,000 U) swish and swallow QID
> *Troche:* 200,000–400,000 U 4–5 times/24 hr

Vaginal:
> *Adolescent and adult:* 1 tab QHS × 14 days

Topical: Apply to affected areas BID-QID

Contraindications: Hypersensitivity to nystatin products.
Warnings/Precautions: Treat until 48–72 hr after resolution of symptoms. Drug is poorly absorbed through the GI tract. **Do not** swallow troches whole (allow to dissolve slowly).
Adverse Effects: May produce diarrhea and GI side effects; especially with large systemic doses. Local irritation, contact dermatitis and Stevens-Johnson syndrome have been reported.
Drug Interactions: None identified.
Drug Administration
> Suspension: Should be swished about the mouth and retained in the mouth as long as possible before swallowing.
> Troche: Dissolve slowly in mouth. **Do not** chew or swallow whole.
> Topical: Apply liberally to affected areas.
> Vaginal: Insert tablet into applicator with the pointed side up. Tablet may be wetted with warm water or water-soluble lubricating gel. Insert applicator into vagina as far as possible and push the plunger all the way in. Remove applicator and wash with warm soapy water.

OFLOXACIN
Floxin, Floxin Otic, Ocuflox, and others
Antibiotic, quinolone

Yes Yes 1 C

Otic solution (Floxin Otic): 0.3% (5, 10 mL)
Ophthalmic solution (Ocuflox): 0.3% (1, 5, 10 mL)
Tabs: 200, 300, 400 mg
Prediluted injection in D$_5$W: 200 mg/50 mL, 400 mg/100 mL

Otitis externa:
> *1–12 yr:* 5 drops to affected ear(s) BID × 10 days
> *≥12 yr:* 10 drops to affected ear(s) BID × 10 days

O

OFLOXACIN *continued*

Chronic suppurative otitis media:
≥**12 yr:** 10 drops to affected ear(s) BID × 14 days
Acute otitis media with tympanostomy tubes:
1–12 yr: 5 drops to affected ear(s) BID × 10 days
Ophthalmic use:
>1 yr: 1–2 drops to affected eye(s) Q2–4 hr × 2 days, then QID for an
additional 5 days
Systemic use (adult; see remarks):
Lower respiratory tract and skin infections: 400 mg PO/IV Q12 hr × 10 days
UTI: 200 mg PO/IV Q12 hr × 10 days
Prostatitis: 300 mg PO/IV Q12 hr × 6 wk; **maximum** IV use at 10 days, convert
to PO

Contraindications: Hypersensitivity to ofloxacin or other fluoroquinolones.
Warnings/Precautions: Use with caution in children <18 yr, seizures,
diabetes, proarrhythmic conditions, and in patients receiving Class Ia or Class
III antiarrhythmics. Like other quinolones, there is concern regarding development of
arthropathy. Use with corticosteroids may increase risk for tendon rupture. **Not
recommended** for gonorrhea because of potential resistance.
Adjust dose in severe renal (see Chapter 3) or hepatic impairment (**max. dose:**
400 mg/24 hr) with systemic use.
Levofloxacin, the S-isomer of ofloxacin, has replaced systemic ofloxacin because
of a more favorable side effect profile.
Adverse Effects: Pruritus, rash, GI disturbances, dizziness, headache and insomnia
are common with systemic use. Pruritus, local irritation, taste perversion, dizziness,
earache have been reported with otic use. Ocular burning/discomfort is frequent with
ophthalmic use.
Drug Interactions: Inhibits CYP 450 1A2. May increase effects/toxicity of
cyclosporine, theophylline, methylxanthines, warfarin, and glyburide. Antacids
containing aluminum, magnesium, and/or calcium, sucralfate, metal cations (e.g.,
zinc, iron) and didanosine decreases ofloxacin's absorption. Probenecid may increase
ofloxacin levels. See Warnings/Precautions section.
Drug Administration
PO: Administer oral doses on an empty stomach. If administering with iron, zinc,
aluminum or magnesium containing products, sulcralfate or buffered didanosine,
administer dose 2 hr before or after.
IV: For intermittent infusion, infuse over 60 min at a concentration of 4 mg/mL.
Otitic Solution: Warm solution by holding the bottle in the hand for 1–2 min.
Cold solutions may result in dizziness. For otitis externa, patient should lie with
affected ear upward before instillation and remain in the same position after dose
administration for 5 min to enhance drug delivery. For acute otitis media with
tympanostomy tubes, patient should lie in the same position prior to instillation
and the tragus should be pumped 4 times after the dose to assist in drug delivery
to the middle ear.
Ophthalmic Drops: Apply finger pressure to lacrimal sac during and for 1–2 min
after dose application. Remove contact lenses prior to administration. Lenses may
be reinserted 15 min after administration.

OSELTAMIVIR PHOSPHATE
Tamiflu
Antiviral

No   Yes   ?   C

Caps: 75 mg
Oral suspension: 12 mg/mL (25 mL); contains saccharin and sodium benzoate

 Treatment of influenza (initiate therapy within 2 days of onset of symptoms):
   Child ≥1 yr: See following table

Weight (kg)	Dosage for 5 Days	Volume of Oral Suspension (mL)
≤15	30 mg PO BID	2.5
>15–23	45 mg PO BID	3.75
>23–40	60 mg PO BID	5
>40	75 mg PO BID	6.25

   ≥12 yr and adult: 75 mg PO BID × 5 days.
Prophylaxis of influenza (see remarks):
   ≥13 yr and adult: 75 mg PO QD for a minimum of 7 days and up to 6 wk;
   initiate therapy within 2 days of exposure.

Contraindications: Hypersensitivity to oseltamivir or any other component of
the product.
   Warnings/Precautions: Currently indicated for the treatment of influenza A and
B strains. **Do not** use in children <1 yr due to concerns of fatalities related to
excessive CNS penetration in 7-day-old rats. Self-injury and delirium in children have
been reported. **Adjust dose in renal impairment; see Chapter 3.** Dosage adjustments
in hepatic impairment, severe renal impairment (GFR <10 mL/min) and dialysis have
not been established for either treatment or prophylaxis use. The safety and efficacy
of repeated treatment or prophylaxis courses have **not** been evaluated.
Prophylaxis Use: Oseltamivir is not a substitute for annual flu vaccination. Safety and
efficacy have been demonstrated for ≤6 wk; duration of protection lasts for as long
as dosing is continued. Adjust prophylaxis dose if GFR is 10–30 mL/min to 75 mg
PO QOD.
Adverse Effects: Nausea and vomiting generally occur within the first 2 days and are
the most common adverse effects. Insomnia, vertigo, seizures, neuropsychiatric
events (may result in fatal outcomes), arrhythmias, rash, and toxic epidermal
necrolysis have also been reported.
Drug Interactions: Probenecid increases oseltamivir levels. Oseltamivir decreases the
efficacy of the nasal influenzae vaccine (fluMist); discontinue oseltamivir 48 hr before
and do not restart for at least 1–2 wk after fluMist administration.
Drug Administration: Doses may be administered with or without food.

FORMULARY

OXACILLIN
Various generic brands
Antibiotic, penicillin (penicillinase resistant)

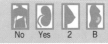

| No | Yes | 2 | B |

Oral solution: 250 mg/5 mL (100 mL); contains 0.8 mEq Na per 250 mg drug and may contain saccharin
Injection: 0.5, 1, 2, 10 g
Injection, premixed in iso-osmotic dextrose: 1 g/50 mL, 2 g/50 mL
Injectable products contain 2.8–3.1 mEq Na per 1 g drug

Neonate: IM/IV:
  ≤7 days:
    <1.2 kg: 50 mg/kg/24 hr ÷ Q12 hr
    <1.2–2 kg: 50–100 mg/kg/24 hr ÷ Q12 hr
    ≥2 kg: 75–150 mg/kg/24 hr ÷ Q8 hr
  >7 days:
    <1.2 kg: 50 mg/kg/24 hr ÷ Q12 hr
    1.2–2 kg: 75–150 mg/kg/24 hr ÷ Q8 hr
    ≥2 kg: 100–200 mg/kg/24 hr ÷ Q6 hr
Infant and child:
  Oral: 50–100 mg/kg/24 hr ÷ Q6 hr
  IM/IV: 100–200 mg/kg/24 hr ÷ Q4–6 hr
  Max. dose: 12 g/24 hr
Adult:
  Oral: 500–1000 mg/dose Q4–6 hr
  IM/IV: 250–2000 mg/dose Q4–6 hr

Contraindications: Hypersensitivity to oxacillin and penicillin products.
Warnings/Precautions: Use with caution with cephalosporin allergy and renal impairment **(adjust dose in renal failure; see Chapter 3).** Use the lower end of the usual dosage range for patients with creatinine clearances <10 mL/min. CSF penetration is poor unless meninges are inflamed.
Adverse Effects: Rash and GI disturbances are common. Leukopenia, reversible hepatotoxicity, and acute interstitial nephritis have been reported. Hematuria and azotemia have occurred in neonates and infants with high doses. May cause false-positive urinary and serum proteins.
Drug Interactions: Probenecid increases serum oxacillin levels. Tetracycline may antagonize the bacteriacidal effects of oxacillin.
Drug Administration
  PO: Should be administered on an empty stomach.
  IV: For IV push, infuse over 10 min at a concentration ≤100 mg/mL. For intermittent infusion, infuse over 15–30 min at a concentration ≤40 mg/mL.
  IM: Dilute with sterile water to 167 mg/mL and inject dose into a large muscle mass.

OXICONAZOLE
Oxistat
Antifungal agent, imidazole

| No | No | ? | B |

Cream: 1% (15, 30, 60 g)
Lotion: 1% (30 mL)
Both preparations contain propylene glycol, cetyl alcohol, stearyl alcohol, and 0.2% benzoic acid.

Continued

OXICONAZOLE *continued*

Pityriasis versicolor: Apply cream to affected and surrounding areas QD × 2 wk.
Tinea corporis, tinea cruris, and tinea pedis: Apply cream or lotion to affected and surrounding areas QD-BID; treat tinea corporis and tinea cruris for 2 wk and tinea pedis for 1 mo.

Contraindications: Hypersensitivity to oxiconazole or any other components in the formulation.
Warnings/Precautions: Discontinue use when experiencing a reaction suggesting of sensitivity, chemical or epidermal irritation.
Hyper- or hypo-pigmented patches on the trunk extending to the neck, arms and upper thighs may occur with pityriasis versicolor. Pigment restoration may take months after successful therapy.
Adverse Effects: Erythema, pruritus, and burning/stinging sensation are common. Folliculitis, papules, fissure, maceration, rash and nodules have been reported.
Drug Interactions: None identified.
Drug Administration: Avoid contact to eyes, vagina and other mucous membranes. Wash hands after applying dose.

PALIVIZUMAB
Synagis
Monoclonal antibody

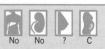

| No | No | ? | C |

Injection, solution: 100 mg/mL (0.5, 1 mL; single use); contains glycine and histidine.

RSV prophylaxis (see latest edition of the AAP Red Book for most recent indications):
Chronic lung disease ≥2 yr, premature infants (≤ 28 wk gestation) <12 mo of age, premature infants (29–32 wk gestation) <6 mo of age, or hemodynamicallly significant cyanotic and acyanotic congenital heart disease ≤2 yr: 15 mg/kg/dose IM Q monthly just prior to and during the RSV season.

Contraindications: History of a severe reaction to palivizumab or other components in the product.
Warnings/Precautions: Use with caution in patients with thrombocytopenia or any coagulation disorder because of IM route of administration. IM is currently the only route of administration. RSV season is typically November through April in the northern hemisphere but may begin earlier or persist later in certain communities. Palivizumab is currently indicated for RSV prophylaxis in high-risk infants only. Efficacy and safety have **not** been demonstrated for treatment of RSV.
Adverse Effects: Rhinitis, rash, pain, increased liver enzymes, pharyngitis, cough, wheeze, diarrhea, vomiting, conjunctivitis and anemia have been reported at slightly higher incidences when compared to placebo. Anaphylaxis and acute hypersensitivity reactions have been reported.
Drug Interactions: Does **not** interfere with the response to routine childhood vaccines (e.g., measles, mumps, rubella, and varicella).
Drug Administration: Each dose should be administered IM in the anterolateral aspect of the thigh. Divide doses with total injection volumes >1 mL. **Avoid** injection in the gluteal muscle because of risk for damage to the sciatic nerve.

PARA-AMINOSALICYLIC ACID
Paser Granules, Aminosalicylic acid, PAS
Antituberculosis agent

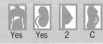

| Yes | Yes | 2 | C |

Oral granules, delayed-release: 4 g/packet; does not contain any sodium or sugar

Tuberculosis:
    Child: 150 mg/kg/24 hr PO ÷ TID; **max. dose:** 12 g/24 hr
    Adult: 4 g PO TID

Contraindications: Hypersensitivity to aminosalicylic acid products and end-stage (severe) renal disease.
Warnings/Precautions: **Not recommended** in patients with severe renal failure. **Use with caution** in hepatic insufficiency (drug not well tolerated), peptic ulcer disease, and impaired renal function. Consider maintenance vitamin B_{12} for therapies ≥1 mo. Crystalluria may be prevented by the maintaining a neutral or an alkaline pH of the urine. **Do not use** product if the package is swollen or the granules are dark brown or purple.
Adverse Effects: GI disturbances are common. Immune hypersensitivity reaction, rash with fever, thrombocytopenia and hepatotoxicity have been reported.
Drug Interactions: May reduce the metabolism of isoniazid and decrease the levels of digoxin, rifampin and vitamin B_{12}.
Drug Administration: Sprinkle oral granules on applesauce or yogurt, or mix granules in a glass with an acidic drink such as tomato or orange juice. **Do not use** if packet is swollen or the granules have lost their tan color, turning dark brown or purple. Store granules in the refrigerator or freezer.

PAROMOMYCIN SULFATE
Humatin
Amebicide, antibiotic (aminoglycoside)

| No | No | 1 | C |

Caps: 250 mg

Intestinal amebiasis (Entamoeba histolytica), Dientamoeba fragilis, and Giardia lamblia infection:
    Child and adult: 25–35 mg/kg/24 hr PO ÷ Q8 hr × 7 days
Tapeworm (T. saginata, T. solium, D. latum, and D. caninum):
    Child: 11 mg/kg/dose PO Q15 min × 4 doses
    Adult: 1 g PO Q15 min × 4 doses
Tapeworm (Hymenolepis nana):
    Child and adult: 45 mg/kg/dose PO QD × 5–7 days
Cryptosporidial diarrhea:
    Adult: 1.5–2.25 g/24 hr PO ÷ 3–6 × daily. Duration varies from 10–14 days to 4–8 wk. Maintenance therapy has also been used. Alternatively, 1 g PO BID × 12 wk in conjunction with azithromycin 600 mg PO QD × 4 wk has been used in patients with AIDS.

Contraindications: History of hypersensitivity reactions to paromomycin products and intestinal obstruction.
Warnings/Precautions: **Use with caution** in ulcerative bowel lesions to avoid renal toxicity via systemic absorption. Drug is generally poorly absorbed and therefore **not indicated** for sole treatment of extraintestinal amebiasis.

Continued

PAROMOMYCIN SULFATE *continued*

Adverse Effects: GI disturbances are common. Hematuria, rash, ototoxicity and hypocholesterolemia have been reported. Bacterial overgrowth of nonsusceptible organisms, including fungi, may occur.
Drug Interactions: May decrease the effects of digoxin.
Drug Administration: Administer doses with or after meals.

PENCICLOVIR
Denavir
Antiviral, topical

No　No　?　B

Cream: 1% (1.5 g); contains propylene glycol

Herpes labialis:
≥12 yr and adult: Apply to affected areas Q2 hr while awake × 4 days. Initiate therapy ASAP (during the prodrome or when lesions appear).

Contraindications: Hypersensitivity to the penciclovir, famciclovir, or any of its components.
　Warnings/Precautions: Not recommended for use on mucous membranes due to the lack of data. **Avoid** contact with eyes since it can cause irritation. Efficacy has **not** been evaluated in immunocompromised patients and children <12 yr.
Adverse Effects: Headache and erythema are common. Application site reaction, rash, taste perversion, and hypesthesia have been reported.
Drug Interactions: None identified.
Drug Administration: Apply topically to affected lesions of the lips and surrounding skin and rub gently until the cream disappears.

PENICILLIN G PREPARATIONS—
AQUEOUS POTASSIUM AND SODIUM
Pfizerpen and others
Antibiotic, aqueous penicillin

No　Yes　2　B

Injection (K⁺): 5, 20 million units (contains 1.7 mEq K and 0.3 mEq Na/1 million units Pen G)
Premixed frozen injection (K⁺): 1 million units in 50 mL dextrose 4%; 2 million units in 50 mL dextrose 2.3%; 3 million units in 50 mL dextrose 0.7% (contains 1.7 mEq K and 0.3 mEq Na/1 million units Pen G)
Injection (Na⁺): 5 million units (contains 2 mEq Na/1 million units Pen G)
Conversion: 250 mg = 400,000 U

Neonate (IM/IV):
≤7 days:
　　≤2 kg: 50,000–100,000 U/kg/24 hr ÷ Q12 hr
　　>2 kg: 75,000–150,000 U/kg/24 hr ÷ Q8 hr
>7 days:
　　<1.2 kg: 50,000–100,000 U/kg/24 hr ÷ Q12 hr
　　1.2–2 kg: 75,000–150,000 U/kg/24 hr ÷ Q8 hr
　　≥2 kg: 100,000–200,000 U/kg/24 hr ÷ Q6 hr
Group B streptococcal meningitis:
　　≤7 days: 250,000–450,000 U/kg/24 hr ÷ Q8 hr
　　>7 days: 450,000–500,000 U/kg/24 hr ÷ Q4–6 hr
Congenital syphilis: 150,000 U/kg/24 hr ÷ Q12 hr

PENICILLIN G PREPARATIONS—AQUEOUS POTASSIUM AND SODIUM *continued*

Infant and child (IM/IV): 100,000–400,000 U/kg/24 hr ÷ Q4–6 hr; **max. dose:** 24 million U/24 hr.

    Congenital syphilis and neurosyphilis: 200,000–300,000 U/kg/24 hr ÷ Q4–6 hr; **max. dose:** 24 million U/24 hr. Duration: × 10 days for congenital syphilis and × 10–14 days for neurosyphilis

Adult (IM/IV): 4–24 million U/24 hr ÷ Q4–6 hr

    Neurosyphilis: 18–24 million U/24 hr ÷ Q4 hr × 10–14 days

---

Contraindications: Hypersensitivity to penicillin or any of its components.

Warnings/Precautions: **Use with caution** in cephalosporin hypersensitivity. For meningitis, use higher daily dose at shorter dosing intervals. For the treatment of anthrax (*Bacillus anthracis*), see www.bt.cdc.gov for additional information. Use penicillin V potassium for oral use. **Adjust dose in renal impairment (see Chapter 3).** Consider the amount of potassium and/or sodium to be provided with the corresponding dosage. Preparations contain potassium and/or sodium salts which may alter serum electrolytes.

Adverse Effects: Eosinophilia is common. Anaphylaxis, urticaria, hemolytic anemia, seizures (renal failure, infants, meningitis and seizure history) and interstitial nephritis, and Jarisch-Herxheimer reaction (syphilis) have been reported.

Drug Interactions: Tetracyclines, chloramphenicol and erythromycin may antagonize penicillin's activity.

    Probenecid increases penicillin levels. May cause false-positive or negative urinary glucose (Clinitest method), false-positive direct Coombs' test, and false-positive urinary and/or serum proteins.

Drug Administration

    IV: For intermittent infusion, infuse over 15–30 min at a concentration 50,000 U/mL for neonates and infants and 100,000–500,000 U/mL for older patients.

    IM: Dilute with sterile water or NS to 50,000–1,000,000 U/mL.

**PENICILLIN G
PREPARATIONS—BENZATHINE**
Bicillin L-A
Antibiotic, penicillin (very long-acting IM)

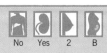

No   Yes   2   B

Injection: 600,000 U/mL (1, 2, 4 mL); contains parabens and povidone
Injection should be IM only.

Group A streptococci:
Infant and child: 25,000–50,000 U/kg/dose IM × 1. **Max. dose:** 1.2 million U/dose
    OR
    >1 mo and <27 kg: 600,000 U/dose IM × 1
    ≥27 kg and adult: 1.2 million U/dose IM × 1

Rheumatic fever prophylaxis:
Infant and child: 25,000–50,000 U/kg/dose IM Q3–4 wk. **Max. dose:** 1.2 million U/dose
Adult: 1.2 million U/dose IM Q3–4 wk or 600,000 U/dose IM Q2 wk

Syphilis:
Neonate, asymptomatic congenital syphilis: 50,000 U/kg/dose IM × 1
Infant and child:
    Congenital syphilis: 50,000 U/kg/dose IM Q wk × 3 doses to be given following a 10 day course of aqueous penicillin (immediate release) IV. Some

Continued

PENICILLIN G PREPARATIONS—BENZATHINE *continued*

experts recommend the aforementioned IM regimen to patients with minimal clinical manifestations (normal CSF and negative VDRL test of CSF).
Primary, secondary, and early latent syphilis: 50,000 U/kg/dose IM × 1; **max. dose:** 2.4 million U/dose
Late latent syphilis or latent syphilis of unknown duration: 50,000 U/kg/dose IM Q wk × 3 doses; **max. dose:** 2.4 million U/dose
Adult:
Primary, secondary, and early latent syphilis: 2.4 million U/dose IM × 1; divide dose into 2 injection sites
Late latent syphilis or latent syphilis of unknown duration: 2.4 million U/dose IM Q wk × 3 doses; divide dose into 2 injection sites

Contraindications: Hypersensitivity to any of the penicillins or any other components in the formulation.
Warnings/Precautions: Use with caution in renal failure. **For intramuscular use only. Use with caution** in asthma, significant allergies and cephalosporin hypersensitivity. Provides sustained levels for 2–4 wk.
Adverse Effects: Rash, urticaria, injection site reaction, fever and Jarisch-Herxheimer reaction (syphilis) are common.
Drug Interactions: Tetracyclines, chloramphenicol and erythromycin may antagonize penicillin's activity. Probenecid increases penicillin levels. May cause false-positive or negative urinary glucose (Clinitest method), false-positive direct Coombs' test, and false-positive urinary and/or serum proteins.
Drug Administration: **Deep IM administration only. Do not administer intravenously (cardiac arrest and death may occur) and do not inject into or near an artery or nerve (may result in permanent neurological damage).** Administer in the midlateral aspect of the thigh for neonates, infants, and small children. Administer in the upper quadrant of the buttock for adults.

PENICILLIN G PREPARATIONS—PENICILLIN G BENZATHINE AND PENICILLIN G PROCAINE

No   Yes   2   B

Bicillin C-R, Bicillin C-R 900/300
Antibiotic, penicillin (very long-acting IM)

Bicillin CR: 300,000 U Pen G procaine + 300,000 U Pen G benzathine/mL to provide 600,000 U penicillin per 1 mL (1, 2 mL tubex, 4 mL syringe)
Bicillin CR (900/300): 150,000 U Pen G procaine + 450,000 U Pen G benzathine/mL (2 mL tubex)
All preparations contain parabens and povidone.
Injection should be for IM use only.

Dosage based on total amount of penicillin.
Group A streptococci:
Child < 14 kg: 600,000 U/dose IM × 1
Child 14–27 kg: 900,000–1,200,000 U/dose IM × 1
Child >27 kg and adult: 2,400,000 U/dose IM × 1

PENICILLIN G PREPARATIONS—PENICILLIN G BENZATHINE AND PENICILLIN G PROCAINE *continued*

Contraindications: Hypersensitivity to procaine or to any penicillin.
Warnings/Precautions: Use with caution in renal failure, asthma, significant allergies, and cephalosporin hypersensitivity. **Do not use** this product to treat syphilis because of potential treatment failure. The addition of procaine penicillin has not been shown to be more efficacious than benzathine alone. However, it may reduce injection discomfort.
For intramuscular use only; do not administer IV. This preparation provides early peak levels in addition to prolonged levels of penicillin in the blood.
Adverse Effects: Injection site reaction is common. Immune hypersensitivity reaction has been reported.
Drug Interactions: Tetracyclines, chloramphenicol and erythromycin may antagonize penicillin's activity. Probenecid increases penicillin levels. May cause false-positive or false-negative urinary glucose (Clinitest method), false-positive direct Coombs' test, and false-positive urinary and/or serum proteins.
Drug Administration: **Deep IM administration only. Do not administer intravenously (cardiac arrest and death may occur) and do not inject into or near an artery or nerve (may result in permanent neurologic damage).** Administer in the midlateral aspect of the thigh for neonates, infants, and small children. Administer in the upper quadrant of the buttock for adults.

PENICILLIN G PREPARATIONS—PROCAINE
Wycillin and others
Antibiotic, penicillin (long-acting IM)

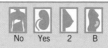

| No | Yes | 2 | B |

Injection: 600,000 U/ml (1, 2 mL); may contain parabens, phenol, povidone, and formaldehyde
Contains 120 mg procaine per 300,000 U penicillin.
Injection should be for IM use only.

Newborn (see remarks): 50,000 U/kg/dose IM QD
    Congenital syphilis: 50,000 U/kg/dose IM QD × 10 days
    Infant and child: 25,000–50,000 U/kg/24 hr ÷ Q12–24 hr IM. **Max. dose:** 4.8 million U/24 hr
Adult: 0.6–4.8 million U/24 hr ÷ Q12–24 hr IM
    Neurosyphilis: 2.4 million U IM QD and probenecid 500 mg Q6 hr PO × 10–14 days (both medications).

Contraindications: Hypersensitivity to penicillin/sulfites or procaine.
Warnings/Precautions: Use with caution in renal failure, neonates (higher incidence of sterile abscess at injection site and risk of procaine toxicity), cephalosporin hypersensitivity, asthma and significant allergies. No longer recommended for empiric treatment of gonorrhea due to resistant strains. Provides sustained levels for 2–4 days. **For intramuscular use only; do not administer IV.**
Adverse Effects: Injection site reaction, rash and urticaria are common. Immune hypersensitivity reaction has been reported.
Drug Interactions: Tetracyclines, chloramphenicol and erythromycin may antagonize penicillin's activity.

Continued

PENICILLIN G PREPARATIONS—PROCAINE *continued*

Probenecid increases penicillin levels. May cause false-positive or false-negative urinary glucose (Clinitest method), false-positive direct Coombs' test, and false-positive urinary and/or serum proteins.

Drug Administration: **Deep IM administration only. Do not administer intravenously (cardiac arrest and death may occur) and do not inject into or near an artery or nerve (may result in permanent neurologic damage).** Administer in the midlateral aspect of the thigh for neonates, infants, and small children. Administer in the upper quadrant of the buttock for adults.

PENICILLIN V POTASSIUM
Veetids and others
Antibiotic, penicillin

No Yes 2 B

Tabs: 250, 500 mg
Oral solution: 125 mg/5 mL, 250 mg/5 mL (100, 200 mL); may contain saccharin
Contains 0.7 mEq potassium/ 250 mg drug
250 mg = 400,000 U

Child: 25–50 mg/kg/24 hr ÷ Q6–8 hr PO. **Max. dose:** 3 g/24 hr
Adolescent and adult: 250–500 mg/dose PO Q6–8 hr
Acute group A streptococcal pharyngitis (see remarks):
  Child <27 kg: 250 mg PO BID–TID × 10 days
  ≥27 kg, adolescent and adult: 500 mg PO BID–TID × 10 days
Rheumatic fever prophylaxis, and pneumococcal prophylaxis for sickle cell disease and functional or anatomical asplenia (regardless of immunization status):
  2 mo–<3 yr: 125 mg PO BID
  3–5 yr: 250 mg PO BID; for sickle cell and asplenia, use may be discontinued after 5 yr of age if child received recommended pneumococcal immunizations and did not experience invasive pneumococcal infection.
Recurrent rheumatic fever prophylaxis:
  Child and adult: 250 mg PO BID

Contraindications: Hypersensitivity to penicillins.
Warnings/Precautions: **Use with caution** with cephalosporin hypersensitivity. Penicillin will prevent rheumatic fever if started within 9 days of the acute illness. The BID regimen for streptococcal pharyngitis should be used only if good compliance is expected. **Adjust dose in renal failure (see Chapter 3).** GI absorption is better than penicillin G.
Adverse Effects: Rash and GI disturbances are common. Hemolytic anemia and immune hypersensitivity reaction have been reported.
Drug Interactions: Tetracyclines, chloramphenicol and erythromycin may antagonize penicillin's activity.

Probenecid increases penicillin levels. May cause false-positive or false-negative urinary glucose (Clinitest method), false-positive direct Coombs' test, and false-positive urinary and/or serum proteins.
Drug Administration: Should be taken 1 hr before or 2 hr after meals. May be administered with food to decrease GI upset.

PENTAMIDINE ISETHIONATE
Pentam 300, NebuPent
Antibiotic, antiprotozoal

No   Yes   ?   C

Injection (Pentam 300 and others): 300 mg
Inhalation (NebuPent): 300 mg

Treatment:
Pneumocystis carinii: 4 mg/kg/24 hr IM/IV QD × 14–21 days (IV is the preferred route)
Trypanosomiasis (T. gambiense, T. rhodesiense): 4 mg/kg/24 hr IM QD × 10 days
Visceral Leishmaniasis (L. donovani, L. infantum, L. chagasi): 4 mg/kg/dose IM QD or QOD × 15–30 doses
Cutaneous Leishmaniasis (L. (V.) panamensis): 2–3 mg/kg/dose IM QD or QOD × 4–7 doses
Prophylaxis:
   Pneumocystis carinii:
      IM/IV: 4 mg/kg/dose Q2–4 wk
      Inhalation
         ≥5 yr: 300 mg in 6 ml H_2O via inhalation Q month. Use with a Respigard II nebulizer.
Max. single dose: 300 mg

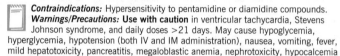

Contraindications: Hypersensitivity to pentamidine or diamidine compounds.
Warnings/Precautions: **Use with caution** in ventricular tachycardia, Stevens Johnson syndrome, and daily doses >21 days. May cause hypoglycemia, hyperglycemia, hypotension (both IV and IM administration), nausea, vomiting, fever, mild hepatotoxicity, megaloblastic anemia, nephrotoxicity, hypocalcemia and granulocytopenia.
Adjust dose in renal impairment (see Chapter 3) with systemic use.
Adverse Effects: Rash, nausea, loss of appetite, increased LFTs and nephrotoxicity (see Drug Interactions) are common with systemic use. Sterile abscess may occur at IM injection site. Aerosol administration may cause bronchospasm, cough, oxygen desaturation and dyspnea. See Warnings/Precautions section.
Drug Interactions: A substrate to CYP 450 2C19. Additive nephrotoxicity with aminoglycosides, amphotericin B, cisplatin and vancomycin may occur.
Drug Administration
   IV: Infuse over 1–2 hr to reduce risk of hypotension at a concentration ≤ 6 mg/mL.
   IM: Reconsititue 300 mg vial with 3 mL of sterile water and administer calculated dose by deep IM injection.
   Inhalation: Administer with an appropriate sized (pediatric vs. adult) nebulizer face mask and the Respigard II nebulizer.

PENTOSTAM

See *Stibogluconate*

PERMETHRIN
Elimite, Acticin, Nix, and others
Scabicidal agent

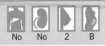

No	No	2	B

Cream (Elimite, Acticin): 5% (60 g);contains 0.1% formaldehyde
Liquid cream rinse (Nix-OTC): 1% (60 mL with comb); contains 20% isopropyl alcohol
Lotion (OTC): 1% (60 mL with comb)

Pediculus capitis, Phthirus pubis:
Head lice: Saturate hair and scalp with 1% cream rinse after shampooing, rinsing, and towel drying hair. Leave on for 10 min, then rinse. May repeat in 7–10 days. May be used for lice in other areas of the body (e.g., pubic lice) in same fashion.
Scabies (see remarks): Apply 5% cream from neck to toe (head to toe for infants and toddlers) wash off with water in 8–14 hr. May repeat in 7 days.

Contraindications: Hypersensitivity to permethrin or chrysanthemums.
Warnings/Precautions: May exacerbate pruritus, edema, and erythema. Ovicidal activity generally makes single-dose regimen adequate. However, resistance to permethrin has been reported. For either lice or scabies, instruct patient to launder bedding and clothing. For lice, treat symptomatic contacts only. For scabies, treat all contacts even if asymptomatic. The 5% cream has been used safely in children <1 mo with neonatal scabies (a 6-hr application time was utilized). Topical cream dosage form contains formaldehyde, a contact allergen.
Adverse Effects: May cause pruritus, hypersensitivity, burning, stinging, erythema, and rash.
Drug Interactions: None identified.
Drug Administration: Shake well before using. **Avoid** contact with eyes or mucous membranes during application. Dispense 60 g cream per 1 adult or 2 small children.

PHENAZOPYRIDINE HCL
Pyridium, Azo-Standard [OTC], and many others
Urinary analgesic

No	Yes	?	B

Tabs: 95 mg [OTC], 97.2 mg, 100 mg [OTC and Rx], 200 mg
Oral suspension: 10 mg/mL

UTI (use with an appropriate antibacterial agent):
Child 6–12 yr: 12 mg/kg/24 hr ÷ TID PO until symptoms of lower urinary tract irritation are controlled or 2 days.
Adult: 100–200 mg TID PO until symptoms are controlled or 2 days.

Contraindications: Hypersensitivity to phenazopyridine products and renal insufficiency (GFR <50 mL/min).
Warnings/Precautions: Medication is an urinary analgesic and does **not** treat infections. **Adjust dose in mild renal impairment (see Chapter 3)** and **avoid use** in moderate/severe impairment (GFR <50 mL/min).
Adverse Effects: Pruritus, rash, GI distress, headache are common. Colors urine orange and stains clothing. May also stain contact lenses. Anaphylactoid-like reaction, methemoglobinemia, hemolytic anemia, renal and hepatic toxicity have been reported, usually at overdosage levels.

FORMULARY

PHENAZOPYRIDINE HCL *continued*

Drug Interactions: May interfere with urinalysis tests (false-negative) based on spectrometry or color reactions.
Drug Administration: Give doses after meals.

PIPERACILLIN
Pipracil and others
Antibiotic, penicillin (extended spectrum)

| No | Yes | 2 | B |

Injection: 2, 3, 4, 40 g
Contains 1.85 mEq Na/g drug

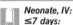

Neonate, IV:
  ≤7 days:
      ≤36 wk gestation: 150 mg/kg/24 hr ÷ Q12 hr
      >36 wk gestation: 225 mg/kg/24 hr ÷ Q8 hr
  >7 days:
      ≤36 wk gestation: 225 mg/kg/24 hr ÷ Q8 hr
      >36 wk gestation: 300 mg/kg/24 hr ÷ Q6 hr
Infant and child:
  200–300 mg/kg/24 hr IM/IV ÷ Q4–6 hr; **max. dose:** 24 g/24 hr
Cystic fibrosis:
  350–600 mg/kg/24 hr IM/IV ÷ Q4–6 hr; **max. dose:** 24 g/24 hr
Adult: 2–4 g/dose IV Q4–6 hr or 1–2 g/dose IM Q6 hr; **max. dose:** 24 g/24 hr

Contraindications: Hypersensitivity to piperacillin, penicillins, or any other components in the formulation.
  Warnings/Precautions: **Use with caution** in cephalosporin hypersensitivity. Discontinue use if bleeding manifestations should occur. **Adjust dose in renal impairment (see Chapter 3).** Cystic fibrosis patients have an increased risk for fever and rash. Like other penicillins, CSF penetration occurs only with inflamed meninges.
Adverse Effects: Thrombophlebitis, injection site pain, rash, diarrhea, headache and fever are common. Seizures (higher doses), prolonged bleeding time, bone marrow suppression, LFT elevations and acute interstitial nephritis have been reported. See Warnings/Precautions section.
Drug Interactions: Probenecid increases serum piperacillin levels. May prolong the neuromuscular blockade effects of vecuronium. May falsely lower aminoglycoside serum levels if the drugs are infused close to one another; allow a minimum of 2 hr between infusions to prevent this interaction. Coagulation parameters should be tested more frequently and monitored regularly with high doses of heparin, warfarin, or other drugs affecting blood coagulation or thrombocyte function.
Drug Administration
  IV: For IV push, infuse over 3–5 min at a concentration ≤200 mg/mL. For intermittent infusion, infuse over 30–60 min at a concentration ≤20 mg/mL.
  IM: Dilute to 400 mg/mL with sterile water, NS, or 0.5 or 1% lidocaine **without** epinephrine. Assess the potential risk/benefit for using lidocaine as a diluent.

For explanation of icons, see p. 306.

PIPERACILLIN/TAZOBACTAM
Zosyn
Antibiotic, penicillin (extended spectrum with beta-lactamase inhibitor)

No   Yes   2   B

8:1 ratio of piperacillin to tazobactam.
Injection, powder: 2 g piperacillin and 0.25 g tazobactam; 3 g piperacillin and 0.375 g tazobactam; 4 g piperacillin and 0.5 g tazobactam; 36 g piperacillin and 4.5 g tazobactam
Injection, premixed in iso-osmotic dextrose: 2 g piperacillin and 0.25 g tazobactam in 50 mL; 3 g piperacillin and 0.375 g tazobactam in 50 mL; 4 g piperacillin and 0.5 g tazobactam in 100 mL
Contains 2.35 mEq Na/g piperacillin

All doses based on piperacillin component.
Infant <6 mo: 150–300 mg/kg/24 hr IV ÷ Q6–8 hr
Infant >6 mo and children: 300–400 mg/kg/24 hr IV ÷ Q6–8 hr
Adult:
Intra-abdomininal or soft tissue infections: 3 g IV Q6 hr
Nosocomial pneumonia: 4 g IV Q6 hr
Cystic fibrosis: See Piperacillin

Contraindications: Hypersensitivity to piperacillin, tazobactam, penicillins or any other components in the formulation.
Warnings/Precautions: **Use with caution** in cephalosporin hypersensitivity or other beta-lactamase inhibitors. **Adjust dose in renal impairment (see Chapter 3).** Abnormal platelet aggregation and prolonged bleeding has been reported in patients with renal failure. Cystic fibrosis patients have an increased risk for fever and rash. Tazobactam is a beta-lactamase inhibitor, thus extending the spectrum of piperacillin. Like other penicillins, CSF penetration occurs only with inflamed meninges.
Adverse Effects: GI disturbances, pruritus, rash and headache are common. See Piperacillin and Warnings/Precautions section.
Drug Interactions: Probenecid increases serum piperacillin levels. May prolong the neuromuscular blockade effects of vecuronium. May falsely lower aminoglycoside serum levels if the drugs are infused close to one another; allow a minimum of 2 hr between infusions to prevent this interaction. Coagulation parameters should be tested more frequently and monitored regularly with high doses of heparin, warfarin, or other drugs affecting blood coagulation or thrombocyte function.
Drug Administration: IV: Infuse over 30 min at a concentration ≤200 mg/mL (piperacillin component); however, concentrations ≤20 mg/mL (piperacillin component) are preferred.

PODOFILOX
Condylox and others
Keratolytic agent

No   No   ?   C

Topical gel: 0.5% (3.5 mL); contains alcohol
Topical solution: 0.5% (3.5 mL); contains 95% alcohol

 Condyloma acuminatum (external and perianal; see remarks): Apply to affected areas Q12 hr (morning and evening) × 3 consecutive days, then withhold use for 4 consecutive days. This 1-week cycle of treatment may be repeated until there is no

PODOFILOX *continued*

visible wart tissue for a **maximum** of 4 cycles. **Limit treatment area to no more than 10 cm² and no more than 0.5 g/24 hr.**

Contraindications: Hypersensitivity or intolerance to podofilox or to any component of the formulation.

Warnings/Precautions: **Do not** exceed the recommended method of application, frequency of application and duration of usage. Safety and efficacy are **not** established for the treatment of mucous membrane warts and in pediatric patients. **Avoid** contact with the eyes.

Adverse Effects: Pruritus, superficial ulcer of skin, pain, burning sensation, headache and inflammation are common.

Drug Interactions: None identified.

Drug Administration: Use the minimum amount necessary to cover lesion by minimizing application to surrounding tissue; allow to dry thoroughly.

Topical Gel: Apply with appilcator tip or finger. Wash hands thoroughly before and after each application.

Topical Solution: Apply with supplied cotton-tip applicator. Wash hands thoroughly after each application. Use protective occlusive dressing around wart to prevent contact with unaffected skin.

PODOPHYLLIN/PODOPHYLLUM RESIN
Podocon-25, Podofin
Keratolytic agent

| No | No | X | X |

Topical liquid: 25% podophyllum resin in tincture of benzoin (15 mL)

Podophyllin 25% solution should be applied by a physician and not dispensed to a patient. Dilute straight 25% solution with alcohol by one-third to one-half when applying near mucous membranes. Use concentrations of 5%–10% for very large lesions (>10–20 cm) to minimize toxicity risk.

Adult:

Genital warts: Apply 10%–25% solution sparingly to warts, avoiding contact with healthy tissue. For the first application, leave in contact with skin for no more than 30–40 min; subsequent applications, leave on skin for minimum time to achieve desired results (1–4 hr). After treatment, remove dried medication thoroughly with soap and water or alcohol.

Contraindications: Diabetics, patients using steroids, or with poor blood circulation. **Do not** use on bleeding warts, moles, birthmarks or unusual warts with hair growing from them. **Use is not recommended during pregnancy.**

Warnings/Precautions: **For external use only.** Podophyllum is caustic and a severe irritant; **avoid contact with the eyes. Do not** use for perianal or mucous membrane warts. Differentiate wart from squamous cell carcinoma and Bowenoid papulosis; podophyllum is not indicated.

Adverse Effects: Pruritus, superficial skin ulceration, burning sensation, inflammatory disorder and localized pain are common.

Drug Interactions: None identified.

Drug Administration: Thoroughly cleanse affected area. Use applicator to apply sparingly to lesion. **Avoid** contact with healthy tissue, eyes, or mucous membranes. After treatment, remove dried medication thoroughly with soap and water or alcohol. Use protective occlusive dressing around wart to prevent contact with unaffected skin.

FORMULARY

For explanation of icons, see p. 306.

POLYMYXIN B SULFATE AND BACITRACIN

See *Bacitracin ± Polymyxin B*

POLYMYXIN B SULFATE AND TRIMETHOPRIM SULFATE

Polytrim Ophthalmic Solution and various
Topical antibiotic (ophthalmic preparations listed)

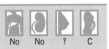

No   No   ?   C

Ophthalmic solution: Polymyxin B sulfate 10,000 U, trimethoprim sulfate 1 mg/mL (10 mL); some preparations may contain 0.04 mg/mL benzalkonium chloride

 ≥2 mo and adult: Instill 1 drop in the affected eye(s) Q3 hr (**maximum of 6 doses/24 hr**) × 7–10 days.

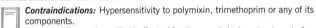

Contraindications: Hypersensitivity to polymixin, trimethoprim or any of its components.
Warnings/Precautions: **Not indicated** for the prophylaxis or treatment of ophthalmia neonatorum.
Adverse Effects: Local irritation consisting of redness, burning, stinging, and/or itching is common. Hypersensitivity reactions consisting of lid edema, itching, increased redness, tearing, and/or circumocular rash have been reported.
Drug Interactions: None identified.
Drug Administration: For ophthalmic use only. **Avoid** contaminating the applicator tip. Apply finger pressure to lacrimal sac during and for 1–2 min after dose application.

POLYMYXIN B SULFATE, NEOMYCIN SULFATE, AND HYDROCORTISONE

Cortisporin Otic, AK-Spore H.C. Otic, PediOtic, and many others
Topical antibiotic (otic and ophthalmic preparations listed)

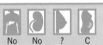

No   No   ?   C

Otic solution or suspension: Polymyxin B sulfate 10,000 U, neomycin sulfate 5 mg (3.5 mg neomycin base), hydrocortisone 10 mg/mL (10 mL); some preparations may contain thimerosol and metabisulfite.
Ophthalmic suspension: Polymyxin B sulfate 10,000 U, neomycin sulfate 5 mg (3.5 mg neomycin base), hydrocortisone 10 mg/mL (7.5 mL); may contain thimerosol and propylene glycol

 Otitis externa:
    ≥2 yr–adult: 3–4 drops TID-QID × 7–10 days; see remarks for drug administation.
Ophthalmic:
    Adolescent and adult: Instill 1–2 drops into the affected eye(s) Q3–4 hr

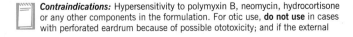

Contraindications: Hypersensitivity to polymyxin, neomycin, hydrocortisone or any other components in the formulation. For otic use, **do not use** in cases with perforated eardrum because of possible ototoxicity; and if the external

POLYMYXIN B SULFATE, NEOMYCIN SULFATE, AND HYDROCORTISONE
continued

auditory canal disorder is suspected or known to be due to cutaneous viral infection (e.g., HSV or varicella).

Warnings/Precautions: Neomycin may cause sensitization. Prolonged treatment may result in overgrowth of nonsusceptible organisms and fungi.

Otic: **Use with caution** in chronic otitis media and when the integrity of the tympanic membrane is in question. Metabisulfite-containing products may cause allergic reactions to susceptible individuals.

Ophthalmic: **Use with caution** in glaucoma.

Adverse Effects: May cause cutaneous sensitization.

Otic: Hypersensitivity (itching, skin rash, redness, swelling, or other sign of irritation in or around the ear) may occur.

Ophthalmic: Blurred vision, burning and stinging may occur. Increased intraocular pressure and mycosis may occur with prolonged use.

Drug Interactions: None identified.

Drug Administration: Shake suspension well before use.

Otic: Warm the medication to body temperature prior to use. Instill drops directly into the affected ear(s). Alternatively, if preferred, a cotton wick may be saturated and inserted into ear canal. Moisten wick with antibiotic every 4 hr. Change wick Q24 hr.

Ophthalmic: **Avoid** contact/contamination with eye dropper tip. Apply finger pressure to lacrimal sac during and for 1–2 min after dose application.

POLYTRIM OPHTHALMIC SOLUTION

See *Polymyxin B Sulfate and Trimethoprim Sulfate*

POSACONAZOLE
Noxafil
Antifungal, triazole

Yes   No   ?   C

Oral suspension: 40 mg/mL; with calibrated dosing spoon marked for doses of 2.5 and 5 mL

Treatment of oropharyngeal candidiasis:
    Adult: 100 mg (2.5 mL) PO BID × 1 day, followed by 100 mg PO QD × 13 days.

Treatment of oropharyngeal candidiasis refractory to fluconazole and/or itraconazole:
    Adult: 400 mg (10 mL) PO BID; duration of therapy should be based on severity of the patient's underlying disease and clinical response.

Prophylaxis of disseminated candidiasis or aspergillus infection in severely immunocompromised patients:
    ≥13 yr and adult: 200 mg (5 mL) PO TID; duration of therapy should be based on recovery from neutropenia or immunosuppression.

Contraindications: Hypersensitivity to posaconazole or to any of the excipients. **Avoid** coadministration with ergot alkaloids; and **avoid** CYP 3A4 substrates (e.g., terfenadine, astemizole, cisapride, pimozide, halofantrine, or quinidine) because this may increase the plasma concentrations of the drugs, leading to QTc prolongation and rare occurrence of torsades de pointes.

Warnings/Precautions: **Use with caution** hepatic impairment (studies have not been completed), hematologic malignancies (may precipitate severe hepatic reactions),

Continued

For explanation of icons, see p. 306.

POSACONAZOLE *continued*

hypersensitivity to other azoles, and patients with potentially proarrhythmic conditions. Monitor hepatic function at the start and during the course of therapy. Active against Zygomycetes.

Adverse Effects: Abdominal pain, diarrhea, nausea and vomiting are common. Prolonged QT interval, adrenal insufficiency, cholestasis, hyperbilirubinemia, increased LFTs, liver failure and seizures have been reported.

Drug Interactions: Drug is an ihhibitor of the CYP 450 3A4 isoenzyme; may increase the effects/toxicity of HMG-CoA reductase inhibitors (e.g., atorvastatin), cyclosporine, sirolimus, tacrolimus, phenytoin, midazolam, rifabutin. vincristine and vinblastine. See Contraindications section for additional interactions. Drug is primarily metabolized via UDP glucuronidation and a substrate for p-glycoprotein (P-gp) efflux. Rifabutin, phenytoin and cimetidine may decrease posaconazole levels and use should be **avoided** unless benefit outweighs the risks.

Drug Administration: Shake oral suspension well before each use. Administer each dose with a full meal or liquid nutritional supplement for optimal absorption. Consider an alternative antifungal agent if patient is unable to eat a full meal or tolerate an oral nutritional supplement. Use the provided measuring spoon and rinse with water after each use.

POTASSIUM IODIDE
Iostat, Pima, SSKI, ThyroShield, and many others
Antithyroid agent

No   Yes   2   D

Tabs (Iostat): 65, 130 mg
Syrup (Pima): 325 mg/5 mL (473 mL, 4000 mL); contains 249 mg iodine per 5 mL
Solution (ThyroShield) [OTC]: 65 mg/mL (30 mL); contains parabens
Saturated solution (SSKI): 1000 mg/mL (30, 240 mL); 10 drops = 500 mg potassium iodide
Lugol's (Strong Iodine) Solution: Potassium iodide 100 mg per mL in combination with iodine 50 mg per mL (120, 473 mL)
Potassium content: 6 mEq (234 mg) K^+/gram potassium iodide

Cutaneous or lymphocutaneous sporotrichosis (see remarks):
Child and adult: Start with 250 mg PO TID. Doses may be gradually increased as tolerated to the following **maximum** doses:
   Child maximum: 1250–2000 mg PO TID
   Adult maximum: 2000–2500 mg PO TID

Contraindications: Pregnancy, iodide hypersensitivity, hyperkalemia, hypothyroidism, and iodine-induced goiter.

Warnings/Precautions: **Use with caution** in thyroid disease, cardiac disease and renal failure. May cause acne flare-up. Monitor thyroid function tests. Use in breastfeeding may cause transient hypothyroidism to infant.

   For sporotrichosis, treat for 4–6 wk after lesions have completely healed. Increase dose until either maximum dose is achieved or signs of intolerance appear.

Adverse Effects: GI disturbance, metallic taste, rash, salivary gland inflammation, headache, lacrimation and rhinitis are symptoms of iodism. Paresthesia and immune hypersensitivity reaction have been reported.

Drug Interactions: Lithium carbonate and iodide-containing medications may have synergistic hypothyroid activity. Potassium-containing medications, potassium-sparing diuretics, and ACE inhibitors may increase serum potassium levels.

Drug Administration: Dilute strong iodine solution with large amounts of water, milk, broth or fruit juice to improve taste. Give with milk or water after meals.

PRAZIQUANTEL
Biltricide
Anthelmintic

Yes   No   3   B

Tab: 600 mg (tri-scored)

Child and adult:
Schistosomiasis:
   S. haematobium, S mansoni: 20 mg/kg/dose PO BID × 1 day
   S. japonicum, S. mekongi: 20 mg/kg/dose PO TID × 1 day
Flukes:
   Clonorchis sinensis, Fasciolopsis buski, Heterophyes heterophyes,
   Metagonimus yokogawai, Metrochis conjunctus, Opisthorchis viverrini: 25
   mg/kg/dose PO Q8 hr × 1 day
   Nanophyetus salmincola: 20 mg/kg/dose PO Q8 hr × 1 day
   Paragonimus westermani: 25 mg/kg/dose PO Q8 hr × 2 days
Cysticercosis (Taenia solium): 50–100 mg/kg/24 hr PO ÷ Q8 hr × 30 days
(dexamethasone may be added to regimen for 2–3 days to minimize
inflammatory response)
Tapeworms:
   Diphyllobothrium latum, Taenia saginata, Taenia solium, Dipylidium
   canium: 5–10 mg/kg/dose PO × 1 dose
   Hymenolepis nana: 25 mg/kg/dose PO × 1 dose

Contraindications: Hypersensitivity to praziquantel or ocular cysticercosis.
Warnings/Precautions: **Use with caution** in patients with severe hepatic
disease, history of seizures, or cardiac irregularities. Hospitalize patients being
treated for schistosomiasis or fluke infection associated with cerebral cysticercosis.
Adverse Effects: Abdominal pain, dizziness, drowsiness, headache and malaise are
common. Seizures, cardiac dysrhythmia, heart block, intracranial hypertension and
increased CSF protein have been reported. Hyperthermia has occurred in patients
treated for neurocysticercosis.
Drug Interactions: Carbamazepine, phenytoin, rifampin and chloroquine may
decrease praziquantel's effects. Cimetidine may increase praziquantel's effects.
Alcohol may increase CNS depression.
Drug Administration: Take with food. **Do not** chew tablets due to bitter taste.

PRIMAQUINE PHOSPHATE
Various generic brands
Antimalarial

No   No   ?   C

Tabs: 26.3 mg (15 mg base)

Doses expressed in mg of primaquine base.
Malaria:
   Prevention of relapses for P. vivax or P. ovale only (initiate therapy during
   the last 2 wk of, or following a course of, suppression with chloroquine or
   comparable drug):
      Child: 0.5 mg/kg/dose (**max. dose:** 30 mg/dose) PO QD × 14 days
      Adult: 30 mg PO QD × 14 days

Continued

PRIMAQUINE PHOSPHATE *continued*

> *Prevention of chloroquine-resistant strains (initiate 1 day prior to departure and continue until 3–7 days after leaving endemic area):*
> *Child:* 0.5 mg/kg/dose PO QD; **max. dose** 30 mg/24 hr
> *Adult:* 30 mg PO QD
> *Pneumocystis carinii pneumonia (in combination with clindamycin):*
> *Adult:* 30 mg PO QD × 21 days

Contraindications: Granulocytopenia (e.g., rheumatoid arthritis, lupus erythematosus) and bone marrow suppression. **Avoid use** with quinacrine and with other drugs which have a potential for causing hemolysis or bone marrow suppression.

Warnings/Precautions: **Use with caution** in G6PD and NADH methemoglobin-reductase deficient patients due to increased risk for hemolytic anemia and leukopenia, respectively. Use in pregnancy is **not recommended** by the AAP Red Book. Cross sensitivity with iodoquinol.

Adverse Effects: May cause headache, visual disturbances, nausea, vomiting and abdominal cramps. Hemolytic anemia, leukopenia and methemoglobinemia have been reported.

Drug Interactions: Quniacrine may increase primaquine toxicity; **avoid use**.

Drug Administration: Administer all doses with food to mask bitter taste.

PYRANTEL PAMOATE
Antiminth, Reese's Pinworm, Pamix, Pin-Rid, and Pin-X
Anthelmintic

Yes	No	?	C

Oral suspension (OTC): 50 mg/mL pyrantel base (144 mg/mL pyrantel pamoate) (30, 60 mL)
Liquid (OTC): 50 mg/mL pyrantel base (144 mg/mL pyrantel pamoate) (30 mL); may contain parabens
Caps (OTC) and tabs (OTC): 62.5 mg pyrantel base (180 mg pyrantel pamoate)

All doses expressed in terms of pyrantel base.
Child and adult:
> *Ascaris (roundworm) and Trichostrongylus:* 11 mg/kg/dose PO × 1
> *Enterobius (pinworm):* 11 mg/kg/dose PO × 1. Repeat same dose 2 wk later.
> *Hookworm or eosinophilic enterocolitis:* 11 mg/kg/dose PO QD × 3 days
> *Moniliformis:* 11 mg/kg/dose PO × 1. Repeat twice 2 wk apart.
> **Max. dose (all indications):** 1 g/dose

Contraindications: Hypersensitivity to pyrantel or any of its components. **Do not** use in combination with piperazine because of antagonism.

Warnings/Precautions: **Use with caution** in liver dysfunction, anemia, severe malnutrition and pregnancy. Limited experience in children <2 yr.

Adverse Effects: May cause nausea, vomiting, anorexia, transient AST elevations, headaches, rash, and muscle weakness.

Drug Interactions: May increase theophylline levels. See Contraindications section.

Drug Administration: Drug may be mixed with milk or fruit juices and may be taken with food.

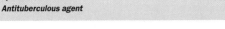

P

FORMULARY

PYRAZINAMIDE
Pyrazinoic acid amide
Antituberculous agent

 Yes   Yes   ?   C

Tab: 500 mg
Oral suspension: 10, 100 mg/mL
In combination with isoniazid and rifampin (Rifater):
   Tab: 300 mg with 50 mg isoniazid and 120 mg rifampin; contains povidone and propylene glycol

---

Tuberculosis: Use as part of a multi-drug regimen for tuberculosis. See latest edition of the AAP Red Book for recommended treatment for tuberculosis.
   Child:
      Daily dose: 20–40 mg/kg/24 hr PO ÷ QD-BID; **max. dose:** 2 g/24 hr
      Twice-weekly dose: 50 mg/kg/dose PO 2 times/wk; **max. dose:** 2 g/dose
   Adult:
      Daily dose: 15–30 mg/kg/24 hr PO ÷ QD-QID; **max. dose:** 2 g/24 hr
      Twice-weekly dose: 50–70 mg/kg/dose PO 2 times/wk; **max. dose:** 4 g/dose
Mycobacterium tuberculosis in HIV, prophylaxis to prevent first episode:
   Adolescent and adult: 15–20 mg/kg/24 hr PO QD × 2 mo in combination with either rifampin 600 mg PO QD × 2 mo or rifabutin 300 mg PO QD × 2 mo.

Contraindications: Hypersensitivity to pyrazinamide products, acute gout and severe hepatic damage.
Warnings/Precautions: **Use with caution** in patients with renal failure (dosage reduction has been recommended), liver disease, gout or diabetes mellitus. Monitor liver function tests (baseline and periodic) and serum uric acid. The CDC and ATS **do not** recommend the combination of pyrazinamide and rifampin for latent TB infections. For HIV mycobacterium tuberculosis prophylaxis and treatment, see www.aidsinfo.nih.gov for latest recommendations.
Adverse Effects: Hepatoxicity (dose related, dosages ≤30 mg/kg/24 hr minimizes effect), hyperuricemia, GI disturbances and arthralgia are common. Maculopapular rash, fever, acne, porphyria, dysuria and photosensitivity may occur.
Drug Interactions: May decrease isoniazid levels. **Severe and fatal hepatic toxicity may occur when used with rifampin.** May interfere with Acetest and Ketostix urine test to produce a pink-brown color.
Drug Administration: May be taken with or without food or milk. If using the fixed-combination product (Rifater), give 1 hr before or 2 hr after a meal with a full glass of water.

PYRETHRINS
Tisit, A-200, Pronto, RID, and others
Pediculicide

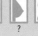 No   No   ?   C

All products are available without a prescription.
Lotion (Tisit): 0.3% pyrethrins and 2% piperonyl butoxide (59, 118 mL); contains petroleum distillate and equivalent to 1.6% ether
Gel (Tisit): 0.3% pyrethrins and 3% piperonyl butoxide (30 mL)
Shampoo (Tisit, RID, Pronto, A-200): 0.33% pyrethrins and 4% piperonyl butoxide (60, 120, 240 mL); may contain alcohol
Mousse (RID): 0.33% pyrethrins and 4% piperonyl butoxide (165 mL); contains alcohol

Continued

PYRETHRINS *continued*

 Pediculosis: Apply to hair or affected body area for 10 min, then wash thoroughly and comb with fine-tooth comb or nit-removing comb; repeat in 7–10 days.

 Contraindications: Ragweed hypersensitivity; drug is derived from chrysanthemum flowers.
Warnings/Precautions: **Do not use** near eyes, mouth, nose or vagina. Low ovicidal activity requires repeat treatment. Dead nits require mechanical removal. Wash bedding and clothing to eraticate infestation.
Adverse Effects: Local irritation including erythema, pruritus, urticaria, edema, and eczema may occur. Rare immune hypersensitivity reaction has been reported.
Drug Interactions: None identified.
Drug Administration: For topical use only. **Avoid** vaginal, eye or facial contact and PO intake. **Avoid** repeat applications in <24 hr.

PYRIMETHAMINE ± SULFADOXINE
Daraprim; in combination with sulfadoxine: Fansidar
Antiparasitic agent ± sulfonamide antibiotic

Yes Yes 2 C

Tabs: 25 mg
Oral suspension: 2 mg/mL
In combination with sulfadoxine:
　Tabs (Fansidar): Pyrimethamine 25 mg and sulfadoxine 500 mg

 PYRIMETHAMINE:
Congenital toxoplasmosis (administer with sulfadiazine; see remarks):
　Load: 2 mg/kg/24 hr PO ÷ Q12 hr × 2 days
　Maintenance: 1 mg/kg/24 hr PO QD × 2–6 mo, then 1 mg/kg/24 hr 3 times/wk to complete total 12 mo of therapy.
Toxoplasmosis (administer with sulfadiazine or trisulfapyrimidines)
　Child:
　　Load: 2 mg/kg/24 hr PO ÷ BID × 3 days; **max. dose:** 100 mg/24 hr
　　Maintenance: 1 mg/kg/24 hr PO ÷ QD-BID × 4 wk; **max. dose:** 25 mg/24 hr
　　Adults: 50–75 mg/24 hr × 3–4 wk depending on response. After response, decrease dose by 50% and continue for an additional 4–5 wk.
Toxoplasma gondii (see remarks):
　First episode prophylaxis:
　　Child ≥1 mo: 1 mg/kg/dose (**max. dose:** 25 mg) PO QD with dapsone 2 mg/kg PO QD plus leucovorin 5 mg PO Q3 days.
　　Adolescent and adult: 75 mg PO Q7 days with dapsone 200 mg PO Q7 days plus leucovorin 25 mg PO Q7 days.
　Recurrence prophylaxis:
　　Child ≥1 mo: 1 mg/kg/dose (**max. dose:** 25 mg) PO QD with sulfadiazine 85–120 mg/kg/24 hr PO ÷ BID-QID plus leucovorin 5 mg PO Q3 days.
　　Adolescent and adult: 25–50 mg PO QD with sulfadiazine 500–1000 mg PO QID, OR clindamycin 300–450 mg PO Q6–8 hr, plus leucovorin 10–25 mg PO QD.
Pneumocystis carinii:
　First episode or recurrence prophylaxis:
　　Adolescent and adult: 50–75 mg PO Q7 days with dapsone (50 mg PO QD or 200 mg PO Q7 days) plus leucovorin 25 mg PO Q7 days.

FORMULARY

PYRIMETHAMINE ± SULFADOXINE *continued*

PYRIMETHAMINE AND SULFADOXINE:
Malaria treatment (acute uncomplicated P. falciparum with suspected chloroquine resistance) >2 mo of age as a single dose PO:
    Child:
        5–10 kg: one-half tab
        11–20 kg: 1 tab
        21–30 kg: 1.5 tabs
        31–45 kg: 2 tabs
        >45 kg: 3 tabs
    Adult: 2–3 tabs
Malaria prophylaxis (for areas of chloroquine-resistant P. falciparum used as a single dose for self-treatment of febrile illness when medical care is not immediately available):
    Child:
        2–11 mo: one-fourth tab
        1–3 yr: one-half tab
        4–8 yr: 1 tab
        9–14 yr: 2 tabs
        >14 yr: 3 tabs
    Adult: 3 tabs

Contraindications: Hypersensitivity to pyrimethamine products, and megaloblastic anemia secondary to folate deficiency.
    Pyrimethamine and Sulfadoxine: In addition to preceding remarks, sulfa hypersensitivity, porphyria, severe renal or hepatic impairment, infants <2 mo, and pregnancy at term.
Warnings/Precautions: **Use with caution** in G6PD deficiency, malabsorption syndromes, alcoholism, pregnancy, and renal or hepatic impairment. Pyrimethamine is a folate antagonist. Supplementation with folinic acid leucovorin at 5–15 mg/24 hr is recommended. For congenital toxoplasmosis, see *Clin Infect Dis* 1994; 18:38–72. Most cases of acquired toxoplasmosis **do not** require specific antimicrobial therapy.
Pyrimethamine and Sulfadoxine: Effective against certain strains of *P. falciparum* that are resistant to chloroquine. Resistance has been reported in Southeast Asia, the Amazon basin, sub-Saharan Africa, Bangladesh, and Oceania.
Adverse Effects: Rash is common. Glossitis, bone marrow suppression, seizures, and photosensitivity may occur.
Pyrimethamine and Sulfadoxine: Additionally, may cause erythema multiforme, Stevens-Johnson syndrome, toxic epidermal necrolysis, GI disturbances, elevated ALT and AST and renal impairment.
Drug Interactions: Aurothioglucose, trimethoprim, and sulfamethoxazole may increase risk for blood dyscrasias. Zidovudine, methotrexate may increase risk for bone marrow suppression.
Pyrimethamine and Sulfadoxine: Aminobenzoic acid (PABA), benzocaine and tetracaine may decrease the effects of sulfadoxine.
Drug Administration: Administer doses with meals; single agent and combination product. Drink plenty of fluids when taking pyrimethamine and sulfadoxine.

For explanation of icons, see p. 306.

QUINIDINE GLUCONATE
Quinidine gluconate and various generic brands
Antiarrhythmic, class Ia

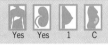

Yes   Yes   1   C

Injection: 80 mg/mL (50 mg/mL quinidine); contains phenol
Slow-release tablets: 324 mg
Quinidine gluconate salt contains 62% quinidine base

All doses expressed as salt forms.
Malaria (see remarks):
  Child and adult (give IV as gluconate; see remarks):
    Loading dose: 10 mg/kg/dose (**max. dose:** 600 mg) IV in NS over 1–2 hr followed by maintenance dose. Omit or decrease load if patient has received quinine or mefloquine.
    Maintenance dose: 0.02 mg/kg/min IV as continuous infusion until oral therapy can be initiated. If more than 48 hr of IV therapy is required, reduce dose by 30%–50%.

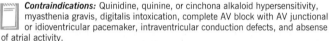

Contraindications: Quinidine, quinine, or cinchona alkaloid hypersensitivity, myasthenia gravis, digitalis intoxication, complete AV block with AV junctional or idioventricular pacemaker, intraventricular conduction defects, and absense of atrial activity.

Warnings/Precautions: **Use with caution** in renal insufficiency (15%–25% of drug is eliminated unchanged in the urine), myocardial depression, sick sinus syndrome, G6PD deficiency and hepatic dysfunction. Continuous monitoring of ECG, blood pressure and serum glucose are recommended; especially in pregnant women and young children.

To assess for possible idiosyncratic reaction to quinidine, the following test dose of **quinidine sulfate salt** administered several hours before full doses has been recommended.
    Child: 2 mg/kg PO × 1
    Adult: 200 mg PO × 1
Toxicity indicated by increase of QRS interval by ≥0.02 sec (skip dose or stop drug).

Adverse Effects: May cause GI symptoms, hypotension, tinnitus, TTP, rash, heart block and blood dyscrasias. When used alone, may cause 1:1 conduction in atrial flutter leading to ventricular fibrillation. Idiosyncratic ventricular tachycardia may occur with low levels, especially when initiating therapy. Myelosuppression, hepatotoxicity, cardiac dysrhythmia, SLE and kidney disease have been reported.

Drug Interactions: Quinidine is a substrate of cytochrome P 450 3A3/4 and 3A5–7 enzymes, and inhibitor of cytochrome P 450 2D6 and 3A3/4 enzymes. Can cause increase in digoxin levels. Quinidine potentiates the effect of neuromuscular blocking agents, beta-blockers, anticholinergics and warfarin. Amiodarone, antacids, delavirdine, diltiazem, grapefruit juice, saquinavir, ritonavir, verapamil or cimetidine may enhance the drug's effect. Barbiturates, phenytoin, cholinergic drugs, nifedipine, sucralfate, or rifampin may reduce quinidine's effect.

Drug Administration
  IV: Dilute to a concentration ≤16 mg/mL and administer at a rate ≤0.25 mg/kg/min. IV tubing length should be minimized to minimize drug adsorption to PVC tubing.
  PO: Administer with water on an empty stomach. May give with food or milk to reduce GI upset. **Avoid** administration with grapefruit juice and **do not** chew or crush slow-release tabs.

Q

QUININE SULFATE
Qualaquin and various generic products
Antimalarial agent

Yes   Yes   1   D

Caps: 200, 260, 324 (Qualaquin), 325 mg
Tabs: 260 mg

Malaria (chloroquine-resistant; in combination with doxycycline, tetracycline or clindamycin):
    Child: 30 mg/kg/24 hr PO ÷ Q8 hr × 3–7 days; **max. dose:** 2 g/24 hr
    Adult: 650 mg PO Q8 hr × 3–7 days
Babesiosis (in combination with clindamycin):
    Child: 25 mg/kg/24 hr PO ÷ Q8 hr × 7–10 days; **max. dose:** 650 mg/dose
    Adult: 650 mg PO Q8 hr × 7–10 days

Contraindications: Hypersensitivity to quinine, mefloquine or quinidine; prolonged QT interval; G6PD deficiency; myasthenia gravis; and optic neuritis.
Warnings/Precautions: **Use with caution** in asthma, heart disease, blackwater fever, tinnitus and hepatic disease. Monitor CBC, platelets, LFTs, blood glucose and administer ophthalmologic examination. **Reduce dosage** in severe chronic renal failure by administering a single load of 648 mg followed 12 hr by maintenance doses of 324 mg Q12 hr in adults for malaria (10 mg/kg/dose load followed by 5 mg/kg/dose Q12 hr in children).
Adverse Effects: Rash, hypoglycemia, headache and GI disturbances are common. DIC, thrombocytopenia, hepatotoxicity, ototoxicity, HUS and interstitial nephritis have been reported.
Drug Interactions: Quinine is a substrate and inhibitor of cytochrome P 450 3A3/4. May increase levels/effects of digoxin, neuromuscular blocking agents and oral anticoagulants. Cimetidine, ritonavir, verapamil and amiodarone may increase serum quinine levels/effects. Urinary alkalinizers and mefloquine may increase toxicity of quinine. Aluminum-containing antacids decrease quinine absorption.
Drug Administration: **Do not** crush tablets or capsule because of bitter taste. Take with food or milk to minmize GI irritation.

QUINUPRISTIN WITH DALFOPRISTIN
Synercid
Antibiotic, streptogramin

Yes   No   ?   B

Injection: 500 mg (150 mg quinupristin and 350 mg dalfopristin)

Doses expressed in mg of combined quinupristin and dalfopristin.
Child <16 yr (limited data), ≥16 yr and adult:
    Vancomycin-resistant Enterococcus faecium (VREF): 7.5 mg/kg/dose IV Q8 hr
    Complicated skin infections: 7.5 mg/kg/dose IV Q12 hr for at least 7 days
Peritonitis associated with CAPD (≥16 yr and adult): 5–10 mg/kg/dose IV Q12 hr × 14 days

Contraindications: Hypersensitivity to quinupristin/dalfopristin or prior hypersensitivity to other streptogramins.
Warnings/Precautions: **Not active** against *Enterococcus faecalis*. **Use with caution** in hepatic impairment; dosage reduction may be necessary especially with

Continued

QUINUPRISTIN WITH DALFOPRISTIN *continued*

hepatic cirrhosis (Child Pugh A or B). **Pediatric studies are incomplete.** Drug is an inhibitor to the cytochrome P 450 3A4 isoenzyme (see Drug Interactions section).
Adverse Effects: Pain, burning, inflammation and edema at the IV infusion site, thrombophlebitis, and thrombosis, GI disturbances, rash, arthralgia, myalgia, increased liver enzymes, hyperbilirubinemia, and headache are common. Dose frequency reductions (Q8 hr to Q12 hr) or discontinuation can improve severe cases of arthralgia and myalgia.
Drug Interactions: **Avoid use** with cytochrome P 450 3A4 substrates which can prolong QTc interval (e.g., cisapride). May increase the effects/toxicity of cyclosporine, tacrolimus, sirolimus, delavirdine, nevirapine, indinavir, ritonavir, diazepam, midazolam, carbamazepine, methylprednisolone, vinca alkaloids, docetaxel, paclitaxel, quinidine and some calcium channel blockers.
Drug Administration: Drug is compatible with D_5W and incompatible with saline and heparin (avoid using NS or heparin flushes). Infuse each dose over 1 hr using the following **maximum** IV concentrations: peripheral line: 2 mg/mL, central line: 5 mg/mL. If injection site reaction occurs, dilute infusion to <1 mg/mL.

RABIES IMMUNE GLOBULIN
BayRab, Imogam Rabies-HT
Immune globulin, rabies (high titer)

| No | No | 3 | C |

Injection: 150 IU/mL (2, 10 mL)

Rabies post-exposure passive immunization (with rabies vaccine and thorough wound treatment):
Child and adult: 20 IU/kg/dose × 1. See Drug Administration section in remarks for method of administration. Dose **must** be administered with or within 7 days of the first dose of rabies vaccine. Individuals previously immunized with rabies vaccine (with good titers) should **not** receive rabies immune globulin. **Do not** repeat dose of rabies immune globulin.

Contraindications: **Should not** be administered in repeated doses once vaccine treatment has been initiated. Repeating the dose may interfere with maximum active immunity expected from the vaccine.
Warnings/Precautions: **Use with caution** in patients with prior systemic reaction to other human immunoglobulin preparations, thrombocytopenia or coagulation disorders and isolated immunoglobulin A deficiency.
Adverse Effects: Injection site pain, immune hypersensitivity reaction, headache and fever are common.
Drug Interactions: Rabies immune globulin and rabies vaccine should **not** be mixed in the same syringe or injected at the same site. Response of live virus vaccines (e.g., MMR, varicella) may be reduced with rabies immune globulin; **do not** administer live vaccines within 4 mo after rabies immune globulin and revaccination is necessary in patients receiving live vaccine within 14 days before rabies immune globulin.
Drug Administration: **Do not** administer IV. **Do not** mix or inject at the same site with rabies vaccine. If possible, infiltrate the entire dose in the area around and into the wound; give the remainder of dose IM distant from vaccine administration.

RALTEGRAVIR
Isentress
HIV-1 integrase strand transfer inhibitor (HIV-1 INSTI)

No   No   3   C

Tabs: 400 mg

 Adult: 400 mg PO BID

Contraindications: Have **not** been determined.
Warnings/Precautions: **Use with caution** when using concurrent medications causing myopathy or rhabdomyolysis or in patients at risk for these effects. See Drug Intractions section for additional information. Immune reconstitution syndrome during the initial treatment period may cause an inflammatory response to indolent or residual opportunistic infections (e.g., MAC, CMV, PCP, VZV). Currently used in treatment-experienced adult patients who have HIV strains resistant to multiple antiretroviral agents. Dosing in hepatic and renal impairment have **not** been determined.
Adverse Effects: Nausea, headache, diarrhea and pyrexia are common. Myocardial infarction, anemia, neutropenia and renal failure have been reported.
Drug Interactions: Stong inducers of uridine diphosphate glucuronosyltransferase (UGT) 1A1 (e.g., rifampin) may decrease raltegravir levels.
Drug Administration: May be taken with or without food.

RETAPAMULIN
Altabax
Antibacterial, pleuromutilin

No   No   ?   B

Ointment: 1% (5, 10, 15 g)

 Impetigo due to S. aureus (methicillin susceptible) or S. pyogenes:
 ≥9 mo and adult: Apply a thin layer to affected area BID × 5 days.
Maximum dose:
 Child: 2% of total body surface area
 Adult: 100 cm² of total area

Contraindications: Have **not** been determined.
Warnings/Precautions: **Discontinue** use if sensitization or severe local irritation occurs. **For external use only; not for** intranasal, ophthalmic or intravaginal use.
Adverse Effects: Application site irritation is common. Pruritus, headache and diarrhea have been reported.
Drug Interactions: Retapamulin is a CYP 3A4 substrate.
Drug Administration: Apply a thin layer to affected area. Treated area may be covered with a sterile bandage or gauze dressing.

RIBAVIRIN
Oral: Rebetol, Copegus, Ribaspheres, and others
Inhalation: Virazole
Antiviral agent

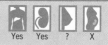
Yes   Yes   ?   X

Oral solution (Rebetol): 200 mg/5 mL (100 mL); contains sodium benzoate
Oral caps (Rebetol, Ribaspheres): 200 mg
Tabs (Copegus, Ribaspheres): 200, 400, 600 mg
Aerosol (Virazole): 6 g

Hepatitis C (PO, see remarks):
Child (≥3 yr, in combination with interferon alfa-2b at 3 million units 3 ×
per week SC using oral solution or capsule):
    25–36 kg: 200 mg BID
    37–49 kg: 200 mg QAM and 400 mg QPM
    50–61 kg: 400 mg BID
    >61 kg: Use adult dose
Dosage modification for toxicity: See remarks.
    Adult:
        Oral capsules in combination with interferon alfa-2b at 3 million units 3 ×
        per week SC:
            ≤75 kg: 400 mg QAM and 600 mg QPM
            >75 kg: 600 mg BID
        Oral capsules in combination with Peginterferon alfa-2b: 400 mg BID
        Oral tablets in combination with Peginterferon alfa-2a for hepatitis C
        genotype 1, 4:
            ≤75 kg: 500 mg BID × 48 wk
            >75 kg: 600 mg BID × 48 wk
        Oral tablets in combination with Peginterferon alfa-2a for genotype 2, 3:
        400 mg BID × 24 wk
        Dosage modification for toxicity: See remarks.
Inhalation:
    Continuous: Administer 6 g by aerosol over 12–18 hr QD for 3–7 days. The 6 g
    ribavirin vial is diluted in 300 mL preservative-free sterile water to a final
    concentration of 20 mg/mL. Must be administered with Viratek Small Particle
    Aerosol Generator (SPAG-2).
    Intermittent (for nonventilated patients): Administer 2 g by aerosol over 2 hr TID
    for 3–7 days. The 6 g ribavirin vial is diluted in 100 mL preservative-free sterile
    water to a final concentration of 60 mg/mL. The intermittent use is **not**
    recommended in patients with endotracheal tubes.

Contraindications
    Oral Ribavirin: Pregnancy, significant or unstable cardiac disease,
    autoimmune hepatitis, hepatic decompensation (Child-Pugh score >6;
    class B or C), hemoglobinpathies, and creatinine clearance <50 mL/min.
    Inhaled Ribavirin: Pregnancy and hypersensitivity to ribavirin or its components.
Warnings/Precautions
    Oral Ribavirin: Used in combination with a specific interferon alfa injection
    product for hepatitis C. **Use with caution** in pre-exisiting cardiac disease,
    pulmonary disease and sarcoidosis. Suicidal ideation has been reported to be
    higher in adolescent and pediatric patients. Reduce or discontinue dosage for
    toxicity as follows:

RIBAVIRIN *continued*

Patient with no cardiac disease:
  Hgb <10 g/dL and ≥8.5 g/dL:
    Child: 7.5 mg/kg/dose PO QD
    Adult:
      Capsule or solution: 600 mg PO QD
      Tablet: 200 mg PO QAM and 400 mg PO QPM
  Hgb <8.5 g/dL: Discontinue therapy permanently.
Patient with cardiac disease:
  ≥2 mg/dL decrease in Hgb during any 4 wk period during therapy:
    Child: 7.5 mg/kg/dose PO QD
    Adult:
      Capsule or solution: 600 mg PO QD
      Tablet: 200 mg PO QAM and 400 mg PO QPM
  Hgb <12 g/dL after 4 wk of reduced dose: Discontinue therapy permanently
Inhaled Ribavirin: Use for RSV is controversial and not routinely indicated.
Aerosol therapy may be considered for selected infants and young children at
high risk for serious RSV disease (see recommendations in *Pediatrics* 1996;
97:137–140 and most recent edition of the AAP Red Book). **Avoid** unnecessary
occupational exposure to ribavirin due to its teratogenic effects. Drug can
precipitate in the respiratory equipment especially with mechanical ventilators.
Sudden deterioration of respiratory function has been reported.

Adverse Effects
  Oral Ribavirin: Anemia (see dose modification for toxicity), insomnia, depression,
  anxiety, irritability, fatigue and GI disturbances are common. Suicidal behavior
  has been reported. Tinnitus, hearing loss, vertigo and severe hypertriglyceridemia
  have been reported in combination with interferon. Dry mouth and
  dental/periodontal disorders have been reported with long-term use.
  Inhaled Ribavirin: Worsening respiratory distress, rash, conjunctivitis, mild
  bronchospasm, hypotension, anemia and cardiac arrest may occur.

Drug Interactions: Oral Ribavirin: May decrease the effects of zidovudine, stavudine;
and increase risk for lactic acidosis with nucleoside analogues (adefovir, didanosine,
lamivudine, stavudine, zalcitabine, or zidovudine).

Drug Administration
  Oral Ribavirin: Administer tablets with food. Capsules and oral solution may be
  administered with or without food.
  Inhaled Ribavirin: Administer with SPAG-2 small particle aerosol generator in a
  well ventilated room (≥6 changes/hr). **Do not** mix with other aerosolized
  medications. Use of one-way valves in inspiratory lines, breathing circuit filter in
  the expiratory line and frequent monitorin and filter replacement have been
  recommended for mechanically ventillated patients.

RIFABUTIN
Mycobutin
Antituberculous agent, rifamycin

   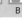

| No | Yes | 3 | B |

Caps: 150 mg
Suspension: 10, 20 mg/mL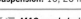

> *MAC prophylaxis for first episode and recurrence of opportunistic disease in HIV*
> *(may be in combination with a macrolide antibiotic; see www.aidsinfo.nih.gov/*
> *guideline):*
>   *<6 yr:* 5 mg/kg/24 hr PO QD; **max. dose:** 300 mg/24 hr

Continued

RIFABUTIN *continued*

>**≥6 yr and adult:** 300 mg PO QD; doses may be administered as 150 mg PO BID if GI upset occurs.

MAC prophylaxis for recurrence of opportunistic disease in HIV (in combination with ethambutol and a macrolide antibiotic):
>*Infant and child:* 5 mg/kg/24 hr PO QD; **max. dose:** 300 mg/24 hr
>*Adolescent and adult:* 300 mg PO QD

MAC treatment:
>*Child:* 5–10 mg/kg/24 hr PO QD; **max. dose:** 300 mg/24 hr as part of a multi-drug regimen.
>*Adult:* 300 mg PO QD; may be used in combination with azithromycin and ethambutol.
>>*In combination with non-nucleoside reverse transcriptase inhibitors:*
>>>*With efavirenz:* 450 mg PO QD or 600 mg PO 3 × per wk
>>>*With nevirapine:* 300 mg PO 3 × per wk
>>*In combination with protease inhibitors:*
>>>*With amprenavir, indinavir, or nelfinavir:* 150 mg PO QD or 300 mg PO 3 × per wk.
>>>*With ritonavir boosted regimens (e.g., saquinavir/ritonavir, or lopinavir/ritonavir):* 150 mg PO QOD or 150 mg PO 3 × per wk

Contraindications: Clinically significant hypersensitivity to rifabutin or to any other rifamycins.

Warnings/Precautions: Should **not** be used for MAC prophylaxis with active TB. **Use with caution** in renal failure. **Adjust dose in renal impairment (see Chapter 3).**

Adverse Effects: GI distress, discoloration of skin and body fluids (brown-orange color) and rash are common. May permanently stain contact lenses. Uveitis can occur when using high doses (>300 mg/24 hr in combination with macrolide antibiotics. Bone marrow suppression and SLE have been reported.

Drug Interactions: Induces cytochrome P 450 3A iso-enzyme and is structurally similar to rifampin (similar drug interactions, see Rifampin). Clarithromycin, fluconazole, itraconazole, nevirapine and protease inhibitors increase rifabutin levels. Efavirenz may decrease rifabutin levels. May decrease effectiveness of dapsone, delavirdine, nevirapine, amprenavir, indinavir, nelfinavir, saquinavir, itraconazole, warfarin, oral contraceptives, digoxin, cyclosporin, ketoconazole and narcotics.

Drug Administration: Doses may be administered with food if patient experiences GI intolerance.

RIFAMPIN
Rimactane, Rifadin, and others
Antibiotic, antituberculous agent, rifamycin

Yes Yes 1 C

Caps: 150, 300 mg
Oral suspension: 10, 15, 25 mg/mL
Injection: 600 mg

Staphylococcus aureus infections (as part of synergistic therapy with other anti-staphylococcal agents):
>*0–1 mo:*
>>*IV:* 10–20 mg/kg/24 hr ÷ Q12 hr
>>*PO:* 10–20 mg/kg/dose Q24 hr
>*>1 mo:* 10–20 mg/kg/24 hr ÷ Q12 hr IV/PO; **max. dose:** 600 mg/24 hr
>*Adult:* 300–600 mg Q12 hr IV/PO

FORMULARY

RIFAMPIN *continued*

Prosthetic valve endocarditis: 300–400 mg Q8 hr IV/PO in combination with antistaphylococcal penicillin with or without gentamicin

Tuberculosis: (see latest edition of the AAP Red Book, for duration of therapy and combination therapy). Twice weekly therapy may be used after 1–2 mo of daily therapy

    Child:
        Daily therapy: 10–20 mg/kg/24 hr ÷ Q12–24 hr IV/PO
        Twice weekly therapy: 10–20 mg/kg/24 hr PO twice weekly
        Max. daily dose: 600 mg/24 hr
    Adult:
        Daily therapy: 10 mg/kg/24 hr QD PO
        Twice weekly therapy: 10 mg/kg/24 hr QD twice weekly
        Max. daily dose: 600 mg/24 hr

Prophylaxis for N. meningitidis (see latest edition of the AAP Red Book for additional information):
    0–1 mo: 10 mg/kg/24 hr ÷ Q12 hr PO × 2 days
    >1 mo: 20 mg/kg/24 hr ÷ Q12 hr PO × 2 days
    Adult: 600 mg PO Q12 hr × 2 days
    Max. dose (all ages): 1200 mg/24 hr

Prophylaxis for H. influenzae (see latest edition of the AAP Red Book for additional information):
    0–1 mo: 10 mg/kg/dose Q24 hr PO × 4 days
    >1 mo: 20 mg/kg/dose (**max. dose:** 600 mg) Q24 hr PO × 4 days
    Adult: 600 mg PO Q24 hr × 4 days

Contraindications: Hypersensitivity to rifampin or other rifamycins.
Warnings/Precautions: **Never use** as monotherapy except when used for prophylaxis. Patients with latent tuberculosis infection should **not** be treated with rifampin and pyrazinamide because of the risk of severe liver injury. Use is **not** recommended in porphyria. Penetrates well into body fluids (see Adverse Effects), including CSF. **Adjust dose in renal failure (see Chapter 3).** Reduce dose in hepatic impairment.

Adverse Effects: May cause GI irritation, allergy, headache, fatigue, ataxia, confusion, fever, hepatitis, blood dyscrasias, interstitial nephritis, and elevated BUN and uric acid. Causes red discoloration of body secretions such as urine, saliva and tears (which can permanently stain contact lenses).

Drug Interactions: Induces hepatic enzymes (CYP 450 2C9, 2C19, and 3A4) which may decrease plasma concentration of digoxin, corticosteroids, buspirone, benzodiazepines, fentanyl, calcium channel blockers, beta-blockers, cyclosporine, tacrolimus, itraconazole, ketoconazole, voriconazole, oral anticoagulants, barbiturates and theophylline. May reduce the effectiveness of oral contraceptives and antiretroviral agents (protease inhibitors and nonnucleoside reverse transcriptase inhibitors). Hepatotoxicity is a concern when used in combination with pyrazinamide.

Drug Administration
    IV: For intermittent infusion, infuse over 0.5–3 hr at a concentration ≤6 mg/mL. **Do not** administer IM or SQ.
    PO: Give 1 hr before or 2 hr after meals. Contents of the oral capsule may be mixed with applesauce or jelly.

For explanation of icons, see p. 306.

RIFAPENTINE
Priftin
Antibiotic, antituberculosis agent, rifamycin

Yes   No   ?   C

Tabs: 150 mg

Pulmonary tuberculosis:
≥12 yr and adult:
> *Intensive phase:* 600 mg PO twice weekly (with an interval of no less than 72 hr between doses) × 2 mo in combination with other susceptible antitubercular drugs
> *Continuation phase:* 600 mg PO Q7 days × 4 mo in combination with other susceptible antitubercular drugs

Contraindications: History of hypersensitivity to any rifamycins (e.g., rifampin and rifabutin).
Warnings/Precautions: Hepatotoxicity of other antituberculosis drugs (e.g., isoniazid, pyrazinamide) used in combination should be taken into account. **Use with caution** in liver disease, abnormal LFTs, and hyperbilirubinemia. The CDC does **not** recommend use with HIV infected patients because of increased risk for TB relapse. Use is **not** recommended in porphyria. Discolors body fluids/tissues red-orange; stains contact lenses and dentures. Drug is extensively protein bound; primarily to albumin.
Adverse Effects: Hyperuricemia, arthralgia, pyogenic proteinuria, elevated ALT/AST and red/orange body fluid discoloration are common.
Drug Interactions: Induces CYP 450 3A4 and 2C8/9 isoenzymes. May decrease the effects of antiretroviral protease inhibitors, oral and other systemic hormonal contraceptives (use alternative non-hormonal contraception), carbamazepine, chloramphenicol, corticosteroids, cyclosporine, delavirdine, fluconazole, voriconazole, warfarin and other CYP 450 3A4 substrates.
Drug Administration: Take with or without food.

RIMANTADINE
Flumadine
Antiviral agent

Yes   Yes   3   C

Syrup: 50 mg/ 5 mL (240 mL); contains saccharin and parabens
Tabs: 100 mg

Influenza A prophylaxis (for at least 10 days after known exposure; usually for 6–8 wk during influenza A season or local outbreak):
Child:
> *1–9 yr:* 5 mg/kg/24 hr PO QD; **max. dose:** 150 mg/24 hr
> **≥10 yr:**
>> *<40 kg:* 5 mg/kg/24 hr PO ÷ QD-BID; **max. dose:** 150 mg/24 hr
>> **≥40 kg:** 100 mg/dose PO BID
Adult: 100 mg PO BID
Influenza A treatment (within 48 hr of illness onset):
> Use the above prophylaxis dosage × 5–7 days.

RIMANTADINE *continued*

> **Contraindications:** Amantadine or rimantadine hypersensitivity.
> **Warnings/Precautions:** Individuals immunized with live attenuated influenza vaccine (e.g., FluMist) should not receive rimantadine prophylaxis for 14 days after the vaccine. Chemoprophylaxis does not interfere with immune response to inactivated influenza vaccine. **Use with caution** in seizures and in renal or hepatic insufficiency; dosage reduction may be necessary. **A dosage reduction of 50% has been recommended in severe hepatic or renal impairment; see Chapter 3.** Has not been fully evaluated in children <1 yr. Use is recommended in stem cell transplant patients and treatment indication in children <13 yr despite insufficient data and lack of FDA approval, respectively.
>
> **Adverse Effects:** GI disturbance, xerostomia, dizziness, headace, insomnia and nervousness are common. CNS disturbances are less than with amantadine. Urinary retention may occur.
>
> **Drug Interactions:** Anticholinergic agents and CNS stimulants may increase adverse effects.
>
> **Drug Administration:** May give with or without food.

RITONAVIR
Norvir
Antiviral, protease inhibitor

Yes   No   3   B

Caps, soft gel: 100 mg; contains alcohol
Oral solution: 80 mg/mL (240 mL); contains alcohol and saccharin

> **Child ≥1 mo:** Start at 250 mg/m^2/dose Q12 hr PO, then increase dose by 50 mg/m^2/dose Q12 hr increments at 2- to 3-day intervals up to 400 mg/m^2/dose Q12 hr as tolerated. Usual dosage range: 350–400 mg/m^2/dose Q12 hr.
> **Max. dose:** 600 mg/dose BID
>
> **Adolescent and adult:** Start at 300 mg/dose Q12 hr PO. To minimize nausea and vomiting, increase by 100 mg increments up to 600 mg/dose Q12 hr over 5 days as tolerated.
>
> If used in combination with other protease inhibitors as a pharmacokinetic enhancer, 100–400 mg/dose Q12 hr PO.

> **Contraindications:** Hypersensitivity to ritonavir or or any other components in the formulation. Coadministration of the following drugs that could result in potential serious and/or life-threatening reactions such as cardiac arrhythmias, prolonged or increased sedation, and respiratory depression: alfuzosin, amiodarone, bepridil, flecainide, propafenone, quinidine, astemizole, terfenadine, ergot derivatives, cisapride, pimozide, midazolam and triazolam. Significantly reduces voriconazole levels.
>
> **Warnings/Precautions: Use with caution** in liver impairment. Dose titration schedule is recommended to minimize risk for side effects. Non-compliance can quickly promote resistant HIV strains. **Avoid** using oral liquid dosage form with amprenavir solution because of large amounts of ethanol and propylene glycol. Use **not** recommended with fluticasone propionate, sildenafil, vardenafil, tadalafil, disopyramide, mexiletine, fluoxetine (serotonin syndrome), nefazodone, beta-blockers, lovastatin, simvastatin and other HMG-CoA reductase inhibitors because of increased risk of toxicity and side effects. Significant drug-drug interactions exist, see Contraindications and Drug Interactions sections.
>
> Adolescent Dosing: Patients in early puberty (Tanner I–II) should be dosed with pediatric regimens and those in late puberty (Tanner IV) should be dosed with adult regimens. Adolescents who are at the midst of their growth spurt (Tanner III females

Continued

RITONAVIR *continued*

and Tanner IV males) can be dosed by either pediatric or adult regimen with close monitoring of efficacy and toxicity.

Adverse Effects: Nausea, vomiting, diarrhea, headache, abdominal pain, anorexia, asthenia and paresthesias are common. Increases in liver enzymes, triglycerides, cholesterol, serum glucose may also occur. Spontaneous bleeding in hemophiliacs, pancreatitis, Stevens-Johnson syndrome and other severe allergic reactions, and hepatitis have been reported.

Drug Interactions: Inhibits and is metabolized by the CYP 450 2D6 and 3A4 microsomal enzymes to cause many drug interactions. Drug may increase the levels and side effects of carbamazepine, clarithromycin, calcium channel blockers, digoxin, cyclosprorine, tacrolimus, sirolimus, desipramine, ketoconazole, rifabutin, trazodone, warfarin, digoxin and other protease inhibitors. St. John's wort and rifampin may reduce the effects of ritonavir. Theopylline, methadone, ethinyl estradiol (PO or transdermal contraception), phenytoin, and valproic acid, lamotrigine, and atovaquine levels may be reduced. **Always check the potential for other drug interactions when either initiating therapy or adding new drugs onto an existing regimen.** See Contraindications and Warnings/Precautions sections for additional interactions.

Drug Administration: Administer doses with food to assure absorption. If didanosine is included in the antiretroviral regimen, space the administration of two drugs by 2 hr. Store both capsules and oral solution in the refrigerator. Oral solution can be kept at room temperature if used within 30 days. Oral solution must be kept in original container. Administering doses with milk, chocolate milk, pudding, or ice cream can enhance compliance in children.

SAQUINAVIR MESYLATE
Invirase
Antiviral agent, protease inhibitor

Yes   No   3   B

Caps, hard gel (Invirase): 200 mg
Tabs: 500 mg

Child: Clinical trials are currently under way to evaluate the administration of saquinavir in combination with other protease inhibitors.
Adolescent (≥16 yr) and adult:
  In combination with ritonavir 100 mg PO BID: 1000 mg PO BID
  In combination with lopinavir 400 mg and ritonavir 100 mg PO BID: 1000 mg PO BID

Contraindications: Saquinavir products and their components and severe hepatic impairment. Coadministration of the following drugs that could result in potential serious and/or life-threatening reactions such as cardiac arrhythmias, prolonged or increased sedation, and respiratory depression: amiodarone, flecainide, propafenone, quinidine, astemizole, terfenadine, ergot derivatives, cisapride, pimozide, midazolam and triazolam. Rifampin may result in treatment failure and hepatotoxicity.

Warnings/Precautions: **Use with caution** in hepatic failure. Use **only** in combination with ritonavir or ritonavir/lopinavir. Use **not** recommended with St. John's wort, lovastatin, simastatin or garlic capsules. Significant drug-drug interactions exist, see Contraindications and Drug Interactions sections. Non-compliance can quickly promote resistant HIV strains. Use sunscreen or protective clothing to prevent photosensitivity reactions. When using in combination with ritonavir, doses >400 mg PO BID for either ritonavir or saquinavir may be associated with risk for increased

SAQUINAVIR MESYLATE *continued*

adverse effects. Soft gelatin capsules (Fortavase) are **not bioequivalent** to the hard gel capsules and tablets and cannot be used interchangeably.

Adolescent Dosing: Patients in early puberty (Tanner I–II) should be dosed with pediatric regimens and those in late puberty (Tanner IV) should be dosed with adult regimens. Adolescents who are at the midst of their growth spurt (Tanner III females and Tanner IV males) can be dosed by either pediatric or adult regimen with close monitoring of efficacy and toxicity.

Adverse Effects: Diarrhea, GI discomfort, nausea, paresthesias, skin rash, lipid abnormalities and headache are common. Spontaneous bleeding in hemophiliacs, hyperglycemia, exacerbation of chronic liver disease and body fat redistribution without serum lipid abnormalities have been reported.

Drug Interactions: Drug inhibits and is metabolized by the CYP 450 3A4 drug metabolizing enzyme and is a p-glycoprotein substrate. Increased levels and/or toxicity may occur with the following concurrent medications: calcium channel blockers, clindamycin, cyclosporine, lidocaine, tacrolimus, dapsone and quinidine. Rifabutin, niveraphine, carbamazepine, dexamethasone, phenobarbital and phenytoin can decrease saquinavir levels. Delavirdine, ketoconazole, grapefruit juice and other protease inhibitors may increase saquinavir levels. **Always carefully review patient's medication profile for other potential drug-drug interactions.**

Drug Administration: Administer doses with food or within 2 hr after a meal.

SELENIUM SULFIDE
Selsun and others
Topical antiseborrheic agent

No   No   ?   C

Lotion/shampoo: 1% [OTC] (210, 325, 400 mL)
Lotion: 2.5% (120 mL)

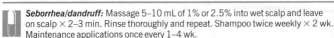

Seborrhea/dandruff: Massage 5–10 mL of 1% or 2.5% into wet scalp and leave on scalp × 2–3 min. Rinse thoroughly and repeat. Shampoo twice weekly × 2 wk. Maintenance applications once every 1–4 wk.

Tinea versicolor: Apply 2.5% lotion to affected areas of skin. Allow to remain on skin × 30 min. Rinse thoroughly. Repeat QD × 7 days. Follow with monthly applications for 3 mo to prevent recurrences.

Contraindications: Hypersensitivity to selenium sulfide or any other components in the formulation.

Warnings/Precautions: **Do not** use for tinea versicolor during pregnancy. Safety of the 2.5% lotion has **not** been established in infants. **Avoid** contact with eyes, genital areas and skin folds. Shampoo may be used for tinea capitis to reduce risk of transmission to others (does **not** eradicate tinea infection).

For tinea versicolor, 15% to 25% sodium hyposulfite or thiosulfate (Tinver lotion) applied to affected areas BID × 2–4 wk is an alternative. Topical antifungals (e.g., clotrimazole, miconazole) may be used for small, focal infections.

Adverse Effects: Local irritation, hair loss, mild contact dermatitis, and hair discoloration are common.

Drug Interactions: None identified.

Drug Administration: For topical use; **do not** use on broken or inflamed areas. Rinse hair and skin thoroughly after use and discontinue use if sensitivity reactions occur. **Avoid** contact with eyes, genital areas and skin folds. Rinse hands and body well after treatment.

SILVER SULFADIAZINE
Silvadene, Thermazene, SSD Cream, SSD AF Cream
Topical antibiotic

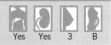

Yes	Yes	3	B

Cream: 1% (20, 25, 50, 85, 400, 1000 g); contains methylparabens

Cover affected areas completely QD–BID. Apply cream to a thickness of ¹⁄₁₆ inch using sterile technique.

Contraindications: Hypersensitivity to silver, sulfonamide products, or any other components in the formulation. Premature infants and infant ≤ 2 mo of age due to concerns of kernicterus; and pregnancy (approaching term).
Warnings/Precautions: Use with caution in G6PD deficiency and renal and hepatic impairment. Significant systemic absorption may occur in severe burns.
Adverse Effects: Pruritus, rash and local skin irritation are common. Bone marrow suppression, hemolytic anemia and interstitial nephritis have been reported.
Drug Interactions: None identified.
Drug Administration: Apply under sterile conditions for topical use to affected areas. Whenever necessary, reapply cream to any areas from which it has been removed by patient activity. Dressings may be used but are **not** necessary. **Not** for ophthalmic use. Discard product if cream has darkened.

SPECTINOMYCIN
Trobicin
Antibiotic, aminoglycoside

No	Yes	?	B

Injection: 2 g with 3.2 mL diluent which contains 0.9% benzyl alcohol

Uncomplicated gonorrhea (in combination with a macrolide):
    Children <45 kg: 40 mg/kg IM × 1; **max. dose:** 2 g/dose
    ≥45 kg and ≥8 yr: 2 g IM × 1
Disseminated gonorrhea (for patients allergic to beta-lactams and fluoroquinolones):
    ≥45 kg and ≥8 yr: 2 g IM Q12 hr × 7 days. Alternatively may treat × 24–48 hr and switch to oral alternative.

Contraindications: Hypersensitivity to spectinomycin or any other components in the formulation.
Warnings/Precautions: Not effective for syphilis. Drug is primarily used to treat gonorrhea in patients who cannot tolerate beta-lactams or fluoroquinolones. **Not** recommended for treatment of pharyngeal infections. Repeat dosing will accumulate in renal failure. See latest edition of the AAP Red Book.
Adverse Effects: Vertigo, malaise, nausea, anorexia, chills, fever, urticaria and injection site pain may occur.
Drug Interactions: None identified.
Drug Administration: IM use only. Inject deep into the upper outer quadrant of the gluteal muscle with a 20-gauge needle is recommended.

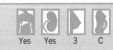

S

FORMULARY

STAVUDINE
Zerit, d4T

Antiviral agent, nucleoside analogue reverse transcriptase inhibitor

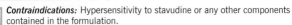

Yes   Yes   3   C

Caps: 15, 20, 30, 40 mg
Oral solution: 1 mg/mL (200 mL); contains methylparabens and propylparabens

Neonate ≤ 13 days old: 0.5 mg/kg/dose PO Q12 hr
Neonate ≥14 days old, infant, and child <30 kg: 1 mg/kg/dose PO Q12 hr;
    max. dose: 30 mg PO Q12 hr
Adolescent ≥30 kg and adult:
    30–60 kg: 30 mg PO Q12 hr
    >60 kg: 40 mg PO Q12 hr

Contraindications: Hypersensitivity to stavudine or any other components
contained in the formulation.
Warnings/Precautions: Fatal lactic acidosis with hepatic steatosis with or
without pancreatitis has been reported with use of nucleoside analogue alone or in
combination therapy. The combination of stavudine and didanosine in pregnant
women may result in fatal lactic acidosis or pancreatitis. **Adjust dosage in renal
impairment (see Chapter 3).**
Adverse Effects: Headache, GI discomfort, lipoatrophy, and rash are common.
Peripheral neuropathy, pancreatitis, lipodystrophy, lactic acidosis, severe
hepatomegaly and elevated liver enzymes have been reported.
Drug Interactions: Should **not** be given in combination with zidovudine (AZT) because
of poor antiviral effect. Drugs associated with peripheral neuropathy (e.g.,
chloramphenicol, dapsone, metronidazole) may increase risk of this side effect. See
Warnings/Precautions.
Drug Administration: Doses may be administered with or without food.
    Oral Solution: Shake well before measuring each dose and keep refrigerated (30
    day stability after initial reconstitution).

STIBOGLUCONATE
Pentostam, pentavalent antimony

Antiparasitic agent (leishmaniasis)

Yes   Yes   ?   ?

AVAILABLE FROM THE U.S. CENTERS FOR DISEASE CONTROL AND PREVENTION
(404-639-3670 Monday-Friday 8:00 am–4:30 pm EST or 404-639-2888 evenings,
weekends or holidays)
Injection: 100 mg of pentavalent antimony/mL; contains sodium

Leishmaniasis:
Child and adult: 20 mg/kg/24 hr IM/IV QD with the following durations of
therapy:
    Cutaneous: For 20 days
    Visceral and mucosal: For 28 days

Contraindications: Hypersensitivity to stibogluconate.
Warnings/Precautions: **Use with caution** in mild/moderate renal or hepatic
insufficiency, pneumonia, cardiac disease, tuberculosis and EKG abnormalities.
Avoid concomitant use of alcohol and medications that are hepatotoxic or cause QT

Continued

STIBOGLUCONATE *continued*

interval prolongation. Majority of dose excreted in urine; no specific renal impairment guidelines exist. Monitor baseline and weekly EKG, creatinine, transaminase, lipase, amylase and CBCs. Hold therapy if QTc >0.5 sec, transaminase ≥4–5 times upper normal limit, and moderately severe clinical pancreatitis.

Adverse Effects: Myalgia/arthralgia (use nonsteroidal anti-inflammatory agent), nausea, vomiting, abdominal pain, fatigue, elevated LFTs, T-wave changes on EKG, and depressed levels of hemoglobin, WBC and platelets are common. Rare severe cardiotoxicity has been reported.

Drug Interactions: None identified.

Drug Administration

    IM: Give undiluted drug (100 mg/mL) IM.

    IV: Dilute patient specific dose with 50 mL of D_5W or NS; smaller volumes of diluent may be used for smaller drug doses. Administer over at least 10 min.

STREPTOMYCIN SULFATE
Various
Antibiotic, aminoglycoside; antituberculous agent

No   Yes   1   D

Injection: 400 mg/mL (2.5 mL)
Powder for injection: 1 g

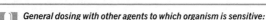

General dosing with other agents to which organism is sensitive:
    Newborn: 10–20 mg/kg/24 hr IM ÷ Q12–24 hr
    Infant: 20–30 mg/kg/24 hr IM ÷ Q12 hr
    Child: 20–40 mg/kg/24 hr IM ÷ 6–12 hr
    Adult: 1–2 g/24 hr IM ÷ 6–12 hr; **max. dose:** 2 g/24 hr
Tuberculosis (use as part of multi-drug regimen; see latest edition of AAP Red Book):
    Infant, child, and adolescent:
        Daily therapy: 20–40 mg/kg/24 hr IM QD
            Max. daily dose: 1 g/24 hr
        Twice weekly therapy: 20–40 mg/kg/dose IM twice weekly
            Max. daily dose: 1.5 g/24 hr
    Adult:
        Daily therapy: 15 mg/kg/24 hr IM QD
            Max. daily dose: 1 g/24 hr
        Twice weekly therapy: 25–30 mg/kg/dose IM twice weekly
            Max. daily dose: 1.5 g/24 hr
Brucellosis (see latest edition of the AAP Red Book):
    Child ≥7 yr: 1 g/dose IM QD (15 mg/kg/dose if ≤50 kg) × 14 days with doxycycline 100 mg PO BID (5 mg/kg/dose if ≤40 kg) × 45 days.
    Adult: 15 mg/kg/dose (**max. dose:** 1 g/dose) IM QD × 2–3 wk in combination with doxycycline 100 mg PO BID × 4–6 wk
Tularemia:
    Child: 30 mg/kg/24 hr IM ÷ Q8–12 hr; **max. dose:** 2 g/24 hr × 10–14 days
    Adult: 1–2 g/24 hr IM ÷ Q8–12 hr × 7–14 days and until afebrile for 5–7 days
Plague:
    Child and adult: 30 mg/kg/24 hr IM ÷ Q8–12 hr; **max. dose:** 2 g/24 hr × 10–14 days

---

Contraindications: Hypersensitivity to streptomycin, aminoglycosides and sulfites.

    Warnings/Precautions: **Use with caution** in pre-existing vertigo, tinnitus, hearing loss and neuromuscular disorders. Monitor auditory status. Concomitant neurotoxic, ototoxic, or nephrotoxic drugs and dehydration may increase risk factors

STREPTOMYCIN SULFATE *continued*

for toxicity. Concomitant use of anesthesia or muscle relaxants increases risk for neuromuscular blockade and respiratory paralysis. **Adjust dose in renal failure (see Chapter 3).**

Therapeutic Levels: Peak 15–40 mg/L, trough: <5 mg/L. Recommended serum sampling time at steady state: trough within 30 min prior to the third consecutive dose and peak 30–60 min after the administration of the third consecutive dose. Therapeutic levels are not achieved in CSF.

Adverse Effects: Drug-induced eosinophilia, facial paresthesia and fever are common. May cause bone marrow suppression, other neurologic problems, CNS depression (in infants with dosages exceeding recommended limits), nephrotoxicity, ototoxicity, myocarditis and serum sickness.

Drug Interactions: Ototoxicity is potentiated with ethacrynic acid and furosemide. See Warnings/Precautions for additional interactions.

Drug Administration: **Drug is administered via deep IM injection only.** The preferred site is the upper outer quadrant of the buttock (e.g., gluteus maximus) or midlateral thigh.

SULCONAZOLE

Exelderm
Antifungal agent, imidazole

No   No   ?   C

Topical cream: 1% (15, 30, 60 g)
Topical solution: 1% (30 mL)

 Apply sparingly to affected and surrounding areas QD–BID. To reduce the risk of recurrence, tinea cruris, tinea corporis and tinea versicolor should be treated for 3 wk and tinea pedis for 4 wk.

 Contraindications: Hypersensitivity to sulconazole products or any other components in the formulation.

Warnings/Precautions: **Discontinue** use if irritation develops. **External use only;** **avoid** contact with eyes.

Adverse Effects: Itching, burning/stinging and redness are common. Immune hypersensitivity reaction has been reported.

Drug Interactions: None identified.

Drug Administration: Gently massage to affected and surrounding areas; **avoid** contact with the eyes.

SULFACETAMIDE SODIUM, OPHTHALMIC

AK-Sulf, Bleph 10, Ocusulf-10, and various generic products
Ophthalmic antibiotic, sulfonamide derivative

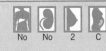

No   No   2   C

Ophthalmic solution: 10% (2, 2.5, 5, 15 mL); may contain methylparaben and propylparben.
Ophthalmic ointment: 10% (3.5 g); may contain phenylmercuric acetate

 Ophthalmic (usual duration of therapy for ophthalmic use is 7–10 days):
>2 mo and adult:
   Ointment: Apply ribbon QID and QHS (5 times/24 hr)
   Drops: 1–2 drops Q2–3 hr to affected eye(s)

Continued

SULFACETAMIDE SODIUM, OPHTHALMIC *continued*

Contraindications: Hypersensitivity to sulfonamides or to any ingredient of the preparation.
Warnings/Precautions: Hypersensitivity reactions between different sulfonamides can occur regardless of route of administration.
Adverse Effects: Local irritation, stinging, burning, conjunctival hyperemia, excessive tear production and eye pain are common. Rare toxic epidermal necrolysis and Stevens-Johnson syndrome have been reported.
Drug Interactions: Sulfacetamide preparations are incompatible with silver preparations.
Drug Administration
   Drops: Apply finger pressure to lacrimal sac during and for 1–2 min after dose application. **Avoid** contact with the tip of the container.
   Ointment: Instill ointment in lower conjunctival sac by avoiding contact of ointment tip with eye or skin.

SULFADIAZINE
Various trade names
Antibiotic, sulfonamide derivative

Yes   Yes   2   C/D

Tabs: 500 mg
Oral suspension: 100 mg/mL

Congenital toxoplasmosis (administer with pyrimethamine and folinic acid; see Pyrimethamine for dosage information; from Clin Infect Dis *18:38, 1994*):
   Infant: 100 mg/kg/24 hr PO ÷ BID × 12 mo
Toxoplasmosis (administer with pyrimethamine and folinic acid; see Pyrimethamine for dosage information):
   Child: 100–200 mg/kg/24 hr ÷ Q6 hr PO × 3–4 wk
   Adult: 4–6 g/24 hr PO ÷ Q6 hr × 3–4 wk
Rheumatic fever prophylaxis:
   ≤27 kg: 500 mg PO QD
   >27 kg: 1000 mg PO QD

Contraindications: Hypersensitivity to sulfadiazine and other sulfonamides, or porphyria.
Warnings/Precautions: Use with caution in premature infants and infants <2 mo because of risk of hyperbilirubinemia, G6PD deficiency, and in hepatic or renal dysfunction (30%–44% eliminated in urine). Maintain hydration to prevent crystalluria and stone formation. Pregnancy category changes from "C" to "D" if administered near term.
Adverse Effects: Fever, rash, photosensitivity, GI disturbances, hepatitis, SLE-like syndrome, vasculitis, bone marrow suppression and hemolysis (patients with G6PD deficiency), and Stevens-Johnson syndrome may occur.
Drug Interactions: May cause increased effects of warfarin, methotrexate, thiazide diuretics, uricosuric agents and sulfonylureas. Large quantities of vitamin C or acidifying agents (e.g., cranberry juice) may cause crystalluria.
Drug Administration: Take on an empty stomach with water (at least 8 ounces for adults).

SULFAMETHOXAZOLE AND TRIMETHOPRIM

Trimethoprim-sulfamethoxazole, Co-trimoxazole,
TMP-SMX; Bactrim, Septra, Sulfatrim, and others
Antibiotic, sulfonamide derivative

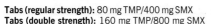 Yes   Yes   1   C/D

Tabs (regular strength): 80 mg TMP/400 mg SMX
Tabs (double strength): 160 mg TMP/800 mg SMX
Suspension: 40 mg TMP/200 mg SMX per 5 mL (20, 100, 150, 200, 480 mL)
Injection: 16 mg TMP/mL and 80 mg SMX/mL; some preparations may contain
propylene glycol and benzyl alcohol (5, 10, 20, 30 mL)

Doses based on TMP component.
Minor/moderate infections (PO or IV):
    Child: 8–12 mg/kg/24 hr ÷ BID
    Adult (>40 kg): 160 mg/dose BID
Severe infections (PO or IV):
    Child and adult: 20 mg/kg/24 hr ÷ Q6–8 hr
UTI prophylaxis:
    Child: 2–4 mg/kg/24 hr PO QD
Pneumocystic carinii pneumonia:
    Treatment (PO/IV): 20 mg/kg/24 hr ÷ Q6–8 hr
    Prophylaxis (PO or IV):
      ≥1 mo and child: 5–10 mg/kg/24 hr ÷ BID or 150 mg/m^2/24 hr ÷ BID for
      3 consecutive days/wk; **max. dose:** 320 mg/24 hr
      Adult: 80–160 mg QD or 160 mg 3 days/wk

Contraindications: Sulfonamide or trimethoprim hypersensitivity, and
megaloblastic anemia due to folate deficiency.
Warnings/Precautions: Use with caution in G6PD deficiency, renal and hepatic
impairment **(reduce dose in renal failure; see Chapter 3)**. Not recommended for use
with infants <2 mo (excluding PCP prophylaxis). **Do not use drug at term during
pregnancy.** Pregnancy risk factor changes to "D" if administered near term. Assure
adequate hydration.
Adverse Effects: May cause kernicterus in newborns. Blood dyscrasias, crystalluria,
glossitis, renal or hepatic injury, GI irritation, rash, Stevens-Johnson syndrome,
hemolysis in patients with G6PD deficiency. Hyperkalemia may appear in HIV/AIDS
patients.
Drug Interactions: Increases effects/toxicity of warfarin, methotrexate and
sulfonylureas, phenytoin, digoxin and thiopental. Decreases cyclosporine levels.
Drug Administration
    IV: For intermittent infusion, infuse over 60–90 min at a concentration 0.64–1.6
    mg/mL. Stability of diluted IV solution is inversely related to concentration,
    ranging from 1–6 hr.
    PO: Administer doses on an empty stomach with adequate hydration.

FORMULARY

SULFISOXAZOLE
Gantrisin and others
Antibiotic, sulfonamide derivative

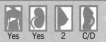

Yes   Yes   2   C/D

Tabs: 500 mg
Suspension: 500 mg/5 mL (480 mL); contains 0.3% alcohol and parabens
Ophthalmic solution: 4% (40 mg/mL) (15 mL)
For combination product with erythromycin, see Erythromycin Ethylsuccinate and Acetylsulfisoxazole.

Child ≥2 mo: 75 mg/kg/dose PO × 1 followed by 120–150 mg/kg/24 hr OR 4 g/m²/24 hr ÷ Q4–6 hr PO; **max. dose:** 6 g/24 hr
   Otitis media prophylaxis: 50 mg/kg/dose QHS PO
   UTI prophylaxis: 10–20 mg/kg/24 hr ÷ Q12 hr
Adult: 2–4 g PO × 1 followed by 4–8 g/24 hr ÷ Q4–6 hr PO
Rheumatic fever prophylaxis:
   <27 kg: 500 mg PO QD
   ≥27 kg: 1000 mg PO QD
Ophthalmic solution (usual duration of therapy is 7–10 days):
   Conjunctivitis or other superficial ocular infections: 1–2 drops Q1–4 hr; increase the time interval between doses as the condition improves.
   Trachoma (with systemic sulfonamide therapy): 2 drops Q2 hr.

Contraindications: Hypersensitivity to sulfonamides, porphyria, urinary obstruction or near-term pregnant.
Warnings/Precautions: **Use with caution** in infants <2 mo, the presence of renal or liver disease, or G6PD deficiency. Maintain adequate fluid intake to prevent crystalluria and stone formation. **Adjust dose in renal impairment with systemic use (see Chapter 3).** Pregnancy category changes to "D" if administered near term in pregnancy.
Adverse Effects: Fever, rash, photosensitivity, GI disturbances, hepatitis, SLE-like syndrome, vasculitis, bone marrow suppression and hemolysis (patients with G6PD deficiency), and Stevens-Johnson syndrome may occur.
Drug Interactions: May cause increased effects of warfarin, methotrexate, thiazide diuretics, uricosuric agents and sulfonylureas. Large quantities of vitamin C or acidifying agents (e.g., cranberry juice) may cause crystalluria. Interferes with folate absorption.
Drug Administration
   PO: Take on an empty stomach with water (at least 8 ounces for adults).
   Ophthalmic Drops: Apply finger pressure to lacrimal sac during and for 1–2 min after dose application. **Avoid** contact with bottle tip.

SURAMIN
Antrypol, Arsobal, Bayer 205, Belganyl, Fourneau
309, Germanin, Mel B, Moranyl, Naphuride
Antiprotozoal, anthelmintic agent

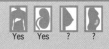

Yes   Yes   ?   ?

AVAILABLE FROM THE U.S. CENTERS FOR DISEASE CONTROL AND PREVENTION (404-639-3670 Monday-Friday 8:00 am–4:30 pm EST or 404-639-2888 evenings, weekends or holidays)
Injection: 1 g

SURAMIN *continued*

Test dose (for all indications):
    Child: 10–20 mg/kg/dose IV × 1; **max. dose:** 200 mg/dose
    Adult: 100–200 mg IV × 1
Typanosomiasis (IV, initiate 24 hr following the adminstration and tolerance of the aforementioned test dose):
    Child: 10–20 mg/kg/dose on days 1, 3, 7, 14 and 21.
    Adult:
        Early stage: 20 mg/kg/dose (**max. dose:** 1 g/dose) on days 1, 3, 7, 14 and 21. Alternatively, 20 mg/kg/dose Q weekly until a total dose of 5 g is achieved may be given. Patients in poor general condition should receive approximately one-quarter of the normal dose.
        Late stage: 10 mg/kg/dose Q5 days for a total of 12 doses. This is given in combination with tryparsamide at a dose of 30 mg/kg/dose (**max. dose:** 2 g/dose) IV Q5 days for 12 doses. If needed, a second treatment course may be repeated 1 mo later.
Onchocerciasis (IV, usually following a 23- to 32-day course of diethylcarbamazine as an alternative to ivermectin):
    Child: Following the administration and tolerance of the aforementioned test dose, initiate 20 mg/kg/dose Q weekly × 5 wk one week after the test dose.
    Adult: Following the administration and tolerance of the aforementioned test dose, treatment with the full dose may be started 1 wk after. A total dose of 66.7 mg/kg should be administered in six incremental weekly doses apportioned as follows: 3.3 mg/kg/dose week one, 6.7 mg//kg/dose week two, 10 mg/kg/dose week three, 13.3 mg/kg/dose week four, 16.7 mg/kg/dose weeks five and six.
Max. daily dose for all indications:
    Child: 20 mg/kg/24 hr
    Adult: 1–1.5 g/24 hr

Contraindications: Hypersensitivity to suramin or any other components in the formulation.
Warnings/Precautions: Administer a test dose before initiating therapy; significant immediate reactions consists of nausea, vomiting, shock, and loss of consciousness (0.1%–0.3% incidence). **Use with caution** in renal and hepatic impairment, peripheral neuritis, and malnourished/debilitated patients. Prolonged use in ocular onchocerciasis may result in degenerative changes to the optic disk and retina.
    Eliminated primarily in the urine very slowly; no specific renal impairment dosing guidelines available. Drug may be absorbed by the liver to cause hepatic damage and is highly protein bound (99.7%). Monitor CBC, creatinine and urinalysis.
Adverse Effects: Arthritis, nephrotoxicity with transient albuminuria, maculopapular eruptions, headache, palmarplantar hyperesthesias, paraesthesias, peripheral neuropathy, pruritus, relative adrenal insufficiency and urticaria are common. Blood dyscrasias, exfoliative dermatitis, hepatitis, jaundice, and ocular effects (e.g., lacrimation, optic atrophy, palpebral edema, photophobia, stomatitis, and prostration) have been reported.
Drug Interactions: None identified.
Drug Administration: Reconstitute vial with sterile water to a 10% (100 mg/mL) concentration and administer by slow IV injection within 30 min of reconstitution.

For explanation of icons, see p. 306.

TENOFOVIR DISOPROXIL FUMARATE
Viread, PMPA, TDF
Antiviral agent, nucleoside analogue reverse transcriptase inhibitor

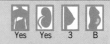

Yes   Yes   3   B

Tabs: 300 mg, equivalent to 245 mg tenofovir disoproxil
Investigational dosage forms:
    Tabs: 75 mg
    Oral powder: In development
In combination with emtricitabine as Truvada:
    Tabs: 300 mg tenofovir disoproxil fumarate and 200 mg emtricitabine
In combination with emtricitabine and efavirenz as Atripla:
    Tabs: 300 mg tenofovir disproxil fumarate, 200 mg emtricitabine and 600 mg efavirenz

---

Dosage based on tenofovir disoproxil fumarate.
Child (dosage from current clinical trials using investigational formulations):
    2–8 yr: 8 mg/kg/dose PO QD
    >8 yr: 210 mg/m^2/dose PO QD; **max. dose:** 300 mg/dose
≥18 and adult: 300 mg PO QD
    Adult in combination with didanosine:
        <60 kg: Didanosine delayed-release capsule 200 mg PO QD is recommended
        ≥60 kg: Didanosine delayed-release capsule 250 mg PO QD is recommended
    Adult in combination with atazanavir: 300 mg atazanavir boosted with 100 mg ritonavir should be used in combination with 300 mg tenofovir, all as PO QD.
Truvada (GFR ≥30 mL/min and not receiving hemodialysis):
    Adult: 1 tab PO QD with or without food
Atripia (GFR ≥50 mL/min):
    Adult: 1 tab PO QD on an empty stomach

Contraindications: Hypersensitivity to tenofovir or any other components in the formulation.
Warnings/Precautions: Lactic acidosis and severe hepatomegaly with steatosis have been reported especially in women with obesity, prior liver disease, or prolonged nucleoside exposure. Severe acute exacerbation of hepatitis may occur in patients with HBV when tenofovir is discontinued. **Use with caution in renal impairment; reduce dose (see Chapter 3).**
Adverse Effects: Nausea, diarrhea, vomiting and flatulence are common. May cause decreased bone mineral density, lactic acidosis, severe hepatomegaly with steatosis (see Warnings/Precautions) and renal tubular dysfunction (monitor renal status).
Drug Interactions: Coadministration with drugs that reduce renal function or compete for active tubular secretion (e.g., cidofovir, acyclovir, valacyclovir, ganciclovir, valganciclovir) may increase tenofovir levels. Tenofovir may increase didanosine levels and decrease atazanavir levels.
Drug Administration: Doses may be administered with or without food; high-fat meals may increase absorption. The combination product, Atripia, should be administered on an empty stomach. When co-administered with didanosine, administer delayed-release didanosine capsules under fasted conditions or with a light meal, and administer buffered didanosine tablets under fasted conditions.

TERBINAFINE
Lamisil, Lamisil AT, DesenexMyax
Antifungal, allylamine

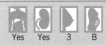

Yes   Yes   3   B

Oral suspension: 25 mg/mL
Oral granules: 125 mg packets, 187.5 mg packets (14s)
Tabs: 250 mg
Topical solution or spray (Lamisil AT) [OTC]: 1% (30 mL); contains propylene glycol
Topical cream (Lamisil AT, DesenexMyax) [OTC]: 1% (12, 24 g); contains benzyl alcohol
Topical gel (Lamisil AT) [OTC]: 1% (6, 12 g); contains benzyl alcohol

Child (dosage is not well established, but the following have been recommended):
"Standard" dose:
  10–20 kg: 62.5 mg PO QD
  20–40 kg: 125 mg PO QD
  >40 kg: 250 mg PO QD
"High" dose:
  10–15 kg: 125 mg PO QD
  16–25 kg: 187.5 mg PO QD
  >25 kg: 250 mg PO QD
Tinea capitis (≥4 yr) using the oral granule dosage form sprinkled on pudding or other soft non-acidic foods (e.g., mashed potatoes; do not use applesauce):
  <25 kg: 125 mg PO QD
  25–35 kg: 187.5 mg PO QD
  >35 kg: 250 mg PO QD
Recommended duration of therapy include tinea capitis for 6 wk or 2–8 wk (Trichophyton species for 2–4 wk, Microsporum species for 2–8 wk) and onychomycosis for 6–12 wk (fingernail for 6 wk, toenail for 12 wk).
Adult: 250 mg PO QD; for fingernail onychomycosis use for 6 wk and for toenail onychomycosis use for 12 wk.
Topical:
 ≥12 yr:
  Tinea pedis: Apply the cream to affected areas BID. Use on interdigital spaces for 1 wk and use on the bottom and sides of the foot for 2 wk.
 Adult:
  Tinea versicolor: Apply the gel to affected areas QD × 7 days; or solution to affected areas BID × 7 days.
  Tinea corporis or tinea cruris: Apply gel to affected areas QD × 7 days.

Contraindications: Hypersensitivity to terbinafine or to any other components of the formulation.
Warnings/Precautions
PO: Rare hepatotoxicity, including hepatic failure, has been reported in patients with or without pre-existing liver disease. Should **not** be used in chronic or active liver disease since the drug is extensively metabolized by the liver and specific hepatic impairment dosing recommendations are **not** currently available. Baseline ALT and AST are recommended.

 Not recommended in patients with GFR <50 mL/min as the drug has extensive renal excretion (no dose modification information available). **Use with caution** in immunodeficiency because of reports of neutropenia (consider monitoring CBC for therapies >6 wk).

Continued

TERBINAFINE *continued*

Topical: **Do not** use on nails, scalp, in or near the mouth or eyes, or for vaginal yeast infections.

Adverse Effects

PO: GI disturbances, headache, abnormal LFTs, rash, urticaria, pruritus and taste disturbances are common and are generally mild and transient. Psoriasiform euptions or exacerbation of psoriasis, acute exanthematous pustulosis, and precipitation and exacerbation of lupus erythematous have been reported. See Warnings/Precautions.

Topical: Localized burning/irritation, itching, skin exfoliation and rash may occur.

Drug Interactions: PO: Cimetidine increases terbinafine levels but rifampin significantly decreases terbinafine levels. Terbinafine may increase the effects/toxicity of dextromethorphan and caffeine but decreases cyclosporine levels. Inhibits CYP 450 2D6 and may increase the effects/toxicity of drugs metabolized by this enzyme (e.g., beta-blockers, class 1C antiarrhythmics, selective serotonin reuptake inhibitors, and MAO inhibitors Type B).

Drug Administration

PO: Take with or without food.

Topical: Clean and dry affected areas prior to dose application. Apply to affected area and surrounding skin. Wash hands after each use.

TERCONAZOLE
Terazol 3, Terazol 7, Zazole, and other generics
Antifungal agent, triazole

No   No   ?   C

Vaginal cream:
   Terazol 7: 0.4% (45 g with or without applicator)
   Terazol 3 or Zazole: 0.8% (20 g with or without applicator)
Vaginal suppository:
   Terazol 3: 80 mg (3s)

Candidal vulvovaginitis:
Cream:
   0.4%: 1 applicator full intravaginally QHS × 7 days
   0.8%: 1 applicator full intravaginally QHS × 3 days
Vaginal suppository: 1 suppository intravaginally QHS × 3 days

---

Contraindications: Hypersensitivy to terconazole or to any of the components of the cream or suppository.

Warnings/Precautions: Avoid use in first trimester of pregnancy. **Do not** use or retreat if sensitization, irritation, fever, chills or flu-like symptoms occur. Components in the suppository dosage form may weaken certain rubber or latex products used in vaginal contraceptive diaphragms and condoms.

Adverse Effects: Abdominal, musculoskeletal and vaginal pain, and headache are common. Fever, chills, and vaginal discomfort may occur.

Drug Interactions: None identified.

Drug Administration: Wash hands prior to use. Gently insert suppository or applicator full of cream high into the vagina at bedtime. Remain lying down for 30 min after administration. Wash applicator with soap and water after each use. Use sanitary napkin or minipad to prevent staining of clothing. **Do not** use tampons.

TETANUS IMMUNE GLOBULIN
BayTet
Immune globulin, tetanus (high titer)

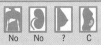

| No | No | ? | C |

Injection, prefilled syringe for IM use only: 250 unit; contains 15%–18% protein

---

Tetanus prophylaxis for patients with incomplete (< 3 doses of absorbed tetanus toxoid) or unknown immunization status:
  <7 yr: 4 units/kg or 250 units IM × 1
  ≥7 yr and adult: 250 units IM × 1
Treatment of active tetanus (early symptoms), see latest AAP Red Book for additional information and alternatives when product is unavailable:
  Child (optimum therapeutic dose has not been established): Some experts recommend 500 units IM × 1, although others have recommended 3000–6000 units IM × 1.
  Adult: 3000–6000 units (30–300 units/kg) IM × 1.

Warnings/Precautions: Use with caution in hypersensitivity to immune globulin products, IgA deficiency (contains trace amounts of IgA), thrombocytopenia, or other contraindications to IM injections. Like other plasma products, the risk for transmission of blood-borne viral agents may occur. **For IM injections only**; intradermal skin tests should **not** be used.
Adverse Effects: Injection site pain is common. Angioedema, nephrotic syndrome and anaphylaxis have been reported.
Drug Interactions: May interfere with the response to live viral vaccines such as measles, mumps, polio, varicella and rubella; defer these vaccines until approximately 3 mo after dose of immune globulin.
Drug Administration: Administer by deep IM injection. Should be administered with Td toxoid but at different extremities and with a separate syringe.

TETRACYCLINE HCL
Sumycin and various generics
Antibiotic

| Yes | Yes | 1 | D |

Caps: 250, 500 mg
Oral suspension: 125 mg/5 mL (480 mL); contains saccharin and sodium metabisulfite

---

Do not use in children <8 yr.
Child ≥8 yr: 25–50 mg/kg/24 hr PO ÷ Q6 hr; **max. dose:** 3 g/24 hr
Adult: 1–2 g/24 hr PO ÷ Q6–12 hr

Contraindications: Hypersensitivity to any tetracycline derivative.
Warnings/Precautions: **Not** recommended in patients <8 yr due to tooth staining and decreased bone growth, and in pregnancy because these side effects may occur in the fetus. The risk for these adverse effects are highest with long-term use. **Avoid** prolonged exposure to sunlight.
Never use outdated tetracyclines because they may cause Fanconi-like syndrome.
Adjust dose in renal failure (see Chapter 3).
Adverse Effects: GI disturbances, rash and photophobia are common. Hepatotoxicity, stomatitis, fever, pseudotumor cerebri and superinfection have been reported.

Continued

For explanation of icons, see p. 306.

TETRACYCLINE HCL *continued*

Drug Interactions: May decrease the effectiveness of oral contraceptives, increase serum digoxin levels, and increase effects of warfarin. Use with methoxyflurane increases risk for nephrotoxicity and use with isotretinoin is associated with pseudotumor cerebri.

Drug Administration: Give 1 hr before or 2 hr after meals.

Do not give with dairy products or with any divalent cations (i.e., Fe^{++}, Ca^{++}, Mg^{++}).

THALIDOMIDE
Thalomid
Immunomodulator

No   No   3   X

Caps: 50, 100, 200 mg

Drug can only be prescribed by health care providers registered with the STEPS program and dispensed by pharmacists registered with the STEPS program at 1-888-423-5436.

Erythema nodosum leprosum:
Adult: 100–300 mg PO QHS and at least 1 hr after the evening meal. Use lower end of dosing range for patients weighing <50 kg. Continue until signs and symptoms have subsided, usually around 2 wk, and dosage may be tapered off in 50 mg decrements at 2 to 4 wk intervals. Patients requiring prolonged maintenance therapy to prevent recurrence or who have failed the tapering process should be maintained on a minimum dose to control symptoms. Tapering should be attempted every 3 to 6 mo in decrements of 50 mg at 2 to 4 wk intervals.

Contraindications: Hypersensitivity to thalidomide products, pregnancy (highly teratogenic), sexually active males not using latex condom (risk to fetus from semen of males taking thalidomide unknown), and women of childbearing potential **not** using two forms of contraception.

Warnings/Precautions: Women of childbearing potential should have a pregnancy test (sensitivity of at least 50 mIU/mL) performed within 24 hr prior to starting therapy and periodically during therapy. Reported teratogenic effects have included amelia, phocomelia, hypoplasticity of the bones, absence of bones, mortality (~40%), external ear abnormalities, congenital heart defects, and alimentary tract, urinary tract, and genital malformations. **Use with caution** in peripheral neuropathy (especially with other medications with the same side effect), seizures, neutropenia, HIV and multiple myeloma. **Avoid** hazardous activities, operating machinery, or driving, as they may cause drowsiness. Patients with neoplastic or infammatory disorders have increased risk for thrombotic events. Dosing in renal or hepatic dysfunction have **not** been established.

Adverse Effects: Edema, rash, hypocalcemia, constipation, nausea, leukopenia, confusion, somnolence and tremor are common. Stevens-Johnson syndrome, TEN, teratogenesis, neutropenia, thrombotic disorder, and peripheral neuropathy may occur. Seizures and pulmonary embolism have been reported.

Drug Interactions: Alcohol, barbiturates, chlorpromazine and reserpine may enhance sedative effects. Dexamethasone may increase risk for TEN. Docetaxel may increase risk for venous thromboembolism. Zoledronic acid may increase risk for renal dysfunction. Darbopoetin alpha increases thrombogenic state in patients with myelodysplastic syndrome.

Drug Administration: Take with water in the evening, at least 1 hr after a meal.

THIABENDAZOLE
Mintezol
Anthelmintic

Yes   Yes   ?   C

Suspension: 500 mg/5 mL
Chewable tabs: 500 mg; contains saccharin
Topical suspension: 10–15%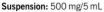
Topical ointment: 10% in white petrolatum

Child and adult: 50 mg/kg/24 hr PO ÷ BID; **max. dose:** 3 g/24 hr
Duration of therapy (consecutive days):
  Strongyloides: × 2 days (5 days for disseminated disease)
  Cutaneous larva migrans: × 2–5 days
  Visceral larva migrans: × 5–7 days
  Trichinosis: × 2–4 days
Angiostrongylosis: 75 mg/kg/24 hr PO ÷ BID-TID × 3 days; **max. dose:** 3 g/24 hr
Dracunculosis: 50–75 mg/kg/24 hr PO ÷ BID × 3 days; **max. dose:** 3 g/24 hr
Topical therapy for cutaneous larva migrans: Apply sparingly to all lesions 4–6 times/24 hr until lesions are inactivated. See *Arch Dermatol* 129:588;1993 for additional information.

Contraindications: Hypersensitivity to thiabendazole and prophylactic treatment for pinworm infestation.
Warnings/Precautions: Clinical experience in children weighing <13.6 kg (30 lb) is limited. **Use with caution** in renal or hepatic impairment. Supportive therapy for malnutrition, anemia, or dehydration is indicated prior to initiation of therapy. **Not** suitable for prophylactic use and for treatment of mixed infections with ascaris. Ocular adverse effects (see below) may persist beyond 1 yr in some instances.
Adverse Effects: GI disturbance, anorexia, drowsiness and vertigo are frequent side effects. May cause abnormal sensation in eyes, xanthopsia, blurred vision, dry mucous membranes, rash, hypersensitivity, erythema multiforme, leukopenia, and hallucinations. Stevens-Johnson syndrome and liver damage have been reported.
Drug Interactions: May increase serum levels of theophylline or caffeine.
Drug Administration: PO: Chew tablet well before swallowing. Give doses after meals.

TICARCILLIN
Ticar
Antibiotic, penicillin (extended spectrum)

Yes   Yes   1   B

Injection: 3 g
Each gram contains 5.2–6.5 mEq Na.

Neonate, IM/IV:
≤7 days:
  <2 kg: 150 mg/kg/24 hr ÷ Q12 hr
  ≥2 kg: 225 mg/kg/24 hr ÷ Q8 hr
>7 days:
  <1.2 kg: 150 mg/kg/24 hr ÷ Q12 hr
  1.2–2 kg: 225 mg/kg/24 hr ÷ Q8 hr
  >2 kg: 300 mg/kg/24 hr ÷ Q6–8 hr

Continued

TICARCILLIN *continued*

Infant and child (IM/IV): 200–300 mg/kg/24 hr ÷ Q4–6 hr; **max. dose:** 24 g/24 hr
Cystic fibrosis (IM/IV): 300–600 mg/kg/24 hr ÷ Q4–6 hr; **max. dose:** 24 g/24 hr
Adult (IM/IV): 1–4 g/dose Q4–6 hr; **max. dose:** 24 g/24 hr

Contraindications: Hypersensitivity to any of the penicillins.
Warnings/Precautions: **Use with caution** with cephalosporin hypersensitivity and CHF (high sodium content). Like other penicillins, CSF penetration occurs only with inflamed meninges. **Do not mix** with aminoglycoside in same solution. Half-life is prolonged with impaired hepatic and/or renal function **(adjust dose in renal failure; see Chapter 3)**.
Adverse Effects: Thrombophlebitis, rash and immune hypersensitivity are common. May cause decreased platelet aggregation, bleeding diathesis, hypernatremia, hematuria, hypokalemia, hypocalcemia, allergy, and increased AST.
Drug Interactions: Probenecid increases ticarcillin levels. May cause false-positive tests for urine protein and serum Coombs' test.
Drug Administration
    IV: For IV push, infuse over 10–20 min at a concentration ≤ 100 mg/mL. For intermittent infusion, infuse over 30–60 min at a concentration ≤ 50 mg/mL. If patient is receiving concomitant aminoglycoside therapy, separate ticarcillin from aminoglycoside by at least 1 hr; separate by at least 2 hr if aminoglycoside serum levels are being sampled before and after an aminoglycoside dosage.
    IM: Dilute with sterile water or lidocaine 1% (without epinephrine) to 385 mg/mL. Assess the potential risk/benefit for using lidocaine as a diluent. Administer by deep IM injection into a large muscle mass.

TICARCILLIN WITH CLAVULANATE
Timentin
Antibiotic, penicillin (extended spectrum with beta-lactamase inhibitor)

Yes   Yes   1   B

Injection: 3.1 g (3 g ticarcillin and 0.1 g clavulanate); contains 4.51 mEq Na$^+$ and 0.15 mEq K$^+$ per 1 g drug
Premixed injection: 3.1 g (3 g ticarcillin and 0.1 g clavulanate) in 100 mL; contains 18.7 mEq Na$^+$ and 0.5 mEq K$^+$ per 100 mL

All doses based on tiarcillin component.
Neonate: See Ticarcillin.
Term neonate and infant <3 mo: 200–300 mg/kg/24 hr IV ÷ Q4–6 hr
Infant ≥3 mo and child:
    Mild/moderate infections: 200 mg/kg/24 hr IV ÷ Q6 hr
    Severe infections: 300 mg/kg/24 hr IV ÷ Q4–6 hr
    Max. dose: 18–24 mg/24 hr
Cystic fibrosis: See Ticarcillin.
Adult: 3 g/dose IV Q4–6 hr IV
    UTI: 3 g/dose IV Q6–8 hr
    Max. dose: 18–24 g/24 hr

Contraindications: Hypersensitivity to penicillins.
Warnings/Precautions: Activity similar to ticarcillin except that beta-lactamase inhibitor broadens spectrum to include *S. aureus* and *H. influenzae*. Like other penicillins, CSF penetration occurs only with inflamed meninges. **Adjust dosage in renal impairment (see Chapter 3).** See Ticarcillin for additional information.

TICARCILLIN WITH CLAVULANATE *continued*

Adverse Effects: Thrombophlebitis, headache and immune hypersensitivity reaction are common. See Ticarcillin for additional adverse effects.

Drug Interactions: Probenecid increases ticarcillin levels. May cause false-positive tests for urine protein and serum Coombs' test.

Drug Administration: For intermittent IV infusion, infuse over 30 min at a concentration ≤100 mg/mL; concentrations ≤50 mg/mL are preferred. If patient is receiving concomitant aminoglycoside therapy, separate ticarcillin/clavulanate from aminoglycoside by at least 1 hr; separate by at least 2 hr if aminoglycoside serum levels are being sampled before and after an aminoglycoside dosage.

TIGECYCLINE
Tygacil
Antibiotic, glycylcycline

Yes   No   ?   D

Injection: 50 mg

 ≥8–16 yr (data limited to single dose pharmacokinetic data; additional studies are ongoing especially for children 8–11 yr where data is extremely limited): 1 mg/kg/dose IV Q12 hr; **max. dose:** 50 mg/dose.

Adult:
Skin, skin structure, or intra-abdominal infection: 100 mg IV × 1, followed by 50 mg IV Q12 hr × 5–14 days.

Contraindications: Hypersensitivity to tigecycline.

Warnings/Precautions: Glycylcycline antibiotics are structurally similar to tetracyclines and may have similar adverse effects. **Not** recommended in patients <8 yr due to tooth staining and decreased bone growth, and in pregnancy because these side effects may occur in the fetus. **Use with caution** with known hypersensitivty to tetracyclines, pancreatitis, and hepatic impairment (Child Pugh C: reduce maintenance dose to 25 mg IV Q12 hr).

Adverse Effects: Diarrhea, nausea and vomiting are common. Injection site reactions, acute pancreatitis, vaginitis, somnolence and taste perversion have been reported.

Drug Interactions: PT and other suitable anticoagulation tests should be monitored if used with warfarin. May reduce the effectiveness of oral contraceptives.

Drug Administration: For intermittent infusion, infuse over 30–60 min at a concentration ≤1 mg/mL.

TINIDAZOLE
Tindamax
Antiprotozoal agent, nitroimidazole

Yes   No   ?   C

Tabs: 250, 500 mg
Oral suspension: 66.7 mg/mL

 Child (≥3 yr):
Amebiasis (Entamoeba histolytica), intestinal: 50 mg/kg/dose PO QD × 3 days
Amebic liver abscess: 50 mg/kg/dose PO QD × 3–5 days
Giardia lamblia: 50 mg/kg/dose PO × 1
Max. dose: 2 g/dose

Continued

TINIDAZOLE *continued*

Adult:
 Amebiasiss (Entamoeba histolytica), intestinal: 2 g PO QD × 3 days
 Amebic liver abscess: 2 g PO QD × 3–5 days
 Giardia lamblia, or Trichomonas vaginalis (treat patient and sexual partner at the same time): 2 g PO × 1

Contraindications: Hypersensitivity to tinidazole or other nitroimidazole derivatives (e.g., metronidazole); and first trimester of pregnancy. For use during lactation, interruption is recommended during therapy and for 3 days following the last dose.

Warnings/Precautions: Use with caution in blood dyscrasia, candidiasis (vaginal candidiasis may develop), CNS disorders and liver dysfunction. If dose is to be administered on day of hemodialysis, give an additional half-dose at the end of hemodialysis. Although there is no data reported specifically with tinidazole, a potential risk for carcinogenicity is based on studies with the chemically related metronidazole in mice and rats.

Adverse Effects: Constipation, epigastric discomfort, indigestion, loss of appetite, nausea, taste sense alterations, vomiting, cramps, asthenia, dizziness, headache, malaise and fatigue are common. Seizures, peripheral neuropathy, urticaria, Stevens-Johnson syndrome, tongue discoloration, darkened urine and palpitations have been reported.

Drug Interactions: Although studies are incomplete and tinidazole is chemically related to metronidazole, may enhance the effects of warfarin and other oral coumarin anticoagulants, alcohols, disulfiram, lithium, phenytoin, cyclosporine, tacrolimus and fluorouracil; and drugs that induce CYP 450 3A4 liver enzymes, cholestyramine, and oxytetracycline may reduce tinidazole's effects. CYP 450 3A4 inhibitors may increase tinidazole's effects/toxicity.

Drug Administration: Give doses with food to minimize GI side effects. **Avoid** consumption of alcoholic beverages and preparations containing ethanol or propylene glycol during therapy and 3 days afterward.

TIOCONAZOLE
Monistat 1, Tioconazole 1, Vagistat-1
Antifungal agent, imidazole

No No ? C

Vaginal ointment (OTC): 6.5% (4.6 g in a prefilled applicator)

≥12 yr and adult: 1 applicator-full (4.6 g of 6.5% ointment) intravaginally once, preferably at bedtime

Contraindications: Hypersensitivity to tioconazole or imidazole antifungal agents.

Warnings/Precautions: Do not use if you are pregnant, have diabetes or HIV. Components in the suppository dosage form may weaken certain rubber or latex products used in vaginal contraceptive diaphragms and condoms. Wait 3 days after treatment to resume use of condoms and diaphragms.

Adverse Effects: Burning, discomfort, rash and itching are common. Abdominal pain, headache, dysuria and nocturia have been reported.

Drug Interactions: Bleeding or bruising may occur when used with warfarin.

TIOCONAZOLE *continued*

Drug Administration: Wash hands prior to use. Gently insert applicator full of cream high into the vagina at bedtime. Remain lying down for 30 min after administration. Use sanitary napkin or minipad to prevent staining of clothing. **Do not** use tampons.

TIPRANAVIR
Aptivus, TPV
Antiviral agent, protease inhibitor

Yes   No   3   C

Caps: 250 mg; contains 7% dehydrated alcohol

 Adult: 500 mg PO BID with ritonavir 200 mg PO BID

Contraindications: Hypersensitivity to tipranavir or other components of the formulation; and moderate/severe hepatic impairment (Child-Pugh Class B or C). Concomitant administration with drugs that are highly dependent on CYP 450 3A clearance such as amiodarone, astemizole, bepridil, cisapride, ergot derivatives, fecainaide, midazolam, pimozide, propafenone, quinidine, terfenadine and triazolam.

Warnings/Precautions: Potential cross-sensitivity with sulfa allergic patients. Co-administration with St. John's wort and HMG-Co-A reductase inhibitors (e.g., lovastatin, simvastatin) are **not** recommended because of causing reductions in tripranavir levels and increasing risk for myopathy and rhabdomyolysis, respectively. Reports of intracranial hemorrhage, hepatitis, and hepatic decompensation have resulted in some fatalities. **Use with caution** in hepatic impairment (primary route of metabolism; no dose reduction recommendations available), hemophilia type A or B, diabetes or hyperglycemia, and in patients at risk for increased bleeding from trauma, surgery, or other medical conditions, or who are receiving medications known to increase the risk of bleeding, such as antiplatelet agents or anticoagulants. Tipranavir should always be administered in combination with ritonavir and is currently indicated in adults who are highly treatment experienced or have HIV-1 strains resistant to multiple protease inhibitors, and who have evidence of viral replication. Liver function tests should be obtained at baseline and monitored frequently.

Adverse Effects: GI disturbances, fatigue, headache, rash, vomiting, and elevated LFTs, cholesterol and triglycerides are common. Fat redistribution, immune reconstitution syndrome, hepatitis, and elevated transaminases and hepatic decompensation in patients with hepatitis B or C or already elevated transaminastes have been reported. See Warnings/Precautions section.

Drug Interactions: Substrate and inhibitor of cytochrome P 450 3A. May reduce levels of valproic acid. Carbamazepine, phenobarbital, and phenytoin may decrease effects of tipranavir. Ritonavir boosts darunavir levels and is also a substrate and inhibitor of CYP 450 3A. See Contraindications and Warnings/Precautions sections. Always check the potential for other drug interactions when either initiating therapy or adding new drugs onto an existing regimen.

Drug Administration: Drug is always given in combination with ritonavir. Administer all doses with a meal or light snack. If given together, separate dose from didanosine by at least 2 hr.

For explanation of icons, see p. 306.

TOBRAMYCIN
Nebcin, Tobrex, AKTob, TOBI and others
Antibiotic, aminoglycoside

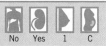

No   Yes   1   C

Injection: 10, 40 mg/mL; may contain phenol and bisulfites
Powder for injection: 1.2 g; preservative free
Ophthalmic ointment (Tobrex, AKTob): 0.3% (3.5 g)
    In combination with dexamethasone (TobraDex): 0.3% tobramycin with 0.1% dexamethasone (3.5 g); contains 0.5% chlorbutanol
Ophthalmic solution (Tobrex): 0.3% (5 mL)
    In combination with dexamethasone: 0.3% tobramycin with 0.1% dexamethasone (2.5, 5, 10 mL); contains 0.01% benzalkonium chloride and EDTA
Nebulizer solution: 300 mg/5 mL (TOBI, preservative free; 56s), 170 mg/3.4 mL (mixed in 0.45% NS, preservative free, use with eFlow nebulizer)

 Neonate, IM/IV (see following table):

Postconceptional Age (wk)	Postnatal Age (days)	Dose (mg/kg/dose)	Interval (hr)
≤29*	0–7	5	48
	8–28	4	36
	>28	4	24
30–33	0–7	4.5	36
	>7	4	24
34–37	0–7	4	24
	>7	4	18–24
≥38	0–7	4	24
	>7	4	12–18

*Or significant asphyxia, PDA, indomethicin use, poor cardiac output, reduced renal function

Child: 7.5 mg/kg/24 hr ÷ Q8 hr IV/IM
Cystic fibrosis: 7.5–10.5 mg/kg/24 hr ÷ Q8 hr IV
Adult: 3–6 mg/kg/24 hr ÷ Q8 hr IV/IM
Ophthalmic:
    Tobramycin:
        Child and adult: Apply thin ribbon of ointment into conjunctival sac(s) BID-TID; or 1–2 drops of solution to affected eye(s) Q4 hr
    Tobramycin with dexamethasone:
        ≥2 yr and adult: Apply ½ inch ribbon of ointment into conjunctival sac(s) TID-QID; or 1–2 drops of solution to affected eye(s) Q2 hr × 24–48 hr, then 1–2 drops Q4–6 hr
Inhalation:
    Cystic fibrosis prophylaxis therapy:
        ≥6 yr and adult:
            TOBI: 300 mg Q12 hr administered in repeated cycles of 28 days on drug followed by 28 days off drug.

TOBRAMYCIN *continued*

>> *Use with eFlow nebulizer:* 170 mg Q12 hr administered in repeated cycles of 28 days on drug followed by 28 days off drug.

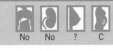

Contraindications: Hypersensitivity to aminoglycosides or any other components in the formulation.

Warnings/Precautions: Use with caution in combination with neurotoxic, ototoxic, or nephrotoxic drugs; anesthetics or neuromuscular blocking agents; pre-existing renal, vestibular or auditory impairment; and in patients with neuromuscular disorders.

Higher doses are recommended in patients with cystic fibrosis, neutropenia, or burns.

Adjust dose in renal failure (see Chapter 3). Monitor peak and trough levels. Therapeutic Peak Levels:

6–10 mg/L in general

8–10 mg/L in pulmonary infections, neutropenia, osteomylitis, and severe sepsis

Therapeutic Trough Levels: <2 mg/L. Recommended serum sampling time at steady state: trough within 30 min prior to the third consecutive dose and peak 30–60 min after the administration of the third consecutive dose.

Adverse Effects: May cause ototoxicity, nephrotoxicity, and neuromuscular blockade. Vertigo, myelotoxicity and hypomagnesemia have been reported. Serious allergic reactions including anaphylaxis and dermatologic reactions including exfoliative dermatitis, toxic epidermal necrolysis, erythema multiforme and Stevens-Johnson syndrome are rare.

Inhalation Use: Transient voice alteration, bronchospasm, dyspnea, pharyngitis and increase cough may occur. Transient tinnitus has been reported.

Drug Interactions: Ototoxic effects synergistic with furosemide. See Warnings/Precautions section.

Drug Administration

IV: Infuse over 30–60 min at a concentration ≤10 mg/mL. Administer beta-lactam antibiotics at least 1 hr before or after tobramycin.

IM: Use either undiluted commercial products of 10 or 40 mg/mL.

Ophthalmic:

Drops: Apply finger pressure to lacrimal sac during and for 1–2 min after dose application.

Ointment: Instill ointment in lower conjunctival sac by avoiding contact of ointment tip with eye or skin.

Inhalation: For use with other medications in cystic fibrosis, use the following order of administration: bronchodilator first, chest physiotherapy, other inhaled medications (if indicated), and tobramycin last.

TOBI: Use PARI LC Plus nebulizer and a DeVilbiss Pulmo-Aide compressor. Treatment period is usually over 20–30 min.

eFlow Nebulizer: Dose may be diluted with NS up to a total volume of 4 mL. Treatment period is usually over 5–7 min.

TOLNAFTATE

Tinactin, Aftate, and many others

Antifungal agent

No	No	?	C

Topical aerosol liquid [OTC]: 1% (60, 120 mL); may contain 36% alcohol
Aerosol powder [OTC]: 1% (100, 105, 150 g); contains 14% alcohol and talc
Cream [OTC]: 1% (15, 21, 30 g)
Gel [OTC]: 1% (15 g)   *Continued*

For explanation of icons, see p. 306.

FORMULARY

TOLNAFTATE *continued*

Topical powder [OTC]: 1% (45, 90 g)
Topical solution [OTC]: 1% (10 mL)

 Child (≥2 yr) and adult:
  Topical: Apply 1–3 drops of solution or small amount of gel, liquid, cream
  or powder to affected areas BID–TID for 2–4 wk.

Contraindications: Hypersensitivity to tolnaftate.
Warnings/Precautions: **Avoid** eye contact. **Do not use** for nail or scalp
infections. **Not** recommended in children less than 2 yr old. **Discontinue use if
sensitization develops.**
Adverse Effects: May cause mild irritation and sensitivity. Contact dermatitis has
been reported.
Drug Interactions: None identified.
Drug Administration: Wash and dry affected area before drug application and **avoid**
contact with eyes. Apply enough medicine to cover affected area. When treating foot
infections, use liberal quantities of powder to affected areas and apply to socks and
shoes. When using the aerosolized liquid or powder dosage form, use a 6–10 inch
distance when applying dose.

TRIFLURIDINE
Viroptic, trifluorothymidine
Antiviral agent, ophthalmic

No No ? C

Ophthalmic solution: 1% (7.5 mL); contains 0.001% thimerosal

Herpes simplex keratitis:
  ≥6 yr and adult: 1 drop onto the cornea of the affected eye(s) Q2 hr while
  awake (**max. dose:** 9 drops/24 hr) until corneal ulcer has completely
re-epithelialized followed by 1 drop Q4 hr while awake (**max. dose:** 5 drops/24 hr)
for an additional 7 days. **Do not exceed** 21 days of continuous therapy.

Contraindications: Hypersensitivity reactions or chemical intolerance to
trifluridine.
Warnings/Precautions: Has **not** shown to be effective in the prophylaxis of
herpes simplex keratoconjunctivitis and epithelial keratitis. Although safety and
efficacy in ophthalmic infections caused by vaccinia virus have not been established,
the drug also is recommended for the treatment and prevention of ocular vaccinia
infections that occur as a complication of smallpox vaccination.
Adverse Effects: May cause mild transient local irritation of the conjunctiva and
cornea and palpebral edema. Superficial punctate keratopathy, epithelial keratopathy,
hypersensitivity reaction, stromal edema and increased intraocular pressure have
been reported.
Drug Interactions: None identified.
Drug Administration: Apply directly onto the cornea and avoid touching the tip of the
dropper. Apply finger pressure to lacrimal sac during and for 1–2 min after dose
application. Store drops in the refrigerator.

TRIMETHOPRIM

Proloprim, Primsol, TMP, and various generics
Anti-infective, folate antagonist

Yes   Yes   1   C

Tabs: 100, 200 mg
Oral solution:
  Primsol: 50 mg/5 mL (473 mL); contains parabens

Acute otitis media:
  ≥6 mo: 10 mg/kg/24 hr ÷ Q12 hr PO × 10 days
UTI:
  Infant and child <12 yr: 4–6 mg/kg/24 hr ÷ Q12 hr PO × 10 days
  ≥12 yr and adult: 100 mg Q12 hr PO or 200 mg Q24 hr PO × 10 days
Pneumocystis carinii pneumonia, mild/moderate:
  ≥12 yr and adult: 15 mg/kg/24 hr ÷ TID PO × 21 days with dapsone (<13 yr: 2 mg/kg/dose PO QD and ≥13 yr: 100 mg PO QD).

Contraindications: Hypersensitivity to trimethoprim and in those with documented megaloblastic anemia due to folate deficiency.
  Warnings/Precautions: Use with caution in patients with possible folate deficiency and impaired hepatic or renal function **(adjust dose in renal failure; see Chapter 3). Discontinue use** if the count of any formed blood element is significantly reduced. Folates may be administered concomitantly without interfering with antibacterial action.
Adverse Effects: Pruritis and rash are common. Fever, headache, bone marrow suppression and elevated liver enzymes, BUN and serum creatinine may occur. Rare immune hypersensitivity reaction (e.g., TEN, Stevens-Johnson syndrome and exfoliative dermatitis) and aseptic meningitis have been reported.
Drug Interactions: Inhibits CYP 450 2C8 and 2C9 isoenzymes. May increase the effects/toxicity of phenytoin, cyclosporine, dapsone, procainamide, rifampin and warfarin. Use with other folate antagonists (e.g., methotrexate, pyrimethamine) may increase risk of megaloblastic anemia. May falsely increase creatinine determination measured by Jaffe alkaline picrate method; and may falsely interfere with serum methotrexate assay (bacterial dihydrofolate reductase methods).
Drug Administration: Give on an empty stomach. If GI upset occurs, give with milk or food.

TRIMETHOPRIM AND SULFAMETHOXAZOLE

See *Sulfamethoxazole and Trimethoprim*

TRIMETREXATE GLUCURONATE

NeuTrexin
Anti-infective agent, folate antagonist

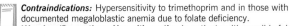

Yes   Yes   ?   D

Injection: 25 mg with or without 50 mg leucovorin

Pneumocystis carinii pneumonia, moderate/severe (limited data in children): 45 mg/m²/dose IV over 60–90 min QD × 21 days with leucovorin 20 mg/m²/dose IV over 5–10 min or PO Q6 hr × 24 days. If using oral leucovorin, round up dose to the next highest 25 mg increment.

Continued

TRIMETREXATE GLUCURONATE *continued*

Alternative trimetrexate and leucovorin dosing by body weight:

Body Weight (kg)	Trimetrexate Glucuronate Dose (mg/kg/dose IV QD)	Leucovorin Dose (mg/kg/dose IV/PO Q6 hr)*
<50	1.5	0.6
50–80	1.2	0.5
>80	1	0.5

*With oral use, round up to the next highest 25 mg increment.

Dose modifications for hematologic toxicity:

HEMATOLOGIC TOXICITY DOSAGE MODIFICATION FOR TRIMETREXATE GLUCURONATE AND LEUCOVORIN

Toxicity Grade	Neutrophils (polys and bands) mm³	Platelets mm³	Trimetrexate Dose (mg/m²/dose IV QD)	Leucovorin Dose (mg/m²/dose IV/PO Q6 hr)*
1	>1000	>75,000	45	20
2	750–1000	50,000–75,000	45	40
3	500–749	25,000–49,999	22	40
4	<500	<25,000	If day 1–9: discontinue**; if day 10–21: interrupt up to 96 hr***	40

* With oral use, round up to the next highest 25 mg increment.

** Maintain leucovorin therapy for an additional 72 hr after discontinuing trimetrexate.

*** If counts recover within 96 hr, resume at trimetrexate dosage at respective toxicity grade level and maintain leucovorin therapy at 40 mg/m2/dose IV/PO Q6 hr. Discontinue trimetrexate if counts do not improve to grade 3 or less within 96 hr of interruption and continue leucovorin therapy for an additional 72 hr after discontinuing trimetrexate.

Contraindications: Clinically significant hypersensitivity to trimetrexate, leucovorin, or methotrexate.
Warnings/Precautions: **Must be used** with concurrent leuovorin to avoid potentially serious or life-threatening toxicities. **Use with caution** in alcoholics, ulcerative disorders of the GI tract, impaired hematologic reserve, receiving myelosuppressive drugs, and impaired hepatic and renal **(adjust dose in renal failure; see Chapter 3)** function.
Adverse Effects: Rash, nausea, vomiting and stomatitis are common. Myelosuppression, hepatotoxicity and nephrotoxicity may occur. Consider alternative safer drugs with pregnancy.

TRIMETREXATE GLUCURONATE *continued*

Drug Interactions: Enzyme inhibiting medications such as erythromycin, cimetidine, rifampin, rifabutin, ketoconazole, clotrimazole, miconazole and fluconazole may increase risk for trimetrexate toxicity. Zidovudine should be discontinued during trimetrexate therapy to allow use of full therapeutic doses.

Drug Administration: For intermittent infusion, infuse over 60–90 min at a concentration 0.25–2 mg/mL diluted in D_5W. Concomitant leucovorin therapy must extend for 72 hr past the last dose of trimetrexate to prevent toxicities.

UNDECYLENIC ACID
Elon Dual Defense Anti-Fungal Formula, Fungoid AF, Goordochom, Caldesene, Cruex, and many others
Antifungal agent

No   No   ?   ?

Topical solution [OTC]: 25% (30 mL); may contain alcohol
Topical powder [OTC]: 10% (45, 60, 120 g), 12% (60 g), 25% (45 g)
Topcial spray [OTC]: 10% (51, 100, 155.9 g), 19% (54, 105,165 g)
Topical cream [OTC]: 20% (15 g)
Soap [OTC]: 97.5 g

Tinea corporis: Apply topically BID to clean dry area × 4 wk.
Tinea pedis: Apply topically BID to clean dry area × 4 wk.

Contraindications: Hypersensitivity to undecylenic acid.
Warnings/Precautions: **For external use only.** Product has **not** been proven effective on the scalp or nail. Cream and solution dosage forms are primarily used. Powders are generally used as adjunctive therapy or as primary therapy for very mild conditions.
Adverse Effects: Skin irritation and rash are common. Hypersensitivity has been reported.
Drug Interactions: None identified.
Drug Administration: **Avoid** contact with eyes or other mucous membranes. **Do not** inhale powder. Clean affected area with soap and warm water and dry thoroughly. Apply thin layer over affected area. For tinea pedis, pay attention to spaces between the toes. **Do not** apply to blistered, raw, or oozing areas of skin or over deep wounds or puncture wounds.

VALACYCLOVIR
Valtrex
Antiviral agent

Yes   Yes   2   B

Tabs: 500, 1000 mg
Oral suspension: 50 mg/mL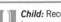

Child: Recommended dosages based on steady-state pharmacokinetic data in immunocompromised children. Efficacy data is incomplete.
To mimic an IV acyclovir regimen of 250 mg/m²/dose or 10 mg/kg/dose TID:
    30 mg/kg/dose PO TID or alternatively by weight:
        4–12 kg: 250 mg PO TID
        13–21 kg: 500 mg PO TID
        22–29 kg: 750 mg PO TID
        ≥30 kg: 1000 mg PO TID

Continued

VALACYCLOVIR *continued*

To mimic a PO acyclovir regimen of 20 mg/kg/dose 4 or 5 times a day:
    20 mg/kg/dose PO TID or alternatively by weight:
        6–19 kg: 250 mg PO TID
        20–31 kg: 500 mg PO TID
        ≥32 kg: 750 mg PO TID
Herpes zoster (see remarks):
    Adult (immunocompetent): 1 g/dose PO TID × 7 days within 48–72 hr of onset of rash.
Genital herpes:
    Adolescent and adult:
        Initial episodes: 1 g/dose PO BID × 10 days.
        Recurrent episodes: 500 mg/dose PO BID × 3 days.
        Suppressive therapy: 500–1000 mg/dose PO QD × 1 yr, then reassess for recurrences. Patients with < 9 recurrences per yr may be dosed at 500 mg/dose PO QD × 1 yr
Herpes labialis (cold sores):
    Adolescent and adult: 2 g/dose PO Q12 hr × 1 day

Contraindications: Hypersensitivity or intolerance to valacyclovir, acyclovir, or any component of the formulation.

Warnings/Precautions: This pro-drug is metabolized to acyclovir and L-valine with better oral absorption than acyclovir. Valacyclovir **cannot** be substituted for acyclovir on a one-to-one basis. **Use with caution** in hepatic or renal insufficiency **(adjust dose; see Chapter 3)**. Thrombotic thrombocytopenic purpura/hemolytic uremic syndrome (TTP/HUS) has been reported in patients with advanced HIV infection and in bone marrow and renal transplant recipients.

For initial episodes of genital herpes, therapy is most effective when initiated within 48 hr of symptom onset; no efficacy data are available if therapy initiated >72 hr after rash onset. Therapy should be initiated immediately after the onset of symptoms in recurrent episodes (no efficacy data when initiating therapy >24 hr after onset of symptoms). Data are not available for use as suppressive therapy for periods >1 yr.

Adverse Effects: Nausea, vomiting and headache are common. See Warnings/Precautions section and Acyclovir for additional information. Aggressive behavior, agitation, mania, sedation and tremors have been reported.

Drug Interactions: Probenecid or cimetidine can reduce the rate of conversion to acyclovir. Use with mycophenolate may increase risk of neutropenia.

Drug Administration: Doses may be given with or without food. Maintain adequate hydration while on therapy.

VALGANCICLOVIR
Valcyte
Antiviral agent

No   Yes   3   C

Tabs: 450 mg
Oral suspension: 60 mg/mL

Neonate and infant:
Symptomatic congenital CMV (from pharmacokinetic (PK) data in 8 infants 4–90 days old, mean: 20 days; and 24 neonates 8–34 days old): 15–16 mg/kg/dose PO BID. Additional PK, safety and efficacy studies are required.

V

VALGANCICLOVIR *continued*

Child:
 CMV prophylaxis in liver transplantation (limited data based on a retrospective review in 10 patients, mean age 4.9 + 5.6 yr): 15–18 mg/kg/dose PO QD × 100 days following transplantation resulted in 1 case of asymptomatic CMV infection detected by CMV antigenemia at day 7 of therapy. This patient then received a higher dose of 15 mg/kg/dose BID until 3 consecutive negative CMV antigenemia were achieved. The dose was switched back to a prophylactic regimen at day 46 post-transplant.

Adolescent and adult:
 CMV retinitis:
  Induction therapy: 900 mg PO BID × 21 days with food
  Maintenance therapy: 900 mg PO QD with food
 CMV prophylaxis in heart, kidney, and kidney-pancreas transplantation: 900 mg PO QD starting within 10 days of transplantation until 100 days posttransplantation.

Contraindications: Hypersensitivity to valganciclovir or ganciclovir; ANC <500 mm³; platelets <25,000 mm³; hemoglobin <8 g/dL; and patients on hemodialysis.

Warnings/Precautions: This pro-drug is metabolized to ganciclovir with better oral absorption than gancicloyor. Valganciclovir **cannot** be substituted for ganciclovir on a one-to-one basis. **Use with caution** in renal insufficiency **(adjust dose; see Chapter 3)**; pre-existing bone marrow supression; or receiving myelosuppressive drugs or irradiation. May impair fertility in men and women; use effective contraception during and for at least 90 days after therapy. **Not** indicated in preventing CMV disease in liver transplant patients.

Adverse Effects: Headache, fever, insomnia, peripheral neuropathy, diarrhea, vomiting, abdominal pain, neutropenia, anemia and thrombocytopenia are common.

Drug Interactions: Immunosuppressive agents may increase hematologic toxicities. May increase the risk for seizures with imipenem/cilastatin. May increase didanosine and zidovudine levels, whereas didanosine and zidovudine may decrease ganciclovir levels. See Ganciclovir for additional information.

Drug Administration: All doses are administered with food. **Do not** break or crush tablet. **Avoid** direct contact with broken or crushed tablets with the skin or mucous membranes.

VANCOMYCIN
Vancocin and others
Antibiotic, glycopeptide

No   Yes   ?   C/B

Injection: 0.5, 1, 5, 10 g
Caps: 125, 250 mg
Oral solution: 1 g (reconstitute to 250 mg/5 mL), 10 g (reconstitute to 500 mg/6 mL)

Neonates, IV (see following table):
Infant and child, IV:
 CNS and serious infections; and non-obese oncology patient without renal impairment: 60 mg/kg/24 hr ÷ Q6 hr
 Other infections: 40 mg/kg/24 hr ÷ Q6–8 hr
 Max. dose: 1 g/dose

Continued

VANCOMYCIN *continued*

Weight (kg)	Postnatal Age	
	<7 Days	**≥7 Days**
<1.2	15 mg/kg/dose Q24 hr	15 mg/kg/dose Q24 hr
1.2–2	10–15 mg/kg/dose Q12–18 hr	10–15 mg/kg/dose Q8–12 hr
>2	10–15 mg/kg/dose Q8–12 hr	15–20 mg/kg/dose Q8 hr

Adult: 2 g/24 hr ÷ Q6–12 hr IV; **max. dose:** 4 g/24 hr
C. difficile colitis:
    Child: 40–50 mg/kg/24 hr ÷ Q6 hr PO × 7–10 days
    Max. dose: 500 mg/24 hr; higher **maximum** of 2 g/24 hr has also been used.
    Adult: 125 mg/dose PO Q6 hr × 7–10 days; dosages as high as 2 g/24 hr ÷ Q6–8 hr have also been used.
Endocarditis prophylaxis for GU or GI (excluding esophageal) procedures (complete all antibiotic dose infusion(s) within 30 min of starting procedure):
    Moderate-risk patients allergic to ampicillin or amoxicillin:
        Child: 20 mg/kg/dose IV over 1–2 hr × 1
        Adult: 1 g/dose IV over 1–2 hr × 1
    High-risk patients allergic to ampicillin or amoxicillin:
        Child and adult: Same dose as moderate-risk patients plus gentamicin 1.5 mg/kg/dose (**max. dose:** 120 mg/dose) IV/IM ×1
Intrathecal/intraventricular (use preservative-free preparation):
    Neonate: 5–10 mg QD
    Child: 5–20 mg QD
    Adult: 10–20 mg QD

Contraindications: Hypersensitivity to vancomycin products.
Warnings/Precautions: **Avoid** IM injection and rapid IV infusions (see Drug Administration). **Use with caution** in renal impairment **(adjust dose; see Chapter 3)**, pre-existing hearing loss, and concomitant nephrotoxic/ototoxic drugs or anesthetics. Low concentrations of the drug may appear in CSF with inflamed meninges.

Metronidazole (PO) is the drug of choice for *C. difficile* colitis; vancomycin should be avoided due to the emergence of vancomycin resistant enterococcus. Pregnancy category "B" is assigned with the oral route of administration.

Measuring serum levels are primarily indicated for enhancing efficacy. Toxicity relationship with serum levels has not been clearly established; earlier impure version of the drug ("Mississippi Mud") may have been more toxic. Although the monitoring of serum levels is controversial, there is a trend toward measuring trough levels in most patients. Therapeutic levels: trough: 5–15 mg/L with the additional suggestions: MRSA pneumonia 15–20 mg/L; CNS infections: 20 mg/L; endocarditis: 10–20 mg/L; and bacteremia: 10–15 mg/L. Peak level measurement (20–50 mg/L) have also been recommended for patients with burns, clinically non-responsive in 72 hr of therapy, persistent positive cultures and CNS infections (≥30 mg/L). See Chapter 6 for additional information.

Recommended serum sampling time at steady-state: trough within 30 min prior to the third consecutive dose and peak 60 min after the administration of the third consecutive dose.

VANCOMYCIN *continued*

Adverse Effects: Nausea, vomiting and drug-induced erythroderma are common. "Red man syndrome" associated with rapid IV infusion may occur. Allergic reactions, neutropenia and immune-mediated thrombocytopenia have been reported.

Drug Interactions: Ototoxicity and nephrotoxicity may occur and may be exacerbated with concurrent use of aminoglycosides, loop diuretics or cisplatin. Use with anesthetics has been associated with erythema and histamine-like flushing in children. May enhance neuromuscular blockade with nondepolarizing muscular relaxants.

Drug Administration

IV: For intermittent infusion, infuse over 60 min or a **maximum rate** of 10 mg/min (whichever is longer) at a concentration ≤5 mg/mL. Infusion may be extended to 120 min if 60 min infusion is not tolerated. Diphenhydramine is used to reverse infusion related red man syndrome.

PO: Oral solution may be further diluted with water or with flavoring syrup to improve taste.

Intrathecal/intraventricular: Dilute 1 g vial with preservative-free NS to a concentration of 20 mg/mL.

VARICELLA-ZOSTER IMMUNE GLOBULIN (HUMAN)

VariZig, VZIG

Hyperimmune globulin, varicella-zoster

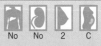

| No | No | 2 | C |

Injection: 125 U; contains 60–200 mg human immunoglobulin G, 0.1 M glycine, 0.04 M sodium chloride, and 0.01% polysorbate 80.

Product is available via an FDA-approved Expanded Access Protocol; see www.fffenterprises.com or call FFF Enterprises at 1-800-843-7477 for additional information.

IM (preferred route) or IV (see remarks):
- **≤ 10 kg:** 125 U
- **10.1–20 kg:** 250 U
- **20.1–30 kg:** 375 U
- **30.1–40 kg:** 500 U
- **>40 kg:** 625 U
- **Max. dose:** 625 U/dose

Contraindications: Hypersensitivity to immune globulin products or any components in the formulation, severe thrombocytopenia (IM injection), IgA deficient individuals, and known immunity to varicella zoster virus.

Warnings/Precautions: Dose should be given within 48 hr of exposure and no later than 96 hr post exposure. See latest AAP Red Book for additional information. As with other products pooled from human plasma, product may contain unknown infectious agents that are not screened for. Hyperviscosity of the blood may increase risk for thrombotic events. IM route is preferred over IV in patients with pre-existing respiratory conditions.

Adverse Effects: Local discomfort, redness and swelling at the injection site, headache, and rash are common. Myalgia, rigors, fatigue, nausea and flushing have been reported.

Drug Interactions: Interferes with immune response to live virus vaccines such as measles, mumps and rubella; defer administration of live vaccines 5 mo or longer after VZIG dose.

Continued

VARICELLA-ZOSTER IMMUNE GLOBULIN (HUMAN) *continued*

Drug Administration

IM: Dilute each vial with 1.25 mL of sterile diluent for a final concentration of 100 U/mL. Administer IM into the anterolateral aspect of the thigh for infants and small children and into the deltoid muscle or anterolateral aspect of the thigh for older children and adults. **Avoid injection** into gluteal region due to risk for sciatic nerve injury. **Do not exceed age specific single maximum IM injection volume.**

IV: Dilute each vial with 2.5 mL of sterile diluent for a final concentration of 50 U/mL. Administer IV dose over 3–5 min. Reconstituted product may be stored up to 12 hr at 2–8°C prior to use.

VORICONAZOLE
Vfend
Antifungal, triazole

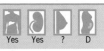

Yes   Yes   ?   D

Tabs: 50, 200 mg; contains povidone
Oral suspension: 40 mg/mL (75 mL); contains sodium benzoate
Injection: 200 mg; contains 3200 mg sulfobutyl ether beta-cyclodextrin (SBECD)

IV (pediatric dosing not well established; see remarks):
    Loading dose: 6 mg/kg/dose Q12 hr × 2 doses.
    Maintenance dose: 4 mg/kg/dose Q12 hr; may be increased to 5 mg/kg/dose Q12 hr if needed or reduced to 3 mg/kg/dose Q12 hr if patient unable to tolerate.

PO, >12 yr (see remarks):
  Invasive aspergillosis/Fusarium/Scedosporium/and other serious infections:
    <40 kg:
      Loading dose: 200 mg PO Q12 hr × 2 doses.
      Maintenance dose: 100 mg PO Q12 hr; dose may be increased to 150 mg PO Q12 hr if response is inadequate.
    ≥40 kg:
      Loading dose: 400 mg PO Q12 hr × 2 doses.
      Maintenance dose: 200 mg PO Q12 hr; dose may be increased to 300 mg PO Q12 hr if response is inadequate.
  Esophageal candidiasis (treat for a minimum of 14 days and until 7 days after resolution of symptoms):
    <40 kg: 100 mg PO Q12 hr
    ≥40 kg: 200 mg PO Q12 hr

Contraindications: Hypersensitivity to voriconazole or its excipients and other azoles. **Do not use** with other CYP 450 3A4 substrates that can lead to prolonged QTc interval (e.g., cisapride, pimozide, and quinidine). Concomitant administration with rifampin, carbamazepine, long-acting barbiturates, ritonavir, efavirenz, and rifabutin can decrease voriconazole levels/effects. Concomitant administration with sirolimus, efavirenz, rifabutin, and ergot alkaloids may result in increased levels/toxicity of these drugs.

Warnings/Precautions: **Use with caution** in severe hepatic disease and galactose intolerance. Avoid strong direct sunlight during therapy and warn patients of potential visual disturbances (blurred vision, photophobia, visual acuity and color changes). **Do not** use IV dosage form for patients with GFR <50 mL/min because of accumulation of the cyclodextrin excipient; switch to oral therapy if possible. Women of child-bearing potential should use effective contraception during treatment. Currently approved for use in invasive aspergillosis, candidal esophagitis, and fusarium and scedosporium apiospermum infections.

VORICONAZOLE *continued*

Adjust dose in hepatic impairment by decreasing only the maintenance dose by 50% for patients with a Child-Pugh Class A or B.

Adverse Effects: Common side effects include GI disturbances, fever, headache, hepatic abnormalities, photosensitivity, rash (6%), and visual disturbances (30%). Serious but rare side effects include anaphylaxis, liver or renal failure, and Stevens-Johnson syndrome.

Drug Interactions: Drug is a substrate and inhibitor for CYP 450 2C9, 2C19 (major substrate), and 3A4 isoenzymes. In addition to the interactions mentioned in the Contraindications section, voriconazole may increase the effects/toxicity of cyclosporine, methadone, tacrolimus, warfarin, coumarin products, statins, benzodiazepines, calcium channel blockers, sulfonylureas, vincristine and vinblastine. Patients receiving concurrent phenytoin should increase their voriconazole maintenance doses (IV: 5 mg/kg/dose Q12 hr; PO: double the usual dose).

Drug Administration: Administer IV over 1–2 hr with a **maximum rate** of 3 mg/kg/hr at a concentration ≤5 mg/mL. Administer oral doses 1 hr before and after meals.

ZALCITABINE
Hivid, dideoxycytidine, ddC
Antiviral agent, nucleoside analogue reverse transcriptase inhibitor

Yes	Yes	3	C

Tabs: 0.375, 0.75 mg

Child < 13 yr: 0.01 mg/kg/dose PO TID
≥13 yr and adult: 0.75 mg PO TID

Contraindications: Hypsensitivity to zalcitabine or any of its components.
Warnings/Precautions: **Use with caution** in patients with liver disease, pancreatitis, pre-existing for neuropathy, or severe myelosuppression. Lactic acidosis and severe hepatomegaly with steatosis, including fatal cases have been reported. Rare cases of hepatic failure and death have been reported in patients with hepatitis B infections. **Discontinue** use of drug if clinical or laboratory evidence of hepatic toxicity develops.

Hemodialysis reduces levels by 50%. **Reduce dose in renal dysfunction (see Chapter 3).**

Adverse Effects: Headaches, GI disturbances and malaise are common side effects. Less common side effects include peripheral neuropathy, bone marrow suppression, hepatitis, pancreatitis, hypertension, rash, oral and esophageal ulcers, myalgias and fatigue. See Warnings/Precautions section for additional information.

Drug Interactions: Amphotericin, cimetidine, foscarnet, probenecid and aminoglycosides may reduce clearance and increase chances of peripheral neuropathy. In addition, drugs which cause peripheral neuropathy (e.g., ddl) should **not** be used in combination with ddC. Concurrent use of IV pentamidine can increase risk of pancreatitis. Antacids can decrease absorption.

Drug Administration: Administer doses on an empty stomach; 1 hr before or 2 hr after meals.

ZANAMIVIR
Relenza
Antiviral

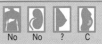

No   No   ?   C

Powder for inhalation: 5 mg/inhalation (5 rotodisks [4 inhalations/rotodisk] with diskhaler); each 5 mg drug contains 20 mg lactose (contains milk proteins)

Treatment of uncomplicated influenza (initiate therapy within 2 days of onset of symptoms):
≥7 yr and adult:
    Day 1: 10 mg inhaled (as two 5 mg inhalations) BID (2–12 hr between the two doses) × 2 doses
    Days 2–5: 10 mg inhaled (as two 5 mg inhalations) Q12 hr × 4 days

Contraindications: Hypersensitivity to any component of the formulation (contains milk proteins).
Warnings/Precautions: Currently indicated for the treatment of influenza A and B strains. **Not recommended** for patients with underlying respiratory diseases (e.g., asthma or COPD) since bronchospasm may occur and efficacy could not be demonstrated. **Discontinue** use if bronchospasm or decline in respiratory function occurs.
Adverse Effects: May cause nasal discomfort, cough, diarrhea, nausea, headache, facial edema, throat/tonsil discomfort and pain. Allergic reactions involving oropharyngeal edema and serious skin rashes have been reported; discontinue therapy if this occurs. See Warnings/Precautions section.
Drug Interactions: None identified.
Drug Administration: See package insert for specific instructions for using the rotodisk/diskhaler system. If patient is concurrently using a bronchodilator, use the bronchodilator before taking zanamivir.

ZIDOVUDINE
Retrovir, AZT
Antiviral agent, nucleoside analogue reverse transcriptase inhibitor

Yes   Yes   3   C

Caps: 100 mg
Tabs: 300 mg
Liquid: 50 mg/5 mL (240 mL); contains 0.2% sodium benzoate
Injection: 10 mg/mL (20 mL)
In combination with lamivudine (3TC) as Combivir:
    Tabs: 300 mg zidovudine + 150 mg lamivudine
In combination with abacavir and lamivudine (3TC) as Trizivir:
    Tabs: 300 mg zidovudine + 300 mg abacavir + 150 mg lamivudine

Dosages may differ in separate protocols.
Neonate–infant <6 wk: See below, Prevention of Vertical Transmission.
Child 6 wk–12 yr:
    PO: 160 mg/m^2/dose Q8 hr. Dose can range from 90–180 mg/m^2/dose Q6–8 hr. Additionally, 180–240 mg/m^2/dose Q12 hr has been used to improve compliance. **Max. dose:** 600 mg/24 hr.
    Intermittent IV: 120 mg/m^2/dose Q6 hr
    Continuous IV infusion: 20 mg/m^2/hr

Continued

ZIDOVUDINE *continued*

≥12 yr and adult:
>   **PO:** 200 mg/dose TID, or 300 mg/dose BID; **max. dose:** 600 mg/24 hr.
>   >   ***Endstage renal disease:*** 100 mg/dose Q6–8 hr.
>   >   ***Combivir:*** 1 tablet PO BID
>   >   ***Trizivir (≥40 kg):*** 1 tablet PO BID
>   **IV:** 1 mg/kg/dose Q4 hr

Prevention of vertical transmission:
>   **14–34 wk of pregnancy:**
>   >   ***Until labor:*** 600 mg/24 hr PO ÷ BID-TID
>   >   ***During labor:*** 2 mg/kg IV over 1 hr followed by 1 mg/kg/hr IV infusion until umbilical cord clamped.
>   ***Neonate–infant <6 wk:*** 2 mg/kg/dose Q6 hr PO or 1.5 mg/kg/dose Q6 hr IV over 60 min. Begin within 12 hr of birth and continue until 6 wk of age.
>   **Premature infant:**
>   >   ***<30 wk gestation:*** 2 mg/kg/dose PO Q12 hr or 1.5 mg/kg/dose IV Q12 hr for first 4 wk of life, then reduce dosing interval to Q8 hr thereafter.
>   >   ***≥30 wk gestation:*** 2 mg/kg/dose PO Q12 hr or 1.5 mg/kg/dose IV Q12 hr for first 2 wk of life, then reduce dosing interval to Q8 hr thereafter. Dosage interval may be further reduced to Q6 hr when the child reaches full term (40 wk postconceptional age).

Needle stick prophylaxis: 200 mg/dose PO TID or 300 mg/dose PO BID × 28 days. Use in combination with lamivudine 150 mg/dose PO BID, and indinavir 800 mg/dose PO TID × 28 days.

Contraindications: Hypersensitivity to zidovudine or any other of its components.
Warnings/Precautions: Use with caution in patients with impaired renal or hepatic function. Neutropenia and severe anemia have occurred in patients with advanced HIV. Lactic acidosis and severe hepatomegaly with steatosis, including fatal cases have been reported. Macrocytosis is noted after 4 wk of therapy and can be used as an indicator of compliance.

Dosage reduction may be necessary in severe renal impairment (GFR <15 mL/min) and in hepatic dysfunction.
Adverse Effects: Most common include: anemia (may require dose interruption), granulocytopenia, nausea and headache (dosage reduction, erythropoietin, filgrastim/GCSF or discontinuance may be required depending on event). Seizures, confusion, rash, myositis, myopathy (use >1 yr), hepatitis and elevated liver enzymes have been reported. See Warnings/Precautions section.
Drug Interactions: Do not use in combination with stavudine because of poor antiretroviral effect. Effects of interacting drugs include: increased toxicity (acyclovir, trimethoprim-sulfamethoxazole); increased hematological toxicity (ganciclovir, interferon-alpha, marrow suppressive drugs); and granulocytopenia (drugs which affect glucuronidation). Methadone, atovaquone, cimetidine, valproic acid, probenecid and fluconazole may increase levels of zidovudine, whereas nelfinavir, ritonavir, rifampin, rifabutin and clarithromycin may decrease levels.
Drug Administration
>   IV: **Do not** administer IM. IV form is incompatible with blood product infusions and should be infused over 1 hr (intermittent IV dosing) at a concentration ≤4 mg/mL diluted in 5% dextrose.
>   PO: Oral doses may be administered with or without food.

REFERENCES

1. Package inserts of medications.
2. Committee on Drugs. The Transfer of Drugs and Other Chemicals into Human Milk. *Pediatrics* 2001;108:776–789.
3. Briggs GG, Freeman RK, Yaffe SJ. A reference guide to fetal and neonatal risk: Drugs in Pregnancy and Lactation, 7th ed. Baltimore, MD: Williams & Wilkins; 2005.
4. Pickering LK, ed. Red Book: 2006 Report of the Committee on Infectious Diseases, 27th ed. Elk Grove Village, IL: American Academy of Pediatrics; 2006.
5. Young TE, Mangum OB. Neofax: A Manual of Drugs Used in Neonatal Care, 20th ed. Raleigh, NC: Acorn Publishing; 2007.
6. McEvoy GK, Snow EK, eds. AHFS Drug Information. Stat! Ref electronic version. Bethesda, MD: American Society of Health-System Pharmacists. www.ahfsdruginformation.com.
7. Facts and Comparisons: CliniSphere 2.0, Electronic Drug Information Service, Facts and Comparisons, St. Louis, MO: Wolters Luwer Health, Inc. www.factsandcomparisons.com.
8. Micromedex Healthcare Series [Internet database]. Greenwood Village, CO: Thomson Healthcare. Updated periodically.
9. Takemoto CK, Hodding JH, Kraus DM. Pediatric Dosage Handbook, 14th ed. Hudson, OH: Lexi-Comp, Inc; 2007.
10. U.S. Department of Health and Human Services. AIDS Information. www.aidsinfo.nih.gov.
11. Physicians' Desk Reference Electronic Drug Information. Greenwood Village, CO: Thomson Healthcare. Updated periodically.
12. Food and Drug Administration Safety Information and Adverse Event Reporting Program. www.fda.gov/medwatch.
13. Jew RK, Mullen RJ, Soo-Hoo W. The Children's Hospital of Philadelphia Extemporaneous Formulations. Bethesda, MD: American Society of Health-System Pharmacists, Inc.; 2003.
14. Marzolini C, Kim RB. Placental transfer of antiretroviral drugs. *Clin Pharmacol Ther* 2005;78:118–122.
15. Pacifici GM. Pharmacokinetics of antivirals in neonate. *Early Hum Dev* 2005;81:773–780.
16. Groll AH, Giri N, Petraitis V, et al. Comparative efficacy and distribution of lipid formulations of amphotericin B in experimental *Candida albacans* infection of the central nervous system. *J Infect Dis* 2000;182:274–282.
17. Groll AH, Piscitelli SC, Walsh TJ. Clinical pharmacology of systemic antifungal agents: a comprehensive review of agents in clinical use, current investigational compounds, and putative targets for antifungal drug development. *Adv Pharmacol* 1998;44:343–500.
18. American Thoracic Society. Targeted tuberculin testing and treatment of latent tuberculosis infection. *Am J of Respir Crit Care Med* 2000;161:1376–1395.
19. Hill DR, Baird JK, Parise ME, et al.: Primaquine: Report from CDC expert meeting on malaria chemoprophylaxis I. *Am J Trop Med Hyg* 2006;75:402–415.

Index

Page numbers followed by f indicate formulary information.

Abacavir sulfate, 317f
administration route for, 224
adverse effects of
CNS, 263, 264
cutaneous, 266
endocrine/metabolic, 271
gastrointestinal, 268–270
hematologic, 262
hepatic, 272
musculoskeletal, 273
contraindications to, in severe hepatic
dysfunction, 175
dosage adjustment, in hepatic dysfunction,
175
mechanism of action of, 224
precautions with, in hepatic dysfunction,
175
tissue distribution, by key organ systems,
191
Abdominal pain, drugs causing, 267–268
Abscess
cerebral, antimicrobial therapy for, 132
dental, antimicrobial therapy for, 119
intra-abdominal, antimicrobial therapy for,
136–137
parapharyngeal, antimicrobial therapy for,
146
peritonsillar, antimicrobial therapy for, 146
pulmonary, antimicrobial therapy for, 128
renal, antimicrobial therapy for, 123
retropharyngeal, antimicrobial therapy for,
146
spinal, antimicrobial therapy for, 125
Absorption (drug), age-dependent physiologic
variables affecting, 153
ABW. *See* Adjusted body weight
Acanthamoeba, 74
Acetaminophen, isoniazid interaction with,
397f
Acetanilide, mechanism of action of, 226
Achromobacter xylosoxidans, 3
Acinetobacter spp., 2
Actinobacillus spp., 2
Actinomyces israeli, 2
Acyclovir, 318f–319f
administration route(s) for, 223
adverse effects of
CNS, 264, 265
cutaneous, 266, 267
gastrointestinal, 268–270
dosage adjustment
in continuous renal replacement therapy,
171
in obesity, 189
in renal failure, 159
for herpes simplex, 50, 51
mechanism of action of, 223
in postexposure prophylaxis of varicella, 287
prophylactic, for prevention of recurrent
herpes simplex, 284
tenofovir interaction with, 472f
tissue distribution, by key organ systems,
191
for varicella, 53
zanamivir interaction with, 495f
Adefovir
for hepatitis B, 49
ribavirin interaction with, 457f
Adjusted body weight, calculation of, 183

Adverse drug effects. *See also* Ototoxicity
cardiovascular, 262
CNS, 263–265
cutaneous, 266–267
endocrine/metabolic, 271
gastrointestinal, 267–271
hematologic, 261–262
hepatic, 272
hypersensitivity reactions as, 273
musculoskeletal, 273
ocular, 273
renal/genitourinary, 271–272
respiratory, 272
Aeromonas hydrophila, 2
Alanine aminotransferase, elevation, drugs
causing, 272
Albendazole, 319f–320f
adverse effects of
CNS, 264
cutaneous, 266
gastrointestinal, 267, 269, 270
hematologic, 261
for *Ancylostoma braziliense,* 74
for *Ancylostoma caninum,* 75
for *Ancylostoma* spp., 75
for *Ascaris lumbricoides,* 76
for *Brachiola vesicularum,* 78
for *Capillaria philippinensis,* 79
for *Clonorchis sinensis,* 79
for *Echinococcus granulosus,* 81
for *Echinococcus multilocularis,* 81
for *Encephalitozoon cuniculi,* 83, 84
for *Encephalitozoon hellem,* 82
for *Encephalitozoon intestinalis,* 83
for *Enterobius vermicularis,* 85
for *Gnathostoma spinigerum,* 86
for *Gongylonema* sp., 86
for *Loa loa,* 89
for *Mansonella perstans,* 89
for *Metrochis conjunctus,* 89
for *Microsporidia,* 90
for *Necator americanus,* 91
for *Oseophagostomum bifurcum,* 91
for *Pleistophora* sp., 95
precautions with, in hepatic dysfunction,
175
for *Strongyloides stercoralis,* 97
for *Taenia solium,* 98
tissue distribution, by key organ systems,
191
for *Toxocara canis/catis,* 98
for *Trachipleistopora* sp., 101
for *Trichinella spiralis,* 101
for *Trichostrongylus,* 101
for *Trichuris trichiura,* 101
for *Uncinaria stenocephala,* 103
for *Vittaforma corneae,* 104
for *Wuchereria bancrofti,* 104
Alcohol (ethyl), interactions, with amprenavir,
toxic effect(s), 248
Alkaline phosphatase, elevation, drugs causing,
272
Allopurinol
amoxicillin interaction with, 323f
cloxacillin interaction with, 361f
Alopecia, drugs causing, 266
Alpha$_1$-agonists, interactions
with furazolidone, toxic effect(s), 251
with linezolid, toxic effect(s), 253

Alpha₂-agonists (ophthalmic), interactions
    with furazolidone, toxic effect(s), 251
    with linezolid, toxic effect(s), 253
Alpha/beta-agonists (indirect-acting), interactions
    with furazolidone, toxic effect(s), 251
    with linezolid, toxic effect(s), 253
Alternaria sp., 54
Amantadine hydrochloride, 320f–321f
    administration route for, 225
    adverse effects of
        cardiovascular, 262
        CNS, 263–265
        gastrointestinal, 268, 269
    dosage adjustment, in renal failure, 159
    mechanism of action of, 225
    precautions with, in hepatic dysfunction, 175
    tissue distribution, by key organ systems, 191
Amikacin sulfate, 321f–322f
    administration route(s) for, 218
    adverse effects of, CNS, 265
    dosage adjustment
        in continuous renal replacement therapy,
            171
        in obesity, 188
        in renal failure, 159
    for *Francisella tularensis*, 17
    high-dose extended-interval dosing of, 239
    mechanism of action of, 218
    for *Morganella*, 21
    for *Mycobacterium abscessus*, 47
    for *Mycobacterium fortuitum*, 46
    for *Mycobacterium tuberculosis*, 42
    nephrotoxicity of, 234
    for *Nocardia brasilensis, asteroides,* spp., 23
    ototoxicity of, 234, 274
    for *Providencia* spp., 25
    serum concentrations
        appropriate times to sample, 234
        and toxicity, 234
    therapeutic drug monitoring goals for, 234
    tissue distribution, by key organ systems, 191
    toxicity of, risk factors for, 234
Aminobenzoic acid, pyrimethamine and
        sulfadoxine interaction with, 451f
Aminoglycosides
    amikacin sulfate interaction with, 322f
    amphotericin B interaction with, 325f
    AUC/MIC, 244, 245
    for *Burkholderia mallei*, 9
    cidofovir interaction with, 355f
    for *Citrobacter* spp., 12
    C_{max}/MIC, 244, 245
    colistimethate sodium interaction with, 362f
    desensitization protocols, 300–302
    dosage adjustment, in obesity, 188
    efficacy relationships in humans, PK/PD
        parameter associated with, 246
    for *Enterobacter* spp., 15
    foscarnet interaction with, 384f
    high-dose extended-interval dosing of, 239
    mechanism of action of, 218
    microbial resistance to, mechanism of, 227,
        228
    for *Mycobacterium bovis*, 43
    for *Mycobacterium tuberculosis*, 40, 41
    pentamidine isethionate interaction with, 439f
    piperacillin interaction with, 441f
    piperacillin/tazobactam interaction with, 442f
    vancomycin interaction with, 491f
    zalcitabine interaction with, 493f
8-Aminoquinolones, mechanism of action of,
        225
Aminosalicylic acid. See para-aminosalicylic
        acid
P-Aminosalicylic acid. See Para-aminosalicylic
        acid
Amiodarone, interactions
    with atazanavir, toxic effect(s), 248
    with fosamprenavir, toxic effect(s), 250
    with indinavir, toxic effect(s), 252
    with lopinavir, 407f

Amiodarone, interactions (*Cont.*)
    with lopinavir/ritonavir, toxic effect(s), 254
    with moxifloxacin, 418f
    with nelfinavir, toxic effect(s), 256
    with quinidine gluconate, 452f
    with quinine sulfate, 453f
    with ritonavir, toxic effect(s), 257
    with saquinavir, toxic effect(s), 257
Amoxicillin, 322f–323f
    administration route for, 219
    adverse effects of
        CNS, 264
        cutaneous, 266
        hypersensitivity, 273
    for *Aeromonas hydrophila*, 2
    for *Borrelia burgdorferi*, 6, 7
    dosage adjustment, in renal failure, 159
    for *Escherichia coli*,
    for *Leptospira interrogans*, 20
    mechanism of action of, 219
    for *Pasteurella multocida*, 23
    prophylactic
        for endocarditis, 277
        for recurrent otitis media, 279
    for *Salmonella typhi* (type D), 26
    for *Streptococci viridans*, 32
    for *Streptococcus* Group A, 31
    for *Streptococcus pneumoniae*, 30
    tissue distribution, by key organ systems, 192
Amoxicillin/clavulanate
    administration route for, 218
    dosage adjustment, in renal failure, 159
    mechanism of action of, 218
    prophylactic
        for animal bite, 276
        for human bite, 276
Amoxicillin with clavulanic acid, 323f–324f
    adverse effects of
        cutaneous, 266
        gastrointestinal, 267–270
        renal/genitourinary, 272
    contraindications to, in hepatic dysfunction,
        176
    tissue distribution, by key organ systems, 192
Amphetamines, interactions
    with furazolidone, toxic effect(s), 251
    with linezolid, toxic effect(s), 253
Amphotericin B, 324f–325f
    for *Acanthamoeba*, 74
    administration route(s) for, 222
    adverse effects of, hematologic, 261
    for *Alternaria* spp., 54
    for *Aspergillus* sp., 54
    for *Bipolaris* sp., 55
    for *Blastomyces dermatitidis*, 56, 57
    for *Candida* sp., 58–61
    cholesteryl sulfate, 325f–326f
        adverse effects of
            cardiovascular, 262
            CNS, 263, 264
            cutaneous, 266
            endocrine/metabolic, 271
            gastrointestinal, 267–269
            hematologic, 261
            renal/genitourinary, 271
            respiratory, 272
        dosage adjustment, in renal failure, 159
        tissue distribution, by key organ systems,
            193
    cidofovir interaction with, 355f
    for *Coccidioides immitis*, 61, 62
    conventional, adverse effects of
        cardiovascular, 262
        CNS, 263–265
        endocrine/metabolic, 271
        gastrointestinal, 267–270
        musculoskeletal, 273
        renal/genitourinary, 271, 272
        respiratory, 272
    for *Cryptococcus neoformans*, 62, 63
    for *Curvularia* sp., 62

Amphotericin B (*Cont.*)
 dosage adjustment
  in obesity, 189
  in renal failure, 159
 for *Exophiala* sp., 63
 for *Exserohilum* sp., 63
 flucytosine interaction with, 382f
 foscarnet interaction with, 384f
 for *Fusarium* sp., 64
 ganciclovir interaction with, 386f
 for *Histoplasma capsulatum*, 64, 65
 for *Leishmania* spp., 87
 lipid complex, 326f
  adverse effects of
   cardiovascular, 262
   CNS, 263–265
   cutaneous, 266
   endocrine/metabolic, 271
   gastrointestinal, 267–270
   renal/genitourinary, 271
   respiratory, 272
  dosage adjustment, in renal failure, 159
  tissue distribution, by key organ systems,
   193
 liposomal, 327f
  adverse effects of
   cardiovascular, 262
   CNS, 263–265
   cutaneous, 266, 267
   endocrine/metabolic, 271
   gastrointestinal, 267–270
   hematologic, 261, 262
   hepatic, 272
   musculoskeletal, 273
   renal/genitourinary, 271
   respiratory, 272
  dosage adjustment, in renal failure, 159
  tissue distribution, by key organ systems,
   193
 for *Madurella* sp., 65
 mechanism of action of, 222
 for *Naegleria fowleri*, 90
 for *Paracoccidiodes brasilensis*, 65
 for *Penicillum marneffei*, 66
 pentamidine isethionate interaction with, 439f
 tissue distribution, by key organ systems, 193
 for *Wangiella* sp., 67
 zalcitabine interaction with, 493f
 for Zygomycetes, 68
Amphotericins, in vivo pharmacodynamic
  characteristics of, in neutropenic mouse
  models, 247
Ampicillin, 327f–328f
 for *Actinomyces israeli* infection, 2
 administration route(s) for, 219
 adverse effects of
  CNS, 265
  cutaneous, 266
  gastrointestinal, 267, 268, 270
  hypersensitivity, 273
 for *Aeromonas hydrophila*, 2
 chloroquine HCl/phosphate interaction with,
  354f
 dosage adjustment
  in continuous renal replacement therapy,
   171
  in obesity, 188
  in renal failure, 159
 for *Eikenella corrodens*, 14
 for *Enterococcus faecalis/faecium*, 15
 for *Erysipelothrix rhusiopathiae*, 15
 for *Haemophilus parainfluenza, haemolyticus,
  aphrophilus,* spp., 18
 for *Heliobacter pylori*, 19
 for *Leuconostoc* spp., 20
 for *Listeria monocytogenes*, 20
 mechanism of action of, 219
 for *Neisseria meninigitidis*, 22
 for *Prevotella* spp., 24
 for *Proteus mirabilis*, 24
 for *Streptobacillus moniliformis*, 29

Ampicillin (*Cont.*)
 for *Streptococci viridans*, 32, 33
 for *Streptococcus* Group B, 31
 tissue distribution, by key organ systems, 193
Ampicillin with sulbactam, 328f–329f
 administration route for, 218
 adverse effects of
  cutaneous, 266, 267
  respiratory, 272
 dosage adjustment
  in obesity, 188
  in renal failure, 160
 mechanism of action of, 218
 tissue distribution, by key organ systems, 193
Amprenavir, 329f–330f
 administration route for, 224
 adverse effects of
  CNS, 263, 264
  cutaneous, 266, 267
  endocrine/metabolic, 271
  gastrointestinal, 268–270
  hepatic, 272
 contraindicated drug interactions, 248
 contraindications to, in hepatic dysfunction,
  176
 dosage adjustment, in hepatic dysfunction,
  176
 interactions, with metronidazole, toxic
  effect(s), 255
 lopinavir interaction with, 407f
 mechanism of action of, 224
 precautions with, in hepatic dysfunction, 176
 tissue distribution, by key organ systems, 193
Anaphylaxis, drugs causing, 273
Anaplasma phagocytophila, 3
Ancylostoma braziliense, 74
Ancylostoma caninum, 75
Ancylostoma spp., 75
Anemia, drugs causing, 261
Angioedema, drugs causing, 266
Angiostrongylus cantonensis, 75
Angiostrongylus costaricensis, 76
Angiotensin-converting enzyme inhibitors,
  potassium iodide interaction with, 446f
Anidulafungin, 330f–331f
 for *Candida* sp., 58, 59
 precautions with, in hepatic dysfunction, 176
 tissue distribution, by key organ systems, 194
Anisakis, 76
Anorexia, drugs causing, 268
Antacids
 atazanavir and, 332f
 cefdinir interaction with, 341f
 cefditoren pivoxil interaction with, 342f
 cefuroxime interaction with, 351f
 chloroquine HCl/phosphate interaction with,
  354f
 clofazimine interaction with, 360f
 delavirdine interaction with, 366f
 ethambutol HCl interaction with, 379f
 levofloxacin interaction with, 404f
 moxifloxacin interaction with, 418f
 ofloxacin interaction with, 429f
 quinidine gluconate interaction with, 452f
 quinine sulfate interaction with, 453f
Anthrax, recommended antimicrobial prophylaxis
  for, 281
Antibacterial agents
 efficacy relationships in humans, PK/PD
   parameter associated with, 246
 mechanism of action of, 218–222
 in vitro resistance relationships, PK/PD
   parameter associated with, 246
Antibiotics, microbial resistance to, common
  mechanisms of, 227–228
Anticholinergics
 amantadine hydrochloride interaction with,
  321f
 nitrofurantoin interaction with, 427f
 quinidine gluconate interaction with, 452f
 rimantadine interaction with, 461f

499

Anticoagulants
  cefazolin and, 340f
  chloramphenicol interaction with, 353f
  neomycin sulfate interaction with, 422f
  quinine sulfate interaction with, 453f
  rifampin interaction with, 459f
Antidepressants, interactions
  with furazolidone, toxic effect(s), 251
  with linezolid, toxic effect(s), 254
Antifolate, mechanism of action of, 225
Antifungal agents
  mechanism of action of, 222–223
  in vivo pharmacodynamic characteristics
    of, in neutropenic mouse models,
    247
Antiherpes virus agents, mechanism of action
  of, 223
Antimetabolites, as antifungals, mechanism of
  action of, 222
Antimycobacterial agents
  efficacy, PK/PD parameter associated with,
    247
  mechanism of action of, 222
Antiparasitic agents
  combination agent, mechanism of action of,
    226
  mechanism of action of, 225–226
Antiretroviral agents, mechanism of action of,
  224
Antiretroviral-nucleoside analogs, mechanism of
  action of, 224
Antiviral agents, mechanism of action of,
  223–225
Anxiety, drugs causing, 263
Arcanobacterium haemolyticum, 3
Area under the serum concentration (AUC),
  245. See also AUC/MIC
Arginase deficiency, aztreonam in, 336f
Aromatic diamidine, mechanism of action of,
  226
Arrhythmia(s) (cardiac), drugs causing, 262
Artemether, for Plasmodium spp., 94
Artesunate, for Plasmodium falciparum, 92
Arthralgia, drugs causing, 273
Arthritis, bacterial, antimicrobial therapy for,
  126
Ascaris lumbricoides, 76
Aseptic meningitis, antimicrobial therapy for,
  134
Aspartate aminotransferase, elevation, drugs
  causing, 272
Aspergillosis, 72
Aspergillus, 54–55, 247
Aspiration pneumonitis, antimicrobial therapy
  for, 128
Astemizole
  amprenavir and, 330f
  atazanavir and, 331f
Ataxia, drugs causing, 263
Atazanavir, 331f–332f
  administration route for, 224
  adverse effects of
    CNS, 263–265
    cutaneous, 266
    endocrine/metabolic, 271
    gastrointestinal, 267–270
    hematologic, 262
    hepatic, 272
    musculoskeletal, 273
  contraindicated drug interactions, 248–249
  dosage adjustment, in hepatic dysfunction,
    176
  mechanism of action of, 224
  precautions with, in hepatic dysfunction,
    176
  tenofovir interaction with, 472f
  tissue distribution, by key organ systems,
    194
Atomoxetine, interactions
  with furazolidone, toxic effect(s), 251
  with linezolid, toxic effect(s), 254

Atorvastatin
  amprenavir and, 330f
  atazanavir and, 331f
  lopinavir interaction with, 407f
Atovaquone
  adverse effects of
    CNS, 263–265
    cutaneous, 266, 267
    endocrine/metabolic, 271
    gastrointestinal, 267–270
    hematologic, 261, 262
  for Babesia microti, 76
  for Microsporidia, 90
  for Plasmodium falciparum, 92
  for Pneumocystis jiroveci, 66
  prophylactic
    for Pneumocystis, 287
    for toxoplasmosis, in HIV-infected patients,
      288
  for Toxoplasma gondii, 99
  zanamivir interaction with, 495f
Atovaquone ± proguanil, 332f–334f
  administration route for, 226
  adverse effects of
    CNS, 263–265
    cutaneous, 267
    gastrointestinal, 267–270
  mechanism of action of, 226
  prophylactic, for malaria, 288
  tissue distribution, by key organ systems, 194
AUC/MIC, 244, 245
Aurothioglucose
  halofantrine interaction with, 390f
  hydroxychloroquine interaction with, 391f
  pyrimethamine interaction with, 451f
Avermectins, mechanism of action of, 225
Azithromycin, 334f–335f
  administration route(s) for, 220
  adverse effects of
    CNS, 264
    gastrointestinal, 267, 269, 270
  for Babesia microti, 76
  for Bartonella henselae, 5
  for Bordetella pertussis, 6
  for Calymmatobacterium granulomatis, 9
  for Campylobacter jejuni, 9
  for Chlamydia trachomatis, 11
  for Chlamydophila pneumoniae, 10
  for Chlamydophila psittaci, 10
  for Cryptosporidium, 79
  dosage adjustment, in obesity, 189
  for Escherichia coli, 17
  for Haemophilus ducreyi, 18
  for Haemophilus influenzae nontypeable, 18
  for Legionella pneumophila, 20
  mechanism of action of, 220
  for Moraxella catarrhalis, 20
  for Mycobacterium avium complex, 43, 44
  for Mycoplasma hominis, 21
  for Mycoplasma pneumoniae, 21
  nelfinavir interaction with, 421f
  for Pasteurella multocida, 23
  precautions with, in hepatic dysfunction, 176
  preventive therapy, after sexual contact/sexual
    assault, 280
  prophylactic
    for endocarditis, in penicillin-allergic
      patient, 277
    for Mycobacterium avium complex, 282
    for Neisseria meningitidis, 283
    for pertussis, 283
  for Salmonella typhi (type D), 26
  for Sappinia diploidea, 96
  for Shigella sonnei, dysenteriae, boydii,
    flexneri, 27, 28
  for Streptococcus Group A, 31
  for Streptococcus pneumoniae, 30
  tissue distribution, by key organ systems, 194
  T > MIC, 244, 245
  for Ureaplasma urealyticum, 35
  for Vibrio cholera, 36

Azotemia, drug causing, 271
Aztreonam, 336f
    administration route for, 220
    adverse effects of
        cutaneous, 266, 267
        gastrointestinal, 268–270
    dosage adjustment
        in obesity, 189
        in renal failure, 160
    mechanism of action of, 220
    tissue distribution, by key organ systems, 195

Babesia microti, 76
Bacillus anthracis, 4. See also anthrax
Bacillus cereus, 4
Bacitracin
    administration route for, 222
    mechanism of action of, 222
Bacitracin ± polymyxin B, 336f–337f
    adverse effects of
        cardiovascular, 262
        CNS, 265
        cutaneous, 266, 267
        gastrointestinal, 268–270
        hypersensitivity, 273
Bacteremia, antimicrobial therapy for, 109
Bacterial infections, 2–37
Bacterial vaginosis
    antimicrobial therapy for, 123
    recommended antibiotic prophylaxis for, 280
Bacteroides: fragilis group, 5
Balamuthia mandrillaris, 77
Balantidium coli, 77
Bartonella bacilliformis, 6
Bartonella henselae, 5–6
Bartonella quintana, 6
Basic peptide, as antimycobacterial agent,
        mechanism of action of, 222
Baylisascaris procyonis, 77
Benzimidazoles, mechanism of action of, 225
Benznidazole, for Trypanosoma cruzi, 102
Benzocaine, pyrimethamine and sulfadoxine
        interaction with, 451f
Benzodiazepines
    rifampin interaction with, 459f
    voriconazole interaction with, 493f
Bepridil, halofantrine interaction with, 390f
Beta-blockers, rifampin interaction with, 459f
Beta-lactamase inhibitors, mechanism of action
        of, 218
Beta-lactams
    dosage adjustment, in obesity, 188–189
    efficacy relationships in humans, PK/PD
        parameter associated with, 246
    mechanism of action of, 218–220
    microbial resistance to, mechanisms of, 227
    T > MIC, 244, 245
Bioavailability, 240
Bipolaris sp., 55
Bismuth, for Heliobacter pylori, 19
Bite
    animal, recommended antimicrobial
        prophylaxis for, 276
    human, recommended antimicrobial
        prophylaxis for, 276
Bithionol
    for Fasciola hepatica, 85
    for Paragonimus westermani, 91
Blastocystis hominis, 77
Blastomyces dermatitidis, 56–57
Blepharitis, antimicrobial therapy for, 115
Blood, adverse drug effects and, 261–262
Blurred vision, drugs causing, 273
Body mass, calculation of, 151
Body mass index, 170
    age percentiles
        for boys 2 to 20 years, 184
        for girls 2 to 20 years, 185
Body surface area
    calculation of, 151
    nomogram for, 151, 152

Bone(s), infections of, antimicrobial therapy for,
        123–128
Bordetella pertussis, 6
Borrelia burgdorferi, 6–7
Borrelia recurrentis, hermsii, turicate, 8
Botulinum immune globulin intravenous,
        human, 337f–338f
    adverse effects of
        cardiovascular, 262
        cutaneous, 266
        endocrine/metabolic, 271
        gastrointestinal, 268, 270
        hematologic, 261
        respiratory, 272
    for Clostridium botulinum, 12
Brachiola vesicularum, 78
Bradycardia, drugs causing, 262
Brain abscess, antimicrobial therapy for, 132
Breast-feeding categories, 307
Bronchiolitis, antimicrobial therapy for, 132
Bronchospasm, drugs causing, 272
Brucella abortus, spp., 8
Brugia malayi, 78
Brugia timori, 79
BSA. See Body surface area
Bupropion, interactions
    with furazolidone, toxic effect(s), 251
    with linezolid, toxic effect(s), 254
Burkholderia cepacia, 9
Burkholderia mallei, 9
Burkholderia pseudomallei, 9
Burn(s), and pharmacokinetic monitoring, 243
Buspirone
    with furazolidone, toxic effect(s), 251
    with linezolid, toxic effect(s), 253
    rifampin interaction with, 459f
Butenafine, 338f
    adverse effects of, cutaneous, 266, 267
    for tinea corporis, 70
    for tinea cruris, 70
Butoconazole, for Candida sp., 60

Caffeine
    ciprofloxacin interaction with, 357f
    terbinafine interaction with, 474f
    thiabendazole interaction with, 477f
Calcium channel blockers
    lopinavir interaction with, 407f
    rifampin interaction with, 459f
    ritonavir interaction with, 462f
    saquinavir interaction with, 463f
    voriconazole interaction with, 493f
Calymmatobacterium granulomatis, 9
Campylobacter jejuni, 9
Campylobacter spp., 10
Candida
    antifungal agents for, in vivo
        pharmacodynamic characteristics of,
        in neutropenic mouse models, 247
    recommended antimicrobial prophylaxis for,
        287
Candida sp., 58–61
Capillaria philippinensis, 79
Capnocytophaga canimorsus, 10
Capnocytophaga ochracea, 10
Capreomycin
    administration route for, 222
    mechanism of action of, 222
Carbamazepine
    clarithromycin interaction with, 358f
    darunavir and, 365f
    delavirdine interaction with, 366f
    doxycycline interaction with, 372f
    erythromycin preparations interaction with,
        378f
    isoniazid interaction with, 397f
    lopinavir interaction with, 407f
    nelfinavir interaction with, 421f
    praziquantel interaction with, 447f
    quinupristin with dalfopristin interaction with,
        454f

Carbamazepine (Cont.)
  rifapentine interaction with, 460f
  ritonavir interaction with, 462f
  saquinavir interaction with, 463f
  tipranavir interaction with, 481f
Carbapenem
  for *Acinetobacter,* 2
  for *Bacteroides:* fragilis group, 5
  for *Campylobacter* spp., 10
  for *Clostridium perfringens,* spp., 13
  dosage adjustment, in obesity, 189
  for *Eikenella corrodens,* 14
  for *Enterobacter* spp., 15
  for *Escherichia coli,* 16
  for *Fusobacterium* spp., 17
  for *Klebsiella* spp., 19
  for *Leuconostoc* spp., 20
  mechanism of action of, 218
  microbial resistance to, mechanism of, 228
  for *Morganella,* 21
  for *Plesiomonas shigelloides,* 23
  for *Prevotella* spp., 24
  for *Proteus vulgaris,* indole positive spp., 25
  for *Pseudomonas aeruginosa,* spp., 25
  for *Streptococcus pneumoniae,* 30
Carbuncles, antimicrobial therapy for, 127
Cardiac glycosides, amphotericin B interaction
    with, 325f
Cardiobacterium hominis, 10
Cardiovascular system, adverse drug effects
    and, 262
Carnitine deficiency, cefditoren pivoxil and, 342f
Caspofungin, 338f–339f
  administration route for, 223
  adverse effects of
    cardiovascular, 262
    CNS, 263–265
    cutaneous, 266, 267
    endocrine/metabolic, 271
    gastrointestinal, 267–270
    hematologic, 261, 262
    hepatic, 272
    musculoskeletal, 273
  for *Aspergillus* sp., 54
  for *Candida* sp., 58, 61
  dosage adjustment, in hepatic dysfunction,
    177
  mechanism of action of, 223
  precautions with, in hepatic dysfunction, 177
  tissue distribution, by key organ systems, 195
Catecholamines, methanamine preparations
    interaction with, 413f
Catheter-related infection, intravascular,
    antimicrobial therapy for, 109
Cefaclor, 339f
  administration route(s) for, 219
  adverse effects of
    cutaneous, 266
    gastrointestinal, 268
    hematologic, 261
    renal/genitourinary, 272
  dosage adjustment, in renal failure, 160
  mechanism of action of, 219
  tissue distribution, by key organ systems, 195
Cefadroxil, 340f
  administration route for, 219
  adverse effects of, gastrointestinal, 268
  dosage adjustment, in renal failure, 160
  mechanism of action of, 219
  prophylactic, for endocarditis, in penicillin-
    allergic patient, 277
  tissue distribution, by key organ systems, 195
Cefazolin, 340f–341f
  administration route(s) for, 218
  adverse effects of
    CNS, 265
    gastrointestinal, 268
  dosage adjustment
    in obesity, 189
    in renal failure, 160
  mechanism of action of, 218

Cefazolin (Cont.)
  precautions with, in hepatic dysfunction, 177
  tissue distribution, by key organ systems, 195
Cefdinir, 341f
  adverse effects of
    CNS, 264
    cutaneous, 266
    gastrointestinal, 267–270
    hematologic, 261
    hepatic, 272
  dosage adjustment, in renal failure, 160
  for *Streptococcus pneumoniae,* 30
  tissue distribution, by key organ systems, 196
Cefditoren pivoxil, 341f–342f
  adverse effects of
    CNS, 264
    endocrine/metabolic, 271
    gastrointestinal, 267–270
  dosage adjustment, in renal failure, 160
  precautions with, in hepatic dysfunction, 177
  tissue distribution, by key organ systems, 196
Cefepime, 342f–343f
  administration route(s) for, 219
  adverse effects of
    CNS, 264
    cutaneous, 266, 267
    gastrointestinal, 268–270
    hematologic, 262
  dosage adjustment
    in continuous renal replacement therapy,
      171
    in obesity, 189
    in renal failure, 160
  efficacy relationships in humans, PK/PD
    parameter associated with, 246
  for *Escherichia coli,* 16
  mechanism of action of, 219
  tissue distribution, by key organ systems, 196
Cefixime, 343f
  administration route for, 219
  adverse effects of, gastrointestinal, 267–269
  dosage adjustment, in renal failure, 161
  mechanism of action of, 219
  for *Neisseria gonorrhea,* 21, 22
  preventive therapy, after sexual contact/sexual
    assault, 280
  for *Shigella sonnei, dysenteriae, boydii,
    flexneri,* 27
  tissue distribution, by key organ systems, 196
Ceftazidime
  for *Achromobacter xylosoxidans,* 3
  for *Burkholderia mallei,* 9
  for *Burkholderia pseudomallei,* 9
Cefoperazone, 343f–344f
  administration route(s) for, 219
  adverse effects of
    cutaneous, 266
    gastrointestinal, 268
    hematologic, 261, 262
    hepatic, 272
  dosage adjustment, in hepatic dysfunction,
    177
  mechanism of action of, 219
  precautions with, in hepatic dysfunction, 177
  tissue distribution, by key organ systems,
    196
Cefotaxime, 344f–345f
  administration route(s) for, 219
  adverse effects of
    cutaneous, 266, 267
    gastrointestinal, 268–270
  for *Citrobacter* spp., 12
  dosage adjustment
    in continuous renal replacement therapy,
      171
    in obesity, 189
    in renal failure, 161
  for *Haemophilus influenzae,* 18
  mechanism of action of, 219
  for *Neisseria gonorrhea,* 21
  tissue distribution, by key organ systems, 197

Cefotaxime *(Cont.)*
  for *Yersinia enterocolitica, pseudotuberculosis,*
    36, 37
Cefotetan, 345f
  administration route(s) for, 219
  adverse effects of, gastrointestinal, 268
  dosage adjustment
    in continuous renal replacement therapy,
     171
    in obesity, 189
    in renal failure, 161
  mechanism of action of, 219
  tissue distribution, by key organ systems, 197
Cefoxitin, 345f–346f
  administration route(s) for, 219
  adverse effects of, gastrointestinal, 268
  for *Bacteroides:* fragilis group, 5
  dosage adjustment
    in continuous renal replacement therapy,
     171
    in renal failure, 161
  for *Escherichia coli,* 16
  mechanism of action of, 219
  for *Mycobacterium abscessus,* 47
  for *Neisseria gonorrhea,* 21
  precautions with, in hepatic dysfunction, 177
  for *Prevotella* spp., 24
  tissue distribution, by key organ systems, 197
Cefpodoxime
  administration route for, 219
  adverse effects of, gastrointestinal, 269
  mechanism of action of, 219
Cefpodoxime proxetil, 346f
  adverse effects of
    cutaneous, 266
    gastrointestinal, 267, 268, 270
  dosage adjustment, in renal failure, 161
  for *Neisseria gonorrhea,* 22
  for *Streptococcus pneumoniae,* 30
  tissue distribution, by key organ systems, 197
Cefprozil, 347f
  administration route for, 219
  adverse effects of
    CNS, 263
    cutaneous, 266
    gastrointestinal, 267–270
    renal/genitourinary, 272
  dosage adjustment, in renal failure, 161
  mechanism of action of, 219
  tissue distribution, by key organ systems, 197
Cefradine
  administration route for, 219
  mechanism of action of, 219
Ceftazidime, 347f–348f
  administration route(s) for, 219
  adverse effects of
    gastrointestinal, 268
    hematologic, 262
  dosage adjustment
    in continuous renal replacement therapy,
     171
    in obesity, 189
    in renal failure, 161
  mechanism of action of, 219
  for *Stenotrophomonas maltophila,* 29
  tissue distribution, by key organ systems, 197
  for *Vibrio vulnificus, parahemolyticus,* spp.,
    36
Ceftibuten, 348f
  administration route for, 219
  adverse effects of
    CNS, 263, 264
    gastrointestinal, 267–270
    hematologic, 261
    hepatic, 272
  dosage adjustment, in renal failure, 161
  mechanism of action of, 219
  tissue distribution, by key organ systems, 197
Ceftibutin
  administration route for, 219
  mechanism of action of, 219

Ceftizoxime, 348f–349f
  administration route(s) for, 219
  adverse effects of
    CNS, 264
    cutaneous, 266, 267
    hematologic, 261
    hepatic, 272
  dosage adjustment, in renal failure, 161
  mechanism of action of, 219
  for *Neisseria gonorrhea,* 21
  tissue distribution, by key organ systems,
    198
Ceftriaxone, 349f–350f
  administration route(s) for, 219
  adverse effects of
    cutaneous, 266
    gastrointestinal, 268
    hematologic, 261
  for *Borrelia burgdorferi,* 7
  for *Citrobacter* spp., 12
  dosage adjustment
    in continuous renal replacement therapy,
     171
    in obesity, 189
  for gonorrhea, preventive therapy, after sexual
    contact/sexual assault, 280
  for *Haemophilus ducreyi,* 18
  for *Haemophilus influenzae,* 18
  for *Haemophilus influenzae* nontypeable, 18
  for *Haemophilus parainfluenza, haemolyticus,*
    aphrophilus, spp., 18
  for *Kingella kingae,* spp., 19
  mechanism of action of, 219
  for *Neisseria gonorrhea,* 21, 22
  for *Nocardia brasilensis, asteroids,* spp., 23
  prophylactic, for *Neisseria meningitidis,* 283
  for *Shigella sonnei, dysenteriae, boydii,*
    flexneri, 27, 28
  for *Streptococci viridans,* 32, 33
  for *Streptococcus* Group A, 31
  for *Streptococcus* Group C, G, 32
  tissue distribution, by key organ systems,
    198
  for *Treponema pallidum,* 35
Cefuroxime (IV, IM)/cefuroxime axetil (PO),
    350f–351f
  administration route(s) for, 219
  adverse effects of
    cutaneous, 267
    hematologic, 261
    hepatic, 272
  for *Borrelia burgdorferi,* 6, 7
  dosage adjustment
    in obesity, 189
    in renal failure, 161
  mechanism of action of, 219
  precautions with, in hepatic dysfunction, 177
  for *Streptobacillus moniliformis,* 29
  for *Streptococcus pneumoniae,* 30
  tissue distribution, by key organ systems,
    198
Cefuroxime sodium, dosage adjustment, in
    continuous renal replacement therapy,
    171
Cellulitis
  antimicrobial therapy for, 127
  orbital, antimicrobial therapy for, 118
  preseptal, antimicrobial therapy for, 118–119
Central nervous system (CNS)
  adverse drug effects and, 263–265
  infections, antimicrobial therapy for, 132–135
Cephalexin, 351f
  administration route for, 218
  adverse effects of, gastrointestinal, 268
  dosage adjustment, in renal failure, 161
  for *Escherichia coli,* 16
  mechanism of action of, 218
  prophylactic, for endocarditis, in penicillin-
    allergic patient, 277
  for *Propionobacterium acnes,* 24
  tissue distribution, by key organ systems, 198

Cephalosporin(s)
  desensitization protocols
    continuous IV infusion, 294–295
    intermittent IV infusion, 294
  dosage adjustment, in obesity, 189
  first generation
    mechanism of action of, 218
    prophylactic, for endocarditis, 277
  fourth generation, mechanism of action of, 219
  second generation, mechanism of action of, 219
  third generation, mechanism of action of, 219
Cephalothin, colistimethate sodium interaction with, 362f
Cephamycin, mechanism of action of, 219
Cephapirin, 351f–352f
  adverse effects of
    cutaneous, 267
    hematologic, 262
  dosage adjustment, in renal failure, 161
  tissue distribution, by key organ systems, 198
Cephradine, 352f
  adverse effects of, gastrointestinal, 268
  dosage adjustment, in renal failure, 161
  tissue distribution, by key organ systems, 198
Cerebrospinal fluid (CSF) isolates, in vitro drug susceptibility and in vivo drug efficacy against, discordance between, 229
Cerebrospinal fluid (CSF) leak, recommended antimicrobial prophylaxis for, 276
Cervastatin
  amprenavir and, 330f
  atazanavir and, 331f
  lopinavir interaction with, 407f
Cervical lymphadenitis, antimicrobial therapy for, 149
Cervicitis, antimicrobial therapy for, 120
Chest pain, drugs causing, 262
Child-Pugh score, 170, 175
Child-Turcotte-Pugh score, 170, 175
Chills, drugs causing, 263
Chlamydia trachomatis, 11
  recommended antibiotic prophylaxis for, 280
Chlamydophila pneumoniaie, 10
Chlamydophila psittaci, 10
Chloramphenicol, 352f–353f
  administration route(s) for, 221
  for Bartonella bacilliformis, 6
  for Borrelia recurrentis, hermsii, turicate, 8
  for Burkholderia pseudomallei, 9
  for Coxiella burnetti, 10
  dosage adjustment, in hepatic dysfunction, 177
  for Francisella tularensis, 17
  for Haemophilus influenzae, 18
  for Leuconostoc spp., 20
  mechanism of action of, 221
  microbial resistance to, mechanism of, 227
  for Mycoplasma hominis, 21
  for Neisseria meningitidis, 22
  for Pediococcus spp., 23
  penicillin G interaction with, 436f
  penicillin V interaction with, 438f
  precautions with, in hepatic dysfunction, 177
  for Prevotella spp., 24
  for Rickettsia akari, 25
  for Rickettsia prowazekii, 26
  for Rickettsia rickettsii, 25
  for Rickettsia spp., 26
  for Rickettsia typhi, 26
  rifapentine interaction with, 460f
  for Salmonella typhi (type D), 26
  serum concentrations
    appropriate times to sample, 235
    and toxicity, 235
  spectinomycin interaction with, 465f
  for Streptococci viridans, 32
  for Streptococcus pneumoniae, 30
  therapeutic drug monitoring goals for, 235
  tissue distribution, by key organ systems, 198

Chloramphenicol (Cont.)
  toxicity of, 235
  for Yersinia enterocolitica, pseudotuberculosis, 36
  for Yersinia pestis, 37
Chlorhexadine gluconate, for Acanthamoeba, 74
Chloroquine HCl/phosphate, 353f–354f
  administration route(s) for, 225
  adverse effects of, gastrointestinal, 268, 269
  ampicillin interaction with, 328f
  dosage adjustment, in renal failure, 161
  for Entamoeba histolytica, 84
  mechanism of action of, 225
  for Plasmodium spp., 94
  praziquantel interaction with, 447f
  precautions with, in hepatic dysfunction, 177
  prophylactic, for malaria, 287
  tissue distribution, by key organ systems, 199
Chlorpromazine, thalidomide interaction with, 476f
Chlorpropamide, chloramphenicol interaction with, 353f
Cholangitis, antimicrobial therapy for, 137
Cholecystitis, antimicrobial therapy for, 137
Cholestyramine, cephalexin interaction with, 351f
Chromobacterium violaceum, 11
Chromomycosis, 72
Chryseobacterium spp., 11
Ciclopirox/ciclopirox olamine, 354f–355f
  adverse effects of
    CNS, 265
    cutaneous, 267
  for Candida sp., 61
  for tinea corporis, 70
  for tinea cruris, 70
Cidofovir, 355f
  administration route(s) for, 224
  adverse effects of
    CNS, 263–265
    cutaneous, 266
    gastrointestinal, 268–270
    hematologic, 261, 262
    renal/genitourinary, 271
  for cytomegalovirus, 48
  mechanism of action of, 224
  tenofovir interaction with, 472f
Cilastatin
  ganciclovir interaction with, 386f
  valganciclovir interaction with, 489f
Cimetidine
  chloroquine HCl/phosphate interaction with, 354f
  praziquantel interaction with, 447f
  quinidine gluconate interaction with, 452f
  quinine sulfate interaction with, 453f
  terbinafine interaction with, 474f
  trimetrexate glucuronate interaction with, 487f
  valacyclovir interaction with, 488f
  zalcitabine interaction with, 493f
  zanamivir interaction with, 495f
Cinchona alkaloids, mechanism of action of, 225
Ciprofloxacin, 355f–357f
  administration route(s) for, 220
  adverse effects of
    CNS, 263–265
    cutaneous, 266
    gastrointestinal, 267–270
    hepatic, 272
  for Bacillus anthracis, 4
  for Bacillus cereus, 4
  for Bartonella bacilliformis, 6
  for Bartonella henselae, 5
  for Burkholderia pseudomallei, 9
  for Calymmatobacterium granulomatis, 9
  for Campylobacter jejuni, 9
  contraindicated drug interactions, 249
  for Cyclospora, 80
  desensitization protocols
    intravenous, 297
    oral, 297–298

Ciprofloxacin (*Cont.*)
  dosage adjustment
    in continuous renal replacement therapy, 172
    in obesity, 189
    in renal failure, 161
  efficacy relationships in humans, PK/PD
      parameter associated with, 246
  foscarnet interaction with, 384f
  for *Francisella tularensis,* 17
  for *Haemophilus ducreyi,* 18
  for *Isospora belli,* 87
  mechanism of action of, 220
  for *Mycobacterium fortuitum,* 46
  prophylactic
    for anthrax, 281
    for *Neisseria meningitidis,* 283
  for *Pseudomonas aeruginosa,* spp., 25
  tissue distribution, by key organ systems, 199
  for *Vibrio cholera,* 36
Cisapride
  amprenavir and, 330f
  atazanavir and, 331f
  halofantrine interaction with, 390f
  interactions
    with amprenavir, toxic effect(s), 248
    with atazanavir, toxic effect(s), 248
    with clarithromycin, toxic effect(s), 249
    with erythromycin ethylsuccinate and
        acetylsulfisoxazole, toxic effect(s), 249
    with erythromycin preparations, toxic
        effect(s), 250
    with fosamprenavir, toxic effect(s), 250
    with indinavir, toxic effect(s), 252
    with lopinavir with ritonavir, toxic effect(s),
        254
    with nelfinavir, toxic effect(s), 256
    with quinupristin, 454f
    with ritonavir, toxic effect(s), 257
    with saquinavir, toxic effect(s), 257
Cisplatin
  pentamidine isethionate interaction with, 439f
  vancomycin interaction with, 491f
Citrobacter, 229
Citrobacter spp., 12
Cl. *See* Clearance (Cl)
Clarithromycin, 357f–358f
  administration route for, 220
  adverse effects of
    CNS, 264
    cutaneous, 266
    gastrointestinal, 267–270
    hematologic, 261
  for *Balamuthia mandrillaris,* 77
  for *Bordetella pertussis,* 6
  for *Chlamydia trachomatis,* 11
  for *Chlamydophila pneumoniaie,* 10
  for *Chlamydophila psittaci,* 10
  contraindicated drug interactions, 249
  dosage adjustment, in renal failure, 162
  for *Haemophilus influenzae* nontypeable, 18
  for *Heliobacter pylori,* 19
  for *Legionella pneumophila,* 20
  lopinavir interaction with, 407f
  mechanism of action of, 220
  for *Moraxella catarrhalis,* 20
  for *Mycobacterium abscessus,* 47
  for *Mycobacterium avium* complex, 43, 44
  for *Mycobacterium chelonae,* 47
  for *Mycobacterium fortuitum,* 46
  for *Mycobacterium marinum,* 45
  for *Mycoplasma pneumoniae,* 21
  precautions with, in hepatic dysfunction, 178
  prophylactic
    for endocarditis, in penicillin-allergic
        patient, 277
    for *Mycobacterium avium* complex, 282
    for pertussis, 283
  ritonavir interaction with, 462f
  for *Streptococcus* Group A, 31
  tissue distribution, by key organ systems, 199
  zidovudine interaction with, 495f

Clavulanate, 478f–479f
  for *Enterobacter* spp., 15
  for *Stenotrophomonas maltophila,* 29
Clearance (Cl), 242
Clindamycin, 358f–359f
  for *Actinomyces israeli,* 2
  administration route(s) for, 221
  adverse effects of
    cardiovascular, 262
    cutaneous, 266, 267
    gastrointestinal, 267–270
  for *Arcanobacterium haemolyticum,* 3
  for *Babesia microti,* 76
  for *Bacillus anthracis,* 4
  for *Bacteroides:* fragilis group, 5
  for *Capnocytophaga canimorsus,* 10
  for *Capnocytophaga ochracea,* 10
  for *Cardiobacterium canimorsus,* 10
  for *Clostridium perfringens,* spp., 13
  contraindicated drug interactions, 249
  for *Corynebacterium jeikeum,* spp., 14
  dosage adjustment
    in hepatic dysfunction, 178
    in obesity, 189
  erythromycin ethylsuccinate and
      acetylsulfisoxazole interactions with,
      249
  erythromycin interactions with, 250
  for *Fusobacterium* spp., 17
  mechanism of action of, 221
  microbial resistance to, mechanism of, 227
  for *Mycoplasma hominis,* 21
  for *Plasmodium falciparum,* 92
  for *Pneumocystis jiroveci,* 66
  precautions with, in hepatic dysfunction, 178
  for *Prevotella* spp., 24
  prophylactic, for endocarditis, in penicillin-
      allergic patient, 277
  for *Propionobacterium acnes,* 24
  saquinavir interaction with, 463f
  for *Staphyloccus aureus;* methicillin-
      susceptible, 28, 29
  for *Streptococcus* Group A, 31
  for *Streptococcus pneumoniae,* 30
  tissue distribution, by key organ systems, 199
  for *Toxoplasma gondii,* 99
Clindamycin/pyrimethamine/leucovorin,
    prophylactic, for toxoplasmosis, in HIV-
    infected patients, 288
Clofazimine, 359f–360f
  adverse effects of
    cutaneous, 266, 267
    endocrine/metabolic, 271
    gastrointestinal, 267–270
  tissue distribution, by key organ systems, 199
Clonorchis sinensis, 79
Clostridium botulinum, 12
Clostridium difficile, 12
  in vitro drug susceptibility and in vivo drug
      efficacy against, discordance between,
      228
Clostridium perfringens, spp., 13
Clostridium tetani, 12
Clotrimazole
  administration route(s) for, 223
  adverse effects of, gastrointestinal, 269, 270
  mechanism of action of, 223
Clotrimazole, 360f–361f
  for *Aspergillus* sp., 55
  for *Candida* sp., 58, 60, 61
  for tinea corporis, 70
  for tinea cruris, 70
  for tinea pedis, 69
  trimetrexate glucuronate interaction with, 487f
Cloxacillin, 361f
  adverse effects of, gastrointestinal, 267–270
  tissue distribution, by key organ systems,
      199
Clozapine, erythromycin preparations interaction
    with, 378f
C_{max}/MIC, 244, 245

Coccidioides immitis, 61–62
Colistimethate sodium
  adverse effects of
    CNS, 263
    renal/genitourinary, 271
  dosage adjustment, in renal failure, 162
  tissue distribution, by key organ systems, 199
Colistimethate sodium, 361f–362f
Colistin
  administration route(s) for, 221
  mechanism of action of, 221
Colitis, drugs causing, 268
Community-acquired pneumonia, antimicrobial
    therapy for, 129
Concentration-dependent antimicrobial activity
    (AUC/MIC or C_{max}/MIC), 244, 245
Concentration-independent antimicrobial activity
    (T > MIC), 244, 245
Confusion, drugs causing, 263
Conivaptan, interactions
  with itraconazole, toxic effect(s), 252
  with ketoconazole, toxic effect(s), 253
  with miconazole, toxic effect(s), 255
Conjunctivitis, bacterial, antimicrobial therapy
    for, 115–116
Constipation, drugs causing, 268
Continuous arteriovenous hemofiltration. *See*
    Continuous renal replacement therapy
Continuous renal replacement therapy
  drug administration to pediatric patients
    receiving, optimal approach for, 158
  drug dosing in, 158, 170–174
  drug removal, with factors affecting, 158
Continuous venovenous hemodiafiltration. *See*
    Continuous renal replacement therapy
Continuous venovenous hemodialysis. *See*
    Continuous renal replacement therapy
Continuous venovenous hemofiltration. *See*
    Continuous renal replacement therapy
Contraceptives, oral
  amoxicillin interaction with, 323f
  ampicillin and, 328f
  amprenavir and, 330f
  cloxacillin interaction with, 361f
  dicloxacillin sodium interaction with, 367f
  fosamprenavir interaction with, 383f
  griseofulvin interaction with, 389f
  nelfinavir interaction with, 421f
  nevirapine interaction with, 425f
  tetracycline interaction with, 476f
Coombs test, positive, drugs causing, 262
Corticosteroids
  for *Aspergillus* sp., 55
  for *Histoplasma capsulatum*, 65
  levofloxacin interaction with, 404f
  methanamine preparations interaction with,
    413f
  rifampin interaction with, 459f
  rifapentine interaction with, 460f
Corynebacterium diphtheriae, 13
Corynebacterium jeikeum, spp., 14
Cotrimoxazole
  administration route(s) for, 221
  contraindicated drug interactions, 249
  dosage adjustment, in renal failure, 162
  lamivudine interaction with, 403f
  mechanism of action of, 221
  precautions with, in hepatic dysfunction, 178
  tissue distribution, by key organ systems, 200
Coxiella burnetti, 14
CrCl. *See* Creatinine clearance
Creatinine clearance
  estimation of, Schwartz method for, 157
  and estimation of glomerular filtration rate,
    156–157
  formula for, 156–157
Crotamiton, 105
CRRT. *See* Continuous renal replacement
    therapy
Cryptococcus neoformans, 62–63
Cryptosporidium, 79

CSF. *See* Cerebrospinal fluid (CSF)
Curvularia sp., 62
Cutaneous candidasis, 72
Cutaneous fungal infections, 72
Cutaneous larva migrans, thiabendazole, 477f
Cyclic peptides, mechanism of action of, 222
Cyclobenzaprine, interactions
  with furazolidone, toxic effect(s), 251
  with linezolid, toxic effect(s), 254
Cycloserine, 363f
  dosage adjustment, in renal failure, 162
  ethionamide interaction with, 379f
  tissue distribution, by key organ systems, 200
Cyclospora, 80
Cyclosporine
  amphotericin B interaction with, 325f
  azithromycin interaction with, 335f
  caspofungin interaction with, 339f
  chloramphenicol interaction with, 353f
  ciprofloxacin interaction with, 357f
  clarithromycin interaction with, 358f
  dirithromycin interaction with, 371f
  erythromycin preparations interaction with,
    378f
  fluconazole interaction with, 381f
  ganciclovir interaction with, 386f
  griseofulvin interaction with, 389f
  lopinavir interaction with, 407f
  nafcillin interaction with, 420f
  norfloxacin interaction with, 427f
  ofloxacin interaction with, 429f
  quinupristin with dalfopristin interaction with,
    454f
  rifampin interaction with, 459f
  rifapentine interaction with, 460f
  ritonavir interaction with, 462f
  saquinavir interaction with, 463f
  terbinafine interaction with, 474f
  tinidazole interaction with, 480f
  trimethoprim interaction with, 485f
  voriconazole interaction with, 493f
Cystic fibrosis
  azithromycin in, 334f
  and pharmacokinetic monitoring, 243
Cytarabine, flucytosine interaction with, 382f
Cytidine analog, mechanism of action of, 225
Cytomegalovirus, 48–49, 284
Cytomegalovirus immune globulin, 262,
    363f–364f
  adverse effects of
    CNS, 263, 264
    gastrointestinal, 269, 270
    musculoskeletal, 273

Dacrocystitis, antimicrobial therapy for, 116
Dalfopristin. *See* Quinupristin with dalfopristin
Dapsone, 364f
  administration route for, 222
  mechanism of action of, 222
  for *Pneumocystis jiroveci*, 66
  prophylactic, for *Pneumocystis*, 287
  saquinavir interaction with, 463f
  spectinomycin interaction with, 465f
  tissue distribution, by key organ systems, 200
  trimethoprim interaction with, 485f
Daptomycin, 365f
  administration route for, 221
  adverse effects of
    cardiovascular, 262
    CNS, 263–265
    cutaneous, 266, 267
    endocrine/metabolic, 271
    gastrointestinal, 267–270
    hematologic, 261
    hepatic, 272
    musculoskeletal, 273
    renal/genitourinary, 271
  dosage adjustment
    in obesity, 189
    in renal failure, 162
  mechanism of action of, 221

Daptomycin *(Cont.)*
  for *Pediococcus* spp., 23
  for *Staphyloccus aureus;* methicillin-
    susceptible, 29
  tissue distribution, by key organ systems,
    200
Darbopoetin, thalidomide interaction with, 476f
Darunavir, 365f–366f
  precautions with, in hepatic dysfunction, 178
  tipranavir interaction with, 481f
Decamethonium, colistimethate sodium
    interaction with, 362f
Dehydration, and pharmacokinetic monitoring,
    243
Delavirdine, 366f
  administration route for, 224
  adverse effects of
    CNS, 263, 264
    cutaneous, 266
    gastrointestinal, 267–270
    hematologic, 261
    hepatic, 272
  contraindicated drug interactions, 249
  mechanism of action of, 224
  nelfinavir interaction with, 421f
  precautions with, in hepatic dysfunction, 178
  quinidine gluconate interaction with, 452f
  quinupristin with dalfopristin interaction with,
    454f
  rifapentine interaction with, 460f
  saquinavir interaction with, 463f
  tissue distribution, by key organ systems,
    200
Dental abscess, antimicrobial therapy for, 119
Depression, drugs causing, 263
Dermatitis, drugs causing, 266
Dermatophytes, 72
Desensitization protocols
  for aminoglycosides, 300–302
  for cephalosporins
    continuous IV infusion, 294–295
    intermittent IV infusion, 294
  for ciprofloxacin
    intravenous, 297
    oral, 297–298
  for fluoroquinolone, 297–298
  for penicillin
    continuous IV infusion, 292–293
    intermittent IV infusion, 292
    oral, 293
  for tobramycin
    inhaled, 301–302
    intravenous, 300–301
  for trimethoprim/sulfamethoxazole
    adverse reactions and response during,
      296
    oral
      for patients with history of typical delayed
        maculopapular reaction, 295–296
      for patients with previous (distant)
        reaction consistent with IgE-mediated
        mechanism, 295
  for vancomycin
    rapid, 298–299
    slow, 299–300
Desipramine, ritonavir interaction with, 462f
Developmental pharmacology, 153–155
Dexamethasone
  albendazole interaction with, 320f
  lopinavir interaction with, 407f
  saquinavir interaction with, 463f
  thalidomide interaction with, 476f
Dexmethylphenidate, interactions
  with furazolidone, toxic effect(s), 251
  with linezolid, toxic effect(s), 253
Dextromethorphan
  interactions
    with furazolidone, toxic effect(s), 251
    with linezolid, toxic effect(s), 254
  terbinafine interaction with, 474f
Dialysis, drug dose adjustment with, 158–169

Diarrhea
  in antibiotic-associated infection, antimicrobial
    therapy for, 138
  drugs causing, 268–269
  in food- or water-borne disease, antimicrobial
    therapy for, 138
  in immunocompromised patient, antimicrobial
    therapy for, 139
  in nosocomial infection, antimicrobial therapy
    for, 139
  in travel-associated infection, antimicrobial
    therapy for, 139
Diazepam
  isoniazid interaction with, 397f
  quinupristin with dalfopristin interaction with,
    454f
Dicloxacillin
  administration route for, 220
  mechanism of action of, 220
Dicloxacillin sodium, 367f
  adverse effects of, gastrointestinal, 267–269
  tissue distribution, by key organ systems, 200
Didanosine, 367f–368f
  administration route for, 224
  adverse effects of
    CNS, 265
    endocrine/metabolic, 271
  dapsone interaction with, 364f
  dosage adjustment, in renal failure, 163
  ganciclovir interaction with, 386f
  levofloxacin interaction with, 404f
  mechanism of action of, 224
  ofloxacin interaction with, 429f
  precautions with, in hepatic dysfunction, 178
  ribavirin interaction with, 457f
  tenofovir interaction with, 472f
  tissue distribution, by key organ systems,
    200
  valganciclovir interaction with, 489f
Dientamoeba fragilis, 80
Diethylcarbamazine, 368f–369f
  administration route for, 225
  for *Brugia malayi,* 78
  for *Brugia timori,* 79
  for *Loa loa,* 88
  for *Mansonella streptocerca,* 89
  mechanism of action of, 225
  tissue distribution, by key organ systems, 200
  for *Wucherheria bancrofti,* 104
Digoxin
  azithromycin interaction with, 335f
  clarithromycin interaction with, 358f
  dirithromycin interaction with, 371f
  erythromycin preparations interaction with,
    378f
  hydroxychloroquine interaction with, 391f
  neomycin sulfate interaction with, 422f
  paromomycin sulfate interaction with, 434f
  quinidine gluconate interaction with, 452f
  quinine sulfate interaction with, 453f
  rifampin interaction with, 459f
  ritonavir interaction with, 462f
  sulfamethoxazole with trimethoprim
    interaction with, 469f
  tetracycline interaction with, 476f
Dihydroergotamine, azithromycin interaction
    with, 335f
Diiodohydroxyquine. *See* iodoquinol
Diloxanide furoate
  administration route for, 226
  for *Entamoeba histolytica,* 84
  mechanism of action of, 226
Diltiazem, quinidine gluconate interaction with,
    452f
Diphtheria, recommended antimicrobial
    prophylaxis for, 281
Diphtheria antitoxin (equine), 369f–370f
  adverse effects of
    CNS, 264
    hypersensitivity, 273
Diphyllabothrium latum, 80

Dipylidium caninum, 80
Dirithromycin, 371f
  administration route for, 220
  adverse effects of
    CNS, 263–265
    cutaneous, 266, 267
    endocrine/metabolic, 271
    gastrointestinal, 267–270
    hematologic, 261
    respiratory, 272
  mechanism of action of, 220
  tissue distribution, by key organ systems, 200
Diskitis, antimicrobial therapy for, 126
Disopyramide, interactions
  with clarithromycin, toxic effect(s), 249
  with erythromycin ethylsuccinate and
    acetylsulfisoxazole, toxic effect(s), 249
  with erythromycin preparations, toxic effect(s),
    250
Distribution (drug), age-dependent physiologic
    variables affecting, 153–154
Disulfiram, interactions
  with amprenavir, toxic effect(s), 248
  with lopinavir with ritonavir, toxic effect(s),
    254
  with ritonavir, toxic effect(s), 257
Dizziness, drugs causing, 263
Docetaxel, 476f
  quinupristin with dalfopristin interaction with,
    454f
Dofetilide, interactions
  with cotrimoxazole, toxic effect(s), 249
  with itraconazole, toxic effect(s), 252
  with ketoconazole, toxic effect(s), 253
  with miconazole, toxic effect(s), 255
  with trimethoprim, toxic effect(s), 258
Doripenem, 371f
  adverse effects of
    CNS, 264
    cutaneous, 266, 267
    gastrointestinal, 269
  dosage adjustment, in renal failure, 163
  tissue distribution, by key organ systems, 200
Doxycycline, 372f–373f
  administration route(s) for, 221
  for *Anaplasma phagocytophila,* 3
  for *Bacillus anthracis,* 4
  for *Bartonella henselae,* 6
  for *Borrelia burgdorferi,* 6, 7
  for *Borrelia recurrentis, hermsii, turicate,* 8
  for *Brucella abortus,* spp., 8
  for *Burkholderia mallei,* 9
  for *Burkholderia pseudomallei,* 9
  for *Calymmatobacterium granulomatis,* 9
  for *Campylobacter jejuni,* 9
  for *Capnocytophaga canimorsus,* 10
  for *Capnocytophaga ochracea,* 10
  for *Cardiobacterium canimorsus,* 10
  for *Chlamydia trachomatis,* 11
  for *Chlamydophila pneumoniaie,* 10
  for *Chlamydophila psittaci,* 10
  for *Chromobacterium violaceum,* 11
  contraindications to, in hepatic dysfunction,
    178
  for *Coxiella burnetti,* 14
  dosage adjustment, in obesity, 189
  for *Ehrlichia chafeensis,* 14
  for *Francisella tularensis,* 17
  for *Legionella pneumophila,* 20
  for *Leptospira interrogans,* 20
  mechanism of action of, 221
  for *Moraxella catarrhalis,* 20
  for *Mycobacterium fortuitum,* 46
  for *Mycobacterium marinum,* 45
  for *Mycoplasma pneumoniae,* 21
  for *Pasteurella multocida,* 23
  for *Plasmodium falciparum,* 92
  for *Plasmodium vivax,* 93
  precautions with, in hepatic dysfunction, 178
  preventive therapy, after sexual contact/sexual
    assault, 280

Doxycycline (*Cont.*)
  prophylactic
    for anthrax, 281
    for malaria, 288
  for *Propionobacterium acnes,* 24
  for *Rickettsia akari,* 25
  for *Rickettsia prowazekii,* 26
  for *Rickettsia rickettsi,* 25
  for *Rickettsia* spp., 26
  for *Rickettsia typhi,* 26
  for *Staphyloccus aureus;* methicillin-
    susceptible, 29
  for *Stenotrophomonas maltophila,* 29
  for *Streptobacillus moniliformis,* 29
  tissue distribution, by key organ systems, 200
  for *Treponema pallidum,* 33, 35
  for *Ureaplasma urealyticum,* 35
  for *Vibrio cholera,* 36
  for *Vibrio vulnificus, parahemolyticus,* spp., 36
  for *Yersinia enterocolitica, pseudotuberculosis,*
    36, 37
  for *Yersinia pestis,* 37
Dracunculus medinensis, 81
Drug interactions, 247
  contraindicated, 247–258
Drug resistance, mechanisms of, 227–228
DTaP, prophylactic, 284
Dyspepsia, drugs causing, 269
Dyspnea, drugs causing, 272

Echinocandins
  mechanism of action of, 223
  in vivo pharmacodynamic characteristics of,
    in neutropenic mouse models, 247
Echinococcus granulosus, 81
Echinococcus multilocularis, 81
Econazole nitrate, 373f
  for *Aspergillus* sp., 55
  for *Candida* sp., 61
  for tinea corporis, 70
  for tinea cruris, 70
  for tinea pedis, 69
Ecthyma gangrenosum, antimicrobial therapy
    for, 128
Edwardsiella tarda, 14
Efavirenz, 373f–374f
  administration route for, 224
  adverse effects of
    CNS, 263–265
    cutaneous, 266, 267
    endocrine/metabolic, 271
    gastrointestinal, 267–270
  amprenavir and, 330f
  atazanavir and, 331f, 332f
  fosamprenavir interaction with, 383f
  idinavir interaction with, 396f
  lopinavir interaction with, 407f
  maraviroc interaction with, 409f
  mechanism of action of, 224
  nelfinavir interaction with, 421f
  precautions with, in hepatic dysfunction, 178
  tissue distribution, by key organ systems, 201
Eflornithine, 103
Eflornithine, for *Trypanosoma brucei gambiense,*
    102, 103
Ehrlichia chafeensis, 14
Ehrlichia phagocytophila. See *Anaplasma*
    phagocytophila
Eikenella corrodens, 14
Elimination (drug), age-dependent physiologic
    variables affecting, 155
Elimination half-life ($T_{1/2}$), 241
  and steady state, 242
Elimination rate constant (Kel), 241
Emtricitabine, 375f
  administration route for, 225
  adverse effects of
    CNS, 263–265
    cutaneous, 266
    endocrine/metabolic, 271
    gastrointestinal, 267–270

Emtricitabine (*Cont.*)
  adverse effects of (*cont.*)
    hepatic, 272
    musculoskeletal, 273
  dosage adjustment, in renal failure, 163
  lamivudine interaction with, 403f
  mechanism of action of, 225
  precautions with, in hepatic dysfunction, 178
  tissue distribution, by key organ systems, 201
Encephalitis, antimicrobial therapy for, 133–134
Encephalitozoon cuniculi, 83–84
Encephalitozoon hellem, 82
Encephalitozoon intestinalis, 83
Endocarditis
  native valve, antimicrobial therapy for, 108
  prosthetic valve, antimicrobial therapy for, 108–109
  recommended antimicrobial prophylaxis for, 277
Endocrine/metabolic system, adverse drug effects and, 271
Endophthalmitis, antimicrobial therapy for, 116–117
Enfuvirtide, 375f–376f
  adverse effects of
    CNS, 265
    endocrine/metabolic, 271
    gastrointestinal, 267–269
    hematologic, 261
    musculoskeletal, 273
  tissue distribution, by key organ systems, 201
Entamoeba dispar, 84
Entamoeba histolytica, 84
Entamoeba polecki, 85
Entecavir, for hepatitis B, 49
Enterobacter, in vitro drug susceptibility and in vivo drug efficacy against, discordance between, 229
Enterobacter spp., 15
Enterobius vermicularis, 85
Enterococcus, in vitro drug susceptibility and in vivo drug efficacy against, discordance between, 228
Enterococcus, vancomycin resistant, 15
Enterococcus faecalis/faecium, 15
Enterocytozoon bieneusi, 85
Eosinophilia, drugs causing, 261
Epididymitis, antimicrobial therapy for, 120
Epiglottitis, antimicrobial therapy for, 145
Epstein-Barr virus, ampicillin and, 328f
Eraxis. *See* Anidulafungin
Ergot alkaloids, clarithromycin interaction with, 358f
Ergotamine, azithromycin interaction with, 335f
Ergot derivatives
  amprenavir and, 330f
  atazanavir and, 331f
  clotrimazole interaction with, 360f
  dirithromycin interaction with, 371f
  interactions
    with amprenavir, toxic effect(s), 248
    with atazanavir, toxic effect(s), 248
    with fosamprenavir, toxic effect(s), 250
    with indinavir, toxic effect(s), 252
    with lopinavir with ritonavir, toxic effect(s), 254
    with nelfinavir, toxic effect(s), 256
    with ritonavir, toxic effect(s), 257
    with saquinavir, toxic effect(s), 257
Ertapenem, 376f
  administration route(s) for, 218
  adverse effects of
    cardiovascular, 262
    CNS, 263–265
    cutaneous, 266, 267
    gastrointestinal, 267–270
    hematologic, 261, 262
    hepatic, 272
    renal/genitourinary, 272
    respiratory, 272

Ertapenem (*Cont.*)
  dosage adjustment
    in obesity, 189
    in renal failure, 163
  mechanism of action of, 218
  tissue distribution, by key organ systems, 201
Erysipelas, antimicrobial therapy for, 127
Erysipelothrix rhusiopathiae, 15
Erythema multiforme, drugs causing, 266
Erythromycin
  administration route(s) for, 220
  adverse effects of
    cutaneous, 267
    gastrointestinal, 267, 269, 270
    hepatic, 272
    hypersensitivity, 273
  dosage adjustment
    in obesity, 189
    in renal failure, 163
  interactions, with clindamycin, toxic effect(s), 249
  mechanism of action of, 220
  prophylactic
    for diphtheria, 281
    for pertussis, 283
    for rheumatic fever, in penicillin-allergic patient, 279
Erythromycin base, preventive therapy, after sexual contact/sexual assault, 280
Erythromycin ethylsuccinate, preventive therapy, after sexual contact/sexual assault, 280
Erythromycin ethylsuccinate and acetylsulfisoxazole
  contraindicated drug interactions, 249
  tissue distribution, by key organ systems, 201
Erythromycin ethylsuccinate and acetylsulfisoxazole, 377f
  for *Calymmatobacterium granulomatis,* 9
Erythromycin ointment, prophylactic, for ophthalmia neonatorum, 279
Erythromycin preparations, 377f–378f
  for *Actinomyces israeli,* 2
  for *Arcanobacterium haemolyticum,* 3
  for *Bartonella henselae,* 6
  for *Bordetella pertussis,* 6
  for *Borrelia burgdorferi,* 6, 7
  for *Borrelia recurrentis, hermsii, turicate,* 8
  for *Calymmatobacterium granulomatis,* 9
  for *Campylobacter jejuni,* 9
  for *Capnocytophaga canimorsus,* 10
  for *Cardiobacterium canimorsus,* 10
  for *Chlamydia trachomatis,* 11
  for *Chlamydophila pneumoniae,* 10
  for *Chlamydophila psittaci,* 10
  contraindicated drug interactions, 250
  contraindications to, in hepatic dysfunction, 178
  for *Corynebacterium diphtheriae,* 13
  for *Corynebacterium jeikeum,* spp., 14
  fosfomycin tromethamine interaction with, 385f
  for *Haemophilus ducreyi,* 18
  for *Legionella pneumophila,* 20
  for *Mycoplasma pneumoniae,* 21
  for *Pediococcus* spp., 23
  penicillin G interaction with, 436f
  penicillin V interaction with, 438f
  precautions with, in hepatic dysfunction, 178
  for *Propionibacterium acnes,* 24
  for *Streptobacillus moniliformis,* 29
  for *Streptococcus* Group A, 31
  tissue distribution, by key organ systems, 201
  trimetrexate glucuronate interaction with, 487f
  for *Ureaplasma urealyticum,* 35
  for *Vibrio cholera,* 36
ESBL. *See* Extended-spectrum beta-lactamase (ESBL)-producing organisms
Escherichia coli, 16–17
  in vitro drug susceptibility and in vivo drug efficacy against, discordance between, 228

Esophagitis, antimicrobial therapy for, 139
Estolate, for *Bordetella pertussis,* 6
Ethacrynic acid, streptomycin sulfate interaction
   with, 467f
Ethambutol HCl, 378f–379f
   administration route for, 222
   adverse effects of
      CNS, 263, 264
      endocrine/metabolic, 271
      gastrointestinal, 267–270
   dosage adjustment, in renal failure, 163
   ethionamide interaction with, 379f
   mechanism of action of, 222
   for *Mycobacterium avium* complex, 43, 44
   for *Mycobacterium kansasii,* 45
   for *Mycobacterium tuberculosis,* 40, 42
   precautions with, in hepatic dysfunction, 178
   tissue distribution, by key organ systems,
      201
Ethanol
   abacavir sulfate interaction with, 317f
   cefoperazone interaction with, 344f
Ethinyl estradiol, ritonavir interaction with, 462f
Ethionamide, 379f
   administration route for, 222
   adverse effects of
      cardiovascular, 262
      CNS, 265
      gastrointestinal, 268–270
      hepatic, 272
   contraindications to, in hepatic dysfunction,
      178
   cycloserine interaction with, 363f
   mechanism of action of, 222
   for *Mycobacterium bovis,* 43
   for *Mycobacterium tuberculosis,* 41
   precautions with, in hepatic dysfunction, 178
   tissue distribution, by key organ systems,
      201
Exophiala sp., 63
Exserohilum sp., 63
Extended-spectrum beta-lactamase (ESBL)-
      producing organisms, in vitro drug
      susceptibility and in vivo drug efficacy
      against, discordance between, 228
Eye(s)
   adverse drug effects and, 273
   infections of, antimicrobial therapy for,
      115–119

Famciclovir, 380f
   administration route for, 223
   adverse effects of
      CNS, 264
      cutaneous, 266, 267
      gastrointestinal, 267–270
      hematologic, 261, 262
      hepatic, 272
   dosage adjustment, in renal failure, 163
   for herpes simplex, 50, 51
   mechanism of action of, 223
   precautions with, in hepatic dysfunction, 178
   prophylactic, for prevention of recurrent
      herpes simplex, 284
   tissue distribution, by key organ systems, 201
   for varicella, 53
Fasciola buski, 85
Fasciola hepatica, 85
Fentanyl
   dirithromycin interaction with, 371f
   econazole nitrate interaction with, 373f
   rifampin interaction with, 459f
Fever, drugs causing, 264
Filaria, 106
Flecainide, interactions
   with lopinavir with ritonavir, toxic effect(s),
      254
   with ritonavir, toxic effect(s), 257
Flucloxacillin
   administration route for, 220
   mechanism of action of, 220

Fluconazole, 380f–382f
   for *Acanthamoeba,* 74
   administration route(s) for, 223
   adverse effects of
      CNS, 264
      cutaneous, 266
      gastrointestinal, 267–270
   for *Balamuthia mandrillaris,* 77
   for *Blastomyces dermatitidis,* 56, 57
   for *Candida* sp., 58–61
   clarithromycin interaction with, 358f
   for *Coccidioides immitis,* 61, 62
   for *Cryptococcus neoformans,* 62, 63
   for *Curvularia* sp., 62
   dosage adjustment
      in continuous renal replacement therapy,
         172
      in obesity, 190
      in renal failure, 163
   for *Histoplasma capsulatum,* 64
   for *Malassezia* sp., 65
   mechanism of action of, 223
   precautions with, in hepatic dysfunction, 178
   prophylactic, for *Candida,* 287
   for *Pseudoallescheria boydii,* 67
   rifapentine interaction with, 460f
   for tinea capitis, 69
   for tinea cruris, 70
   for tinea favosa, 71
   for tinea pedis, 69
   for tinea unguium, 71
   tissue distribution, by key organ systems, 201
   trimetrexate glucuronate interaction with, 487f
   zanamivir interaction with, 495f
Flucytosine, 382f
   adverse effects of
      cutaneous, 266
      gastrointestinal, 267–270
      hematologic, 261, 262
      hepatic, 272
   for *Balamuthia mandrillaris,* 77
   for *Candida* sp., 59
   for *Cryptococcus neoformans,* 62, 63
   dosage adjustment
      in continuous renal replacement therapy,
         172
      in renal failure, 164
   for *Sappinia diploidea,* 96
   serum concentrations
      appropriate times to sample, 235
      and toxicity, 235
   therapeutic drug monitoring goals for, 235
   tissue distribution, by key organ systems, 201
   toxicity of, 235
   in vivo pharmacodynamic characteristics of,
      in neutropenic mouse models, 247
Fluid overload, and pharmacokinetic monitoring,
   243
Flukes, 106
5-Fluorocytosine
   administration route(s) for, 222
   mechanism of action of, 222
   microbial resistance to, mechanism of, 227
Fluoroquinolones
   AUC/MIC, 244, 245
   for *Burkholderia mallei,* 9
   for *Capnocytophaga ochracea,* 10
   for *Chlamydophila pneumoniae,* 10
   for *Chromobacterium violaceum,* 11
   for *Citrobacter* spp., 12
   C_{max}/MIC, 244, 245
   for *Coxiella burnetti,* 14
   desensitization protocols, 297–298
   didanosine interaction with, 368f
   dosage adjustment, in obesity, 189
   efficacy relationships in humans, PK/PD
      parameter associated with, 246
   for *Enterobacter* spp., 15
   for *Enterococcus,* vancomycin resistant, 15
   for *Erysipelothrix rhusiopathiae,* 15
   for *Escherichia coli,* 17

Fluoroquinolones (Cont.)
  for Haemophilus influenzae, 18
  for Haemophilus influenzae-aegypticus, 18
  for Klebsiella spp., 19
  for Legionella pneumophila, 20
  mechanism of action of, 220
  microbial resistance to, mechanisms of, 227,
      228
  for Moraxella catarrhalis, 20
  for Morganella, 21
  for Mycoplasma pneumoniae, 21
  for Pasteurella multocida, 23
  for Plesiomonas shigelloides, 23
  for Proteus mirabilis, 24
  for Proteus vulgaris, indole positive spp., 25
  for Providencia spp., 25
  for Rickettsia prowazekii, 26
  for Salmonella (non-typhi), 27
  for Salmonella typhi (type D), 26
  for Shigella sonnei, dysenteriae, boydii,
      flexneri, 27, 28
  for Vibrio vulnificus, parahemolyticus, spp., 36
  in vitro resistance relationships, PK/PD
      parameter associated with, 246
  for Yersinia enterocolitica, pseudotuberculosis,
      36, 37
Fluorouracil, tinidazole interaction with, 480f
Flushing, drugs causing, 262
Folinic acid
  for Pneumocystis jiroveci, 66
  for Toxoplasma gondii, 99, 100
Folliculitis, antimicrobial therapy for, 127
Fosamprenavir, 382f–383f
  adverse effects of
    CNS, 263, 264
    cutaneous, 266, 267
    endocrine/metabolic, 271
    gastrointestinal, 267, 269, 270
    hematologic, 262
  contraindicated drug interactions, 250
  dosage adjustment, in hepatic dysfunction, 178
  precautions with, in hepatic dysfunction, 178
  tissue distribution, by key organ systems, 202
Foscarnet, 384f
  administration route for, 223
  adverse effects of
    cardiovascular, 262
    CNS, 263–265
    cutaneous, 266, 267
    endocrine/metabolic, 271
    gastrointestinal, 267–270
    hematologic, 261, 262
    musculoskeletal, 273
    ocular, 273
    renal/genitourinary, 271
    respiratory, 272
  contraindicated drug interactions, 250
  for cytomegalovirus, 48
  dosage adjustment, in renal failure, 164
  mechanism of action of, 223
  tissue distribution, by key organ systems, 202
  for varicella, 53
  zalcitabine interaction with, 493f
Fosfomycin tromethamine, 384f–385f
  administration route for, 221
  adverse effects of
    CNS, 263–265
    cutaneous, 266
    gastrointestinal, 267, 269
    renal/genitourinary, 272
  mechanism of action of, 221
  tissue distribution, by key organ systems, 202
Francisella tularensis, 17
Fumagillin
  for Enterocytozoon bieneusi, 85
  for Microsporidia, 90
Fungal genera
  by clinical presentation, 72
  by laboratory report, 72–73
Fungal infections, 54–71
  superficial cutaneous, 69–71

Furazolidone, 385f–386f
  administration route for, 221
  adverse effects of
    CNS, 264
    gastrointestinal, 267, 269, 270
  for Blastocystis hominis, 77
  contraindicated drug interactions, 251
  for Giardia lamblia, 86
  mechanism of action of, 221
  for Vibrio cholera, 36
Furosemide
  aztreonam interaction with, 336f
  streptomycin sulfate interaction with, 467f
  tobramycin interaction with, 483f
Furuncles, antimicrobial therapy for, 127
Fusarium sp., 64
Fusobacterium spp., 17

Gallamine, colistimethate sodium interaction
    with, 362f
Ganciclovir, 386f–387f
  administration route(s) for, 223
  adverse effects of
    CNS, 263–265
    cutaneous, 266, 267
    gastrointestinal, 267, 269, 270
    hematologic, 261, 262
  contraindicated drug interactions, 251
  for cytomegalovirus, 48, 49
  dosage adjustment
    in continuous renal replacement therapy,
        172
    in renal failure, 164
  imipenem-cilastatin interaction with, 392f
  interactions, with imipenem-cilastatin, toxic
      effect(s), 252
  mechanism of action of, 223
  prophylactic, for prevention of CMV
      transmission to transplant recipient,
      284
  tenofovir interaction with, 472f
  tissue distribution, by key organ systems, 202
Gardenerella vaginalis. See bacterial vaginosis
Gastrointestinal tract
  adverse drug effects and, 267–271
  infections, antimicrobial therapy for, 136–141
Gatifloxacin
  for Acinetobacter spp., 2
  administration route(s) for, 220
  mechanism of action of, 220
  precautions with, in hepatic dysfunction, 179
Genitourinary system
  adverse drug effects and, 271–272
  infections, antimicrobial therapy for, 120–123
Gentamicin, 387f–388f
  administration route(s) for, 218
  adverse effects of
    CNS, 265
    cutaneous, 267
    renal/genitourinary, 271
  for Bartonella henselae, 5
  for Brucella abortus, spp., 8
  for Burkholderia mallei, 9
  dosage adjustment
    in continuous renal replacement therapy,
        172
    in obesity, 183, 188
    in renal failure, 164
  for Enterococcus faecalis/faecium, 15
  for Escherichia coli, 16
  for Francisella tularensis, 17
  for Haemophilus influenzae-aegypticus, 18
  for Haemophilus parainfluenza, haemolyticus,
      aphrophilus, spp., 18
  high-dose extended-interval dosing of, 239
  for Kingella kingae, spp., 19
  for Klebsiella spp., 19
  for Listeria monocytogenes, 20
  mechanism of action of, 218
  nephrotoxicity of, 236
  ototoxicity of, 236, 274

Gentamicin (*Cont.*)
  for *Proteus vulgaris,* indole positive spp., 25
  serum concentrations
    appropriate times to sample, 236
    and toxicity, 236
  for *Staphyloccus aureus;* methicillin-
    susceptible, 28
  for *Streptococci viridans,* 32, 33
  for *Streptococcus* Group B, 31
  for *Streptococcus* Group C, G, 32
  therapeutic drug monitoring goals for, 236
  tissue distribution, by key organ systems, 202
  toxicity of, risk factors for, 236
  for *Yersinia pestis,* 37
Gentian violet, 388f–389f
GFR. *See* Glomerular filtration rate
Giardia lamblia, 86
Gingivitis, antimicrobial therapy for, 142
Glomerular filtration rate
  estimation of
    methods for, 156–157
    urinary creatinine method for, 156–157
  normal values for, by age, 156
Glomerular function, determination of, by
    nuclear medicine scans, 157
Glyburide, ofloxacin interaction with, 429f
Glycopeptides
  AUC/MIC, 244, 245
  efficacy relationships in humans, PK/PD
    parameter associated with, 246
  mechanism of action of, 221
  microbial resistance to, mechanism of, 227
  in vitro resistance relationships, PK/PD
    parameter associated with, 246
Gnathostoma spinigerum, 86
Gongylonema sp., 86
Gonorrhea, recommended antibiotic prophylaxis
    for, 280
Gray baby syndrome, 235
Griseofulvin, 389f
  administration route for, 223
  adverse effects of
    CNS, 263–265
    cutaneous, 266
    gastrointestinal, 267, 269, 270
  contraindicated drug interactions, 251
  contraindications to, in hepatic dysfunction,
    179
  mechanism of action of, 223
  precautions with, in hepatic dysfunction, 179
  for tinea capitis, 70
  for tinea corporis, 70
  for tinea cruris, 70
  for tinea favosa, 71
  for tinea pedis, 69
  for tinea unguium, 71
  tissue distribution, by key organ systems, 202

Haemophilus ducreyi, 18
Haemophilus influenzae, 18
Haemophilus influenzae-aegypticus, 18
Haemophilus influenzae nontypeable, 18
Haemophilus influenzae type b, recommended
    antimicrobial prophylaxis for, 281
*Haemophilus parainfluenza, haemolyticus,
    aphrophilus,* spp., 18
H_2 agonists
  atazanavir and, 332f
  cefuroxime interaction with, 351f
  delavirdine interaction with, 366f
Halofantrine, 389f–390f
  adverse effects of
    CNS, 263–265
    cutaneous, 267
    gastrointestinal, 267–270
    musculoskeletal, 273
  for *Plasmodium falciparum,* 92
  for *Plasmodium vivax,* 93
HDEI. *See* High-dose extended-interval dosing
    (HDEI)
Headache, drugs causing, 264

Hearing loss, drugs causing, 274
Heliobacter pylori, 19
Hematuria, drugs causing, 271
Heparin
  piperacillin interaction with, 441f
  piperacillin/tazobactam interaction with, 442f
Hepatic failure, drugs causing, 272
Hepatic insufficiency, drug dosing in, 170,
    175–183
Hepatic toxicity, drugs causing, 272
Hepatitis, drugs causing, 272
Hepatitis A, recommended antimicrobial
    prophylaxis for, 285
Hepatitis A vaccine, for postexposure
    prophylaxis, 285
Hepatitis B, 49
  recommended antibiotic prophylaxis for, after
    sexual contact/sexual assault, 280
  recommended antimicrobial prophylaxis for,
    285
  with needle stick, 278
Hepatitis-B immune globulin, 390f–391f
  adverse effects of
    CNS, 263–265
    cutaneous, 266
    gastrointestinal, 269, 270
    musculoskeletal, 273
  adverse effects of, hypersensitivity, 273
  for postexposure prophylaxis, 285
  prophylactic, after needle stick, 278
Hepatitis B vaccine
  for postexposure prophylaxis, 285
  prophylactic, after needle stick, 278
Hepatitis C, 49
  recommended antimicrobial prophylaxis for,
    with needle stick, 278
Herpes simplex, 50–51
  acyclovir resistant, foscarnet for, 384f
  keratitis, trifluridine for, 484f
  recommended antimicrobial prophylaxis for,
    284
Heterophyes heterophyes, 86
Hexobarbital
  azithromycin interaction with, 335f
  dirithromycin interaction with, 371f
Hidradenitis suppurativa, antimicrobial therapy
    for, 128
High-density lipoproteins (HDL), increased,
    drugs causing, 271
High-dose extended interval dosing (HDEI),
    of aminoglycosides, 239
Histoplasma capsulatum, 64–65
Hives, drugs causing, 266
HIV protease inhibitors, administration routes
    for, 224
Hookworm, 106
Hordeolum, antimicrobial therapy for, 119
Human immunodeficiency virus (HIV)
  maternal-to-child transmission, prevention of,
    285
  postexposure prophylaxis, 285
  recommended antimicrobial prophylaxis for,
    285
  with needle stick, 278–279
Hydroxychloroquine, 391f–392f
  administration route for, 225
  adverse effects of
    CNS, 263, 264
    cutaneous, 266, 267
    gastrointestinal, 267–270
    ocular, 273
  for *Coxiella burnetti,* 14
  mechanism of action of, 225
  for *Plasmodium* spp., 94
  precautions with, in hepatic dysfunction, 179
17-hydroxycorticosteroids, methanamine
    preparations interaction with, 413f
Hymenolepis nana, 86
Hyperbilirubinemia, drugs causing, 272
Hypercholesterolemia, drugs causing, 271
Hyperglycemia, drugs causing, 271

Hyperkalemia, drugs causing, 271
Hypernatremia, drugs causing, 271
Hypersensitivity, adverse drug effects and, 273
Hypertension, drugs causing, 262
Hypertriglyceridemia, drugs causing, 271
Hyperuricemia, drugs causing, 271
Hypoglycemia, drugs causing, 271
Hypokalemia, drugs causing, 271
Hyponatremia, drugs causing, 271
Hypotension, drugs causing, 262

IBW. See Ideal body weight
Ideal body weight
    for boys
        from birth to 24 months, 188
        from 2 to 20 years, 188
    estimation of, for children, 170
    for girls
        from birth to 24 months, 188
        from 2 to 20 years, 188
Idinavir, 395f–396f
    nevirapine interaction with, 425f
    quinupristin with dalfopristin interaction with,
        454f
Imidazoles, mechanism of action of, 223
Imipenem
    for Bacillus cereus, 4
    for Burkholderia mallei, 9
    for Burkholderia pseudomallei, 9
    for Capnocytophaga ochracea, 10
    for Chromobacterium violaceum, 11
    for Citrobacter spp., 12
    for Erysipelothrix rhusiopathiae, 15
    for Francisella tularensis, 17
    ganciclovir interaction with, 251, 386f
    for Klebsiella spp., 19
    for Nocardia brasilensis, asteroids, spp., 23
    for Pasteurella multocida, 23
    for Pediococcus spp., 23
    for Serratis marcesens, 27
    valganciclovir interaction with, 489f
Imipenem-cilastatin, 392f
    administration route for, 218
    adverse effects of
        cardiovascular, 262
        CNS, 265
        cutaneous, 266, 267
        gastrointestinal, 269, 270
    contraindicated drug interactions, 252
    dosage adjustment
        in continuous renal replacement therapy,
            172
        in obesity, 189
        in renal failure, 164
    mechanism of action of, 218
    tissue distribution, by key organ systems, 203
Imiquimod, 392f–393f
    adverse effects of
        cardiovascular, 262
        CNS, 263–265
        cutaneous, 266, 267
        endocrine/metabolic, 271
        gastrointestinal, 269
        musculoskeletal, 273
Immune globulin, 393f–394f
    adverse effects of
        cardiovascular, 262
        CNS, 263
        gastrointestinal, 269
        respiratory, 272
    adverse effects of, hypersensitivity, 273
    botulinum (See botulinum immune globulin
        intravenous, human)
    cytomegalovirus (See cytomegalovirus
        immune globulin)
    hepatitis B (See hepatitis-B immune globulin)
    intramuscular, in postexposure prophylaxis of
        rubella, 286
    for parvovirus, 53
    in postexposure prophylaxis of measles, 286
    in postexposure prophylaxis of varicella, 287

Immune globulin (Cont.)
    rabies (See rabies immune globulin)
    tetanus (See tetanus immune globulin)
    varicella-zoster (See varicella-zoster immune
        globulin (human))
Immunocompromised host, asplenic,
    recommended antimicrobial prophylaxis
    for, 277
Indinavir
    administration route for, 224
    adverse effects of
        CNS, 263–265
        cutaneous, 266, 267
        gastrointestinal, 267–270
        hematologic, 267
        hepatic, 272
    atazanavir and, 331f
    contraindicated drug interactions, 252
    delavirdine interaction with, 366f
    dosage adjustment, in hepatic dysfunction, 179
    efavirenz interaction with, 374f
    mechanism of action of, 224
    precautions with, in hepatic dysfunction, 179
    tissue distribution, by key organ systems, 203
Infection(s)
    of bone, joint, and soft tissue, antimicrobial
        therapy for, 123–128
    of central nervous system, antimicrobial
        therapy for, 132–135
    gastrointestinal, antimicrobial therapy for,
        136–141
    genitourinary, antimicrobial therapy for,
        120–123
    intravascular, antimicrobial therapy for,
        108–114
    lower respiratory tract, antimicrobial therapy
        for, 128–132
    ocular, antimicrobial therapy for, 115–119
    odontogenic, antimicrobial therapy for,
        142–143
    systemic, antimicrobial therapy for, 108–114
    upper respiratory tract, antimicrobial therapy
        for, 143–149
Influenza, recommended antimicrobial
    prophylaxis for, 285
Insomnia, drugs causing, 265
Interferon-alpha
    for hepatitis B, 49
    for hepatitis C, 49
    zanamivir interaction with, 495f
Interstitial nephritis, drugs causing, 271
Intra-abdominal abscess, antimicrobial therapy
    for, 136–137
Intracranial pressure, increased, drug causing,
    264
Intravascular catheter-related infection,
    antimicrobial therapy for, 109
Intravascular infections, antimicrobial therapy
    for, 108–114
Iododeoxyuridine, for herpes simplex, 51
Iodoquinol, 396f
    adverse effects of
        CNS, 263–265
        cutaneous, 266
        gastrointestinal, 267, 269, 270
        ocular, 273
    for Blastocystis hominis, 77
    contraindications to, in hepatic dysfunction,
        179
    for Dientamoeba fragilis, 80
    for Entamoeba histolytica, 84
    precautions with, in hepatic dysfunction, 179
Iron-containing vitamins
    cefdinir interaction with, 341f
    moxifloxacin interaction with, 418f
Isoniazid, 397f
    administration route for, 222
    adverse effects of
        CNS, 263, 265
        gastrointestinal, 267–270
        hepatic, 272

Isoniazid (Cont.)
  contraindicated drug interactions, 252
  contraindications to, in hepatic dysfunction,
    179
  cycloserine interaction with, 363f
  dosage adjustment, in renal failure, 165
  efficacy, PK/PD parameter associated with,
    247
  ethionamide interaction with, 379f
  mechanism of action of, 222
  for Mycobacterium bovis, 43
  for Mycobacterium kansasii, 45
  for Mycobacterium tuberculosis, 38–42
  para-aminosalicylic acid interaction with, 433f
  precautions with, in hepatic dysfunction, 179
  prophylactic, for Mycobacterium tuberculosis,
    282
  pyrazinamide interaction with, 449f
  tissue distribution, by key organ systems,
    203
Isonicotinic acid derivative, mechanism of action
    of, 222
Isospora belli, 87
Isotretinoin
  minocycline interaction with, 417f
  tetracycline interaction with, 476f
Itching, drugs causing, 267
Itraconazole, 398f–399f
  administration route(s) for, 223
  adverse effects of
    cardiovascular, 262
    CNS, 263–265
    cutaneous, 266, 267
    endocrine/metabolic, 271
    gastrointestinal, 267–270
    hepatic, 272
  for Alternaria spp., 54
  for Aspergillus sp., 55
  for Bipolaris sp., 55
  for Blastomyces dermatitidis, 56, 57
  for Candida sp., 59
  for Coccidioides immitis, 61
  contraindicated drug interactions, 252
  for Cryptococcus neoformans, 62, 63
  for Curvularia sp., 62
  dosage adjustment, in continuous renal
    replacement therapy, 173
  for Exserohilum sp., 63
  for Histoplasma capsulatum, 64, 65
  lopinavir interaction with, 407f
  for Madurella sp., 65
  for Malassezia sp., 65
  mechanism of action of, 223
  nevirapine interaction with, 425f
  for Paracoccidiodes brasiliensis, 65
  for Penicillum marneffei, 66
  precautions with, in hepatic dysfunction, 179
  for Pseudoallescheria boydii, 67
  rifampin interaction with, 459f
  for Sappinia diploidea, 96
  for tinea capitis, 69
  for tinea corporis, 70
  for tinea cruris, 70
  for tinea favosa, 71
  for tinea unguium, 71
  tissue distribution, by key organ systems, 204
  for Trichosporon sp., 67
  for Wangiella sp., 67
Ivermectin, 399f–400f
  administration route for, 225
  adverse effects of
    cardiovascular, 262
    CNS, 263
    cutaneous, 267
    gastrointestinal, 269
    hematologic, 261
    hepatic, 272
    musculoskeletal, 273
    ocular, 273
  for Ancylostoma braziliense, 74
  for Gnathostoma spinigerum, 86

Ivermectin (Cont.)
  for Loa loa, 88
  for Mansonella ozzardi, 89
  for Mansonella streptocerca, 89
  mechanism of action of, 225
  for Onchocerca volvulus, 91
  for scabies, 105
  for Strongyloides stercoralis, 97
  tissue distribution, by key organ systems, 204
  for Trichuris trichiura, 101
  for Uncinaria stenocephala, 103
  for Wuchereria bancrofti, 104

Jaundice, drugs causing, 272
Joint(s), infections of, antimicrobial therapy for,
    123–128
Jugular vein septic phlebitis, antimicrobial
    therapy for, 146

Kanamycin, 401f
  administration route(s) for, 218
  adverse effects of
    CNS, 265
    renal/genitourinary, 271
  dosage adjustment, in renal failure, 165
  mechanism of action of, 218
  tissue distribution, by key organ systems, 204
Kaolin, chloroquine HCl/phosphate interaction
    with, 354f
Kawasaki disease, 394f
Kel. See Elimination rate constant (Kel)
Keratitis, antimicrobial therapy for, 117
Ketoconazole
  for Acanthamoeba, 74
  administration route(s) for, 223
  adverse effects of
    CNS, 264
    cutaneous, 266, 267
    gastrointestinal, 267, 269, 270
  for Candida sp., 60, 61
  contraindicated drug interactions, 253
  didanosine interaction with, 368f
  lopinavir interaction with, 407f
  for Malassezia sp., 65
  mechanism of action of, 223
  nevirapine interaction with, 425f
  for Paracoccidiodes brasiliensis, 65
  precautions with, in hepatic dysfunction, 179
  rifampin interaction with, 459f
  ritonavir interaction with, 462f
  saquinavir interaction with, 463f
  for tinea corporis, 70
  for tinea cruris, 70
  tissue distribution, by key organ systems, 204
  trimetrexate glucuronate interaction with, 487f
Ketolides, AUC/MIC, 244, 245
Kidney(s). See also Renal failure
  adverse drug effects and, 271–272
Kingella kingae, spp., 19
Klebsiella, in vitro drug susceptibility and in vivo
    drug efficacy against, discordance
    between, 228
Klebsiella spp., 19
Kunecatechins, 402f
Kunecatechins, adverse effects of
  CNS, 265
  cutaneous, 266, 267

Lamivudine, 402f–403f
  administration route for, 224
  adverse effects of
    CNS, 263–265
    cutaneous, 266
    gastrointestinal, 267–270
    hematologic, 262
    musculoskeletal, 273
  dosage adjustment, in renal failure, 165
  emtricitabine interaction with, 375f
  for hepatitis B, 49
  mechanism of action of, 224
  precautions with, in hepatic dysfunction, 179

Lamivudine (*Cont.*)
  for prevention of mother-infant HIV
    transmission, 285
  ribavirin interaction with, 457f
  tissue distribution, by key organ systems, 204
Lamotrigine, ritonavir interaction with, 462f
Lansoprazole, for *Heliobacter pylori*, 19
Laryngitis, antimicrobial therapy for, 145
Legionella pneumophila, 20
Leishmania spp., 87–88
Lemierre syndrome, antimicrobial therapy for, 146
Leptospira interrogans, 20
Leuconostoc spp., 20
Leucovorin, for *Pneumocystis jiroveci*, 66
Leukopenia, drugs causing, 261
Levofloxacin, 403f–404f
  administration route(s) for, 220
  adverse effects of
    cardiovascular, 262
    CNS, 263–265
    cutaneous, 266, 267
    gastrointestinal, 267–270
    ocular, 273
    renal/genitourinary, 272
    respiratory, 272
  for *Chlamydia trachomatis*, 11
  contraindicated drug interactions, 253
  dosage adjustment
    in obesity, 189
    in renal failure, 165
  efficacy relationships in humans, PK/PD
    parameter associated with, 246
  mechanism of action of, 220
  tissue distribution, by key organ systems, 205
  in vitro resistance relationships, PK/PD
    parameter associated with, 246
Levofloxacin/gatifloxacin, efficacy relationships in
    humans, PK/PD parameter associated
    with, 246
Levomethadyl, halofantrine interaction with, 390f
Lice, 105
Lidocaine
  lopinavir interaction with, 407f
  saquinavir interaction with, 463f
Lincomycin, interactions
  with erythromycin ethylsuccinate and
    acetylsulfisoxazole, toxic effect(s), 249
  with erythromycin preparations, toxic effect(s),
    250
Lincosamides
  interactions
    with erythromycin ethylsuccinate and
      acetylsulfisoxazole, toxic effect(s), 249
    with erythromycin preparations, toxic
      effect(s), 250
  mechanism of action of, 221
Lindane, 404f–405f
  adverse effects of
    CNS, 263, 265
    cutaneous, 266
Linezolid, 405f–406f
  administration route(s) for, 221
  adverse effects of
    CNS, 263–265
    cutaneous, 266
    gastrointestinal, 268–270
    hematologic, 261, 262
  contraindicated drug interactions, 253–254
  dosage adjustment
    in continuous renal replacement therapy,
      173
    in obesity, 190
  for *Enterococcus*, vancomycin resistant, 15
  mechanism of action of, 221
  for *Mycobacterium chelonae*, 47
  for *Pediococcus* spp., 23
  precautions with, in hepatic dysfunction, 179
  for *Staphyloccus aureus*; methicillin-
    susceptible, 28, 29
  for *Streptococcus pneumoniae*, 30
  tissue distribution, by key organ systems, 205

Lipopeptide, mechanism of action of, 221
Listeria monocytogenes, 20
Lithium
  metronidazole interaction with, 415f
  potassium iodide interaction with, 446f
  tinidazole interaction with, 480f
Liver, adverse drug effects and, 272
Loa loa, 88
Loop diuretics
  amikacin sulfate interaction with, 322f
  gentamicin interaction with, 388f
  vancomycin interaction with, 491f
Lopinavir, 406f
  administration route for, 224
  adverse effects of
    cardiovascular, 262
    CNS, 263–265
    cutaneous, 266
    endocrine/metabolic, 271
    gastrointestinal, 267–270
    hematologic, 262
    hepatic, 272
    musculoskeletal, 273
  contraindicated drug interactions, 254–255
  darunavir and, 365f
  maraviroc interaction with, 409f
  mechanism of action of, 224
  precautions with, in hepatic dysfunction, 179
  tissue distribution, by key organ systems, 205
Loracarbef, 408f
  administration route for, 218
  adverse effects of
    CNS, 264, 265
    cutaneous, 266, 267
    gastrointestinal, 267–270
    renal/genitourinary, 272
  dosage adjustment, in renal failure, 165
  mechanism of action of, 218
  tissue distribution, by key organ systems, 205
Lower respiratory tract infection(s), antimicrobial
    therapy for, 128–132
Ludwig's angina, antimicrobial therapy for, 142
Lung abscess, antimicrobial therapy for, 128

Macrolides
  for *Arcanobacterium haemolyticum*, 3
  dosage adjustment, in obesity, 189
  for *Leuconostoc* spp., 20
  mechanism of action of, 220
  microbial resistance to, mechanisms of, 227,
    228
  for *Staphyloccus aureus*; methicillin-
    susceptible, 28
  T > MIC, 244, 245
Madurella sp., 65
Magnesium salts, nitrofurantoin interaction with,
    427f
Maintenance dose, adjustment of
  with dialysis, 158–169
  in renal insufficiency, 157–158
    by dose reduction, 157–158
    by interval extension, 157
    by interval extension and dose reduction,
      158
Malaise, drugs causing, 265
Malaria, recommended antimicrobial prophylaxis
    for, 287–288
Malarone. *See* Atovaquone ± proguanil
Malassezia sp., 65
Malathion, 105
Malathion, 408f–409f
Mansonella ozzardi, 89
Mansonella perstans, 89
Mansonella streptocerca, 89
Maraviroc, 409f
  adverse effects of
    cardiovascular, 262
    CNS, 263–265
    cutaneous, 266, 267
    gastrointestinal, 267–269
    hematologic, 262

Maraviroc (*Cont.*)
  hepatic, 272
  musculoskeletal, 273
  respiratory, 272
Mastoiditis, antimicrobial therapy for, 149
Measles, recommended antimicrobial
    prophylaxis for, 286
Measles vaccine, for postexposure prophylaxis,
    286
Mebendazole, 410f
  administration route for, 225
  adverse effects of, gastrointestinal, 268–270
  for *Ancylostoma caninum*, 75
  for *Ancylostoma* spp., 75
  for *Ascaris lumbricoides*, 76
  for *Capillaria philippinensis*, 79
  for *Echinococcus multilocularis*, 81
  for *Enterobius vermicularis*, 85
  for *Mansonella perstans*, 89
  mechanism of action of, 225
  for *Necator americanus*, 91
  tissue distribution, by key organ systems,
    205
  for *Toxocara canis/catis*, 98
  for *Trichinella spiralis*, 101
  for *Trichostrongylus*, 101
  for *Trichuris trichiura*, 101
Mefloquine, 410f–411f
  administration route for, 225
  adverse effects of
    CNS, 263, 264
    cutaneous, 266
    gastrointestinal, 268–270
    musculoskeletal, 273
  halofantrine interaction with, 390f
  mechanism of action of, 225
  for *Plasmodium falciparum*, 92
  for *Plasmodium vivax*, 93
  precautions with, in hepatic dysfunction, 179
  prophylactic, for malaria, 288
  quinine sulfate interaction with, 453f
  tissue distribution, by key organ systems, 205
Meglumine antimonate, for *Leishmania* spp.,
    87, 88
Melarsoprol, 411f–412f
  adverse effects of
    cardiovascular, 262
    CNS, 263–265
    cutaneous, 266, 267
    hepatic, 272
    musculoskeletal, 273
    renal/genitourinary, 271
  tissue distribution, by key organ systems, 206
  for *Trypanosoma brucei gambiense*, 103
  for *Trypanosoma brucei rhodesiense*, 103
Meningitis
  aseptic, antimicrobial therapy for, 134
  bacterial, antimicrobial therapy for, 134–135
Meperidine, interactions
  with furazolidone, toxic effect(s), 251
  with linezolid, toxic effect(s), 254
Meropenem, 412f
  for *Achromobacter xylosoxidans*, 3
  administration route for, 218
  adverse effects of
    CNS, 264, 265
    cutaneous, 266, 267
    gastrointestinal, 268–270
    hematologic, 261
  for *Bacillus cereus*, 4
  for *Burkholderia cepacia*, 9
  for *Citrobacter* spp., 12
  dosage adjustment
    in continuous renal replacement therapy,
     173
    in obesity, 189
    in renal failure, 165
  for *Escherichia coli*, 16
  for *Klebsiella* spp., 19
  mechanism of action of, 218
  for *Mycobacterium chelonae*, 47

Meropenem (*Cont.*)
  for *Mycobacterium fortuitum*, 46
  for *Serratis marcesens*, 27
  tissue distribution, by key organ systems, 206
Mesoridazine, halofantrine interaction with,
    390f
Metabolism (drug), age-dependent physiologic
    variables affecting, 154–155
Metagonimus yokogawa, 89
Metformin, cephalexin interaction with, 351f
Methadone
  abacavir sulfate interaction with, 317f
  nelfinavir interaction with, 421f
  nevirapine interaction with, 425f
  ritonavir interaction with, 462f
  voriconazole interaction with, 493f
  zanamivir interaction with, 495f
Methanamine preparations, 413f
Methenamine, dosage adjustment, in renal
    failure, 165
Methenamine mandelate
  adverse effects of
    cutaneous, 266
    gastrointestinal, 269, 270
  contraindications to, in hepatic dysfunction,
    180
  precautions with, in hepatic dysfunction, 180
Methicillin
  administration route(s) for, 220
  mechanism of action of, 220
Methicillin-resistant staphylococci, in vitro drug
    susceptibility and in vivo drug efficacy
    against, discordance between, 228
Methotrexate
  ciprofloxacin interaction with, 357f
  cloxacillin interaction with, 361f
  neomycin sulfate interaction with, 422f
  pyrimethamine interaction with, 451f
  sulfadiazine interaction with, 468f
  sulfamethoxazole with trimethoprim
    interaction with, 469f
  sulfisoxazole interaction with, 470f
  trimethoprim interaction with, 485f
Methoxyflurane, tetracycline interaction with,
    476f
Methylphenidate, interactions
  with furazolidone, toxic effect(s), 251
  with linezolid, toxic effect(s), 253
Methylprednisone
  erythromycin preparations interaction with,
    378f
  quinupristin with dalfopristin interaction with,
    454f
Methylxanthines, ofloxacin interaction with,
    429f
Metoclopramide
  atovaquone interaction with, 333f
  fosfomycin tromethamine interaction with,
    385f
Metrochis conjunctus, 89
Metronidazole, 414f–415f
  administration route(s) for, 222
  adverse effects of
    CNS, 263, 264
    gastrointestinal, 268–270
  for *Bacteroides fragilis* group, 5
  for *Blastocystis hominis*, 77
  for *Clostridium difficile*, 12
  for *Clostridium pefringens*, spp., 13
  for *Clostridium tetani*, 12
  contraindicated drug interactions, 255
  for *Dientamoeba fragilis*, 80
  dosage adjustment
    in continuous renal replacement therapy,
     173
    in hepatic dysfunction, 180
    in obesity, 190
    in renal failure, 165
  for *Dracunculus medinensis*, 81
  for *Entamoeba histolytica*, 84
  for *Entamoeba poleckii*, 85

Metronidazole (*Cont.*)
for *Fusobacterium* spp., 17
for *Giardia lamblia*, 86
for *Heliobacter pylori*, 19
interactions, with amprenavir, toxic effect(s), 248
mechanism of action of, 222
microbial resistance to, mechanism of, 227
for *Microsporidia*, 90
precautions with, in hepatic dysfunction, 180
preventive therapy, after sexual contact/sexual assault, 280
for *Prevotella* spp., 24
spectinomycin interaction with, 465f
tissue distribution, by key organ systems, 206
for *Trichomonas vaginalis*, 101
Mezlocillin
administration route(s) for, 220
mechanism of action of, 220
MIC. See Minimum inhibitory concentration (MIC)
Micafungin sodium, 415f–416f
adverse effects of
cardiovascular, 262
CNS, 263–265
cutaneous, 266, 267
endocrine/metabolic, 271
gastrointestinal, 268–270
hematologic, 261, 262
hepatic, 272
for *Candida* sp., 58, 59
precautions with, in hepatic dysfunction, 180
tissue distribution, by key organ systems, 206
Miconazole, 416f–417f
administration route(s) for, 223
adverse effects of
CNS, 263–265
cutaneous, 266, 267
gastrointestinal, 268–270
for *Candida* sp., 60, 61
contraindicated drug interactions, 255
mechanism of action of, 223
for *Naegleria fowleri*, 90
for tinea corporis, 70
for tinea cruris, 70
for tinea pedis, 69
tissue distribution, by key organ systems, 206
trimetrexate glucuronate interaction with, 487f
Microbial resistance, common mechanisms of, 227–228
Microsporidia, 106
Microsporidia, 90
Midazolam
amprenavir and, 330f
atazanavir and, 331f
fluconazole interaction with, 381f
quinupristin with dalfopristin interaction with, 454f
Minimum inhibitory concentration (MIC), 244, 245. *See also* AUC/MIC; C$_{max}$/MIC; T > MIC
Minocycline, 417f–418f
administration route(s) for, 221
adverse effects of, gastrointestinal, 269, 270
for *Burkholderia cepacia*, 9
for *Chryseobacterium* spp., 11
mechanism of action of, 221
precautions with, in hepatic dysfunction, 180
for *Propionobacterium acnes*, 24
for *Stenotrophomonas maltophila*, 29
tissue distribution, by key organ systems, 206
vestibular toxicity of, 274
Mirtazapine, interactions
with furazolidone, toxic effect(s), 251
with linezolid, toxic effect(s), 254
Monobactams, mechanism of action of, 220
Moraxella catarrhalis, 20
Morganella, 21
in vitro drug susceptibility and in vivo drug efficacy against, discordance between, 229

Mosteller formula, for body surface area calculation, 151
Moxifloxacin, 418f
administration route(s) for, 220
adverse effects of, gastrointestinal, 269, 270
contraindicated drug interactions, 255
contraindications to, in hepatic dysfunction, 180
dosage adjustment, in obesity, 189
mechanism of action of, 220
precautions with, in hepatic dysfunction, 180
tissue distribution, by key organ systems, 207
Mucosal fungal infections, 72
Mupirocin, 419f
administration route for, 222
adverse effects of
CNS, 264
cutaneous, 266, 267
gastrointestinal, 270
mechanism of action of, 222
Muscle relaxants, colistimethate sodium interaction with, 362f
Musculoskeletal system, adverse drug effects and, 273
Myalgia, drugs causing, 273
Mycetoma, 72
Mycobacterial infections, 38–47
Mycobacterium abscessus, 47
Mycobacterium avium complex, 43–44
recommended antimicrobial prophylaxis for, 282
Mycobacterium bovis, 43
Mycobacterium chelonae, 47
Mycobacterium fortuitum, 46
Mycobacterium kansasii, 45
Mycobacterium marinum, 45
Mycobacterium tuberculosis, 38–43, 282
Mycobacterium ulcerans, 45
Mycophenolate, valacyclovir interaction with, 488f
Mycoplasma hominis, 21
Mycoplasma pneumoniae, 21
Myocarditis, antimicrobial therapy for, 110

Naegleria fowleri, 90
Nafcillin, 419f–420f
administration route(s) for, 220
adverse effects of, cutaneous, 266
dosage adjustment
in hepatic dysfunction, 180
in obesity, 188
in renal failure, 166
mechanism of action of, 220
precautions with, in hepatic dysfunction, 180
tissue distribution, by key organ systems, 207
Naftifine, 420f
adverse effects of, cutaneous, 267
for *Candida* sp., 61
for tinea corporis, 70
for tinea cruris, 70
Nalidixic acid, for *Shigella sonnei*, *dysenteriae*, *boydii*, *flexneri*, 27, 28
Nanophyetus salmincola, 91
Nausea, drugs causing, 269–270
Necator americanus, 91
Necrotizing fasciitis, antimicrobial therapy for, 123, 140
Needle stick, recommended antimicrobial prophylaxis for, 278
Neisseria gonorrhea, 21–22
Neisseria meningitidis, recommended antimicrobial prophylaxis for, 283
Neisseria meninigitidis, 22
Nelfinavir, 421f
administration route for, 224
adverse effects of
cutaneous, 266
gastrointestinal, 269, 270
hematologic, 262
hepatic, 272
azithromycin interaction with, 335f

Nelfinavir (Cont.)
  contraindicated drug interactions, 256
  efavirenz interaction with, 374f
  mechanism of action of, 224
  precautions with, in hepatic dysfunction, 180
  tissue distribution, by key organ systems, 207
  zanamivir interaction with, 495f
Neomycin/hydrocortisone otic preparations, 422f–423f
Neomycin-polymixin B-gramicidin ophthalmic solution, for *Acanthamoeba,* 74
Neomycin/polymyxin B/± bacitracin, 423f–424f
Neomycin sulfate
  administration route for, 218
  adverse effects of, gastrointestinal, 269, 270
  dosage adjustment, in renal failure, 166
  mechanism of action of, 218
  tissue distribution, by key organ systems, 207
Neomycin sulfate/polymyxin B sulfate/bacitracin, adverse effects of
  cutaneous, 266
  hypersensitivity, 273
  renal/genitourinary, 271
Neonate(s), pharmacokinetic monitoring in, 243
Nephrotoxicity, drugs causing, 271
Nephrotoxic medications, cidofovir interaction with, 355f
Neuraminidase inhibitor, mechanism of action of, 225
Neuromuscular blocking agents
  amphotericin B interaction with, 325f
  quinidine gluconate interaction with, 452f
  quinine sulfate interaction with, 453f
Neuropathy, drugs causing, 265
Neurotoxicity, drugs causing, 265
Neutropenia, drugs causing, 262
Nevirapine, 424f–425f
  administration route for, 224
  adverse effects of
    CNS, 264
    cutaneous, 266
    gastrointestinal, 268–270
    hepatic, 272
  atazanavir and, 332f
  idinavir interaction with, 396f
  lopinavir interaction with, 407f
  mechanism of action of, 224
  nelfinavir interaction with, 421f
  for prevention of mother-infant HIV transmission, 285
  quinupristin with dalfopristin interaction with, 454f
  tissue distribution, by key organ systems, 207
Niclosamide
  for *Diphyllabothrium latum,* 80
  for *Dipylidium caninum,* 80
  for *Taenia saginata,* 97
  for *Taenia solium,* 97
Nifedipine
  micafungin sodium interaction with, 416f
  quinidine gluconate interaction with, 452f
Nifurtimox, 425f
  adverse effects of
    CNS, 263, 264
    cutaneous, 266
    gastrointestinal, 268, 270
  for *Trypanosoma cruzi,* 102
Nitazoxanide, 426f
  adverse effects of
    CNS, 264
    gastrointestinal, 268–270
  for *Blastocystis hominis,* 77
  for *Clostridium difficile,* 12
  for *Cryptosporidium,* 79
  for *Giardia lamblia,* 86
  for *Hymenolepis nana,* 86
  precautions with, in hepatic dysfunction, 180
  tissue distribution, by key organ systems, 207
Nitrofuran, mechanism of action of, 221

Nitrofurantoin, 426f–427f
  administration route for, 221
  adverse effects of
    CNS, 264
    gastrointestinal, 270
  dapsone interaction with, 364f
  for *Enterococcus,* vancomycin resistant, 15
  for *Enterococcus faecalis/faecium,* 15
  for *Escherichia coli,* 16
  long-term use, adverse effects of, respiratory, 272
  mechanism of action of, 221
  norfloxacin interaction with, 427f
  prophylactic, for urinary tract infection, 280
Nitroimidazole, mechanism of action of, 222
Niverapine, saquinavir interaction with, 463f
Nocardia brasilensis, asteroids, spp., 23
Non-nucleoside reverse transcriptase inhibitors, administration routes for, 224
Nonsteroidal anti-inflammatory drugs
  for *Histoplasma capsulatum,* 65
  levofloxacin interaction with, 404f
Norfloxacin, 427f
  administration route for, 220
  adverse effects of
    CNS, 263–265
    gastrointestinal, 268, 270
  contraindicated drug interactions, 256
  dosage adjustment, in renal failure, 166
  mechanism of action of, 220
  tissue distribution, by key organ systems, 207
Normeperidine, acyclovir interaction with, 319f
Nucleoside analog, mechanism of action of, 225
Nucleotide analog reverse transcriptase inhibitors, administration routes for, 224
Nystatin, 428f
  administration route(s) for, 222
  adverse effects of
    cutaneous, 266, 267
    gastrointestinal, 268
  for *Candida* sp., 58, 60, 61
  mechanism of action of, 222

Obesity
  body mass index and, 170
  drug dosing in, 170–183, 188–190
Ocular infections, antimicrobial therapy for, 115–119
Odontogenic infections, antimicrobial therapy for, 142–143
Ofloxacin, 428f–429f
  administration route(s) for, 220
  adverse effects of
    cardiovascular, 262
    CNS, 263–265
    cutaneous, 266, 267
    gastrointestinal, 268–270
    ocular, 273
    renal/genitourinary, 272
  for *Chlamydia trachomatis,* 11
  for *Coxiella burnetti,* 14
  dosage adjustment
    in hepatic dysfunction, 180
    in renal failure, 166
  mechanism of action of, 220
  tissue distribution, by key organ systems, 207
  for *Vibrio cholera,* 36
Omeprazole
  ceftibuten interaction with, 348f
  for *Heliobacter pylori,* 19
Onchocerca volvulus, 91
Oncology, and pharmacokinetic monitoring, 243
Ophthalmia neonatorum
  antimicrobial therapy for, 115
  recommended antimicrobial prophylaxis for, 279
Opisthorchis viverrini, 91
Oral contraceptives
  amoxicillin interaction with, 323f
  ampicillin and, 328f

Oral contraceptives (*Cont.*)
    amprenavir and, 330f
    cloxacillin interaction with, 361f
    dicloxacillin sodium interaction with, 367f
    fosamprenavir interaction with, 383f
    griseofulvin interaction with, 389f
    nelfinavir interaction with, 421f
    nevirapine interaction with, 425f
    tetracycline interaction with, 476f
Orbital cellulitis, antimicrobial therapy for, 118
Oseltamivir phosphate, 430f
    administration route for, 225
    adverse effects of, gastrointestinal, 268, 270
    dosage adjustment, in renal failure, 166
    for influenza, 52
    mechanism of action of, 225
    prophylactic, for influenza, 285
    tissue distribution, by key organ systems, 208
Oseophagostomum bifurcum, 91
Osteomyelitis, antimicrobial therapy for, 124
Otitis externa
    antimicrobial therapy for, 143
    malignant, antimicrobial therapy for, 143
Otitis media
    acute, antimicrobial therapy for, 144
    chronic suppurative (*See* Mastoiditis)
    with effusion, antimicrobial therapy for, 144
    recurrent, recommended antimicrobial
        prophylaxis for, 279
Ototoxicity, drugs causing, 274
Overweight, body mass index and, 170
Oxacillin, 431f
    administration route(s) for, 220
    adverse effects of, gastrointestinal, 269, 270
    dosage adjustment
        in continuous renal replacement therapy,
            173
        in renal failure, 166
    mechanism of action of, 220
    tissue distribution, by key organ systems,
        208
Oxamniquine, for *Schistosoma mansoni*, 96
Oxazolidinone, mechanism of action of, 221
Oxiconazole, 431f–432f
    adverse effects of, cutaneous, 267
    for tinea corporis, 70
    for tinea cruris, 70

Paclitaxel, quinupristin with dalfopristin
    interaction with, 454f
PAE. *See* Postantibiotic effect (PAE)
PAFEs. *See* Post-antifungal effects (PAFEs)
Pain. *See also* Abdominal pain; Chest pain
    drugs causing, 265
Palivizumab, 432f
    adverse effects of
        CNS, 264
        cutaneous, 266
        gastrointestinal, 269
        hematologic, 261
        hepatic, 272
Pancreatitis, drugs causing, 270
Pancuronium, clindamycin interaction with,
    359f
Para-aminosalicylic acid, 433f
    administration route for, 222
    adverse effects of, gastrointestinal, 268–270
    mechanism of action of, 222
    precautions with, in hepatic dysfunction, 180
    tissue distribution, by key organ systems,
        208
Paracoccidioides brasilensis, 65
Paragonimus westermani, 91
Parapharyngeal abscess, antimicrobial therapy
    for, 146
Parasitic infections, 74–105
Paromomycin sulfate, 433f–434f
    adverse effects of, gastrointestinal, 268–270
    for *Cryptosporidium*, 79
    for *Dientamoeba fragilis*, 80
    for *Entamoeba histolytica*, 84

Paromomycin sulfate (*Cont.*)
    for *Giardia lamblia*, 86
    for *Leishmania* spp., 88
    precautions with, in hepatic dysfunction, 180
Parotitis
    acute, antimicrobial therapy for, 145
    antimicrobial therapy for, 119
    subacute/chronic, antimicrobial therapy for,
        145
Parvovirus, 53
Pasteurella multocida, 23
Pediculosis capitis, 105
Pediococcus spp., 23
Pefloxacin
    administration route(s) for, 220
    mechanism of action of, 220
Pelvic inflammatory disease (PID), antimicrobial
    therapy for, 121
Penciclovir
    administration route for, 223
    adverse effects of
        CNS, 264
        cutaneous, 266
    mechanism of action of, 223
Penciclovir, 434f
    famciclovir interaction with, 380f
Penicillin
    for *Bartonella bacilliformis*, 6
    for *Borrelia burgdorferi*, 7
    for *Borrelia recurrentis, hermsii, turicate,* 8
    for *Capnocytophaga canimorsus*, 10
    for *Cardiobacterium hominis*, 10
    desensitization protocols
        continuous IV infusion, 292–293
        intermittent IV infusion, 292
        oral, 293
    dosage adjustment, in obesity, 188
    for *Eikenella corrodens*, 14
    for *Enterococcus faecalis/faecium*, 15
    mechanism of action of, 219
    penicillinase stable, mechanism of action of,
        220
    for *Prevotella* spp., 24
    for Streptococci viridans, 32
    for *Streptococcus* Group A, 31
    for *Streptococcus* Group C, G, 31
Penicillin G
    for *Actinomyces*, 2t
    administration route(s) for, 219
    aqueous potassium and sodium, 434f–435f
    aqueous potassium and sodium, tissue
        distribution, by key organ systems, 208
    benzathine, 435f–436f
        adverse effects of
            CNS, 265
            hypersensitivity, 273
        prophylactic
            for diphtheria, 281
            for rheumatic fever, 279
        tissue distribution, by key organ systems,
            208
    benzathine and penicillin G procaine, tissue
        distribution, by key organ systems, 209
    for *Clostridium perfringens*, spp., 13
    for *Clostridium tetani*, 12
    for *Corynebacterium diphtheriae*, 13
    dosage adjustment
        in obesity, 188
        in renal failure, 166
    for *Erysipelothrix rhusiopathiae*, 15
    for *Fusobacterium* spp., 17
    for *Kingella kingae*, spp., 19
    for *Leptospira interrogans*, 20
    for *Leuconostoc* spp., 20
    mechanism of action of, 219
    for *Neisseria meningitidis*, 22
    for *Pasteurella multocida*, 23
    for *Pediococcus* spp., 23
    penicillin G benzathine and penicillin G
        procaine, 436f–437f
    procaine, 437f–438f

Penicillin G (*Cont.*)
  procaine, adverse effects of, CNS, 265
  for *Propionobacterium acnes*, 24
  for *Streptobacillus moniliformis*, 29
  for *Streptococci viridans*, 33
  for *Streptococcus* Group C, G, 32
  for *Treponema pallidum*, 34, 35
Penicillin V, neomycin sulfate interaction with,
  422f
Penicillin V potassium, 438f
  administration route(s) for, 219
  adverse effects of, gastrointestinal, 269, 270
  dosage adjustment, in renal failure, 166
  mechanism of action of, 219
  prophylactic
    for asplenic patient, 277
    for rheumatic fever, 279
  tissue distribution, by key organ systems, 209
Penicillum marneffei, 66
Pentamidine isethionate, 439f
  for *Acanthamoeba*, 74
  administration route(s) for, 226
  adverse effects of
    cardiovascular, 262
    CNS, 263, 264
    cutaneous, 266
    endocrine/metabolic, 271
    gastrointestinal, 268–270
    hematologic, 261, 262
    renal/genitourinary, 271
    respiratory, 273
  for *Balamuthia mandrillaris*, 77
  contraindicated drug interactions, 256
  dosage adjustment, in renal failure, 166
  for *Leishmania* spp., 87, 88
  mechanism of action of, 226
  for *Pneumocystis jiroveci*, 66
  precautions with, in hepatic dysfunction, 180
  prophylactic, for *Pneumocystis*, 287
  for *Sappinia diploidea*, 96
  tissue distribution, by key organ systems, 209
  for *Trypanosoma brucei gambiense*, 102
  zalcitabine interaction with, 493f
Pentostam. See Stibogluconate
Pericarditis, purulent, antimicrobial therapy for,
  111
Periodontitis, antimicrobial therapy for, 142
Peritonitis, antimicrobial therapy for, 140–141
Peritonsillar abscess, antimicrobial therapy for,
  146
Permethrin, 105, 266, 267, 440f
Pertussis, recommended antimicrobial
  prophylaxis for, 283
Phaeohyphomycosis, 72
Phagocyte function defect, recommended
  antimicrobial prophylaxis for, 278
Pharmacodynamics, 231, 232
Pharmacokinetic/pharmacodynamic (PK/PD)
  antimicrobial relationships, 244–247
  of antifungal agents, and in vivo
    pharmacodynamic characteristics in
    neutropenic mouse models, 247
  of antimycobacterial agents, and efficacy, 247
  common indices of, 244–245
  factors affecting, 244
  in humans, 246
  and in vitro resistance relationships, 246
Pharmacokinetics, 231, 232
  disease-specific factors affecting, 243
  one-compartment first-order elimination model
    of, 240
  patient age and, 243
  terminology for, 240–242
  volume status and, 243
Pharyngitis
  exudative, antimicrobial therapy for, 146
  vesicular, antimicrobial therapy for, 146
Phenazopyridine HCl, 440f–441f
  adverse effects of
    CNS, 263, 264
    gastrointestinal, 268

Phenazopyridine HCl (*Cont.*)
  contraindications to, in hepatic dysfunction,
    180
  dosage adjustment, in renal failure, 167
  precautions with, in hepatic dysfunction, 180
Phenicol, mechanism of action of, 221
Phenobarbital
  chloramphenicol interaction with, 353f
  darunavir and, 365f
  delavirdine interaction with, 366f
  griseofulvin interaction with, 389f
  lopinavir interaction with, 407f
  metronidazole interaction with, 415f
  nelfinavir interaction with, 421f
  saquinavir interaction with, 463f
  tipranavir interaction with, 481f
Phenytoin
  azithromycin interaction with, 335f
  chloramphenicol interaction with, 353f
  clofazimine interaction with, 360f
  cycloserine interaction with, 363f
  darunavir and, 365f
  delavirdine interaction with, 366f
  dirithromycin interaction with, 371f
  doxycycline interaction with, 372f
  fluconazole interaction with, 381f
  isoniazid interaction with, 397f
  lopinavir interaction with, 407f
  metronidazole interaction with, 415f
  nelfinavir interaction with, 421f
  praziquantel interaction with, 447f
  quinidine gluconate interaction with, 452f
  ritonavir interaction with, 462f
  saquinavir interaction with, 463f
  sulfamethoxazole with trimethoprim
    interaction with, 469f
  tinidazole interaction with, 480f
  tipranavir interaction with, 481f
  trimethoprim interaction with, 485f
Phlebitis, drugs causing, 267
Photophobia, drugs causing, 273
PID. See Pelvic inflammatory disease (PID)
Pimozide
  amprenavir and, 330f
  atazanavir and, 331f
  interactions
    with amprenavir, toxic effect(s), 248
    with atazanavir, toxic effect(s), 248
    with clarithromycin, toxic effect(s), 249
    with erythromycin ethylsuccinate and
      acetylsulfisoxazole, toxic effect(s), 249
    with erythromycin preparations, toxic
      effect(s), 250
    with fosamprenavir, toxic effect(s), 250
    with indinavir, toxic effect(s), 252
    with itraconazole, toxic effect(s), 252
    with ketoconazole, toxic effect(s), 253
    with lopinavir with ritonavir, toxic effect(s),
      254
    with miconazole, toxic effect(s), 255
    with nelfinavir, toxic effect(s), 256
    with ritonavir, toxic effect(s), 257
    with saquinavir, toxic effect(s), 258
Piperacillin, 441f
  administration route for, 220
  adverse effects of
    CNS, 265
    cutaneous, 266, 267
    gastrointestinal, 269
  for *Burkholderia cepacia*, 9
  for *Burkholderia pseudomallei*, 9
  dosage adjustment
    in continuous renal replacement therapy,
      173
    in renal failure, 167
  for *Enterobacter* spp., 15
  for *Escherichia coli*, 16
  mechanism of action of, 220
  tissue distribution, by key organ systems, 209
  for *Yersinia enterocolitica, pseudotuberculosis*,
    36, 37

Piperacillin/tazobactam, 442f
   administration route for, 218
   adverse effects of
      cardiovascular, 262
      CNS, 264, 265
      cutaneous, 266, 267
      gastrointestinal, 268–270
      hematologic, 261
   dosage adjustment
      in continuous renal replacement therapy,
         173
      in obesity, 188
      in renal failure, 167
   mechanism of action of, 218
   tissue distribution, by key organ systems, 210
Piperazine derivatives, mechanism of action of,
      225
Plasmodium falciparum, 92
Plasmodium ovale, 95
Plasmodium spp., 94
Plasmodium vivax, 93, 95
Pleistophora sp., 95
Plesiomonas shigelloides, 23–24
Pneumocystis, recommended antimicrobial
      prophylaxis for, 287
Pneumocystis jiroveci, 66
Pneumonia
   antimicrobial therapy for, 129–131
   community-acquired, antimicrobial therapy
      for, 129
   in cystic fibrosis, antimicrobial therapy for,
      130
   in HIV-infected (AIDS) patients, antimicrobial
      therapy for, 131
   in immunocompromised patient, antimicrobial
      therapy for, 130
   in neonate, antimicrobial therapy for, 131
   ventilator-associated, antimicrobial therapy
      for, 131
Podofilox, 442f–443f
   adverse effects of
      CNS, 265
      cutaneous, 267
      gastrointestinal, 270
Podophyllin/podophyllum resin, 443f
Polyenes
   mechanism of action of, 222
   in vivo pharmacodynamic characteristics of,
      in neutropenic mouse models, 247
Polyhexamethylene biguanide, for
      Acanthamoeba, 74
Polymyxin, colistimethate sodium interaction
      with, 362f
Polymyxin B
   administration route for, 221
   mechanism of action of, 221
Polymyxin B sulfate, neomycin sulfate,
      hydrocortisone
   adverse effects of
      CNS, 265
      cutaneous, 266, 267
   contraindicated drug interactions, 256
Posoconazole, 445f–446f
   administration route for, 223
   adverse effects of
      cardiovascular, 262
      CNS, 263–265
      cutaneous, 266, 267
      endocrine/metabolic, 271
      gastrointestinal, 268–270
      hematologic, 261, 262
      hepatic, 272
      musculoskeletal, 273
      ocular, 273
   for Fusarium sp., 64
   halofantrine interaction with, 390f
   mechanism of action of, 223
   precautions with, in hepatic dysfunction, 180
   tissue distribution, by key organ systems, 210
   for Zygomycetes, 68
Postantibiotic effect (PAE), 239, 245

Post-antifungal effects (PAFEs), 247
Potassium iodide, 446f
Praziquantel, 447f
   adverse effects of
      CNS, 263–265
      gastrointestinal, 268, 270
   albendazole interaction with, 320f
   for Clonorchis sinensis, 79
   for Diphyllobothrium latum, 80
   for Dipylidium caninum, 80
   for Fasciola buski, 85
   for Heterophyes heterophyes, 86
   for Hymenolepis nana, 86
   for Metagonimus yokogawa, 89
   for Metrochis conjunctus, 89
   for Nanophyteus salmincola, 91
   for Opisthorchis viverrini, 91
   for Paragonimus westermani, 91
   precautions with, in hepatic dysfunction, 180
   for Schistosoma haematobium, 96
   for Schistosoma japonicum, 96
   for Schistosoma mansoni, 96
   for Schistosoma mekongi, 97
   for Taenia saginata, 97
   for Taenia solium, 97, 98
   tissue distribution, by key organ systems, 210
Prednisone
   isoniazid interaction with, 397f
   for Pneumocystis jiroveci, 66
Pregnancy categories, 307
Preseptal cellulitis, antimicrobial therapy for,
      118–119
Prevotella spp., 24
Primaquine phosphate, 447f–448f
   administration route for, 225
   adverse effects of, gastrointestinal, 268, 270
   dapsone interaction with, 364f
   mechanism of action of, 225
   for Plasmodium vivax, 93, 95
   for Pneumocystis jiroveci, 66
Probenecid
   acyclovir interaction with, 319f
   amoxicillin interaction with, 323f
   aztreonam interaction with, 336f
   cefaclor interaction with, 339f
   cefadroxil interaction with, 340f
   cefazolin interaction with, 340f
   cefdinir interaction with, 341f
   cefditoren pivoxil interaction with, 342f
   cefepime interaction with, 342f
   cefixime interaction with, 343f
   cefotaxime interaction with, 344f
   cefotetan interaction with, 346f
   cefpodoxime proxetil interaction with, 346f
   cefprozil interaction with, 347f
   ceftazidime interaction with, 348f
   ceftriaxone interaction with, 350f
   cephalexin interaction with, 351f
   cephradine interaction with, 352f
   ciprofloxacin interaction with, 357f
   cloxacillin interaction with, 361f
   doripenem interaction with, 371f
   ertapenem interaction with, 376f
   famciclovir interaction with, 380f
   ganciclovir interaction with, 386f
   imipenem-cilastatin interaction with, 392f
   loracarbef interaction with, 408f
   meropenem interaction with, 412f
   nafcillin interaction with, 420f
   nitrofurantoin interaction with, 427f
   norfloxacin interaction with, 427f
   ofloxacin interaction with, 429f
   oseltamvir phosphate interaction with, 430f
   oxacillin interaction with, 431f
   penicillin G interaction with, 436f
   penicillin V interaction with, 438f
   piperacillin interaction with, 441f
   piperacillin/tazobactam interaction with, 442f
   ticarcillin interaction with, 478f, 479f
   for Treponema pallidum, 35
   valacyclovir interaction with, 488f

Probenecid (*Cont.*)
  zalcitabine interaction with, 493f
  zanamivir interaction with, 495f
Procainamide
  moxifloxacin interaction with, 418f
  trimethoprim interaction with, 485f
Proguanil, 332f–334f
  for *Plasmodium falciparum,* 92
Propafenone, interactions
  with lopinavir with ritonavir, toxic effect(s), 255
  with ritonavir, toxic effect(s), 257
Propamidine isethionate, for *Acanthamoeba,* 74
Propionibacterium acnes, 24
Protease inhibitors, interactions, with quinidine
      gluconate, toxic effect(s), 256
Proteus mirabilis, 24–25
  in vitro drug susceptibility and in vivo drug
      efficacy against, discordance between,
      228
Proteus vulgaris, indole positive spp., 25
Prothrombin time (PT), increased, drugs
      causing, 261
Proton pump inhibitors
  atazanavir and, 332f
  cefuroxime interaction with, 351f
Protozoal infections, 74–105
Providencia, in vitro drug susceptibility and in
      vivo drug efficacy against, discordance
      between, 229
Providencia spp., 25
Pruritis, drugs causing, 267
Pseudoallescheria boydii, 67
Pseudomembranous enterocolitis, drugs
      causing, 268
Pseudomonas aeruginosa spp., 25, 229
Pseudomonic acid, mechanism of action of, 222
Pulmonary fibrosis, drug causing, 272
Pulmonary fungal infections, 72
Pyomyositis, antimicrobial therapy for, 125
Pyrantel pamoate, 448f
  adverse effects of, gastrointestinal, 268–270
  for *Ancylostoma* spp., 75
  for *Ascaris lumbricoides,* 76
  for *Enterobius vermicularis,* 85
  for *Necator americanus,* 91
  for *Oseophagostomum bifurcum,* 91
  precautions with, in hepatic dysfunction, 180
  for *Trichostrongylus,* 101
Pyrazinamide, 449f
  administration route for, 222
  adverse effects of
    gastrointestinal, 268, 270
    musculoskeletal, 273
  contraindications to, in hepatic dysfunction,
      180
  dosage adjustment, in renal failure, 167
  ethionamide interaction with, 379f
  mechanism of action of, 222
  for *Mycobacterium tuberculosis,* 39–41
  precautions with, in hepatic dysfunction, 180
  tissue distribution, by key organ systems,
      210
Pyrazinoic acid, mechanism of action of, 222
Pyrethrins, 449f–450f
Pyrethrins/piperonyl butoxide, adverse effects of,
      cutaneous, 267
Pyridoxine, for *Mycobacterium tuberculosis,* 38,
      42
Pyrimethamine
  adverse effects of
    gastrointestinal, 268, 270
    hematologic, 261, 262
Pyrimethamine
  dapsone interaction with, 364f
  for *Isospora belli,* 87
  for *Toxoplasma gondii,* 99, 100
  trimethoprim interaction with, 485f
Pyrimethamine ± sulfadoxine, 450f–451f
  administration route for, 225
  mechanism of action of, 225
  for *Plasmodium falciparum,* 92

Pyrimethamine ± sulfadoxine (*Cont.*)
  precautions with, in hepatic dysfunction, 181
  tissue distribution, by key organ systems, 210
Pyrmethrin, 105
Pyrophosphate analog, mechanism of action of,
      223

QTc prolongation, drugs causing, 262
Quinacrine
  for *Giardia lamblia,* 86
  primaquine phosphate interaction with, 448f
Quinidine
  amantadine hydrochloride interactions with,
      321f
  lopinavir interaction with, 407f
  moxifloxacin interaction with, 418f
  saquinavir interaction with, 463f
Quinidine gluconate, 452f
  adverse effects of
    cardiovascular, 262
    CNS, 263–265
    cutaneous, 266
    gastrointestinal, 268–270
    ocular, 273
  contraindicated drug interactions, 256
  interactions
    with amprenavir, toxic effect(s), 248
    with atazanavir, toxic effect(s), 248
    with fosamprenavir, toxic effect(s), 250
    with indinavir, toxic effect(s), 252
    with lopinavir with ritonavir, toxic effect(s),
        255
    with nelfinavir, toxic effect(s), 256
    with ritonavir, toxic effect(s), 257
    with saquinavir, toxic effect(s), 258
  for *Plasmodium* spp., 94
  precautions with, in hepatic dysfunction, 181
  serum concentrations
    appropriate times to sample, 236
    and toxicity, 236
  therapeutic drug monitoring goals for, 236
  tissue distribution, by key organ systems, 210
  toxicity of, 236
Quinine
  amantadine hydrochloride interaction with,
      321f
  for *Babesia microti,* 76
Quinine dihydrochloride, for *Plasmodium* spp., 94
Quinine sulfate, 453f
  administration route(s) for, 225
  adverse effects of
    CNS, 264
    gastrointestinal, 269, 270
    ocular, 273
  mechanism of action of, 225
  for *Plasmodium falciparum,* 92
  for *Plasmodium vivax,* 93
  precautions with, in hepatic dysfunction, 181
  tissue distribution, by key organ systems, 211
Quinolines, synthetic, mechanism of action of,
      225
Quinolone derivatives, mechanism of action of,
      225
Quinolones, for *Burkholderia cepacia,* 9
Quinupristin with dalfopristin, 453f–454f
  administration route for, 221
  adverse effects of
    CNS, 264, 265
    cutaneous, 266, 267
    endocrine/metabolic, 271
    gastrointestinal, 269, 270
    hematologic, 261
    hepatic, 272
    musculoskeletal, 273
  dosage adjustment
    in hepatic dysfunction, 181
    in obesity, 189
  for *Enterococcus,* vancomycin resistant, 15
  mechanism of action of, 221
  precautions with, in hepatic dysfunction, 181
  tissue distribution, by key organ systems, 211

Rabies immune globulin, 454f
Rabies immune globulin, adverse effects of, CNS, 264, 265
Raltegravir, 455f
  adverse effects of
    CNS, 264
    gastrointestinal, 269, 270
Ranitidine
  ceftibuten interaction with, 348f
  for *Heliobacter pylori*, 19
Ranolazine, interactions
  with itraconazole, toxic effect(s), 252
  with ketoconazole, toxic effect(s), 253
  with miconazole, toxic effect(s), 255
Rapamycin, lopinavir interaction with, 407f
Rash, drugs causing, 266
Renal abscess, antimicrobial therapy for, 123
Renal failure
  drug dosing in, 156–170
  drugs causing, 271
  and pharmacokinetic monitoring, 243
Renal insufficiency. *See* Renal failure
Renal tubular acidosis, drug causing, 272
Reserpine, thalidomide interaction with, 476f
Resistance. *See* Drug resistance; Microbial resistance
Respiratory syncytial virus, 52
Respiratory system. *See also* Lower respiratory tract infection(s); Upper respiratory tract infections
  adverse drug effects and, 272
Retapamulin, 455f
  adverse effects of
    CNS, 264
    cutaneous, 266, 267
    gastrointestinal, 269, 270
Retropharyngeal abscess, antimicrobial therapy for, 146
Reverse transcriptase inhibitors, administration routes for, 224
Rhabdomyolysis, drug causing, 273
Rheumatic fever, recommended antimicrobial prophylaxis for, 279
Rho(D) immune globulin intravenous (human), adverse effects of
  cardiovascular, 262
  CNS, 263–265
  cutaneous, 266, 267
  gastrointestinal, 268–270
  hypersensitivity, 273
  musculoskeletal, 273
  renal/genitourinary, 271
Ribavirin, 456f–457f
  administration route(s) for, 225
  adverse effects of
    CNS, 264, 265
    gastrointestinal, 268, 270
    hematologic, 261
  contraindications to, in hepatic dysfunction, 181
  didanosine interaction with, 368f
  for hepatitis C, 49
  mechanism of action of, 225
  precautions with, in hepatic dysfunction, 181
  for respiratory syncytial virus, 52
  tissue distribution, by key organ systems, 211
Rickettsia akari, 25
Rickettsia prowazekii, 26
Rickettsia rickettsi, 25
Rickettsia spp., 26
Rickettsia typhi, 26
Rifabutin, 457f–458f
  administration route for, 222
  adverse effects of
    CNS, 264
    cutaneous, 266
    gastrointestinal, 268–271
    hematologic, 261, 262
    hepatic, 272
    musculoskeletal, 273
  amprenavir and, 330f

Rifabutin (*Cont.*)
  atovaquone interaction with, 333f
  dapsone interaction with, 364f
  delavirdine interaction with, 366f
  dosage adjustment, in renal failure, 167
  fluconazole interaction with, 381f
  fosamprenavir interaction with, 383f
  idinavir interaction with, 396f
  lopinavir interaction with, 407f
  mechanism of action of, 222
  for *Mycobacterium avium* complex, 43, 44
  nelfinavir interaction with, 421f
  precautions with, in hepatic dysfunction, 181
  prophylactic
    for *Mycobacterium avium* complex, 282
    for *Mycobacterium tuberculosis*, 282
  ritonavir interaction with, 462f
  saquinavir interaction with, 463f
  tissue distribution, by key organ systems, 211
  trimetrexate glucuronate interaction with, 487f
  zidovudine interaction with, 495f
Rifampin, 458f–459f
  for *Acanthamoeba*, 74
  administration route(s) for, 222
  adverse effects of, hepatic, 272
  amprenavir and, 330f
  for *Anaplasma phagocytophila*, 3
  atazanavir and, 332f
  atovaquone interaction with, 333f
  for *Bacillus anthracis*, 4
  for *Bartonella bacilliformis*, 6
  for *Bartonella henselae*, 5, 6
  for *Brucella abortus*, spp., 8
  chloramphenicol interaction with, 353f
  for *Chryseobacterium* spp., 11
  for *Coxiella burnetii*, 14
  dapsone interaction with, 364f
  darunavir and, 365f
  delavirdine interaction with, 366f
  dosage adjustment, in renal failure, 167
  doxycycline interaction with, 372f
  efavirenz interaction with, 374f
  efficacy, PK/PD parameter associated with, 247
  for *Ehrlichia chafeensis*, 14
  ethionamide interaction with, 379f
  fluconazole interaction with, 381f
  fosamprenavir interaction with, 383f
  idinavir interaction with, 396f
  for *Legionella pneumophila*, 20
  lopinavir interaction with, 407f
  mechanism of action of, 222
  metronidazole interaction with, 415f
  for *Mycobacterium avium* complex, 43, 44
  for *Mycobacterium bovis*, 43
  for *Mycobacterium kansasii*, 45
  for *Mycobacterium marinum*, 45
  for *Mycobacterium tuberculosis*, 38–42
  for *Mycoplasma hominis*, 21
  for *Naegleria fowleri*, 90
  nelfinavir interaction with, 421f
  para-aminosalicylic acid interaction with, 433f
  praziquantel interaction with, 447f
  precautions with, in hepatic dysfunction, 181
  prophylactic
    for *Haemophilus influenzae* type b, 281
    for *Mycobacterium tuberculosis*, 282
    for *Neisseria meningitidis*, 283
  pyrazinamide interaction with, 449f
  quinidine gluconate interaction with, 452f
  raltegravir interaction with, 455f
  ritonavir interaction with, 462f
  for *Staphyloccus aureus*; methicillin-susceptible, 29
  for *Streptococcus pneumoniae*, 30
  terbinafine interaction with, 474f
  tissue distribution, by key organ systems, 211
  trimethoprim interaction with, 485f
  trimetrexate glucuronate interaction with, 487f
  zidovudine interaction with, 495f

Rifamycins
mechanism of action of, 222
microbial resistance to, mechanism of, 227
Rifapentine, 460f
administration route for, 222
adverse effects of
cardiovascular, 262
CNS, 263–265
cutaneous, 266, 267
endocrine/metabolic, 271
gastrointestinal, 268–271
hematologic, 261, 262
hepatic, 272
musculoskeletal, 273
mechanism of action of, 222
precautions with, in hepatic dysfunction, 181
Rigors, drugs causing, 263
Rimantadine, 460f–461f
administration route for, 225
adverse effects of
CNS, 263–265
gastrointestinal, 268, 270, 271
dosage adjustment
in hepatic dysfunction, 181
in renal failure, 167
mechanism of action of, 225
precautions with, in hepatic dysfunction, 181
tissue distribution, by key organ systems, 211
Ritonavir, 461f–462f
administration route for, 224
adverse effects of
CNS, 263–265
cutaneous, 266
endocrine/metabolic, 271
gastrointestinal, 268–271
hematologic, 261, 262
musculoskeletal, 273
atazanavir and, 331f, 332f
contraindicated drug interactions, 257
darunavir and, 365f
darunavir interaction with, 366f
dosage adjustment, in hepatic dysfunction, 181
efavirenz interaction with, 374f
interactions, with voriconazole, toxic effect(s), 258
lopinavir and, 406f–407f
maraviroc interaction with, 409f
mechanism of action of, 224
nevirapine interaction with, 425f
precautions with, in hepatic dysfunction, 181
quinidine gluconate interaction with, 452f
quinine sulfate interaction with, 453f
quinupristin with dalfopristin interaction with, 454f
tissue distribution, by key organ systems, 212
zidovudine interaction with, 495f
Rubella, recommended antimicrobial prophylaxis for, 286
Rubella vaccine, for postexposure prophylaxis, 286

St. John's wort
amprenavir and, 330f
atazanavir and, 332f
darunavir and, 365f
interactions
with amprenavir, toxic effect(s), 248
with atazanavir, toxic effect(s), 249
with fosamprenavir, 383f
with fosamprenavir, toxic effect(s), 250
with indinavir, toxic effect(s), 252
with lopinavir, 407f
with lopinavir with ritonavir, toxic effect(s), 255
with nelfinavir, toxic effect(s), 256
with ritonavir, 462f
with ritonavir, toxic effect(s), 257
with saquinavir, toxic effect(s), 258
Salicylic acid, as antimycobacterial agent, mechanism of action of, 222

Salmonella, in vitro drug susceptibility and in vivo drug efficacy against, discordance between, 228
Salmonella (non-typhi), 27
Salmonella typhi (type D), 26
Sappinia diploidea, 96
Saquinavir mesylate
administration route for, 224
adverse effects of
cardiovascular, 262
CNS, 263–265
cutaneous, 266
endocrine/metabolic, 271
gastrointestinal, 268–271
hepatic, 272
contraindicated drug interactions, 257–258
contraindications to, in hepatic dysfunction, 181
mechanism of action of, 224
precautions with, in hepatic dysfunction, 181
tissue distribution, by key organ systems, 212
Saquinavir sulfate, 462f–463f
darunavir and, 365f
delavirdine interaction with, 366f
efavirenz interaction with, 374f
nevirapine interaction with, 425f
quinidine gluconate interaction with, 452f
Sarcoples scabiei, 105
Schistosoma haematobium, 96
Schistosoma japonicum, 96
Schistosoma mansoni, 96
Schistosoma mekongi, 97
Sebhorric dermatitis, ciclopirox/ciclopirox olamine, 354f
Seizures, drugs causing, 265
Selective serotonin reuptake inhibitors, interactions
with furazolidone, toxic effect(s), 251
with linezolid, toxic effect(s), 254
Selenium sulfide, 463f
adverse effects of
cutaneous, 266
gastrointestinal, 268, 271
for Malassezia sp., 65
Sepsis, antimicrobial therapy for, 111–114
Serotonin/norepinephrine reuptake inhibitors, interactions
with furazolidone, toxic effect(s), 251
with linezolid, toxic effect(s), 254
Serratia, in vitro drug susceptibility and in vivo drug efficacy against, discordance between, 229
Serratis marcesens, 27
Serum concentrations. See also Therapeutic drug monitoring
measurement of
methods for, 242–243
in non–steady state, 243
in steady state, 242
therapeutic, 231–233
Serum sickness, drugs causing, 273
Sexual assault, recommended antimicrobial prophylaxis after, 280
Sexual contact, recommended antimicrobial prophylaxis after, 280
Shigella, in vitro drug susceptibility and in vivo drug efficacy against, discordance between, 228
Shigella sonnei, dysenteriae, boydii, flexneri, 27–28
Sibutramine, interactions
with furazolidone, toxic effect(s), 251
with linezolid, toxic effect(s), 254
Sildenafil, nelfinavir interaction with, 421f
Silver nitrate, prophylactic, for ophthalmia neonatorum, 279
Silver sulfadiazine, 464f
adverse effects of
cutaneous, 266, 267
hematologic, 261
hepatic, 272

Sinusitis
  acute, antimicrobial therapy for, 147–148
  chronic, antimicrobial therapy for, 148
Sinusitis fungal infections, 72
Sirolimus
  clotrimazole interaction with, 360f
  micafungin sodium interaction with, 416f
  nelfinavir interaction with, 421f
  quinupristin with dalfopristin interaction with,
    454f
  ritonavir interaction with, 462f
Skin, adverse drug effects and, 266–267
Sodium citrate, colistimethate sodium interaction
    with, 362f
Soft tissue, infections of, antimicrobial therapy
    for, 123–128
Somnolence, drugs causing, 265
Sotalol, moxifloxacin interaction with, 418f
Sparfloxacin
  administration route for, 220
  mechanism of action of, 220
Spectinomycin, 464f
  administration route(s) for, 218
  mechanism of action of, 218
  for Neisseria gonorrhea, 21, 22
Spinal abscess, antimicrobial therapy for, 125
Spinal fusion, infection after, antimicrobial
    therapy for, 125
Spiramycin, for Toxoplasma gondii, 100
Sporotrichosis, 72
Staphyloccus aureus; methicillin-susceptible,
    28–29
Staphylococci (Staphylococcus spp.)
  methicillin-resistant, in vitro drug susceptibility
    and in vivo drug efficacy against,
    discordance between, 228
  in vitro drug susceptibility and in vivo drug
    efficacy against, discordance between,
    229
Statins
  amprenavir and, 330f
  atazanavir and, 331f
  darunavir and, 365f
  voriconazole interaction with, 493f
Stavudine, 465f
  adverse effects of
    CNS, 264, 265
    cutaneous, 266
    gastrointestinal, 269–271
    hepatic, 272
  didanosine interaction with, 368f
  dosage adjustment, in renal failure, 167
  precautions with, in hepatic dysfunction,
    181
  ribavirin interaction with, 457f
  tissue distribution, by key organ systems,
    212
  zanamivir interaction with, 495f
Steady state, 242
Stenotrophomonas maltophila, 29
Stevens-Johnson syndrome, drugs causing, 267
Stibogluconate, 465f–466f
  adverse effects of
    hepatic, 272
    musculoskeletal, 273
  for Leishmania spp., 87, 88
  tissue distribution, by key organ systems,
    212
Stimulants
  amantadine hydrochloride interaction with,
    321f
  rimantadine interaction with, 461f
Stomatitis, antimicrobial therapy for, 142
Streptobacillus moniliformis, 29
Streptococci (Streptococcus spp.), in vitro drug
    susceptibility and in vivo drug efficacy
    against, discordance between, 229
Streptococci viridans, 32–33
Streptococcus Group A, 31
Streptococcus Group B, 31
Streptococcus Group C, G, 31–32

Streptococcus pneumoniae, 30
Streptogramins
  mechanism of action of, 221
  microbial resistance to, mechanism of, 227
Streptomycin sulfate, 466f–467f
  administration route(s) for, 218
  adverse effects of
    CNS, 265
    renal/genitourinary, 271
  for Bartonella bacilliformis, 6
  for Brucella abortus, 8
  for Burkholderia mallei, 9
  dosage adjustment, in renal failure, 167
  for Francisella tularensis, 17
  mechanism of action of, 218
  ototoxicity of, 274
  for Streptobacillus moniliformis, 29
  tissue distribution, by key organ systems, 212
  for Yersinia pestis, 37
Stridor, drugs causing, 272
Strongyloides stercoralis, 97
Stye, antimicrobial therapy for, 119
Subcutaneous fungal infections, 72
Succinylcholine, colistimethate sodium
    interaction with, 362f
Sucralfate, quinidine gluconate interaction with,
    452f
Sulconazole, 467f
  adverse effects of, cutaneous, 267
  for tinea corporis, 70
  for tinea cruris, 70
Sulfacetamide sodium, 467f–468f
  administration route(s) for, 221
  adverse effects of, cutaneous, 267
  mechanism of action of, 221
Sulfadiazine, 468f
  for Acanthamoeba, 74
  administration route(s) for, 221
  adverse effects of
    CNS, 263, 264
    cutaneous, 266, 267
    gastrointestinal, 268–271
    hematologic, 261, 262
    hepatic, 272
  for Balamuthia mandrillaris, 77
  for Burkholderia mallei, 9
  mechanism of action of, 221
  precautions with, in hepatic dysfunction, 181
  prophylactic, for rheumatic fever, 279
  tissue distribution, by key organ systems, 212
  for Toxoplasma gondii, 99, 100
Sulfadiazine/pyrimethamine/leucovorin,
    prophylactic, for toxoplasmosis,
    in HIV-infected patients, 288
Sulfamethasoxazole, dosage adjustment,
    in renal failure, 167
Sulfamethasoxazole/trimethoprim
  for Acanthamoeba, 74
  for Achromobacter xylosoxidans, 3
  adverse effects of
    cutaneous, 266, 267
    gastrointestinal, 268, 270, 271
    hepatic, 272
  for Aeromonas hydrophila, 2
  for Bartonella henselae, 5
  for Bordetella pertussis, 6
  for Brucella abortus, spp., 8
  for Burkholderia cepacia, 9
  for Burkholderia mallei, 9
  for Burkholderia pseudomallei, 9
  for Calymmatobacterium granulomatis, 9
  for Chromobacterium violaceum, 11
  for Chryseobacterium spp., 11
  for Citrobacter spp., 12
  for Coxiella burnetti, 14
  for Cyclospora, 80
  desensitization protocols
    adverse reactions and response during, 296
    oral
      for patients with history of typical delayed
        maculopapular reaction, 295–296

Sulfamethasoxazole/trimethoprim (*Cont.*)
  desensitization protocols (*cont.*)
    oral (*cont.*)
      for patients with previous (distant)
        reaction consistent with IgE-mediated
        mechanism, 295
  dosage adjustment
    in continuous renal replacement therapy,
      174
    in obesity, 190
  for *Eikenella corrodens*, 14
  for *Escherichia coli*, 17
  for *Isospora belli*, 87
  for *Kingella kingae*, spp., 19
  for *Klebsiella* spp., 19
  for *Legionella pneumophila*, 20
  for *Listeria monocytogenes*, 20
  mechanism of action of, 221
  for *Moraxella catarrhalis*, 20
  for *Morganella*, 21
  for *Mycobacterium fortuitum*, 46
  for *Mycobacterium marinum*, 45
  for *Nocardia brasilensis, asteroids*, spp., 23
  for *Pasteurella multocida*, 23
  for *Plesiomonas shigelloides*, 23
  for *Pneumocystis jiroveci*, 66
  prophylactic
    for pertussis, 283
    for phagocyte function defect, 278
    for *Pneumocystis*, 287
    for toxoplasmosis, in HIV-infected patients,
      288
    for urinary tract infection, 280
  for *Proteus mirabilis*, 24
  for *Providencia* spp., 25
  pyrimethamine interaction with, 451f
  for *Salmonella* (non-*typhi*), 27
  for *Salmonella typhi* (type D), 26
  for *Shigella sonnei, dysenteriae, boydii,
    flexneri*, 27, 28
  for *Staphyloccus aureus*; methicillin-
    susceptible, 28, 29
  for *Stenotrophomonas maltophila*, 29
  for *Streptococcus* Group C, G, 31
  for *Vibrio cholera*, 36
  for *Vibrio vulnificus, parahemolyticus*, spp., 36
  for *Yersinia enterocolitica, pseudotuberculosis*,
    36
Sulfisoxazole, 470f
  administration route(s) for, 221
  adverse effects of
    CNS, 263, 264
    cutaneous, 266, 267
    gastrointestinal, 268–271
    hematologic, 261, 262
    hepatic, 272
  dosage adjustment, in renal failure, 167
  for *Escherichia coli*, 16
  mechanism of action of, 221
  precautions with, in hepatic dysfunction, 181
  prophylactic
    for recurrent otitis media, 279
    for rheumatic fever, 279
  tissue distribution, by key organ systems, 212
Sulfonamides
  for *Chlamydia trachomatis*, 11
  mechanism of action of, 221
  microbial resistance to, mechanism of, 227
Sulfone, mechanism of action of, 222
Suramin, 470f–471f
  adverse effects of
    CNS, 264, 265
    cutaneous, 266
    gastrointestinal, 270, 271
    hematologic, 261, 262
    hepatic, 272
    musculoskeletal, 273
    renal/genitourinary, 271
  dosage adjustment, in hepatic dysfunction, 182
  precautions with, in hepatic dysfunction, 182
  tissue distribution, by key organ systems, 212

Suramin (*Cont.*)
  for *Trypanosoma brucei gambiense*, 102
  for *Trypanosoma brucei rhodesiense*, 103
Swimmer's ear, antimicrobial therapy for, 143
Syphilis
  congenital, penicillin G for, 434f, 435f
  latent, penicillin G for, 436f
Systemic febrile illness, antimicrobial therapy
  for, 111–114
Systemic infections, antimicrobial therapy for,
  108–114

$T_{1/2}$. *See* Elimination half-life ($T_{1/2}$)
Tachycardia, drugs causing, 262
Tachypnea, drugs causing, 272
Tacrolimus
  chloramphenicol interaction with, 353f
  clarithromycin interaction with, 358f
  clotrimazole interaction with, 360f
  fluconazole interaction with, 381f
  ganciclovir interaction with, 386f
  lopinavir interaction with, 407f
  nelfinavir interaction with, 421f
  quinupristin with dalfopristin interaction with,
    454f
  rifampin interaction with, 459f
  ritonavir interaction with, 462f
  saquinavir interaction with, 463f
  tinidazole interaction with, 480f
  voriconazole interaction with, 493f
Taenia saginata, 97
Taenia solium, 97–98
Tapeworms, 106
TBW. *See* Total body weight
Td, prophylactic, 284
Tdap, prophylactic, 284
Teicoplanin
  administration route(s) for, 221
  mechanism of action of, 221
Telbivudine, for hepatitis B, 49
Telithromycin, AUC/MIC, 244, 245
Tenofovir, 472f
  acyclovir interaction with, 319f
  administration route for, 224
  adverse effects of
    CNS, 263–265
    cutaneous, 266
    gastrointestinal, 268–271
    hematologic, 262
    musculoskeletal, 273
  atazanavir and, 331f, 332f
  didanosine interaction with, 368f
  dosage adjustment, in renal failure, 167
  mechanism of action of, 224
  precautions with, in renal dysfunction, 182
  tissue distribution, by key organ systems, 213
Terbinafine, 473f–474f
  adverse effects of
    CNS, 263, 264
    cutaneous, 266, 267
    gastrointestinal, 268, 269
    ocular, 273
  contraindicated drug interactions, 258
  dosage adjustment, in hepatic dysfunction,
    182
  precautions with, in hepatic dysfunction, 182
  for tinea capitis, 69
  for tinea corporis, 70
  for tinea cruris, 70
  for tinea favosa, 71
  for tinea pedis, 69
  for tinea unguium, 71
  tissue distribution, by key organ systems, 213
Terconazole, 474f
  adverse effects of
    CNS, 263, 264
    gastrointestinal, 268
  for *Candida* sp., 60
Terfenadine
  amprenavir and, 330f
  atazanavir and, 331f

Tetanus, recommended antimicrobial
  prophylaxis for, 284
Tetanus immune globulin, 475f
  adverse effects of
    CNS, 264, 265
    cutaneous, 266
    hypersensitivity, 273
  prophylactic, 284
Tetanus toxoid, prophylactic, 284
Tetracaine, pyrimethamine and sulfadoxine
  interaction with, 451f
Tetracycline, 475f–476f
  administration route(s) for, 221
  adverse effects of, gastrointestinal, 269, 270
  for Aeromonas hydrophila, 2
  for Anaplasma phagocytophila, 3
  for Arcanobacterium haemolyticum, 3
  atovaquone interaction with, 333f
  for Balantidium coli, 77
  for Bartonella bacilliformis, 6
  contraindications to, in hepatic dysfunction,
    182
  for Dientamoeba fragilis, 80
  dosage adjustment, in renal failure, 167
  for Leuconostoc spp., 20
  mechanism of action of, 221
  oxacillin interaction with, 431f
  penicillin G interaction with, 436f
  penicillin V interaction with, 438f
  for Plasmodium falciparum, 92
  precautions with, in hepatic dysfunction, 182
  tissue distribution, by key organ systems, 213
  for Treponema pallidum, 34, 35
  for Vibrio cholera, 36
  for Vibrio vulnificus, parahemolyticus, spp., 36
  for Yersinia enterocolitica, pseudotuberculosis,
    36, 37
  for Yersinia pestis, 37
Tetracycline ointment, prophylactic, for
  ophthalmia neonatorum, 279
Thalidomide, 476f
  adverse effects of
    cardiovascular, 262
    CNS, 263–265
    cutaneous, 266, 267
    gastrointestinal, 268–270
    hematologic, 261, 262
    hepatic, 272
    musculoskeletal, 273
    respiratory, 272
  contraindicated drug interactions, 258
  precautions with, in hepatic dysfunction, 182
Theophylline
  ciprofloxacin interaction with, 357f
  clarithromycin interaction with, 358f
  erythromycin preparations interaction with,
    378f
  fluconazole interaction with, 381f
  lindane interaction with, 405f
  norfloxacin interaction with, 427f
  ofloxacin interaction with, 429f
  pyrantel pamoate interaction with, 448f
  rifampin interaction with, 459f
  ritonavir interaction with, 462f
  thiabendazole interaction with, 477f
Therapeutic drug monitoring
  abnormal pharmacokinetic parameter
    calculations and, 243
  antimicrobials requiring, 233–238
  assistance with, 244
  benefits of, 233
  challenges to, 243
  drug-drug interactions and, 243
  improper drug administration and, 243
  improper serum sampling and, 243
  inaccurate time documentation of serum
    sampling and/or dose administration
    and, 243
  pharmacokinetic monitoring in, 240–244
  principles of, 231
  reduced drug absorption and, 243

Therapeutic index, 233
Therapeutic range, 231, 232
Therapeutic serum concentrations, 231–233
Thiabendazole, 477f
  administration route for, 225
  adverse effects of
    CNS, 263–265
    cutaneous, 266, 267
    gastrointestinal, 268–271
  for Ancylostoma braziliense, 74
  mechanism of action of, 225
  precautions with, in hepatic dysfunction, 182
  for Strongyloides stercoralis, 97
  tissue distribution, by key organ systems, 213
  for Uncinaria stenocephala, 103
Thiazide diuretics
  sulfadiazine interaction with, 468f
  sulfisoxazole interaction with, 470f
Thiopental, sulfamethoxazole with trimethoprim
  interaction with, 469f
Thioridazine, interactions
  with clarithromycin, toxic effect(s), 249
  with delavirdine, toxic effect(s), 249
  with erythromycin ethylsuccinate and
    acetylsulfisoxazole, toxic effect(s), 249
  with erythromycin preparations, toxic effect(s),
    250
  with foscarnet, toxic effect(s), 250
  with isoniazid, toxic effect(s), 252
  with ketoconazole, toxic effect(s), 253
  with levofloxacin, toxic effect(s), 253
  with lopinavir with ritonavir, toxic effect(s), 255
  with miconazole, toxic effect(s), 255
  with moxifloxacin, toxic effect(s), 255
  with norfloxacin, toxic effect(s), 256
  with pentamidine, toxic effect(s), 256
  with quinidine gluconate, toxic effect(s), 256
  with ritonavir, toxic effect(s), 257
  with terbinafine, toxic effect(s), 258
  with voriconazole, toxic effect(s), 258
Thrombocytopenia
  drugs causing, 262
  HIV associated, immune globulin for, 394f
  idiopathic, immune globulin for, 394f
Thrombophlebitis, drugs causing, 267
Thrush, antimicrobial therapy for, 143
Ticarcillin, 477f–478f
  adverse effects of
    CNS, 265
    cutaneous, 267
    hematologic, 261
  dosage adjustment
    in continuous renal replacement therapy,
      173
    in renal failure, 167
  for Enterobacter spp., 15
  for Stenotrophomonas maltophila, 29
  tissue distribution, by key organ systems, 213
Ticarcillin with clavulanate, 478f–479f
  administration route for, 218
  dosage adjustment
    in continuous renal replacement therapy,
      173
    in obesity, 188
    in renal failure, 168
  mechanism of action of, 218
  tissue distribution, by key organ systems, 213
Tigecycline, 479f
  dosage adjustment
    in hepatic dysfunction, 182
    in obesity, 190
  precautions with, in hepatic dysfunction, 182
  tissue distribution, by key organ systems, 213
Time-independent antimicrobial activity
  (T > MIC), 244, 245
Tinea capitis, 69
Tinea corporis, 70
Tinea cruris, 70
Tinea favosa, 71
Tinea pedis, 69
Tinea unguium, 71

Tinea versicolor, 72
Tinidazole, 479f–480f
    adverse effects of
        CNS, 263–265
        gastrointestinal, 268–271
    for Entamoeba histolytica, 84
    for Giardia lamblia, 86
    precautions with, in hepatic dysfunction, 182
    tissue distribution, by key organ systems, 214
    for Trichomonas vaginalis, 101
Tioconazole, 480f–481f
    adverse effects of, renal/genitourinary, 272
    for Candida sp., 60
Tipranavir, 481f
    contraindications to, in hepatic dysfunction,
        182
    precautions with, in hepatic dysfunction, 182
    tissue distribution, by key organ systems, 214
Tizanidine
    ciprofloxacin interaction with, 357f
    interactions, with ciprofloxacin, toxic effect(s),
        249
T > MIC, 244, 245
TMP-SMX. See
    Sulfamethasoxazole/trimethoprim
Tobramycin, 482f–483f
    administration route(s) for, 218
    adverse effects of
        CNS, 265
        renal/genitourinary, 271
    desensitization protocols
        inhaled, 301–302
        intravenous, 300–301
    dosage adjustment
        in continuous renal replacement therapy,
            174
        in obesity, 188
        in renal failure, 168
    for Haemophilus influenzae-aegypticus, 18
    high-dose extended-interval dosing of, 239
    mechanism of action of, 218
    for Mycobacterium chelonae, 47
    nephrotoxicity of, 237
    ototoxicity of, 237, 274
    serum concentrations
        appropriate times to sample, 237
        and toxicity, 237
    therapeutic drug monitoring goals for, 237
    tissue distribution, by key organ systems, 214
    toxicity of, risk factors for, 237
Tolnaftate, 483f–484f
    adverse effects of, cutaneous, 266, 267
    for tinea corporis, 70
    for tinea cruris, 70
Total body weight, 170
Toxic epidermal necrolysis syndrome, drug
    causing, 267
Toxic shock syndrome, antimicrobial therapy for,
    114
Toxocara canis/catis, 98–99
Toxoplasma gondii, 99–100
Toxoplasmosis, recommended antimicrobial
    prophylaxis for, 288
Tracheitis, antimicrobial therapy for, 147
Trachipleistopora sp., 101
Trazodone, ritonavir interaction with, 462f
Treponema pallidum, 34–35
Triazolam
    amprenavir and, 330f
    atazanavir and, 331f
    clarithromycin interaction with, 358f
Triazoles
    mechanism of action of, 223
    in vivo pharmacodynamic characteristics of,
        in neutropenic mouse models, 247
Trichinella spiralis, 101
Trichomonas vaginalis, 101
Trichomoniasis, recommended antibiotic
    prophylaxis for, 280
Trichosporon sp., 67
Trichostrongylus, 101

Trichuris trichiura, 101
Triclabendazole, for Fasciola hepatica, 85
Tricyclic amines, mechanism of action of, 225
Tricyclic antidepressants, interactions
    with furazolidone, toxic effect(s), 251
    with linezolid, toxic effect(s), 254
Trifluridine, 484f
    for herpes simplex, 51
Trimethoprim-sulfamethoxazole, 444f, 469f,
        485f
    for Achromobacter xylosoxidans, 3
    administration route for, 221
    adverse effects of
        cutaneous, 266
        hematologic, 261
    for Aeromonas hydrophila, 2
    amantadine hydrochloride interaction with,
        321f
    for Bartonella henselae, 5
    for Blastocystis hominis, 77
    for Bordetella pertussis, 6
    for Brucella abortus, spp., 8
    for Burkholderia cepacia, 9
    for Burkholderia mallei, 9
    for Burkholderia pseudomallei, 9
    for Calymmatobacterium granulomatis, 9
    for Chromobacterium violaceum, 11
    for Chryseobacterium spp., 11
    for Citrobacter spp., 12
    contraindicated drug interactions, 258
    for Coxiella burnetti, 14
    for Cyclospora, 80
    dapsone interaction with, 364f
    dosage adjustment, in renal failure, 168
    for Eikenella corrodens, 14
    for Escherichia coli, 16, 17
    for Isospora belli, 87
    for Kingella kingae, spp., 19
    for Klebsiella spp., 19
    for Legionella pneumophila, 20
    for Listeria monocytogenes, 20
    mechanism of action of, 221
    microbial resistance to, mechanism of, 227
    for Moraxella catarrhalis, 20
    for Morganella, 21
    for Mycobacterium fortuitum, 46
    for Mycobacterium marinum, 45
    for Nocardia brasilensis, asteroids, spp., 23
    for Pasteurella multocida, 23
    for Plesiomonas shigelloides, 23
    for Pneumocystis jiroveci, 66
    precautions with, in hepatic dysfunction, 183
    for Proteus mirabilis, 24
    for Providencia spp., 25
    pyrimethamine interaction with, 451f
    for Salmonella (non-typhi), 27
    for Salmonella typhi (type D), 26
    for Shigella sonnei, dysenteriae, boydii,
        flexneri, 27
    for Staphyloccus aureus; methicillin-
        susceptible, 28, 29
    for Stenotrophomonas maltophila, 29
    for Streptococcus Group C, G, 31
    tissue distribution, by key organ systems, 214
    for Vibrio cholera, 36
    for Vibrio vulnificus, parahemolyticus, spp.,
        36
    for Yersinia enterocolitica, pseudotuberculosis,
        36, 37
Trimetrexate glucuronate, 485f–487f
    adverse effects of
        CNS, 263–265
        cutaneous, 266, 267
        endocrine/metabolic, 271
        gastrointestinal, 270, 271
        hematologic, 261, 262
        hepatic, 272
        hypersensitivity, 273
    contraindicated drug interactions, 258
    dosage adjustment, in hepatic dysfunction,
        183

Trimetrexate glucuronate *(Cont.)*
  for *Pneumocystis jiroveci,* 66
  precautions with, in hepatic dysfunction, 183
  tissue distribution, by key organ systems, 214
Trypanosoma brucei gambiense, 102–103
Trypanosoma brucei rhodesiense, 103
Trypanosoma cruzi, 102
Tubocurarine
  clindamycin interaction with, 359f
  colistimethate sodium interaction with, 362f
Typhoid vaccine
  cephapirin interaction with, 352f
  minocycline interaction with, 417f

Uncinaria stenocephala, 103
Undecylenic acid, 487f
  adverse effects of, cutaneous, 266
Upper respiratory tract infections, antimicrobial
        therapy for, 143–149
Ureaplasma urealyticum, 35
Ureidopen
  for *Eikenella corrodens,* 14
  for *Enterobacter* spp., 15
  mechanism of action of, 220
Urethritis, antimicrobial therapy for, 120
Urinary tract infection(s)
  antimicrobial therapy for, 121–122
  recommended antimicrobial prophylaxis for,
        280
UTI. *See* Urinary tract infection(s)

Vaginitis, drugs causing, 272
Valacyclovir, 487f–488f
  administration route for, 223
  adverse effects of
    CNS, 263, 264
    gastrointestinal, 268, 270, 271
    hepatic, 272
    musculoskeletal, 273
  dosage adjustment, in renal failure, 168
  for herpes simplex, 50, 51
  mechanism of action of, 223
  prophylactic, for prevention of recurrent
        herpes simplex, 284
  tenofovir interaction with, 472f
  tissue distribution, by key organ systems, 215
Valganciclovir, 488f–489f
  administration route for, 223
  adverse effects of
    CNS, 263–265
    gastrointestinal, 268–271
    hematologic, 261, 262
  for cytomegalovirus, 48
  dosage adjustment, in renal failure, 169
  mechanism of action of, 223
  prophylactic, for prevention of CMV
        transmission to transplant recipient,
        284
  tenofovir interaction with, 472f
  tissue distribution, by key organ systems, 215
Valproic acid
  ertapenem interaction with, 376f
  isoniazid interaction with, 397f
  mefloquine interaction with, 411f
  meropenem interaction with, 412f
  ritonavir interaction with, 462f
  tipranavir interaction with, 481f
  zanamivir interaction with, 495f
Vancomycin, 489f–491f
  administration route(s) for, 221
  adverse effects of
    cardiovascular, 262
    CNS, 263, 264
    cutaneous, 266
    gastrointestinal, 270, 271
    hematologic, 261, 262
  AUC/MIC, 244, 245
  for *Bacillus anthracis,* 4
  for *Bacillus cereus,* 4
  for *Chryseobacterium* spp., 11
  for *Clostridium difficile,* 12

Vancomycin *(Cont.)*
  for *Corynebacterium jeikeum,* spp., 14
  desensitization protocols
    rapid, 298–299
    slow, 299–300
  dosage adjustment
    in continuous renal replacement therapy,
        174
    in obesity, 190
    in renal failure, 169
  efficacy relationships in humans, PK/PD
        parameter associated with, 246
  for *Enterococcus faecalis/faecium,* 15
  mechanism of action of, 221
  "Mississippi Mud" formulation, 238, 239
  nephrotoxicity of, 239
  ototoxicity of, 240
  pentamidine isethionate interaction with, 439f
  serum concentrations
    appropriate times to sample, 238
    monitoring, controversy about, 240
    and toxicity, 238–240
  for *Staphyloccus aureus;* methicillin-
        susceptible, 28, 29
  for *Streptococci viridans,* 32, 33
  for *Streptococcus* Group A, 31
  for *Streptococcus* Group B, 31
  for *Streptococcus* Group C, G, 31, 32
  for *Streptococcus pneumoniae,* 30
  therapeutic drug monitoring goals for, 238
  tissue distribution, by key organ systems, 215
  T > MIC, 244
  toxicity of, risk factors for, 238
  in vitro resistance relationships, PK/PD
        parameter associated with, 246
Vanillylmandelic acid, methanamine
        preparations interaction with, 413f
Varicella, 53, 287
Varicella immunization, in postexposure
        prophylaxis of varicella, 287
Varicella-zoster immune globulin (human)
  adverse effects of
    CNS, 264, 265
    cutaneous, 266, 267
    gastrointestinal, 270
    hypersensitivity, 273
    musculoskeletal, 273
  in postexposure prophylaxis of varicella, 287
Vd. *See* Volume of distribution (Vd)
Vecuronium, piperacillin interaction with, 441f
Ventilator-associated pneumonia, antimicrobial
        therapy for, 131
Verapamil
  quinidine gluconate interaction with, 452f
  quinine sulfate interaction with, 453f
Vestibular toxicity, drugs causing, 274
Vibrio cholera, 36
Vibrio vulnificus, parahemolyticus, spp., 36
Vidarabine
  administration route(s) for, 223
  for herpes simplex, 51
  mechanism of action of, 223
  tissue distribution, by key organ systems, 215
Vinblastine, voriconazole interaction with, 493f
Vincristine, voriconazole interaction with, 493f
Viral infections, 48–53
Visceral larva migrans, thiabendazole, 477f
Vision
  blurred, drugs causing, 273
  disturbances, drugs causing, 273
Vitamin A, minocycline interaction with, 417f
Vitamin B$_{12}$
  chloramphenicol interaction with, 353f
  neomycin sulfate interaction with, 422f
  para-aminosalicylic acid interaction with,
        433f
Vittaforma cornaea, 104
Volume of distribution (Vd), 241
Volume status, and pharmacokinetic monitoring,
        243
Vomiting, drugs causing, 270–271

Voriconazole, 492f–493f
  administration route(s) for, 223
  adverse effects of
    cardiovascular, 262
    CNS, 263, 264
    cutaneous, 266, 267
    endocrine/metabolic, 271
    gastrointestinal, 268–271
    hematologic, 262
    hepatic, 272
    ocular, 273
  for *Aspergillus* sp., 54
  atazanavir and, 332f
  for *Candida* sp., 58
  contraindicated drug interactions, 258
  for *Curvularia* sp., 62
  dosage adjustment, in hepatic dysfunction,
      183
  for *Exophiala* sp., 63
  for *Exserohilum* sp., 63
  for *Fusarium* sp., 64
  interactions
    with lopinavir with ritonavir, toxic effect(s),
        255
    with ritonavir, toxic effect(s), 257
  mechanism of action of, 223
  precautions with, in hepatic dysfunction, 183
  for *Pseudoallescheria boydii,* 67
  rifampin interaction with, 459f
  rifapentine interaction with, 460f
  tissue distribution, by key organ systems, 215
  for *Trichosporon* sp., 67

Wangiella sp., 67
Warfarin
  azithromycin interaction with, 335f
  ciprofloxacin interaction with, 357f
  clarithromycin interaction with, 358f
  delavirdine interaction with, 366f
  dicloxacillin sodium interaction with, 367f
  doxycycline interaction with, 373f
  efavirenz interaction with, 374f
  fluconazole interaction with, 381f
  levofloxacin interaction with, 404f
  metronidazole interaction with, 415f
  miconazole interaction with, 417f
  minocycline interaction with, 417f
  nafcillin interaction with, 420f
  norfloxacin interaction with, 427f
  ofloxacin interaction with, 429f
  piperacillin interaction with, 441f
  piperacillin/tazobactam interaction with, 442f
  proguanil and, 332f
  quinidine gluconate interaction with, 452f
  rifapentine interaction with, 460f
  ritonavir interaction with, 462f
  sulfadiazine interaction with, 468f
  sulfamethoxazole with trimethoprim
      interaction with, 469f
  sulfisoxazole interaction with, 470f
  tetracycline interaction with, 476f
  tigecycline interaction with, 479f
  tinidazole interaction with, 480f
  tioconazole interaction with, 480f
  trimethoprim interaction with, 485f
  voriconazole interaction with, 493f
Weakness, drugs causing, 265

Weight-for-length percentiles
  for boys, from birth to 36 months, 186
  for girls, from birth to 36 months, 187
Wuchereria bancrofti, 104

Yersinia enterocolitica, pseudotuberculosis,
    36–37t
Yersinia pestis, 37

Zalcitabine, 493f
  administration route for, 224
  adverse effects of
    CNS, 263–265
    cutaneous, 266, 267
    endocrine/metabolic, 271
    gastrointestinal, 268, 269, 271
    hematologic, 261
    hepatic, 272
    musculoskeletal, 273
  didanosine interaction with, 368f
  dosage adjustment, in renal failure, 169
  lamivudine interaction with, 403f
  mechanism of action of, 224
  precautions with, in hepatic dysfunction, 183
  ribavirin interaction with, 457f
  tissue distribution, by key organ systems, 215
Zanamivir, 494f
  administration route for, 225
  adverse effects of
    CNS, 263–265
    gastrointestinal, 268–271
    musculoskeletal, 273
  for influenza, 52
  mechanism of action of, 225
  prophylactic, for influenza, 285
  tissue distribution, by key organ systems, 215
Zidovudine, 494f–495f
  administration route(s) for, 224
  adverse effects of
    cardiovascular, 262
    CNS, 263–265
    cutaneous, 266, 267
    gastrointestinal, 269–271
    hematologic, 261
    hepatic, 272
    hypersensitivity, 273
    musculoskeletal, 273
    ocular, 273
    respiratory, 272
  dapsone interaction with, 364f
  ganciclovir interaction with, 386f
  mechanism of action of, 224
  precautions with, in hepatic dysfunction, 183
  for prevention of mother-infant HIV
      transmission, 285
  pyrimethamine interaction with, 451f
  ribavirin interaction with, 457f
  spectinomycin interaction with, 465f
  tissue distribution, by key organ systems, 215
  trimetrexate glucuronate interaction with, 487f
  valganciclovir interaction with, 489f
  zanamivir interaction with, 495f
Ziprasidone, halofantrine interaction with, 390f
Zoledronic acid, thalidomide interaction with,
    476f
Zygomycetes, 68
Zygomycosis, 72